SECOND EDITION

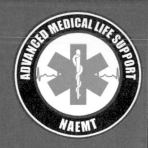

AMLS

Advanced Medical Life Support

AN ASSESSMENT-BASED APPROACH

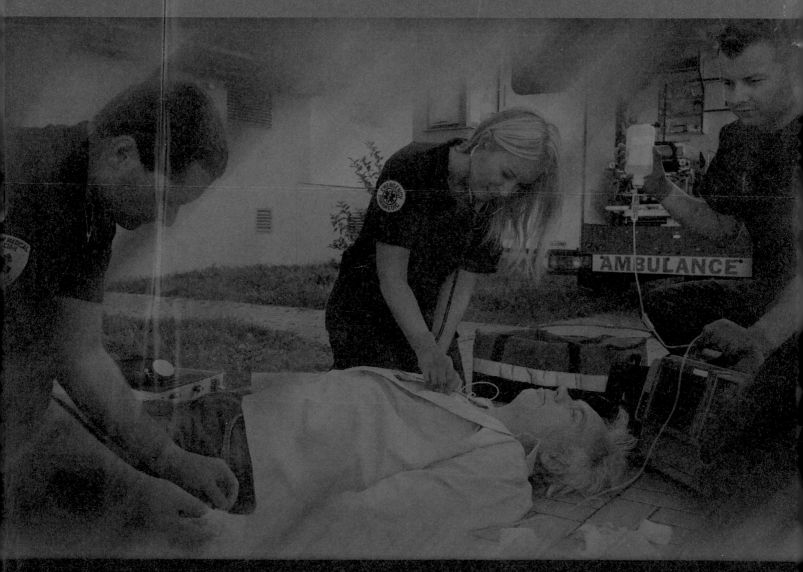

SECOND EDITION

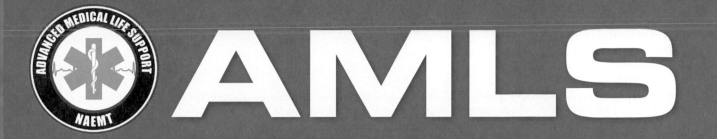

AMLS

Advanced Medical Life Support

AN ASSESSMENT-BASED APPROACH

Advanced Medical Life Support
Committee of the National Association
of Emergency Medical Technicians

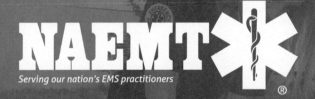

Serving our nation's EMS practitioners

Endorsed by

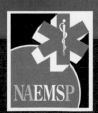

NAEMSP

Published by

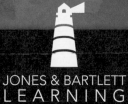

JONES & BARTLETT
LEARNING

World Headquarters
Jones & Bartlett Learning
5 Wall Street
Burlington, MA 01803
978-443-5000
info@jblearning.com
www.jblearning.com

Jones & Bartlett Learning books and products are available through most bookstores and online booksellers. To contact Jones & Bartlett Learning directly, call 800-832-0034, fax 978-443-8000, or visit our website, www.jblearning.com.

Substantial discounts on bulk quantities of Jones & Bartlett Learning publications are available to corporations, professional associations, and other qualified organizations. For details and specific discount information, contact the special sales department at Jones & Bartlett Learning via the above contact information or send an email to specialsales@jblearning.com.

10760-9

Production Credits
General Manager: Doug Kaplan
General Manager and Executive Publisher—Public Safety: Kimberly Brophy
VP, Product and Executive Editor: Christine Emerton
Senior Editor: Barbara Scotese
Senior Production Editor: Jessica deMartin
VP, Sales—Public Safety Group: Matthew Maniscalco
Director of Sales, Public Safety Group: Patricia Einstein

VP, Marketing: Alisha Weisman
VP, Manufacturing and Inventory Control: Therese Connell
Rights and Media Specialist: Rob Boder
Composition: diacriTech
Cover and Interior Design: Kristin E. Parker
Cover Image: © CandyBox Images/Shutterstock
Printing and Binding: RR Donnelley
Cover Printing: RR Donnelley

Library of Congress Cataloging-in-Publication Data
AMLS : advanced medical life support : an assessment-based approach/Advanced Medical Life Support Committee of the National Association of Emergency Medical Technicians. -- Edition 2.
    p.; cm.
  Advanced medical life support : an assessment-based approach
  Includes bibliographical references and index.
  ISBN 978-1-284-04092-0
  I. National Association of Emergency Medical Technicians (U.S.). Advanced Medical Life Support Committee. II. Title: Advanced medical life support : an assessment-based approach.
  [DNLM: 1. Advanced Trauma Life Support Care–methods. 2. Emergencies. 3. Emergency Medical Services.
4. Emergency Medical Technicians. 5. Needs Assessment. WX 162]
  RA645.5
  362.18--dc23
                                                                                                                2015029163

6048

Printed in the United States of America
20 19 18 17 16   10 9 8 7 6 5 4 3 2

CONTENTS

CHAPTER 8   Infectious Diseases 284

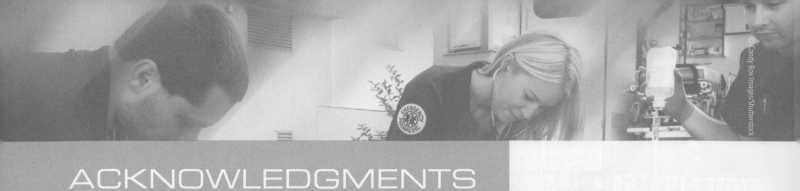

ACKNOWLEDGMENTS

The Advanced Medical Life Support Committee offers our gratitude to the many individuals who devoted countless hours of time in the development of the second edition of AMLS. It is with great pleasure that the AMLS Committee, with support from the National Association of Emergency Medical Technicians (NAEMT) and in partnership with Jones & Bartlett Learning, have developed this textbook and instructor resources. Such collaboration has ensured that this edition remains true to the AMLS philosophy and has allowed the development of more dynamic and informative components for the book and program. AMLS has taken on a broader audience of participants from all around the world as they engage in teaching one of the only programs that focuses on critical thinking, history taking, and physical exam to develop a list of potential differential diagnoses. Following the AMLS Assessment Pathway ensures a more likely process for identifying a differential diagnosis that will assist in guiding your treatment.

The individuals who offered contributions possess an unrelenting commitment for excellence. The hard work and fortitude of the many authors, reviewers, editors, and videographers provided the foundation for all the components of the book and program. The National Association of EMS Physicians (NAEMSP) has supported the participation of their members, Dr. Vincent Mosesso and Dr. Angus Jameson, which we really appreciate. The Committee provided a conscious effort throughout the process to ensure the AMLS program is consistent with all NAEMT education program policies and procedures so that participants, instructors, course coordinators, and affiliate faculty find ease in teaching and dissemination of the AMLS program.

We welcomed the expertise and support of our publisher, Jones & Bartlett Learning. Our editorial team, headed by Barb Scotese, worked efficiently to ensure the content was revised and formatted, the illustrations were accurate and relevant, and the book was printed on schedule. It is with sincere gratitude that we also thank Tracy Foss, NAEMT Education Development Manager, and Corine Curd, NAEMT Education Services Manager, for their day-to-day commitment to AMLS and support of the Committee on not only this publication but for assisting in the growth of the AMLS program.

It has been a pleasure to work with everyone involved in bringing the second edition to publication. The AMLS Committee is excited with the revisions of the chapters, the new chapter on environmental-related emergencies, as well as new lectures and scenarios. Our hope is that these revisions and new editions continue to make the AMLS Course the premiere course for addressing common medical complaints.

Jeff J. Messerole, EMT-P
Chair, AMLS

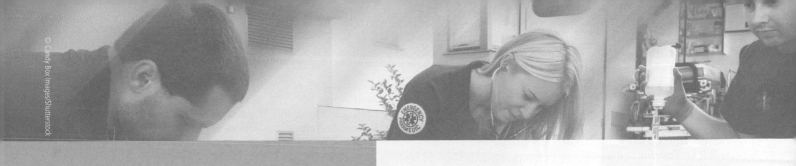

CONTRIBUTORS

Editors-in-Chief

Jeff J. Messerole, EMT-P
Committee Chair, AMLS
Clinical Instructor
Spencer Hospital
Spencer, Iowa

Vince N. Mosesso, Jr, MD
Medical Director, AMLS
Associate Chief, Division of EMS
Professor of Emergency Medicine
University of Pittsburgh School of Medicine
Medical Director, Prehospital Care Department
University of Pittsburgh Medical Center
Pittsburgh, Pennsylvania

Editors

Linda M. Abrahamson, MA, RN, EMTP, NCEE
AMLS Committee
Paramedic Program Director
Advocate Christ Medical Center EMS Academy
Oak Lawn, Illinois

Les R. Becker, PhD, MS.MedL, NRP, CHSE
Vice-Chair, AMLS Committee
Maryland PHTLS State Coordinator
Clinical Educator, Simulation Training & Education Lab of
    MedStar Health
Washington, DC

Ann Bellows, RN, REMT-P, EdD
AMLS Committee
University of New Mexico EMS Academy
Las Cruces, New Mexico

Angus Jameson, MD, MPH
Associate Medical Director, AMLS Committee
Medical Director, Pinellas County EMS
Largo, Florida

Jeri Smith, EMT-P
EMS Director
Arkansas City Fire/EMS Department
Arkansas City, Kansas

Contributors

Leslie P. Hernandez, MaEd, NRP, FP-C
Director, Community Education
Emergency Health Sciences Department
School of Health Professions
University of Texas Health Science Center at
    San Antonio
San Antonio, Texas

Peter Laitinen, RN, BSN, NREMT-P, EMT-I/C
Northeastern University
Burlington, Massachusetts

Michael Lynch, MD
Medical Director, Pittsburgh Poison Center
Assistant Professor
Division of Medical Toxicology, Department of
    Emergency Medicine
Divisions of Adolescent and Pediatric
    Emergency Medicine, Department of Pediatrics
University of Pittsburgh School of Medicine
Pittsburgh, Pennsylvania

Dawn Poetter, Paramedic
Portland Community College
Vernonia, Oregon

Lee Richardson, BS, CEMSO, NR-P, CCP, TP-C
Mercy College of Health Sciences—EMS Program
Des Moines, Iowa

Kristin Spencer, MS, NREMT-P, I/C/E
Crowder College
Neosho, Missouri

Reviewers

Rosemary Adam, RN, PM
The University of Iowa Hospitals' EMS Learning Resources
    Center
Iowa City, Iowa

Michael Arinder, NRP
American Medical Response
Jackson, Mississippi

Tracy Davis, MSN, RN, LP, ACAGNP-BC
Wilson, Texas

Anne Austin Ellerbee, AAS, NRP
H.E.R.O. Training Company
The Rock, Georgia

Major Mary Finn, MD, USAF, MC
UT Health Science Center at San Antonio
San Antonio, Texas

Matt Fults, NRP, CCP
University of Iowa EMSLRC
Iowa City, Iowa

Craig Manifold, DO
Clinical Assistant Professor
Department of Emergency Health Sciences
EMS Medical Director
UT Health Science Center
San Antonio, Texas

Terrence J. McGregor, Paramedic
Lancaster County Emergency Services
Gloucester, Virginia

Steven Mountfort, CCEMTP, NCEE
Florida Hospital EMS
Orlando, FL

Robert H. Quinn, MD, FAAOS
Chair, Professor, Residency Program Director
Department of Orthopaedic Surgery
University of Texas Health Science Center San Antonio
San Antonio, Texas

Lee Richardson, BS, CEMSO, NR-P, CCP, TP-C
Mercy College of Health Sciences—EMS Program
Des Moines, Iowa

Mark Seliga
Adjunct EMS Instructor
Advocate Christ Medical Center EMS Academy
Monee Fire Protection District
Mokena, Illinois

Christopher J. Van Houten, Paramedic
Medford, NY

International Reviewers

Michael Brand, Nurse Manager
GHR Mulhouse Sud-Alsace
FAEMT Member
Coordinator AMLS France
Geispitzen, France

John (Greg) Clarkes, EMT-P, NRP, MICP
Canadian College of EMS
Edmonton, Alberta, Canada

Jan Filippo, RN
EMS RAV Flevoland, Department of Education
Regionale Ambulance Voorziening
Almere, The Netherlands

Chris O'Connor, MSc, Dip. EMT, NREMT-P (USA), NQEMT-AP
Education and Practice Development Manager
Medicall Ambulance Service
Dublin, Ireland

Magnus Simonsson, MD
Central Hospital
Kristianstad, Sweden

Mark Tappenden
Senior Education Manager
Education, Development & Training
South East Coast Ambulance Service NHS Trust
Surrey, UK

AMLS Committee

Linda M. Abrahamson, MA, RN, EMTP, NCEE
AMLS Committee
Paramedic Program Director
Advocate Christ Medical Center EMS Academy
Oak Lawn, Illinois

Les R. Becker, PhD, MS.MedL, NRP, CHSE
Vice-Chair, AMLS Committee
Maryland PHTLS State Coordinator
Clinical Educator, Simulation Training & Education Lab of MedStar Health
Washington, DC

Ann Bellows, RN, REMT-P, EdD
AMLS Committee
University of New Mexico EMS Academy
Las Cruces, New Mexico

Angus Jameson, MD, MPH
Associate Medical Director, AMLS Committee
Medical Director, Pinellas County EMS
Largo, Florida

Peter Laitinen, RN, BSN, NREMT-P, EMT-I/C
Northeastern University
Burlington, Massachusetts

Jeff J. Messerole, EMT-P
Committee Chair, AMLS
Clinical Instructor
Spencer Hospital
Spencer, Iowa

Vince N. Mosesso, Jr, MD
Medical Director, AMLS
Associate Chief, Division of EMS
Professor of Emergency Medicine
University of Pittsburgh School of Medicine
Medical Director, Prehospital Care Department
University of Pittsburgh Medical Center
Pittsburgh, Pennsylvania

NAEMT Officers

Conrad T. "Chuck" Kearns, *President*
Dennis Rowe, *Present-Elect*
Bruce Evans, *Secretary*
Scott A. Matin, *Treasurer*
Don Lundy, *Immediate Past President*

NAEMT Board of Directors

Sean J. Britton, *Director Region I*
Robert Luckritz, *Director Region I*

Chad E. McIntyre, *Director Region II*
Cory S. Richter, *Director Region II*
Aimee Binning, *Director Region III*
Jason Scheiderer, *Director Region III*
Terry David, *Director Region IV*
D. Troy Tuke, *Director Region IV*
Ben Chlapek, *At-Large Director*
Matt Zavadsky, *At-Large Director*
Paul Hinchey, MD, *Medical Director*

AMLS Regional Coordinators

Jason McKay, MPA, NRP, *Region I*
Eric Bauer, BS, FP-C, CCP-C, *Region II*
Lee Richardson, BS, CEM SO, NR-P, CCP, TP-C, *Region III*
Jeri Smith, EMT-P, *Region IV*

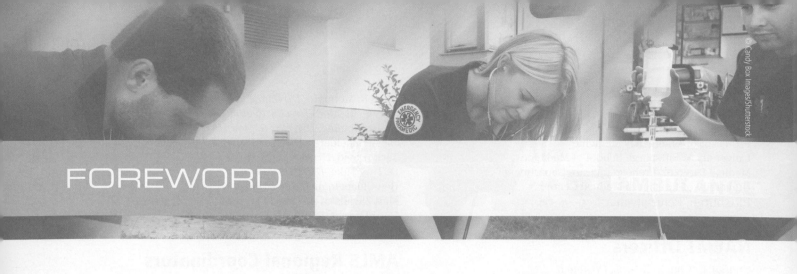

FOREWORD

One of the most difficult tasks in prehospital medicine is the urgent assessment of our patients. Medical patients, in particular, comprise the greatest number of cases in both the prehospital and hospital environments, and pose some of the greatest challenges to healthcare providers at all levels.

Caring for medical patients requires effective communication with the patient, family, friends, coworkers, and bystanders to piece together the critical information needed to understand what led to the call for help. It requires we use all of our senses in examining our patients to detect and decipher the often subtle clues of a patient's condition. It requires us to focus intently on our patient in an uncontrolled environment where noise, peripheral movement, environmental extremes, and even violence can be present.

The medical patient challenges our diagnostic capabilities and demands our best critical thinking skills and therapeutic interventions. The second edition of the *Advanced Medical Life Support* (AMLS) textbook is the foundational component of a comprehensive course that offers a unique "think outside the box" process designed to strengthen and refine the assessment and diagnostic skills of prehospital practitioners.

The authors and editors have incorporated the latest evidence-based information into this text to provide students with the best information available regarding the care of the medical patient. A refined AMLS Assessment Pathway; additional content on highly critical patients, environmental-related disorders, and infectious diseases; and the integration of the BLS provider with ALS throughout the assessment process are all new in this second edition.

Emergency medical care is a continuum requiring a dedicated team effort. Prehospital practitioners provide a critical role in the transition of care in the emergency department and has a direct impact on the follow-up care during hospital admission. Actions we take in the prehospital environment affect the treatment decisions during emergency evaluation and inpatient hospital care. Students who take the AMLS second edition course, both prehospital and in-hospital, can help ensure the best possible experience and outcomes for their medical patients. Our collaborative efforts will save lives and serve our communities in ways that truly make a difference.

I congratulate the authors and editors of the second edition of *Advanced Medical Life Support* and encourage all emergency healthcare providers to include AMLS as part of their continuing education. My hope is with successful completion of this course, you will enhance your ability to provide compassionate care and service excellence to your patients!

Craig Manifold, DO
Clinical Assistant Professor
Department of Emergency Health Sciences
EMS Medical Director
UT Health Science Center
San Antonio, Texas

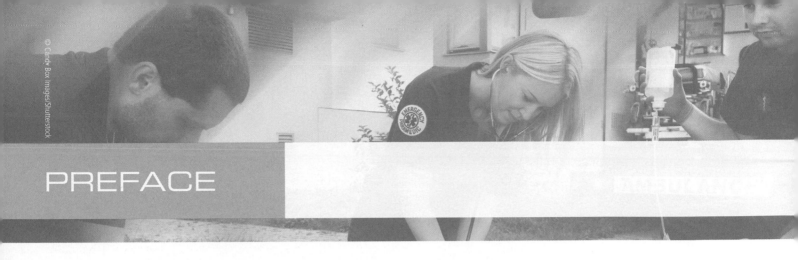

PREFACE

Taught throughout the world since 1999, Advanced Medical Life Support (AMLS) was the first EMS education program that fully addresses how to best manage patients in medical crises. AMLS continues to be the leading course for prehospital practitioners in the assessment and treatment of medical conditions. This new, second edition of the AMLS program remains true to the AMLS philosophy and of using critical thinking when assessing patients and formulating treatment plans. The case-based lecture presentations provide interactive discussion with students. Practical skill stations challenge students to apply their knowledge to realistic situations.

Endorsed by the National Association of EMS Physicians (NAEMSP), the AMLS course emphasizes the use of the AMLS pathway, a systematic assessment tool that enables EMS practitioners to diagnose medical patients with urgent accuracy. The AMLS assessment pathway emphasizes early identification of a patient's cardinal presentation or chief complaint. In addition to the pathway, AMLS provides (1) a foundation of anatomy, physiology, pathophysiology, and (2) an efficient and thorough evaluation of historical, physical exam, and diagnostic findings, which enhances the ability of students to narrow down the patient's differential diagnoses. The healthcare provider's expertise in clinical reasoning and decision making are essential skills in accurately determining diagnoses and initiating treatment. All aspects of AMLS are focused on an assessment-based approach to reduce morbidity and mortality and improve positive outcomes in medical patients.

AMLS incorporates the 2015 American Heart Association Guidelines for Cardiopulmonary Resuscitation and Emergency Cardiovascular Care. Although the AMLS program remains an advanced course, emergency medical technicians (EMTs) are able to participate in the program.

This textbook is a required component for the AMLS program and an invaluable reference for a variety of medical emergencies. The book and the course are informative resources for all healthcare practitioners in emergency care.

The first chapter, Advanced Medical Life Support Assessment for the Medical Patient, introduces the AMLS assessment pathway and provides a step-by-step walk-through of the thorough, comprehensive assessment process. This chapter discusses the cardinal presentation and chief complaint, pattern recognition, clinical reasoning, clinical decision making, and therapeutic communication skills.

Respiratory Disorders, Chapter 2, includes discussion on common respiratory complaints and reviews airway management adjuncts and strategies. Additional chapters discuss the etiology, assessment, basic and advanced diagnostic findings, and effective treatment options for cardiovascular disorders, shock, neurologic disorders, abdominal disorders, endocrine and metabolic disorders, infectious diseases, environmental-related disorders, and toxicology/hazardous materials/weapons of mass destruction.

Textbook features such as Rapid Recall Boxes, tables, and graphs are included throughout the book to serve as learning tools. Scenarios and Chapter Review Questions assist in testing the student's knowledge.

New Features

- A revised AMLS assessment pathway flow chart.
- New and expanded content on SARS, RSV, Chikungunya, Chagas disease, viral hemorrhagic fevers, seizures/epilepsy, carbon monoxide exposure, the progression of shock, the treatment of stroke, acid-base balance, hepatitis C, and drugs of abuse, including flakka.
- New chapter on Environmental-Related Disorders.
- Updated recommendations based on the 2015 American Heart Association ILCOR guidelines.
- Access to eBook and mobile-ready content before and during the course, such as the AMLS assessment pathway flow chart, 12-lead placement information, 12-lead electrocardiogram review, airway procedures, and cardiovascular procedures.
- New, updated case-based lecture presentations.
- New scenarios with debriefing content and explanation of diagnoses.

The AMLS Committee and NAEMT hope you find that the information you have read and studied in the textbook and AMLS program enhances your knowledgeabout the variety of medical emergencies your patients encounter, better preparing you to serve your EMS communities.

Jeff J. Messerole, EMT-P
Chair, AMLS

All levels of healthcare providers, both prehospital practitioners and in-hospital practitioners, encounter patients who present with a variety of subtle medical complaints. In the assessment process, these vague presentations offer many challenges to enable an accurate diagnosis and optimum care. The need for additional education on medical emergencies has been identified on certification and licensure exams for prehospital healthcare providers. AMLS is designed to enhance the knowledge base for assessment and management of medical emergencies, and it does so by building on the healthcare provider's clinical background, foundation of knowledge, and skills through case-based presentations and practical applications covering a variety of etiologies that cause medical complaints. AMLS recognizes that scene safety and early identification and management in life-threatening situations are critical initial interventions that can support positive outcomes in patients. The AMLS philosophy supports education that builds on the healthcare provider's current knowledge and scope of practice to work as a member of a team of healthcare professionals to improve patient outcomes. The combination of understanding the pathophysiology of the many medical disease processes, identifying cardinal presentations or chief complaints, and applying clinical reasoning skills assists the provider in performing efficient, accurate assessments. The AMLS assessment pathway process is not rigid; rather, it is a dynamic and ongoing process. It is not necessarily a critical action to alter the pathway if the patient's complaint or assessment findings necessitate doing so. The patient is always the priority, not the process. The order of the components of the assessment can be modified as long as all the components are evaluated.

We understand that the science and practice of medicine are in a constant state of change. In the next decade, we look forward to a future of growth, both domestically and abroad. AMLS is committed to providing technology-enhanced resources to encourage an interactive educational experience for course participants and faculty.

NAEMT

The NAEMT provides the administrative structure for the AMLS program. All proceeds, surcharges, royalties, and fees from the textbook and ancillary materials go directly to NAEMT. No editor or contributing author receives proceeds from these revenues. The monies received serve as an asset to NAEMT and are used for future educational projects and issues that are relevant to their membership.

International AMLS

Thanks to the success across the nation and abroad of NAEMT's inaugural continuing education program, Prehospital Trauma Life Support (PHTLS), our colleagues from around the world have easily integrated AMLS as a standard in their educational programs. Our U.S. Armed Forces have trained servicemen and women abroad serving our country in trauma response and AMLS.

To date, AMLS healthcare providers in the following countries are participating in and teaching AMLS programs: Argentina, Aruba, Austria, Belgium, Brazil, Colombia, Costa Rica, Ecuador, France, Germany, Greece, Ireland, Italy, Japan, Mexico, Netherlands, Norway, Panama, Peru, Saudi Arabia, Spain, Sweden, Switzerland, and the United Kingdom.

AMLS and NAEMT appreciate the support of not only the AMLS programs but of the NAEMT mission. We are proud to assist in establishing education standards for healthcare providers around the globe.

Comments and Suggestions

We encourage your comments and suggestions on the second edition and for future AMLS content. We are committed to providing the most current information within an interactive, effective learning process. Please send your comments to:

The National Association of EMTs
c/o Corine Curd, Education Services Manager
PO Box 1400
Clinton, MS 39056
You can also reach the AMLS Executive Committee via e-mail at: info@naemt.org
Visit Jones and Bartlett Learning
website at: www.jblearning.com

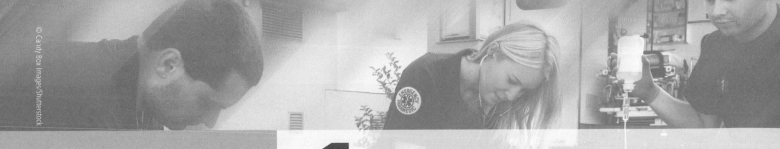

CHAPTER 1

Advanced Medical Life Support Assessment for the Medical Patient

In this chapter, providers will apply their knowledge of anatomy, physiology, pathophysiology, and epidemiology to the comprehensive, efficient AMLS assessment process, using their clinical reasoning to determine a list of differential diagnoses and formulate management strategies for a variety of medical emergencies.

LEARNING OBJECTIVES

At the conclusion of this chapter, you will be able to:

- Identify safety concerns in the prehospital and in-hospital situations that compromise the safety of the healthcare providers and patients.

- Understand the AMLS assessment pathway to identify emergent, nonemergent, potential, or actual life-threatening patient presentations.

- Identify the components of the first impression and the elements of the primary survey for patients with a variety of medical emergencies.

- Apply the AMLS assessment pathway to rule in or out differential diagnoses, based on a patient's initial presentation, assessment, and diagnostic findings.

- Integrate the patient's history (OPQRST and SAMPLER), pain assessment, and physical examination and diagnostic findings to determine working diagnoses and treatment interventions.

- Select appropriate diagnostic assessment tools, from basic to advanced, for a variety of medical emergencies.

- Correlate the symptoms of a patient's cardinal presentation to the appropriate body system to assess various emergent and nonemergent potential diagnoses.

- Discuss how cultural awareness can help counter any unconscious prejudices that might impede the assessment process.

- Compare and contrast the assessment concepts of clinical decision making, pattern recognition, and clinical reasoning.

- Understand how basic life support (BLS) assessment and treatment combined with advanced life support (ALS) assessment and treatment management supports an integrated team approach to patient care.

EMS responds to a residence to care for an 86-year-old man. Dispatch indicates the patient is experiencing fatigue and feels faint when standing up from a sitting position. This patient was transported twice last week by EMS to the local hospital for vague, but similar complaints. On examination, the patient responds to verbal stimuli. He remains seated in a chair during the assessment and says he is unusually tired and agitated. He is not feeling any better after several days. His body positioning is not concerning, but you notice a walker beside the chair. No difficulty in breathing is noted. He slowly answers questions regarding his current symptoms, but is unsure if he took his medications today. His daughter provides his medications for hypertension and constipation. She tells you that "he takes some sort of blood thinner for an irregular heartbeat." When obtaining vital signs, the EMT and paramedic notice the patient's skin is pale and clammy. The patient's respirations are 22 breaths/min and regular, his blood pressure is 110/84 mm Hg, and his pulse rate is 126 beats/min and irregular. The providers determine differential diagnoses and begin the focused assessment.

- How will the provider's comprehensive assessment be complicated by the patient's age?
- Which conditions are you going to consider as possible diagnoses based on your findings in the primary survey?
- Which additional assessments will you perform based on this patient's chief complaint and the history you have obtained?
- Which concerns might the provider encounter as a result of the age of the patient?

This chapter provides guidance for all levels of healthcare providers on how to apply their knowledge of anatomy, physiology, pathophysiology, and epidemiology to the Advanced Medical Life Support (AMLS) assessment process. An accurate patient assessment relies not only on a provider's foundational knowledge and experience, but also on therapeutic communication techniques, clinical reasoning, and clinical decision-making skills.

An organized, systematic evaluation of the patient's initial presentation, medical history, physical exam findings, and diagnostic test results is essential. These findings help determine the criticality of the patient's condition, working diagnoses, and management strategies. The ability of the healthcare provider to communicate effectively and use clinical reasoning enables the provider to consider all the possible etiologies related to the presenting symptoms. A thorough patient assessment ensures appropriate interventions and better patient outcomes.

It is important to understand the foundation of the AMLS assessment pathway is based on effective therapeutic communication skills, keen clinical reasoning abilities, and expert clinical decision making. BLS and ALS providers working together efficiently as a team enhance the timeliness and quality of care of the patient. Let's take a look at each of these elements.

Therapeutic Communication

Therapeutic communication uses various communication techniques and strategies, both verbal and nonverbal, to encourage patients to express how they are feeling and to achieve a positive, empathetic relationship with the patient. Obtaining a comprehensive medical history and being able to perform a thorough physical examination depend on good therapeutic interpersonal communication techniques. To obtain critical information about the patient's condition, BLS and ALS providers need to effectively communicate with the patient, family, bystanders, and the entire healthcare team. The information obtained can often provide clues to help identify the specific injuries sustained or to point toward a particular diagnosis.

Effective Verbal and Nonverbal Communication

Effective verbal communication is a dynamic process. According to the Bayer Institute for Health Care Communication, EMS providers carry out four principal communication tasks called the four *E*s: engagement, empathy, education, and enlistment.

- *Engagement* is the connection between you and your patients. You must establish a comfortable rapport with patients in order to keep them calm and elicit a thorough, accurate history. Your words and actions convey your genuine concern. Failing to introduce yourself, grilling patients with aggressive, rapid-fire questions, and interrupting them when they are talking undermines the bond you need to develop and may cause the patient to disengage. When making contact with patients and their loved ones, be sure to introduce yourself, if circumstances allow. Developing a rapport with patients also assists in building their confidence in the healthcare provider and facilitates open communication. Make a positive first impression.
- *Empathy* refers to your sincere identification with the patient's feelings of anxiety, pain, fear, panic, or loss. Empathy is rooted in a sense of compassion for what the patient is going through. Acknowledge to the patient what you hear and understand by summarizing or paraphrasing the information the patient has shared.

Accept what the patient tells you, regardless of the circumstances surrounding the call. Empathy is especially important in situations such as suicide attempts, accidental drug overdoses, and cases of domestic assault.

- *Patient education* fortifies your bond by letting patients know what is happening and what you are doing. Begin by asking what the patient already knows, and follow up with questions until you have all the information you need. Keep patients informed during the entire call. Describe tests and procedures in simple, straightforward terms, which will help minimize the patient's anxiety.

- *Enlistment* involves encouraging patients to participate in their own care and treatment decisions. When you ask for a patient's consent for treatment, be sure to explain fully any possible side effects or potential adverse outcomes associated with the intervention. For example, before giving the patient a nitroglycerin tablet, explain the purpose of the medication or intervention and that headaches are a frequent side effect of the medication. Explain to the patient how the benefits of the intervention outweigh the risks.

Nonverbal communication, which includes facial expressions, body language, and eye contact, is a powerful form of communication. It is important that you are aware of your own body language and the body language of your patients. Your gestures, body movements, and attitude toward the patient are critically important in gaining the trust of each patient and his or her family. Look for nonverbal behaviors, such as facial affect and body positioning, that indicate whether the patient feels at ease. These findings can be key indicators of the levels of discomfort, pain or fear. Keep in mind that patients may present with comorbid conditions that can complicate assessment and delay implementation of appropriate management strategies. Patience is essential when such a complex assessment must be made.

Therapeutic communication is a skill that is developed over time. To assist in developing these skills, the following verbal and nonverbal communication techniques are important to incorporate into your daily interactions.

- Talk with the patient at the patient's eye level and maintain good eye contact while talking. This is especially important with patients who are frightened, hard of hearing, or elderly.
- Speak clearly and slowly. If the patient has a hearing impairment, only raise your voice if the patient asks.
- Maintain an open, attentive body position during the interview. Try not to appear rushed or flustered.
- Acknowledge your understanding of what the patient is saying by nodding and paraphrasing the patient's words.
- Avoid distracting mannerisms such as writing while the patient is talking, tapping or clicking a pen, or fidgeting with keys or coins in your pocket.
- Your nonverbal language should reassure patients that you are there to help.

- Inform patients of what you and your colleagues are doing and why. Tell them where they are being transported and what to expect when they arrive.
- Ask "what" questions because "why" questions can sound accusatory to patients and their families.
- Show empathy by acknowledging the patient's pain, distress, anger, and other feelings. Answer the patient's questions to assist in decreasing anxiety and fear.
- Respond to and reinforce empathetic and caring behavior.
- Respect the patient's right to confidentiality by keeping your voice down as much as possible in public or semiprivate settings, such as at the scene and in the receiving facility.
- Protect the patient's modesty by keeping the patient covered as much as possible during the physical examination. Doing so will increase the patient's level of trust in the care you are providing and make the patient more willing to share pertinent health information.
- If you suspect a patient may become violent, interact with the patient in a calm, reassuring manner and call for additional resources. Do not try to handle a violent patient alone.

Communicating in Special Situations

Adjustments in your communication technique or asking for assistance may be required in special situations, such as when sign language is necessary for a deaf patient. As a general rule, communicate with patients using terminology matched to their knowledge and understanding. For example, it may be more appropriate to ask the patient about a history of "heart problems" rather than asking about "previous episodes of myocardial infarction."

Cultural and Language Differences

All healthcare providers encounter patients from diverse cultural backgrounds, including ethnicity, race, religion, or sexual orientation. For example, some cultures encourage people to express their emotions, whereas others see it as a sign of weakness. In some cultures, body odor and close proximity indicate acceptance and familiarity, while others may be offended or intimidated. Some providers may consciously or subconsciously force their cultural values onto their patient because they believe their values are better. This attitude can bias your approach to treatment and impair developing a rapport with the patient and family, resulting in ineffective communication or even miscommunication and poor treatment.

In many areas, particularly large urban centers, major segments of the population may not speak English. It would be beneficial for you to learn some common words and phrases in the language spoken. Bilingual family members or bystanders may be able to offer assistance and interpret for you.

Hearing-Impaired Patients

People who are hearing impaired may communicate through sign language, gestures, writing, or lip reading—any or all of which may be difficult to do when they are ill or injured. Some people with deafness have partial speech or hearing. Try to determine what the patient's abilities are to communicate as effectively as possible.

The patient's family members or friends may be able to help. In addition, learning how to ask a few basic questions in sign language, and interpret the answers, can be helpful. You may also be able to exchange written questions and answers with the patient.

Clinical Reasoning

Most healthcare providers would agree that skills proficiency alone cannot ensure quality care. **Clinical reasoning** skills are also essential. Clinical reasoning involves good judgment combined with a knowledge of anatomy, physiology, and pathophysiology seasoned by clinical experience to direct questioning about the patient's complaints. An understanding of the epidemiology of human disease processes is essential for early diagnosis, particularly when the patient's signs and symptoms do not point to an obvious cause. Elements that contribute to clinical reasoning are as follows:

- Knowledge in medical sciences
- Ability to gather and organize data
- Ability to focus on specific and multiple data
- Ability to identify medical ambiguity
- Ability to understand relevant/irrelevant data
- Ability to analyze and compare situations
- Ability to explain reasoning

As the interview questions are answered by your patient, you begin to analyze the answers based on your underlying medical knowledge. Once the chief complaint, history of the present illness, past medical history, and review of body systems have been completed, you can begin to formulate a **differential diagnosis**, which is a working hypothesis of the nature of the problem. As historical information, assessment findings, and test results are evaluated, a number of illnesses or conditions can be ruled out. The differential diagnosis therefore becomes narrowed until the provider formulates a **working diagnosis**—the presumed cause of the patient's condition. The working diagnosis becomes a definitive diagnosis pending confirmation by further diagnostic tests, usually performed at the receiving facility.

Scope of Clinical Reasoning

Creation of a mental list of differential diagnoses is not a static process. Vital signs, lung sounds, neurologic examination findings, oxygen saturation measurements, response to interventions, laboratory and radiographic test results, and other information are used to evaluate potential diagnoses. When you are developing differential diagnoses, start with broad possibilities—that is, which body systems might be contributing to the patient's complaint. For example, chest pain could involve the cardiac, respiratory, or gastrointestinal systems. This approach will help you to avoid tunnel vision, which is defined as locking into a diagnosis

early before considering all the possibilities. Because chest pain could involve multiple systems, it is important for providers to consider all the possible diagnoses and rule each one out systematically in order to determine a diagnosis.

You should begin by considering the patient's chief complaint. A significant number of illnesses or injuries can be ruled out quickly by just determining the chief complaint. For example, suppose your patient reports chest pain. Your knowledge gives insight into the potential problems that can cause chest pain. Your differentials might include heart attack, gastroesophageal reflux, pulmonary embolism, or aortic dissection. A patient reporting chest pain is not likely to have gastrointestinal bleeding; therefore, you can use the chief complaint to immediately narrow the diagnosis. In addition to the chief complaint, the associated signs and symptoms along with the history will narrow the possible causes even further.

The physical exam (discussed in detail later in the chapter) is another important aspect of clinical reasoning. Tenderness or other specific exam findings that point you toward specific anatomic locations can help refine your diagnostic possibilities. Once you are able to identify the possible organ systems involved, you can use your knowledge of pathophysiology to determine the most likely diagnosis.

Of course, clinical reasoning is not an exact science. Just like a scientist, however, you can test your differential diagnosis to determine whether it holds true. This is accomplished through further assessment and testing. This process evolves as different questions are asked based on the patient's answers. You may use various diagnostics to test these theories, such as a glucose check or a 12-lead electrocardiograph (ECG). The additional information is combined with the existing knowledge, and your differential diagnosis can be confirmed or modified.

To provide the best quality care for the patient, every provider must possess the core knowledge required in his or her level of training (**Figure 1-1**). This knowledge should be enhanced with experience and common sense to develop reliable clinical reasoning skills. A provider must be able to think and perform quickly and effectively under extreme pressure using critical

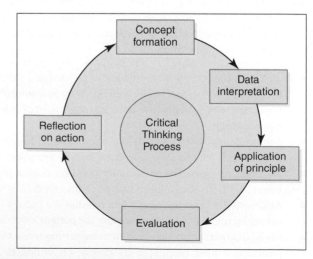

Figure 1-1 Critical thinking process.

Reproduced from Sanders MJ: *Mosby's paramedic textbook, revised reprint,* ed 3, St Louis, 2007, Mosby.

reasoning to determine an accurate working diagnosis and treatment plan based on patient care protocols or standing orders.

Clinical Decision Making

Clinical decision making is a process where decisions are made about a patient's healthcare problems and appropriate therapeutic interventions are considered and implemented to improve the patient's outcome. Like clinical reasoning, clinical decision making is an ongoing process that takes place at every stage of care, beginning with the creation of the differential diagnosis. Both require a sufficient knowledge of anatomy, physiology, and pathophysiology; an ability to perform specific assessment skills; and the resourcefulness to apply complex diagnostic tools to a broad range of medical emergencies. A pivotal skill necessary for effective clinical decision making is pattern recognition.

Pattern Recognition

Pattern recognition is a process of recognizing and classifying data (patterns) based on past knowledge and experience. The provider compares the patient's presentation with similar patient presentations encountered in the past. Analyzing similar diagnoses and which strategies were effective and which were not is a useful foundation for clinical decision making. One's clinical decision making and pattern recognition skills become more and more reliable with experience. The combination of well-honed therapeutic communication techniques, the ability to recognize patterns, and dependable clinical reasoning skills enables prudent clinical decision making, allowing providers to gauge the severity of the patient's illness or injury and initiate appropriate, timely interventions.

The ability to modify a systematic approach to patient assessment relies on clinical reasoning, pattern recognition, and decision-making skills. Using the six *R*s can help the provider put it all together and make better judgments under pressure (Rapid Recall box). The AMLS assessment pathway gives you an efficient process to apply your clinical reasoning and clinical decision making skills to effectively manage your patients.

RAPID RECALL   © HunThomas/ShutterStock, Inc.

The Six Rs

1. **R**ead the scene—Observe environmental conditions, safety hazards, and likely mechanisms of injury.
2. **R**ead the patient—Assess the patient's condition, take his or her vital signs, treat life threats, review the chief complaint, and record your general impression.
3. **R**eact—Manage life threats (ABCs) in the order in which they're discovered, and treat the patient based on his or her cardinal presentation.
4. **R**eevaluate—Reassess vital signs, and reconsider the patient's initial medical management.
5. **R**evise management plan—On the basis of your reevaluation and additional historical data, physical examination findings, diagnostic test results, and the patient's response to early interventions, revise your management plan to accord with the patient's new clinical picture.
6. **R**eview performance—Critiquing the call or patient encounter gives you a chance to reflect on your clinical decision making and target areas in which more advanced skills or a deeper level of knowledge are needed.

AMLS Assessment Pathway

The **Advanced Medical Life Support (AMLS) assessment pathway** is a reliable process for reducing patient morbidity and mortality by identifying a broad range of medical emergencies early and managing them effectively. Determination of an accurate field or in-hospital diagnosis and initiation of a timely, effective management plan hinges on a reliable patient assessment process.

The success of the AMLS pathway depends on the integration of BLS patient assessment and interventions and the early integration of ALS assessment and interventions. Taken together, the patient's initial presentation, history, chief complaint, physical exam findings, and diagnostic results should begin to suggest possible diagnoses. For example, if the chief complaint is low back pain, the provider should pursue that lead by asking patients follow-up questions such as:

- Have you recently sustained any injuries?
- Are you having weakness or numbness in your extremities?
- Have you had a fever?
- Does the pain seem to move around or radiate anywhere?
- What makes it better or worse?
- Have you recently called EMS for these symptoms?

The presence or absence of pertinent signs and symptoms associated with the initial presentation is equally important. Information gleaned from the patient's answers will help providers prioritize various differential diagnoses by using pattern recognition skills. When providers have seen what a condition looks like repeatedly based on experience, they can pick out the pattern almost immediately. Active listening and attention to pattern recognition will help build your knowledge of characteristic presentations that can be used to evaluate the current patient's presentation. A healthcare provider's knowledge of pathophysiology and the knowledge gained from patient care experience enhance the effectiveness of pattern recognition skills.

As providers talk to the patient to obtain a history and perform a physical exam, they are looking for critical life-threatening and non–life-threatening problems that must be managed within their scope of practice and adherence to medical protocols and guidelines. They are also forming a general impression of the patient's condition. Of course, all findings should be thoroughly documented and clearly communicated to the receiving facility.

The AMLS assessment pathway supports **assessment-based patient management**. This process is not driven by rote performance skills. Instead, the AMLS pathway recognizes that although all components of the assessment process (**Figure 1-2**) are important to patient care, they are conducted based on the patient's unique presentation. For example, if you have a high index of suspicion that the patient has sustained an injury, performing a rapid physical exam may be a higher priority than obtaining a past medical history. The history is not omitted, however; it's given a lower priority during the assessment process. The opposite is also true. With a medically ill patient it may be more appropriate to immediately obtain a history of the patient's present illness and a past medical history and perform the physical exam en route to the receiving facility. The physical exam and present and past medical history are not segregated entities. They are typically evaluated in tandem.

During the secondary survey, the healthcare provider should follow a dynamic, flexible approach to the patient assessment process. The process should be systematic, but it must remain dynamic and adaptable in order to confirm or eliminate diagnoses as more findings are noted and the patient's therapeutic response is observed.

Although the AMLS assessment pathway supports flexibility in deciding when to obtain specific details of a patient's history and physical exam, one important principle is that the initial observations at the scene must be made to ensure the scene is safe before the **primary survey** is performed so that any life-threatening medical emergencies can be identified and managed without delay. The discussion of the AMLS pathway that follows reflects the algorithm in Figure 1-2.

▼ Initial Observations
Scene Safety Considerations

Prehospital providers reach the scene or situation before they reach the patient. For prehospital personnel, this gives them a moment to integrate what the dispatcher has stated with their own judicious observation of the scene. The scene and the potential for safety hazards or threats are continually evaluated until patient care has been transferred (**Figure 1-3**). In-hospital environments may also place patients in an unsafe set of circumstances, such as when side rails are left down and the patient has an altered level of consciousness.

Prehospital providers enter the patient's environment, which may be a home, office, or vehicle. Anger or anxiety may be part of that environment, particularly when a stressful event such as an injury or assault has just occurred. The presence of EMS, law enforcement, or fire department personnel may make a violent person feel threatened. Behavioral red flags may precede an angry outburst or assault. Staying alert to potential or real threats of violence is equally as important in any healthcare institution, even if there are security personnel on site. All healthcare personnel must be aware of a gradual acceleration of emotion or concerning behavioral clues, such as pacing, gesturing, and hostile words that indicate an escalation of a dangerous situation.

Before approaching the patient, survey the environment and the patient's affect. This vigilance is essential in out-of-hospital and in-hospital situations. Determine the number of patients, family members, or bystanders present and whether any additional resources are needed, such as more ambulances, law enforcement, and fire or hazardous materials (hazmat) assistance. Evidence of weapons, alcohol, or drug paraphernalia can be an early indicator that the situation is unsafe and law enforcement backup is needed. Assess the situation for assistive devices, such as canes, wheelchairs, and oxygen concentrators, which indicate chronic conditions with the potential for poor perfusion presentations. In the prehospital setting, ominous background noise such as people arguing should cause enough concern for you to contact law enforcement to assist at the scene. Less menacing distractions such as televisions should be turned off or otherwise eliminated.

It is important to protect the integrity of the crime scene and preservation of associated evidence, as well as the safety of the victim. Work with your colleagues to keep the scene safe. Designate one person to have contact with the patient while the other remains alert for problems, a practice followed in law enforcement (**Figure 1-4**). Keep your communication equipment with you. On calls involving overdose, violent crime, or potential hazardous materials exposure, stage at a reasonable distance and wait for law enforcement to advise you that the scene is safe. Listen to your instincts—if the situation doesn't feel right, leave, if appropriate, and call for help. Always follow local or institutional protocols for such situations. Ensure documentation is timely and is an accurate reflection of the situation.

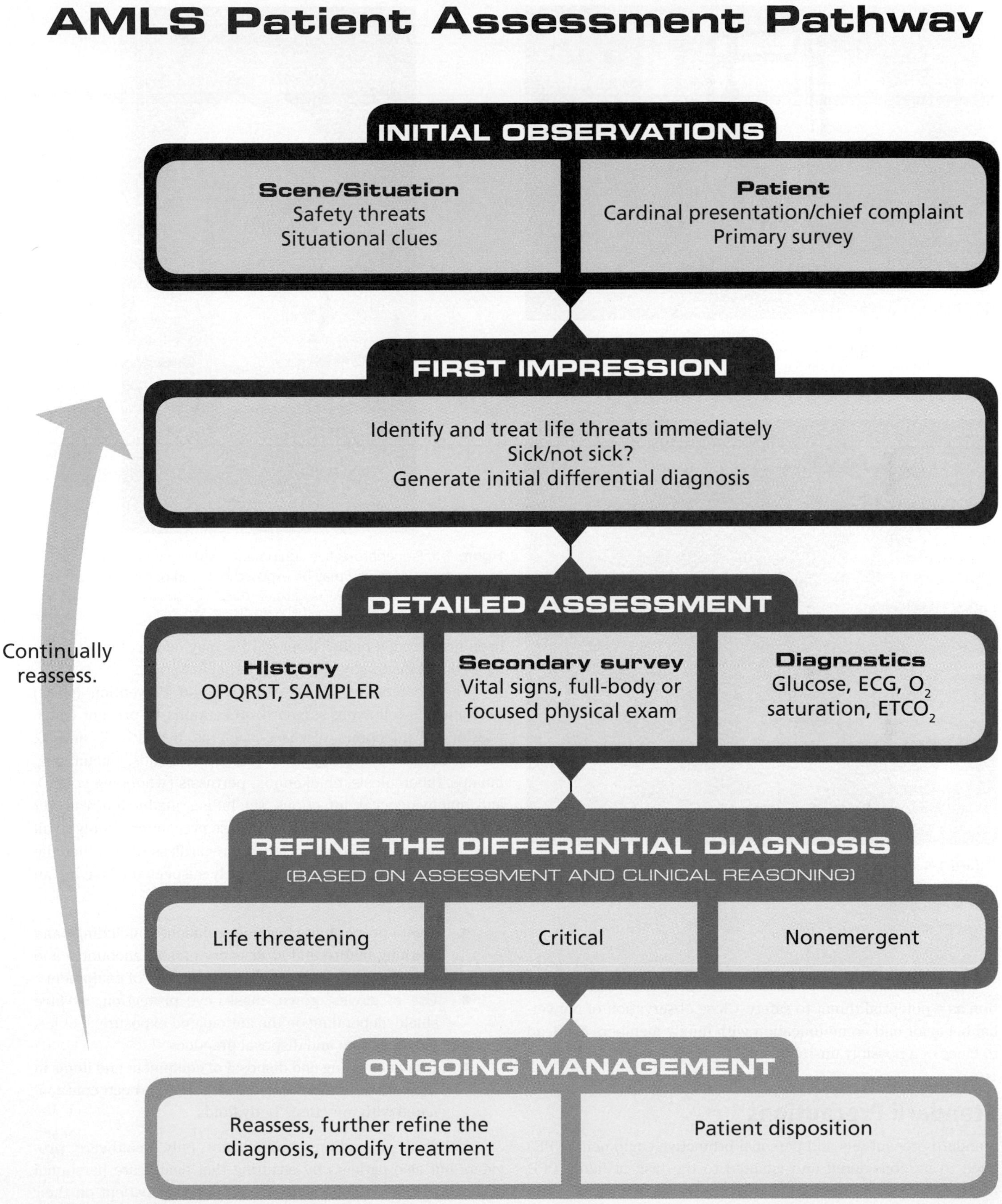

AMLS Patient Assessment Pathway

INITIAL OBSERVATIONS

Scene/Situation	**Patient**
Safety threats	Cardinal presentation/chief complaint
Situational clues	Primary survey

FIRST IMPRESSION

Identify and treat life threats immediately
Sick/not sick?
Generate initial differential diagnosis

Continually
reassess.

DETAILED ASSESSMENT

| **History** | **Secondary survey** | **Diagnostics** |
| OPQRST, SAMPLER | Vital signs, full-body or focused physical exam | Glucose, ECG, O_2 saturation, $ETCO_2$ |

REFINE THE DIFFERENTIAL DIAGNOSIS
(BASED ON ASSESSMENT AND CLINICAL REASONING)

| Life threatening | Critical | Nonemergent |

ONGOING MANAGEMENT

| Reassess, further refine the diagnosis, modify treatment | Patient disposition |

Figure 1-2 Algorithm for AMLS patient assessment.

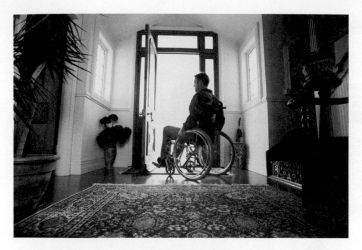

Figure 1-3 Throw rugs are a hazard; it is important to evaluate the safety of the patient's residence.
© Michael Pole/CORBIS/Flirt/Alamy

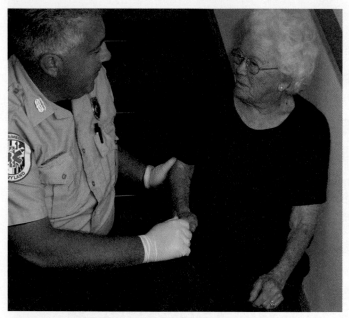

Figure 1-4 When providing care at a possible crime scene, one provider should care for the patient while another provider remains alert for problems.
© Jones & Bartlett Publishers. Courtesy of MIEMSS.

All personnel should evaluate each scene and patient situation as a potential threat to safety. Close observation of nonverbal behavior and communication with family members can lead to clues of a possibly unstable environment.

Standard Precautions

Standard precautions and personal protective equipment (PPE) need to be considered and adapted to the task at hand. PPE includes gloves, protective eyewear, gowns, face masks, and respirators (HEPA and N-95) (**Figure 1-5**). If weapons of mass destruction have been used or other hazardous materials have

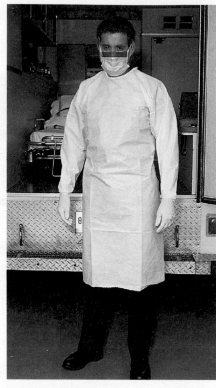

Figure 1-5 Proper protective equipment is vital when you are called to a scene in which you may be exposed to blood or other body fluids.
Reprinted with permission from Crosby LA, Lewallen DG (eds): Emergency Care and Transportation of the Sick and Injured, ed 6. Rosemont, IL, American Academy of Orthopaedic Surgeons, 1995.

been dispersed, a higher level of PPE may be necessary to prevent contamination by potentially lethal materials.

The Centers for Disease Control and Prevention (CDC) recommends following standard precautions to prevent transmission of infectious diseases such as hepatitis B and C, human immunodeficiency virus (HIV), meningitis, pneumonia, mumps, tuberculosis, chickenpox, pertussis (whooping cough), and staphylococcal infections (including methicillin-resistant *Staphylococcus aureus* [MRSA]). These precautions apply to all patients in every healthcare setting, regardless of whether the patient is known to be infected or only suspected of having an infection. Standard precautions include:

- Use of proper hand hygiene techniques, including hand washing before and after every patient encounter and after removal of gloves and disinfection of equipment
- Use of gloves, gown, mask, eye protection, or face shield, depending on the anticipated exposure
- Safe injection and disposal practices
- Proper cleaning and disposal of equipment and items in the patient's environment likely to have been contaminated with infectious body fluids

Standard precautions protect not only healthcare providers but also patients by ensuring that healthcare personnel do not carry infectious agents from patient to patient on their hands or transmit them via equipment used during patient care (**Figure 1-6**). An exposure can occur by contact with blood

Levels of Personal Protective Equipment

PPE is categorized by the Environmental Protection Agency (EPA) according to the level of protection it offers. Levels C, B, and A require specialized training before use. You should select a level higher than D if skin-damaging agents, such as corrosive substances, are or may be present. Emission of gases or vapors also requires a higher level of protection.

If you begin performing a different task at the same scene that brings you in closer contact with hazardous materials, you will need to upgrade your PPE accordingly. But you don't have to have a reason—if you feel uncomfortable using a lower level of protection, you should be allowed to upgrade on request.

A—Offers the greatest skin, eye, respiratory system, and mucous membrane protection.

B—Offers the highest level of respiratory system protection but less skin and eye protection. At least this level of protection should be selected until a reliable site analysis can be completed.

C—Used when the type and concentration of particulate matter are known, the criteria for using air-purifying respirators have been met, and skin and eye exposure are unlikely.

D—Used when no special protection from contaminants or hazards is needed; it is essentially a uniform consisting of coveralls and safety shoes or boots. It offers no protection from respiratory or skin hazards.

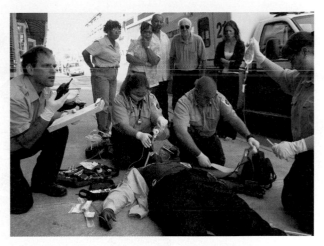

Figure 1-6 Standard precautions require that all healthcare personnel do not carry infectious agents on their hands. Gloves are essential.
© Jones & Bartlett Learning. Courtesy of MIEMSS.

or through inhalation or ingestion of respiratory secretions, airborne droplets, or saliva. Occupational Safety and Health Administration (OSHA) regulations specify training requirements, mandatory vaccinations, exposure control plans, and PPE. The Rapid Recall box is a reminder of the levels of PPE.

Other Hazards

Assess the scene for other hazards such as downed electrical lines, fires, imminent structural collapse, and presence of hazardous materials (**Figure 1-7**). Animals should be secured in advance of your entry. If you do receive an animal bite, contact local animal control authorities so the animal can be confined and tested for diseases. If toxic substances are present or you can't rule out the possibility, call in the hazmat team. If you can do so at a safe distance, find out the name of the toxic substance from the Material Safety Data Sheet (MSDS) or placard numbers on containers. Networks such as WISER (Wireless Information System for Emergency Responders), from the National Library

of Medicine, can provide suggestions for evacuating and information on medical toxidromes and treatments, depending on the kind of hazard present.

Patient Cardinal Presentation/Chief Complaint

The chief complaint is what the patient, family member, or friend reports to you as his or her primary concern. The chief complaint answers the question, "Why did you call for help?" Cardinal presentations are conditions and complaints recognized by medical providers as key concerns. Usually this will be based on the chief complaint, but sometimes will reflect your recognition of what is the most critical condition that must be evaluated.

With a responsive medical patient, you must first identify the chief complaint. In most cases, some type of pain, discomfort, or body dysfunction prompts the call for help. In some cases, the complaint may be vague. Vague complaints also challenge you to ask the right questions and be a patient listener as you obtain the information you need to make appropriate care decisions.

Primary Survey

The primary survey identifies life-threatening presentations and establishes immediate management strategies. To conduct this assessment and continue to formulate an initial impression of the patient's condition, determine whether the patient's condition is emergent (the patient is injured or ill and in need of immediate medical attention) or nonemergent (the patient is not in need of immediate medical attention).

To determine the patient's status, providers must evaluate the patient's level of consciousness (LOC) and identify any airway, breathing, or circulation problems. If a life threat is identified, immediate interventions must be initiated before further

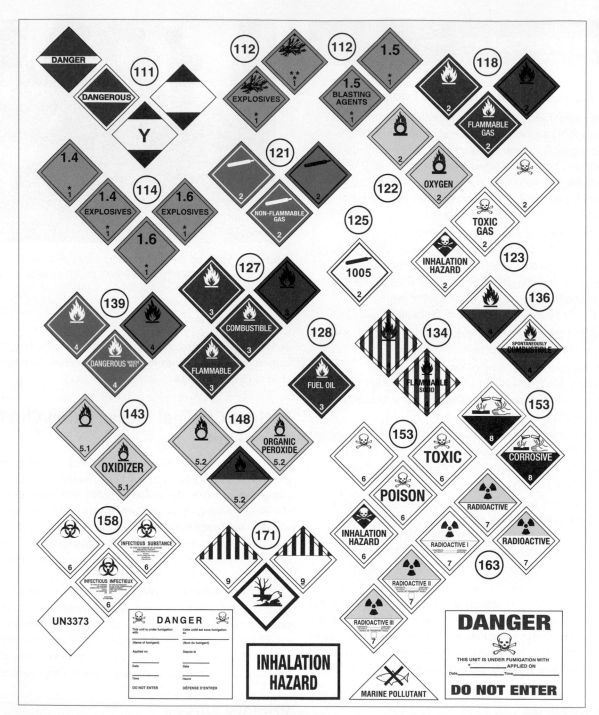

Figure 1-7 The Department of Transportation uses labels, placards, and markings to give responders a general idea of the hazard inside a particular container or cargo tank.

assessment is performed. The remaining history taking and physical exam can be performed en route to the receiving facility.

The prehospital emergency medical team must then make transport decisions. Is the patient to be transported by ground or air? What are the implications of either mode of transportation? Which is the closest, most appropriate medical center?

If the assessment does not reveal an immediate life threat, the patient should be evaluated for critical or emergent conditions. An emergent patient has a poor general impression or decreased level of consciousness, is unresponsive, shows signs and symptoms of shock, complains of severe pain, has sustained multiple injuries, or is having trouble breathing, has chest pain with a systolic blood pressure of less than 100, or has uncontrolled bleeding.

At this point in the assessment process, providers may not be able to pinpoint a working diagnosis, but differential diagnoses should begin to be formulated. Keep in mind the various possible causes of the patient's signs and symptoms as further assessment data become available and are interpreted.

Level of Consciousness

Assessment of the patient's mental status, or level of consciousness (LOC), involves evaluation of brain function. As providers approach the patient, they need to carefully observe the patient's LOC to immediately determine any potential life-threatening presentations. Observation of the patient's LOC is an important assessment tool. For example, if the patient is conscious, note the patient's responsiveness. A patient with a limited attention span or a patient who seems to be daydreaming should be assessed for hypoglycemia, dehydration, cardiovascular compromise, stroke, or head trauma.

LOC is associated with the function of the reticular activating system (RAS) and the cerebral hemispheres. The RAS is located in the upper brainstem and is responsible for maintenance of consciousness, specifically a person's level of arousal. The cerebral hemispheres are responsible for awareness and understanding. Reacting to the environment occurs through the cerebral hemispheres. The RAS alerts the cerebral hemispheres so they activate a response to the stimulus, such as an emotional or physical reaction. Coma can be caused by dysfunction of the RAS or both cerebral hemispheres.

The quickest and simplest way to assess the patient's LOC is to use the AVPU process:

- A *Alert* to person, place, and day
- V Responsive to *verbal* stimuli
- P Responsive to *pain*
- U *Unresponsive*

When you are classifying the response to stimuli, grade the patient according to the best response you can elicit. For example, a patient passed out on the street who moans in response to a loud shout from the provider would score a V on the AVPU scale. Response to tactile stimuli, such as pinching a nail bed, would be graded a P. No response to verbal or tactile stimuli would be classified as U. Table 1-1 discusses the AVPU process in greater detail.

Awareness is a high-level neurologic function and demonstrates a response to person, place, and time. This is more commonly referred to as *alert and oriented ×3*, or *AO×3*. A patient who is not AO×3 might be described as drowsy, confused, or disoriented. Of course, a patient can be awake but disoriented (not aware), indicating adequate RAS function but cerebral hemisphere dysfunction.

The Glasgow Coma Scale (GCS), used to assess victims of trauma or critical medical illness, is an effective tool for assessing neurologic function and is particularly important in establishing the patient's baseline LOC (Table 1-2). The score is also helpful in providing additional information on patients with changes in mental status. Documented changes in the GCS score that indicate diminishing neurologic function guide in-hospital diagnostic testing and inpatient placement.

GCS evaluates the patient's response to eye opening and best verbal and motor responses. The score for each

Table 1-1 Mental Status and AVPU		
AVPU Level	**Assessment Findings**	
Alert	Responds spontaneously; further define mental status	
	Alert and oriented × 3	Person, place, and time
	Alert and oriented × 2	Person and place
	Alert and oriented × 1	Person
Verbal	Responds to verbal stimuli	
Pain	Responds to painful stimuli	
Unresponsive	Does not respond to stimuli	

© Jones & Bartlett Learning

of these responses should be documented (for example, E = 3, V = 4, M = 4, for a total GCS score of 11). A score of 8 or less often indicates the need for aggressive airway management. Although 15 is the highest score possible, this does not mean the patient has full mental capacity. Definitive care should not be determined on the GCS findings alone but in conjunction with other diagnostic and historical data obtained.

Assessment of LOC helps determine whether the patient's neurologic and perfusion status are stable and allows life-threatening conditions to be identified and managed early. Patients with difficulties in mentation should receive a complete neurologic examination.

If the patient is unresponsive and flaccid with no signs of life, you should immediately check for the presence of a pulse. If you cannot detect a pulse within 10 seconds or if uncertain, begin chest compressions immediately and proceed with cardiopulmonary resuscitation.

Airway and Breathing

After assessing LOC and ensuring the patient has a pulse, the patient's airway status must be rapidly evaluated. Airway patency must be established and maintained. A patent airway allows good airflow and is free of fluids, secretions, teeth, and other types of foreign bodies (such as food or dentures) that may obstruct airflow. A patient's inability to maintain a patent airway is a life-threatening emergency and necessitates emergency interventions and immediate transport to an appropriate medical facility. Assessment of a patient's airway is completed in the same way regardless of the patient's age. In responsive patients of any age, talking or crying will give clues about the adequacy of the airway. For all unresponsive patients, you must establish responsiveness and assess breathing. Open the airway and observe the

Table 1-2 **Glasgow Coma Scale**					
Eye Opening	**Score**	**Best Verbal Response**	**Score**	**Best Motor Response**	**Score**
Spontaneous	4	Oriented and converses	5	Follows commands	6
To verbal command	3	Disoriented conversation	4	Localizes pain	5
To pain	2	Speaking but nonsensical	3	Withdraws to pain	4
No response	1	Moans or makes unintelligible sounds	2	Decorticate flexion	3
		No response	1	Decerebrate extension	2
				No response	1

Scores:
15: Indicates no neurologic disabilities
13–14: Mild dysfunction
9–12: Moderate to severe dysfunction
8 or less: Severe dysfunction (The lowest possible score is 3.)

mouth and upper airway for air movement. Performing a jaw-thrust maneuver on a trauma patient is appropriate if the potential for head, neck, or spine injury is noted. In cases of suspected trauma, manually protect the cervical spine from movement by positioning the patient in a neutral, in-line position. Look for evidence of upper airway problems, such as facial trauma, and check for the presence of vomitus and blood.

During the assessment of a patient's airway, BLS and ALS providers work together to observe the patient's position or posture to gather clues that will help determine which interventions are most appropriate. Is the patient lying in an unnatural position on the ground or in bed? Does the patient seem to favor an upright position or the tripod position? Certain positions maximize airflow and indicate increased work of breathing and respiratory fatigue, distress, and imminent failure.

A compromised airway may require suctioning or removal of a foreign object. In the case of obstruction, such as by food, BLS procedures to clear the obstruction require no equipment and can be done quickly. Suctioning, however, may be necessary to clear the airway. Suctioning takes longer (because of the need to set up and use the equipment) and is a more complicated procedure than positioning a patient to improve airflow. If you suction the patient for too long, you may create new problems, such as hypoxia and bradycardia secondary to vagal stimulation.

If a mechanical means is required to keep the airway open and patent, you must choose an airway adjunct. If you decide to place an oropharyngeal or nasopharyngeal airway, you must measure and choose the right size for the specific patient, and then properly insert the airway. If you determine that the patient cannot maintain his or her airway and you cannot maintain it by any other means, you need to use a more invasive technique, such as endotracheal intubation. BLS and ALS adjuncts include the following:

- Basic life support adjuncts
  - Suction
  - Manual maneuvers
  - Oropharyngeal/nasopharyngeal device
  - Supraglottic airway devices (Combitube, laryngeal mask airway, or king LT)
- Advanced life support adjuncts
  - Intubation (oral, nasal)
  - Chest de compression
  - Needle or surgical cricothyrotomy

Initial BLS interventions can be used and, when appropriate, progress to definitive ALS interventions. A thorough assessment will determine the urgency of airway management and suggest which devices are most likely to be effective.

A person's breathing status is directly related to the adequacy of his or her airway. Breathing rate, rhythm, and effort are evaluated in the primary survey. A normal respiratory rate varies widely in adults, ranging from 12 to 20 breaths/min. Children breathe at even faster rates, 15 to 30 breaths/min. The provider assesses the patient's rate of breathing. With practice, you will be able to estimate the rate and determine whether it is too fast or too slow. Lung sounds may be auscultated in the primary survey if labored respirations are noted. Inadequate respiratory rates or irregular breathing patterns may require the application of supplemental oxygen devices. The patient's respiratory rhythm should be easy, regular, and pain free. Painful or irregular breaths may indicate a medical or trauma related emergency and should be evaluated further to determine the cause of the abnormal breathing pattern. Symmetry of the chest rise and utilization of accessory muscles should be noted. Nasal flaring, agitation, and the ability to speak only two or three words without stopping for a breath are indications of distress and compromised air exchange (Table 1-3).

Conditions and injuries that cause a life-threatening compromise of the patient's ability to breathe include bilateral pneumothorax, tension pneumothorax, flail chest, cardiac tamponade,

Table 1-3 Irregular Breathing Patterns

Pattern	Description	Cause	Comments*
Tachypnea	Increased respiratory rate	Fever Respiratory distress Toxins Hypoperfusion Brain lesion Metabolic acidosis Anxiety	One of the body's coping mechanisms, but it can have a harmful effect by promoting respiratory acidosis. Because of the rapid respiratory rate, the body does not complete oxygen/carbon dioxide exchange in the alveoli. Consequently, the patient may require both oxygen and ventilatory assistance.
Bradypnea	Slower-than-normal respiratory rate	Narcotic/sedative drugs, including alcohol Metabolic disorders Hypoperfusion Fatigue Brain injury	In addition to bradypnea, the patient may have episodes of apnea. The patient may require both oxygen and ventilatory assistance.
Cheyne-Stokes respiration	A respiratory pattern with alternating periods of increased and decreased rate and depth with brief periods of apnea	Increased intracranial pressure Congestive heart failure Renal failure Toxin Acidosis	Repeating pattern. May indicate spinal injury.
Biot's respiration	Similar to Cheyne-Stokes but with an irregular pattern instead of a repeating pattern	Meningitis Increased intracranial pressure Neurologic emergency	Think of it as the atrial fibrillation of the respiratory system (irregularly irregular).
Kussmaul's respiration	Deep and fast breaths lacking any apneic periods	Metabolic acidosis Renal failure Diabetic ketoacidosis	Deep, labored breathing that indicates severe acidosis.
Apneustic	A long, gasping inspiration followed by a very short expiration in which the breath is not completely expelled. The result is chest hyperinflation.	Brain lesion	Causes severe hypoxemia.
Central neurogenic hyperventilation	A very deep, rapid respiratory rate (> 25 breaths/min)	Tumor or lesion of the brainstem that causes increased intracranial pressure or direct injury to the brainstem Stroke	CNS acidosis triggers rapid, deep breathing leading to systemic alkalosis.

* NOTE: Record the patient's airway status, breathing rate, rhythm, and breath sounds.

pulmonary embolus, or any other condition that diminishes tidal and minute volume and increases the work and effort of breathing.

Respiratory distress can result from hypoxia, a condition in which too little oxygen is available to the body's tissues. Hypoxia can be caused by any of the aforementioned conditions or by asthma, chronic obstructive pulmonary disease (COPD), airway obstruction, or any condition that restricts normal gas exchange by the alveoli, such as pneumonia, pulmonary edema, or abnormal mucous secretions.

When the patient's chief complaint is respiratory distress, another possible syndrome is hyperventilation, which will lead to respiratory alkalosis. Hyperventilation may be compensating for metabolic acidosis, anxiety, fear, or CNS insult. Working diagnoses may include possible causes such as stroke and diabetic ketoacidosis.

An elevated level of carbon dioxide in the blood caused by hypoventilation is called hypercarbia. Hypercarbia occurs when the body cannot rid itself of carbon dioxide, causing it to build up in the bloodstream, leading to respiratory failure. Hypercarbia should be considered in every patient with decreased mental status, especially if the patient appears somnolent or very fatigued. In the primary survey, midaxillary lung sounds are auscultated if the patient presents with a diminished level of consciousness, difficulty in breathing, or poor perfusion. Audible respiratory sounds such as wheezing are an important clinical finding. Gurgling and stridor are upper airway sounds (above the carina), and the other abnormal breath sounds are lower airway sounds. Abnormal breath sounds are as follows:

- *Gurgling.* A hollow bubbling sound.
- *Stridor.* A harsh, high-pitched sound heard during inhalation; indicates narrowing, usually as a result of swelling.
- *Wheezing.* High-pitched, whistling sounds made by air being forced through narrowed airways, which makes them vibrate, much like the reed in a musical instrument; wheezing suggests the bronchi are swollen and constricted, such as in patients with asthma and foreign body obstruction.
- *Crackles.* Typically described as the sound of hair rolling between your fingers.
- *Rhonchi.* Low-pitched crackles caused by secretions in the larger airways; rhonchi can be a sign of chronic obstructive pulmonary disease or an infectious process such as bronchitis.

Accessory muscle use and retraction can be seen at the suprasternal notch, beneath and between the ribs. If the work of breathing is increased, or the patient's breathing becomes progressively more difficult, the patient should be monitored for respiratory distress and imminent collapse. The combination of abnormal breath sounds and accessory muscle use or retraction is a more ominous sign than abnormal breath sounds alone. When you are assessing breathing, you must obtain the following information:

- Respiratory rate
- Rhythm, regular or irregular
- Quality/character of breathing
- Depth of breathing

As you assess the patient's breathing, ask yourself the following questions:

- Does the patient appear to be choking?
- Is the respiratory rate too fast or too slow?
- Are the patient's respirations shallow or deep?
- Is the patient cyanotic?
- Do you hear abnormal sounds when listening to the lungs?
- Is the patient moving air into and out of the lungs on both sides equally?

Other important questions the patient may be able to answer include:

- Did the difficulty breathing come on suddenly or get worse over several days?
- Is this problem chronic?
- Do you have any associated symptoms, such as a productive cough, chest pain, or a fever?
- Did you try to treat the condition on your own? If so, how?

Compromising breathing patterns should be identified and managed in the primary survey. If a patient seems to experience difficulty breathing after your primary assessment, you should immediately reevaluate the airway. Remember that air exchange is a critical issue, not the number of breaths.

Circulation/Perfusion

Assessing circulation helps you to evaluate how well blood is circulating to the major organs, including the brain, lungs, heart, kidneys, and the rest of the body. The patient's pulse rate, quality, and regularity should be obtained. Palpating the radial, carotid, or femoral artery is essential. An apical pulse can be auscultated at the apex of the heart near the fifth intercostal space, a landmark known as the point of maximum impulse (PMI), but this does not allow assessment of pulse strength. The normal resting pulse rate for an adult is between 60 and 100 beats/min and could be as much as 100 beats/min in geriatric patients. In pediatric patients, the younger the patient, the faster the pulse will be.

Pulse quality is described as absent, weak, thready, bounding, or strong. A weak pulse may indicate poor perfusion. A bounding pulse may indicate increased pulse pressures, such as with aortic regurgitation or elevated systolic blood pressure. Factors that can decrease myocardial contractility include hypoxia, hyperkalemia, and hypercarbia. Early identification of irregular, weak, or thready pulses in the primary survey indicates poor perfusion and may prompt urgent application and interpretation of ECG findings.

The pulse should also be evaluated to determine whether it is regular or irregular. A normal rhythm is regular, like the ticking of a clock. If some beats come early or late or are skipped, the pulse is considered irregular. An irregular heartbeat may have a cardiac or respiratory cause, or it may be brought on by a toxic substance such as a drug.

If a patient has inadequate circulation, you must take immediate action to restore or improve circulation, control severe bleeding, and improve oxygen delivery to the tissues. At this point, perform a rapid exam to identify any major external bleeding. The rapid exam is a quick, thorough palpation of the body. You will take about 60 to 90 seconds and perform a rapid exam of the patient's body to identify injuries that must be managed and/or protected immediately. This is an abbreviated exam as opposed to the more focused physical examination that will be performed during the secondary assessment.

Once the pulse rate, quality, and regularity have been assessed, the skin needs to be assessed for color, temperature, moisture, and capillary refill. Capillary refill time is often evaluated to determine the status of the cardiovascular system. To perform this test, pressure is applied to the nail bed until it turns white. The provider then measures the time it takes for normal color to return. A blanching time of more than 2 seconds is considered an indicator that capillary blood is being inappropriately shunted. This test can be unreliable in adult patients for several reasons. Older adults, especially those who take many medications and those with immune system or renal disease, tend to have poor perfusion. The temperature of the environment can also reduce the accuracy of the capillary refill test. Cooler environments cause vasoconstriction as a compensatory mechanism and may give a false impression of poor perfusion status.

Pulse pressure is calculated by subtracting diastolic blood pressure from systolic blood pressure (110 [systolic] − 70 [diastolic] = 40 [pulse pressure]. Normal pulse pressure is 30 to 40 mm Hg. If pulse pressure is low (less than 25% of systolic blood pressure), the cause may be low stroke volume or increased peripheral resistance. A narrowing pulse pressure may indicate shock or cardiac tamponade. Identification of pulse pressure changes are used to identify increased intracranial pressure. Observation of hypertension with a widening pulse pressure, bradycardia, and an irregular breathing pattern is a key indicator and is identified as Cushing's triad.

Information from dispatch, the initial observations, the patient's chief complaint, patency of the airway and breathing, and circulation/perfusion status should suggest potential underlying diagnoses and initiate appropriate initial treatment interventions. Diagnoses and patient management are dynamic throughout the call. They are continually reevaluated and modified as additional patient history, physical exam findings, and diagnostic results are obtained. The patient's response to treatment is also considered a priority in modifying ongoing treatment.

▼ First Impression

More often than not, you will form the first impression of your patient based on the **initial patient presentation** and chief complaint. Visual, olfactory, and kinesthetic observations at the scene will add valuable information to your patient assessment process to help determine the patient's differential diagnosis.

Visual Observation

You should think of your initial impression of the patient as a visual assessment (**Figure 1-8**). Extrinsic clues can include body positioning, expressions of pain, and abnormal breath sounds, which are all cause for concern. In adults, a decorticate or decerebrate posture, tripod position, or fetal body position can be signs of a life-threatening condition. Visual indications of extreme distress, such as a patient guarding his chest or abdomen or a chest pain patient holding a fist on the chest, known as Levine sign, indicate an emergent situation.

Look around for assistive devices that could indicate a chronic disease process. Walkers, canes, wheelchairs, oxygen concentrators, portable nebulizer devices, and hospital beds in private residences (**Figure 1-9**) are examples. Prosthetic and mobility devices indicate possible mobility problems that may be associated with chronic respiratory, cardiovascular, musculoskeletal, or neurologic deficits.

Decorticate posturing indicates dysfunction of the cerebral cortex. In this rigid body position, the patient's elbows are bent, the arms are held close to the chest, and the fists are clenched. The toes point down, and the legs are extended (**Figure 1-10**). Decorticate posturing may progress to decerebrate posturing, a grave sign indicating significant brain injury. This body position is also characterized by rigidity. The patient's arms and legs are extended, the toes point downward, and the head and neck are arched (**Figure 1-11**).

Oxygen in the home can be stored as compressed gas or liquid oxygen or may be generated with an oxygen concentrator. Oxygen may be delivered by nasal cannula, oxygen mask, tracheostomy, ventilator, continuous positive airway pressure (CPAP), or biphasic positive airway pressure (BiPAP; **Figure 1-12**).

The care of patients dependent on technology such as ventilators can be complicated by chronic illness and poor perfusion. Some patients will require automatic transport ventilators. These ventilators should be identified on arrival. Patients are placed on these ventilators to provide extended positive-pressure

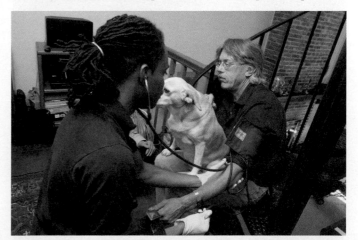

Figure 1-8 Be aware that each patient will have different ways of dealing with his or her immediate situation. Some may be relieved to talk openly about how they feel, while others may have a greater sense of privacy or stoicism.
© Jones & Bartlett Learning. Courtesy of MIEMSS.

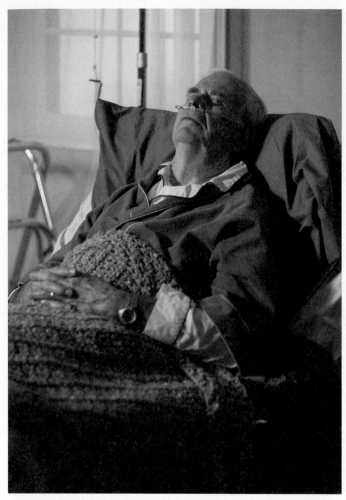

Figure 1-9 An elderly person on home oxygen indicates a chronic disease process.
© Photodisc/Photodisc/Getty

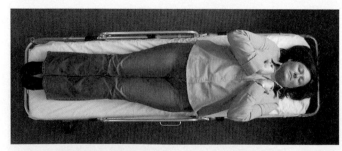

Figure 1-10 Decorticate posturing.
Courtesy of Chuck Sowerbrower MEd, NREMT-P

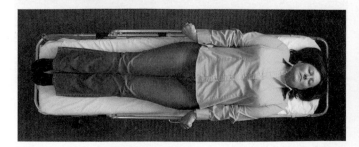

Figure 1-11 Decerebrate posturing.
Courtesy of Chuck Sowerbrower MEd, NREMT-P

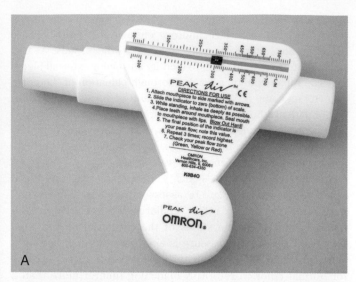

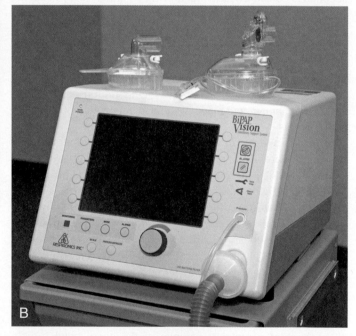

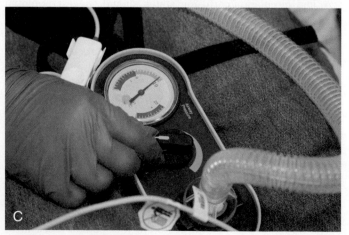

Figure 1-12 **A.** A peak flow meter. **B.** BiPAP machine. **C.** CPAP flow generator.

ventilation. To ensure quality continuity of care, prehospital providers should disclose technology-dependent patient information to the receiving facility as soon as it is identified.

Olfactory Observation

Odors can also serve as warning signs of an unsafe environment even before patient contact is established. Evidence of gas fumes, especially with multiple patients complaining of similar distressing symptoms, indicates the need for immediate evacuation. Odors associated with spoiled food, mold, or insect or rodent infiltration may indicate an unhealthy environment for the patient and family members. This type of environment may indicate failure to thrive or may be evidence of neglect or domestic abuse. This observation should be reported to the proper authorities per local protocols and statutory requirements.

Also note unusual patient odors. Certain smells are associated with various acute or chronic disease processes, such as a fruity acetone breath odor with diabetic ketoacidosis. Observation of any excreted patient fluids such as blood, vomitus, urine, or feces may indicate dysfunction of the central nervous system (CNS). Other odors, such as a musty breath odor, can point toward chronic liver dysfunction. Significant body odor and uncleanliness may be evidence that the patient can no longer perform the activities of daily living without assistance.

Kinesthetic Observation

The sense of touch also gives clues to the patient's condition. Patients may have skin that feels cool, cold, warm, hot, or sweaty. Excessively warm or hot skin may indicate an elevated core body temperature. A hot day with high humidity can lead to hyperthermia. Intrinsic causes of hot skin include stroke, fever, and heat stroke.

Likewise, an extremely cold environment may cause hypothermia. However, in older adult patients, hypothermia can occur even in a warm environment. Immobility, compromised cardiovascular and neurologic systems, inappropriate clothing, drug toxicities, and comorbid conditions cause poor perfusion and diminished compensatory mechanisms. Cool, clammy skin can also be the result of shock or compensatory mechanisms such as vasoconstriction.

Moist or wet skin is typically found in patients with heat exhaustion, exertion, or drug toxicity. Patients with cardiovascular compromise that leads to poor perfusion also present with moist skin. Patients who are dehydrated will have dry skin. Deterioration of thirst and taste mechanisms often accompany advancing age, so it is especially important to evaluate older adult patients for dry skin and dehydration.

Touch also provides essential assessment information by allowing you to feel the patient's pulse and determine the rate—too fast or too slow, weak, thready, or bounding. Touch can help identify an irregular pulse, which may indicate cardiovascular compromise.

In addition to obtaining information from initial sensory observations, the provider should ascertain the patient's reason for asking for medical assistance. Asking the patient what seems to be wrong (e.g., area of pain, discomfort, or abnormality), the chief complaint, assists in prioritizing the approach to obtaining historical and physical exam information. The patient may describe symptoms—chest pain or difficulty breathing—or an observed event such as syncope. Address any life-threatening problems immediately. Building on dispatch information, initial observations, and the patient's chief complaint, providers can begin to focus on the primary survey and continue to determine what happened.

▼ Detailed Assessment

History Taking

For patients with medical emergencies, historical information can be obtained before the physical exam is performed. Modifying the approach to obtaining historical information before performing a physical exam is dependent on the patient's initial presentation. Many diagnostic assessments are ordered on the basis of additional information obtained during the patient interview. An efficient, systematic, comprehensive interview, then, can help providers eliminate differential diagnoses, establish a working diagnosis, and determine treatment interventions.

History of the Present Illness

The history of the present illness can be obtained by using the mnemonic *OPQRST*, which is summarized in the Rapid Recall

RAPID RECALL © HunThomas/ShutterStock, Inc.

History of the Present Illness: OPQRST

To assess the cause of a patient's injury or illness, providers need to know what brought it on and when, where it hurts, and how badly. The OPQRST mnemonic will help you remember which questions to ask in order to elicit the most pertinent answers from the patient:

- **O**nset—What were you doing when the pain started? Did the pain start all of a sudden or come on over a period of time?
- **P**alliation/provocation—Does anything make the pain go away or feel better or feel worse?
- **Q**uality—Describe the pain (burning, sharp, dull, ache, stabbing).
- **R**egion/radiation/referral—Can you point to the place where it hurts? Does the pain stay there or go somewhere else?
- **S**everity—On a scale of 1 to 10, with 1 being very minor and 10 the worst pain you have ever felt, how would you rate this?
- **T**ime/duration—How long have you felt this way?

box. This tool helps analyze the patient's complaint by focusing on obtaining a clear, chronologic account of the symptoms the patient is experiencing.

Onset

First, determine the time of onset and origin of the pain or discomfort. Find out what the patient was doing when symptoms began. Ask about any similar episodes the patient may have had. Obtaining the following information will assist you in determining a differential diagnosis:

- What the patient was doing when symptoms began. Pain or discomfort that occurs on exertion may have a different origin than pain or discomfort occurring at rest.
- Whether the onset of symptoms was gradual or sudden.
- Any associated complaints, which may suggest the severity of the problem and indicate that multiple body systems are involved. Associated symptoms of importance are:
  - Trouble breathing
  - Shortness of breath
  - Pain on deep inspiration
  - Chest pain or pressure
  - Palpitations
  - Nausea or vomiting
  - Syncope (fainting)
  - Numbness or tingling
  - Indigestion (epigastric pain, abdominal pain, or bloating)
  - Confusion or disorientation
  - General feeling of illness or being out of sorts
- Any information offered by bystanders.
- Whether the patient has experienced similar symptoms before. Ask whether the patient is under a doctor's care, and if so, when the last visit was. Inquire about medications prescribed and other treatments given.

Palliation Provocation

Palliation and provocation refer to factors that make the patient's symptoms better (palliate them) or worse (provoke them). A patient whose chief complaint is dizziness, for example, might say that the symptoms are better when lying down (palliation) and worse with movement, such as suddenly trying to get out of bed (provocation).

Quality

The patient's perception of the quality of the pain or discomfort can be an important diagnostic clue. Ask for a description of the type of pain or discomfort. Some common descriptions include terms such as *sharp*, *dull*, *tearing*, *ripping*, *crushing*, *pressure*, and *stabbing*. The patient's description can suggest whether the pain is of visceral or somatic origin, which will help in determining the differential diagnosis. Visceral pain is from internal organs and often vague and difficult to localize, whereas somatic pain can be precisely located and more likely to be sharp or stabbing in nature. Assessing whether the discomfort is constant or occurs only intermittently, either randomly or with certain breathing patterns or movements, can be a key indicator of the body system involved and the severity of the etiology. Along with palliation and provocation, how a patient describes the quality of the pain or discomfort can also indicate the underlying body system affected. In quotation marks, document exactly how patients describe their symptoms.

Region/Radiation/Referral

Region, radiation, and referral are all associated with the location of the pain or discomfort. Ask the patient to point to where it hurts or indicate whether the pain seems to radiate or move anywhere else (Table 1-4). Try to ascertain whether the pain is referred, such as abdominal distention with pain in the shoulder (Kehr sign).

Severity

The majority of patients seen by healthcare providers have experienced either acute or chronic pain or discomfort. Pain and discomfort can result from infection, inflammation, and neurologic dysfunction. Injury and overuse of muscles and the skeletal system can generate acute or chronic pain. Organs in every body system can elicit pain and discomfort. Activation of nociceptive pain fibers is the root cause of both chronic and acute pain.

Table 1-4 Referred Pain	
Location	**Organ**
Left shoulder pain	Diaphragm irritation (blood or air from rupture of other abdominal structures such as ovaries), ruptured spleen, myocardial infarction
Right shoulder pain	Liver irritation, gallbladder pain, diaphragm irritation
Right scapular pain	Liver and gallbladder
Epigastric	Stomach, lung, cardiac
Umbilical	Small intestine, appendix
Back	Aorta, stomach, pancreas
Flanks to groin	Kidney, ureter
Perineal	Bladder
Suprapubic	Bladder, colon

When the fibers are stimulated, the pain impulse will travel via nerve fibers to the spinal cord to the brain.

Pain or discomfort can present with very vague signs and symptoms, especially in patients who are poor historians, as in the elderly. Oftentimes, patients are taking over-the-counter (OTC) medications, self-remedies, or multiple medications. Whether medications are OTC or prescribed, their effects may mask the quality and severity of pain. Historical information regarding pain may present differently based on the patient's cultural background and religious belief systems, making the assessment and management challenging.

Any and all complaints of pain or discomfort must be taken seriously. Exercise patience in determining the location, severity, and quality of pain. Precise patient descriptions of the pain can help you differentiate pain associated with a life-threatening medical emergency from less critical pain and allow you to provide appropriate pain management.

Ask the patient to rate the level of the pain or discomfort on a scale from 1 to 10, with 1 being the least discomfort or pain and 10 the highest. This numeric scale is commonly used by both EMS and hospital personnel. Not only will the patient's report of the severity of the pain help narrow down its source, but it might also set a useful baseline by which to gauge whether the patient's condition is improving or worsening. The Wong-Baker Faces pain scale is a useful alternative for children or patients who may not be able to communicate verbally (**Figure 1-13**).

A variety of pain remedies may be encountered. Non-narcotic analgesics that control pain or diminish the perception of pain—acetaminophen (Tylenol), nonsteroidal anti-inflammatory drugs (NSAIDs) such as ibuprofen (Motrin/Advil), and naproxen (Aleve)—are typical OTC medications taken by patients. Opioid analgesics, such as morphine, hydrocodone, and oxycodone, are prescribed for acute and chronic pain.

Obtain as much information as possible on which pain medications the patient has been taking and whether self-administration of those medications has been optimal. From the additional information gathered in the present illness history, diagnoses and treatment are evaluated and modified.

Time/Duration

Finally, ask patients how long (time/duration) they have had the pain or discomfort. If the patient can't respond or isn't sure, ask a family member or a bystander to tell you exactly how long ago the patient last seemed to be feeling normal. Narrowing down the time frame of the discomfort may become crucial for sound medical decision making about certain conditions, such as deciding whether to administer fibrinolytic agents to a stroke patient or whether to catheterize a patient with suspected myocardial infarction (MI).

Past Medical History

The past medical history gives the provider an opportunity to learn about any pertinent or chronic underlying medical conditions the patient may have. Whereas not all aspects of the past history may seem important at the present time, a careful and thorough history will help paint a clear picture of the patient's overall health status. The SAMPLER mnemonic, summarized in the Rapid Recall box, can also be useful in the interviewing process.

RAPID RECALL © HunThomas/ShutterStock, Inc.

The SAMPLER Approach to Past Medical History

The SAMPLER mnemonic represents a sensible approach to inquiring about a patient's medical conditions:

Signs/symptoms

Allergies

Medications

Pertinent past medical history

Last oral intake (what and when)

Events preceding the current illness or injury

Risk factors

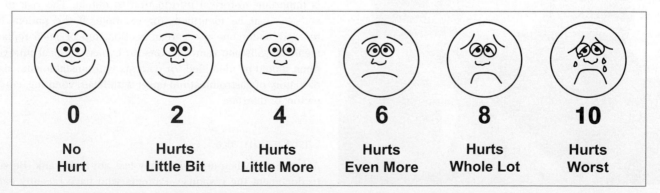

Figure 1-13 Wong-Baker FACES Pain Rating Scale. To use this scale, point to each face and use the words to describe the pain intensity. Ask the patient to choose the face that best describe his or her own pain, and document the number.

Signs and Symptoms

Symptoms are the subjective perceptions of what the patient feels, such as nausea, or has experienced, such as a sensation of seeing flashing lights. **Signs** are objective data that you or another healthcare professional have observed, felt, seen, heard, touched, or smelled and usually measured, such as data that indicate tachycardia. A symptom reported by the patient, such as diarrhea, becomes a sign as well when observed by a healthcare provider. All signs and symptoms should be well documented (**Figure 1-14**).

In awake and alert patients with no cognitive deficits, it is appropriate to use open-ended questions when asking how they are feeling. Such patients are able to process the question and give a reply. Patients with speech, hearing, or cognitive difficulties may respond more easily to yes-or-no questions. Often a simple head nod or shake can communicate effectively enough to help you complete the history. For patients who are disabled and for older adults who are frail, use patience when obtaining information. Allowing enough time for the patient to answer the question can often be challenging. Rushing a patient's verbal response, however, will inhibit rapport, might be frustrating or intimidating, and could impede the willingness to share information. Use appropriate therapeutic communication techniques to obtain information from the patient.

Allergies

Many patients have allergies to prescribed or OTC medications, animals, or food. Ask the patient about any known causes of allergic reactions and which symptoms are normally experienced, such as hives or trouble breathing. Find out how quickly the symptoms tend to develop.

Some symptoms are more worrisome than others. A patient who breaks out in a slight rash when around cats raises

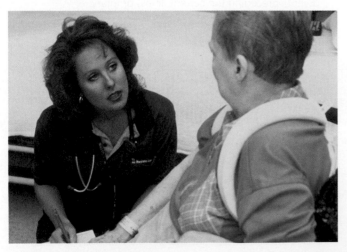

Figure 1-14 Be especially patient when you are obtaining information about a patient's symptoms.

fewer concerns than a patient who develops stridor when a particular food is eaten. Some untoward responses are adverse reactions rather than true allergic responses. Many patients may misinterpret hypersensitivity to a food, animal, or medication as an allergy, so it becomes important to evaluate exactly how the patient responds to contact with the reported allergen or irritant. This information will help distinguish a hypersensitivity response from an allergic or anaphylactic reaction.

Medications

In written documentation, include a record of all medications the patient takes regularly—OTC drugs and medications prescribed by all the patient's doctors. Healthcare providers may or may not know what the patient's physician may have prescribed. Drug interactions and adverse reactions must be considered in the overall medication profile.

Some patients also take OTC drugs or dietary supplements, also known as holistic, herbal, or alternative medications. Trends in legalization of cannabis indicate inclusion of additional patient questioning regarding the use of cannabis for recreational or medicinal use. Remember to ask about liquid OTC drinks and herbal teas that may have a high content of caffeine, vitamins, or other ingredients that might be causing the patient's signs and symptoms. Hypertensive patients who take OTC medications, such as cough suppressants or antitussive agents that contain dextromethorphan or guaifenesin, in conjunction with monoamine oxidase inhibitors (MAOIs) or selective serotonin reuptake inhibitors (SSRIs) can experience elevations in blood pressure.

Pertinent Past Medical History

Try to discern which medical history is pertinent to the presenting complaint. If the patient is having chest pain and had a stent recently placed, for example, that information is pertinent. A femur fracture that occurred 2 years ago is most likely not essential information.

A description of past surgeries, especially recent ones, is important historical information to obtain. The risk of an embolus can be identified, for example, if the patient has recently undergone a cesarean section, hip or knee replacement, or gallstone removal. Gastric bypass surgical interventions should be identified for patients with unstable vital signs or history of gastrointestinal upset with fever, vomiting, constipation, or diarrhea.

Last Oral Intake

Ask patients when and what they last ate and drank. Be sure to document the response. Patients who have recently eaten or had something to drink may aspirate stomach contents into the lungs if they become unconscious and vomit or have to be anesthetized for emergency surgery and vomit while under anesthesia.

Events Preceding the Current Illness or Injury

Find out which events led to the decision to request an ambulance or go to the hospital. Ask the patient, bystanders, and family the following questions: What happened today? Why did you call EMS? What has made the discomfort better or worse? This last question is appropriate when the events elapsed slowly, such as when a patient has trouble breathing all night but doesn't call EMS or obtain medical care until symptoms begin to worsen.

Risk Factors

Risk factors for a patient's given condition can be environmental, social, psychological, or familial. Is the patient living alone and at risk for falls? Does the residence contain any fall-related hazards? Is the patient confined to bed and dependent on someone else for meals and care? Other significant risk factors for medical problems include recent travel, surgeries, diabetes, hypertension, gender, race, age, smoking, and obesity.

Does the patient adhere to a prescribed medication regimen? Is the patient able to differentiate medications and take them properly? Is there a list of medications, and is the dispensing routine clear to the patient? An often helpful suggestion for patients taking several medications is to compile a complete list and post it in a visible place for themselves and their families. Doing so can reduce the likelihood of medication error and decrease the risk of drug toxicity.

Current Health Status

The personal habits of patients relevant to their overall health history can be important in determining the acuity of the current complaint. Frequent visits to their physician or emergency department for similar complaints may indicate the need for evaluation of a chronic condition and change in treatment regimens.

Alcohol or Substance Abuse and Tobacco Use

Asking patients about their use of drugs (licit or illicit, including the use of prescription drugs not prescribed to them), tobacco products, and alcohol may elicit important information about the potential for multiple underlying etiologies. Assure the patient of confidentiality when making such inquiries. The CAGE questionnaire, summarized in the Rapid Recall box, can be used to help identify alcohol abuse patterns of behavior. Such evaluation can indicate a chronic versus acute illness with the potential for traumatic injury. For example, a chronic alcoholic is at increased risk for subdural bleeding due to falling while intoxicated.

RAPID RECALL © HunThomas/ShutterStock, Inc.

CAGE Questionnaire

C: Have you ever been concerned about your own or someone else's drinking? Have you ever found the need to cut down on drinking?

A: Have you ever felt annoyed by criticism of your drinking?

G: Have you ever felt guilty about your drinking? Have you ever felt guilty about something you said or did while you were drinking?

E: Have you ever felt the need for a morning eye opener?

Modified from Ewing JA: Detecting alcoholism: the CAGE questionnaire, *JAMA* 252:1905, 1984.

Immunizations

Information about current screening tests and an immunization record help identify patients at risk for communicable diseases. Recent travel history outside the country or immigration status is also helpful in identifying conditions that should be included in the differential diagnosis.

Family History

Family history may be important if the differential diagnosis includes inherited conditions such as sickle cell disease or tuberculosis. Asking about family members with the following diseases may indicate high risk factors for the patient, aiding clinical reasoning and leading to more rapid diagnosis and treatment:

- Arthritis
- Cancer
- Headaches
- Hypertension
- Stroke
- Lung disease
- Tuberculosis
- Communicable and autoimmune diseases

Healthcare providers are patient advocates by seeking out family and friends who are supportive and may help the patient improve the safety of the home environment. Asking patients what they need to get through a difficult physical or psychological emergency is an empathetic and compassionate approach to patient care.

Patients who are able to develop a rapport with providers feel more trusting in answering questions and accepting decisions made about their care. Fostering an open, positive patient experience will help limit the associated stress of an illness or injury and make it easier for providers to obtain an accurate history, establish a working diagnosis, and begin prompt treatment. Therapeutic communication plays an important role in developing a rapport with your patients.

Once the patient's historical information is obtained, additional underlying etiologies and diagnoses should be modified and either disregarded or considered. Does the patient's response to initial treatment warrant modification? Let's look at the information you can obtain from the physical exam.

Secondary Survey

The **secondary survey** (also known as the physical exam) consists of two elements—obtaining vital signs that measure overall body function and performing a head-to-toe survey that evaluates the workings of specific body organ systems. The survey is done in a sequential manner, starting with the head, moving down to the toes, ensuring that every aspect of the body's function is evaluated. Of course, the conditions in the prehospital setting may determine precisely how the secondary survey is performed. Sometimes, it may be condensed. For example, for an unresponsive medical patient or a trauma patient with a significant mechanism of injury, there may only be time to perform a rapid exam. The amount of time spent on this exam and its thoroughness will be directly related to your scope of practice as a healthcare provider, the patient's status, and the diagnostic assessment tools available (e.g., reflex hammer, otoscope, ophthalmoscope).

In medical patients, vital signs are taken and a history is often obtained before a physical exam is performed. Depending on the severity of the patient's condition, the availability of healthcare personnel, and the estimated transport time to the appropriate healthcare facility, the physical exam may be performed either at the scene or en route to the receiving facility.

Vital Signs

Health care is a team effort, whether it is provided before the patient reaches the hospital or when the patient is in the hospital. Therefore, several healthcare providers can be involved simultaneously in the patient's assessment, obtaining diagnostic information, and providing patient care. Vital signs are generally the first component of the secondary survey. Vital signs traditionally include pulse rate, regularity, and quality; respiratory rate, regularity, and quality; blood pressure; and body temperature. You should measure these parameters frequently and continually. Even if the patient's initial presentation doesn't suggest an immediate life threat, the patient's condition may deteriorate. Establishing baseline vital signs and being alert for trends during ongoing monitoring can aid in early identification of any adverse change. Even if the patient's condition remains stable and nonemergent, vital signs are indispensable to sound medical decision making. They guide providers in establishing a specific diagnosis and formulating a treatment plan likely to be effective.

Pulse

Patients with suspected medical emergencies should be assessed for both central and peripheral pulses. The rate, regularity, and quality should be reevaluated, as previously discussed. Abnormal findings can lead to early application of ECG monitoring.

Respiration

The work of breathing should be assessed for symmetry, depth, rate, and quality (**Figure 1-15**). For a detailed discussion of breathing, see the earlier section.

Blood Pressure

Evaluation of this vital sign provides an estimate of the patient's perfusion status and can identify pulsus paradoxus and pulse pressure. **Blood pressure** is the tension exerted by blood on

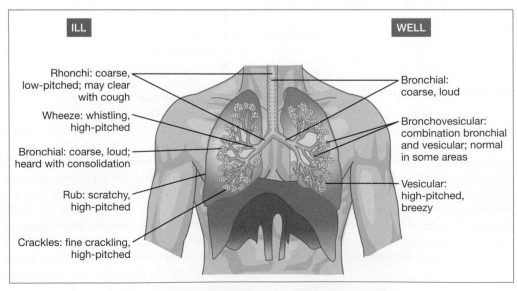

Figure 1-15 Lung sounds that may be heard in an ill patient (at left) and a well patient (at right).

the arterial walls. Blood pressure is calculated using the following equation:

$$\text{Blood pressure} = \text{Flow} \times \text{Resistance}$$

If flow or resistance is altered, blood pressure will increase or decrease. Resistance is altered when vessels narrow, increasing resistance and raising pressure, and when vessels dilate, decreasing resistance and lowering pressure.

In patients with cardiovascular disease or a life-threatening pulmonary condition, such as a pulmonary embolus or tension pneumothorax, pulsus paradoxus will be seen. Pulsus paradoxus is an irregularity that occurs when systolic blood pressure falls more than 10 mm Hg on inspiration. It is caused by differences in intrathoracic pressure with respiration, such as back flow of blood into the lungs as a result of heart failure.

A baseline blood pressure should be taken during initial contact with the patient. Measure blood pressure a minimum of two times while treating the patient in the prehospital environment. Ideally, the second blood pressure reading is obtained once the patient has been secured in the ambulance or other transport vehicle. Depending on the status of the patient and transport time, a third measurement is taken en route to the receiving facility. An initial blood pressure should be taken manually, and reassessment of blood pressure can be done using an automated device (**Figure 1-16**). Generally, vital signs for patients in stable condition are obtained every 15 minutes. Vital signs for patients in unstable condition are obtained every 5 minutes.

Temperature

Oral, rectal, tympanic, or axillary temperature measurements may be taken, depending on the patient's injuries, age, and LOC. Some patients with a decreased LOC may be too agitated for an oral measurement. Facial or other injuries may also preclude use of an oral thermometer. Another way to assess temperature is simply by touching the skin.

Be sure to inspect the skin for diaphoresis (sweating) and assess the color of the skin and nail beds. The skin should be dry to the touch and feel neither cool nor hot. If the patient has anything but dry, pink, warm skin, you should look for the cause of the altered perfusion.

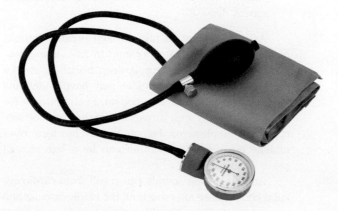

Figure 1-16 A blood pressure device.
© WizData, Inc/Shutterstock

Hyperthermia can be caused by sepsis (infection) or by medications such as antibiotics, narcotics, barbiturates, and antihistamines. Other causes of fever include heart attack, stroke, heat exhaustion, heatstroke, and burns. Hypothermia can be caused by exposure, shock, alcohol or other drug use, or hypothyroidism, and it can occur in patients who are severely burned and unable to regulate their body temperature. The environment, whether too warm, cold, or humid, may affect the patient's skin temperature and should be considered when evaluating skin vital signs.

The vital signs should offer important information to help you formulate a more in-depth impression about the patient's health status and treatment needs. In patients with alterations in mentation, also assess the pupils and perform an abbreviated neurologic exam during the assessment of vital signs. Motor and sensory function, distal pulses, and capillary refill should be evaluated as well. In addition, blood glucose levels should be obtained.

Confirming or ruling out whether life threats, emergent, or nonemergent conditions exist are core considerations for initiating care at the scene, prior to packaging for transport. Modifying or establishing a new care regimen will be based on continued information gathering during the secondary survey.

Physical Exam

The physical examination of a patient in the prehospital setting is the most important skill a healthcare provider can master. This ability is first developed as an EMT and should be refined as an advanced practitioner. The exam can be a full-body head-to-toe exam or a focused exam. The goal of this process is to identify hidden injuries or identify causes that may not have been found during the 60- to 90-second rapid scan that took place during the primary survey. The healthcare provider must determine, based on the acuity of the patient, which exam is most appropriate. In most emergency response situations, a focused exam is appropriate in conscious patients. A full-body head-to-toe exam is necessary in patients who are unconscious or have a diminished LOC and in those whose presentation indicates possible substance abuse or toxicity. Detailed physical exams may be more practical in the hospital, although a detailed exam may be performed by prehospital personnel if transport time allows.

The physical exam findings should augment the historical data and diagnostic assessment information already obtained to rule in or rule out certain differential diagnoses. As information is gathered and critically evaluated, an appropriate treatment pathway will be identified and implemented.

Stethoscopes, otoscopes, and ophthalmoscopes are common equipment used to gather valuable information when performing a physical exam, but the tools are only as good as the examiner's scope of practice and observation skills. Therefore, inspection, auscultation, palpation, and percussion are critical components of the assessment process. The physical examination will help identify life threats in the primary or secondary survey. In an unconscious patient, the physical exam may be the only way to obtain clues to identify the problem.

In many medical patients, historical information is obtained before the physical exam is performed. Altering the order of the components of the assessment is dependent on the severity of symptoms, the criticality of the patient's status, and the initial presentation up to this point. The physical exam during the primary survey may be performed prior to obtaining the history or simultaneously with obtaining the history if enough personnel are present. The physical exam findings enable to provider to rule in or rule out conditions that make up the differential diagnosis constructed during the history taking. The opposite may be true of traumatic injuries. In trauma patients, a rapid physical exam may be carried out before medical information is obtained.

Examination Techniques

- Inspection is the visual assessment of the patient to look for abnormalities. You begin observing visual clues to the patient's condition during the initial observation period. This preliminary inspection can reveal the implications of the environment and the severity of the patient's condition before the history is taken or the physical exam performed. Other aspects that may be readily apparent and worth noting include dress, hygiene, expression, overall size, posture, untoward odors, and overall state of health.

    Significant injury should be identified during your visual exam. Bruising, abrasions, surgical scars (particularly evidence of previous surgeries such as cardiac surgery or lung removal, because they may be pertinent to dyspnea or other respiratory distress), and rashes should be noted. Note whether a stoma is present. Read and document any medical alert tags.

    The trachea should be observed and potentially palpated to be midline. The shape of the patient's chest can offer the first clue to chronic lung disease. A barrel chest can indicate underlying COPD such as emphysema or chronic bronchitis.

    A patient in a supine position with flattened neck veins may have hypovolemia. Look for any unusual neck masses, jugular venous distention (JVD), and swelling. JVD with diminished or absent breath sounds may indicate tension pneumothorax and cardiac tamponade.

    Assess the patient for vascular assistive devices (VAD) that indicate chronic disease processes and the need for nutritional support or long-term vascular access, as in the case of chemotherapy regimens or frequent blood samples.

    Tracheal tugging and use of intercostal and neck muscles are a sign of distress. Asymmetry, grunting, and deep or shallow respiratory movement are abnormal. Immediate intervention should be initiated to improve oxygenation and ventilation, stabilize the work of breathing, and promote adequate perfusion.

    In patients with chronic renal failure, especially those on dialysis, you may note grafts or fistulas. Patients who receive peritoneal dialysis at home will have evidence of an abdominal catheter. In addition, a gastric tube may be used in the home setting to remove fluids and gas, instill irrigation solutions or medications, or administer enteral feedings. Be alert for the possibility the patient has aspirated gastric contents, and make sure the device is working properly.

    With keen observation, providers will note any kyphosis (spinal curvature), pressure ulcers, moles, abrasions, rashes, ecchymosis or hematoma, bleeding, needle or track marks, and discoloration.

- Auscultation is the use of a stethoscope or just your ears to evaluate the sounds the body makes, such as the flow of blood against the brachial artery with the head of the stethoscope. This is auscultation of blood pressure. Lung sounds, heart sounds, and bowel sounds can also be evaluated using auscultation.

    The lungs initially should be auscultated in the upper and lower lung fields, both anteriorly and posteriorly. If the patient's initial presentation is dyspnea or respiratory distress, lung sounds can be auscultated in the midaxillary position (**Figure 1-17**). Performing auscultation early in the assessment can reveal life-threatening respiratory compromise attributable to acute asthma or pulmonary edema.

    Lung sounds vary based on the part of the airway over which you are auscultating and the presence of abnormal conditions (see Figure 1–15).

- Vesicular lung sounds are auscultated over the anterior and posterior part of the chest. Normally these sounds are soft, low-pitched sounds heard over healthy lung tissue.
- Bronchovesicular sounds are auscultated over the main bronchi. These sounds are lower than the vesicular sounds and have a medium pitch.
- Bronchial sounds are heard over the trachea, near the manubrium of the sternum. They are typically high pitched.
- A sandpaper-like sound is an indication that the visceral and parietal pleura are rubbing together. This sign is called a friction rub and is associated with pulmonary diseases such as pleurisy.
- Adventitious lung sounds are audible sounds heard over the normal, nearly inaudible sound of breathing. They include crackles, rhonchi, and wheezing, each of which reveals valuable clues about lower airway disease.

Ask the patient to take a deep breath. Patients having acute asthma attacks tend to have more trouble exhaling than inhaling. If deep breathing causes pain or discomfort, the patient may have underlying pleurisy or a pulmonary embolism. Feel the torso for instability of bony structures. Palpate the chest for subcutaneous emphysema. Palpate the trachea for proper midline positioning. Deviation can be a late sign of pneumothorax.

Abnormal lung sounds can result from cardiovascular compromise affecting both the cardiovascular and respiratory systems. Crackles, for example, can signal pulmonary congestion from ventricular heart failure.

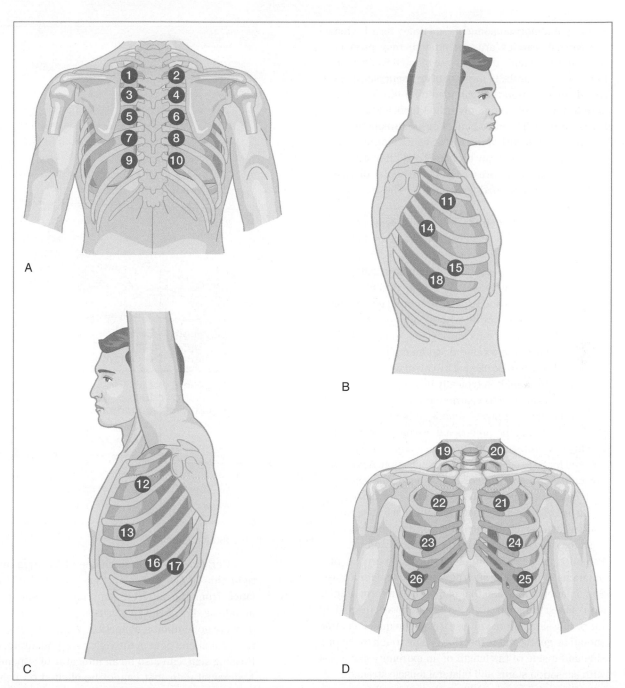

Figure 1-17 When you are listening to lung sounds, listen to one lung and then the other lung at the same location. Listen to at least one full inhalation and exhalation at each location—posterior chest **(A)**, right lateral chest **(B)**, left lateral chest **(C)**, and anterior chest **(D)**.

Using the proper assessment tools will help you confirm or eliminate differential diagnoses related to the respiratory system. The findings of such supplemental assessments will aid your clinical reasoning and ensure that your medical decision making is well informed and accurate.

As noted earlier in the chapter, some patients transported by prehospital personnel may require special transport ventilators. They may be intubated or have other preexisting respiratory system needs that will significantly affect EMS management and prehospital care.

Heart tones are auscultated for loudness (intensity), length (duration), pitch (frequency), and timing of the cardiac cycle. When listening at the fifth intercostal space, toward the apex of the heart, the normal heart sounds of S_1 and S_2 can be heard. These sounds are caused by heart valves closing and are best heard if the patient is leaning forward, sitting up, or in a left lateral recumbent position (and even supine). Positioning is best when the heart is closer to the left anterior chest wall. To better hear S_1, ask the patient to breathe normally, then hold his or her breath on expiration. To better hear S_2, ask the patient to breathe normally, then hold his or her breath on inspiration.

Abnormal heart sounds, such as murmurs, indicate a problem with the blood flow in and out of the heart.

Bruits are abnormal sounds sometimes heard when the carotid arteries are auscultated; they produce high-pitched sounds that indicate blood flow obstruction in those vessels. In the case of an aneurysm, a fine tremor or vibration that can identify a blockage can be felt; these are commonly called thrills. Murmurs, bruits, and thrills can be benign or life threatening.

In patients with a history of heart failure, additional heart sounds can be heard. Additional heart sounds occur in the presence of ventricular disease and are often identified as S_3 and S_4. These sounds are called gallops.

The S_3 sound, identified as a third heart sound, is an early clue to a diagnosis of left heart failure. Difficult to detect, it can be referred to as a gallop, which would sound similar to a horse's gallop. It appears approximately 0.12 to 0.16 second after the second heart sound and results from rapid expansion of the ventricles as they fill with blood.

The S_4 sound occurs during the second phase of ventricular filling when the atrium contracts. This sound is thought to be caused by valvular and ventricular wall vibration. It is typically heard when there is increased resistance to ventricular filling.

Auscultation of bowel sounds, although not often performed during the prehospital evaluation, can help identify bowel obstruction. Bowel sounds should be auscultated for 30 to 60 seconds before palpation. A normal bowel makes a gurgling noise and sounds the same in each quadrant. High-pitched hyperactive bowel sounds in the presence of a distended abdomen may give early warning of a bowel obstruction. An obstruction or accumulation of gases can rupture the intestinal wall.

■ Palpation is physical touching for the purpose of obtaining information, such as when you feel for a pulse. Some patients may feel that palpation is a form of invasion of their personal space, so be sure to ask the patient for permission before you use this technique. Palpation should be gentle and respectful. A light touch to the outside and inside of the length of an extremity can assist with sensation status and bilateral muscle strength.

The abdomen should be palpated in all four quadrants. It should be soft and nontender, with no tension, swelling, or masses. Muscle guarding is an abnormal finding that indicates pain and possible underlying injury. Abdominal rigidity is a sign of a life threat, such as internal bleeding. Upper right quadrant tenderness that worsens with inspiration, known as Murphy sign, is an indication of the presence of gallstones and cholecystitis (**Figure 1-18**).

The quadrant with the most reported discomfort should be palpated last. Palpation should be used to evaluate pain when gentle pressure is applied. It is also a means of identifying an increase in pain on removal of gentle pressure, known as rebound tenderness. This sign is a red flag for peritonitis.

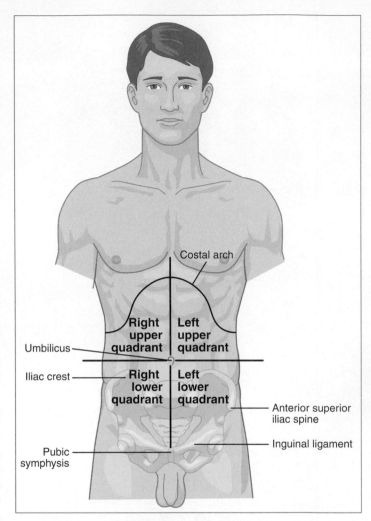

Figure 1-18 The four quadrants.

McBurney point is the name of the area over the right side of the abdomen that is a third of the distance from the anterior superior iliac spine to the umbilicus. Localized tenderness in this area is a sign of acute appendicitis. Palpation of the left lower quadrant that elicits pain in the right lower quadrant, called Rovsing sign, can also be an indicator of appendicitis. Abdominal pain that cannot be elicited on palpation can be caused by renal calculi or a urinary tract infection. Flank and back pain often accompany both of these diagnoses.

■ Percussion entails gently striking the surface of the body, typically where it overlies various body cavities. Sound waves are heard as percussion tones, which change according to the density of the tissue.

Percussion is not typically performed in the prehospital environment. However, this assessment provides important information regarding the abdominal cavity. If a dullness is heard during percussion, an abundance of fluid may be accumulating in this cavity, as occurs in liver failure. A hyperresonant sound may indicate that air, as opposed to fluid, is abundant (**Table 1-5**).

Table 1-5 Percussion Tones and Examples

Percussion Tone	Example
Tympany (the loudest)	Gastric bubble
Hyperresonance	Air-filled lungs (COPD, pneumothorax)
Resonance	Healthy lungs
Dullness	Liver
Flat (the quietest)	Muscle

The Full-Body Physical Exam

The full-body physical exam is a systematic head-to-toe physical examination. Like the rapid exam, the full-body exam includes looking, listening where appropriate, and palpating. Any patient who has sustained a significant mechanism of injury, is unresponsive, or is in critical condition should receive this type of examination. To perform this physical exam of a patient with no suspected spinal injuries, follow the steps listed. If your patient has sustained significant trauma, be sure that spinal immobilization is in place.

1. Look at the face for obvious swelling, lacerations, bruises, fluids, and deformities.
2. Inspect the area around the eyes and eyelids.
3. Examine the eyes for redness, contact lenses, and yellow or reddened sclera. Assess the pupils using a penlight.
4. Look behind the patient's ears to assess for bruising (the Battle sign).
5. Use the penlight to look for drainage of spinal fluid or blood in the ears.
6. Look for bruising and lacerations about the head. Palpate for tenderness, depressions of the skull, and deformities.
7. Palpate the zygomas for tenderness, symmetry, and instability.
8. Palpate the stability of the maxillae.
9. Check the nose for blood, drainage, or nasal flaring.
10. Palpate the stability of the mandible.
11. Assess the mouth for cyanosis, foreign bodies (including loose or broken teeth or dentures), bleeding, lacerations, and deformities.
12. Check for unusual odors on the patient's breath.
13. Look at the neck for obvious lacerations, bruises, and deformities. Observe for jugular venous distention and/or tracheal deviation.
14. Palpate the front and the back of the neck for tenderness and deformity. Auscultate for bruits if perfusion is compromised.
15. Look at the chest for obvious signs of injury before you begin palpation. Be sure to watch for movement of the chest with respirations. Assess for neck chains, bruising,

and scars as evidence of a previous surgery. Observe placement of central line catheters, such as a peripheral inserted central catheter (PICC) or a Hickman, Broviac, or Groshong catheter. Assess the work of breathing.

16. Gently palpate over the ribs to assess structural integrity and elicit tenderness. Avoid pressing over obvious bruises and fractures.
17. Listen for breath sounds over the midaxillary and midclavicular lines—a minimum of four fields if you check the anterior chest, and six fields if you are assessing the posterior chest.
18. Lung assessment must include the bases and apices of the lungs. At this point, also assess the back for tenderness and deformities, so that you logroll the patient only once. Remember, if a spinal cord injury is suspected, use spinal precautions as you logroll the patient.
19. Look at the abdomen and pelvis for obvious lacerations, bruises, and deformities. Gently palpate the abdomen for pain on pressure or rebound tenderness. Observe for tenderness, guarding, rigidity, and pulsating masses.
20. Gently compress the pelvis and iliac crest from the sides to assess for tenderness, instability, and/or crepitus.
21. Inspect all four extremities for lacerations, bruises, swelling, deformities, ports or fistulas, and medical alert anklets or bracelets. Also assess distal pulses and motor and sensory function in all extremities. Compare right and left sides to determine strength and weakness variances.

The Focused Physical Assessment

A focused physical assessment is generally performed on patients who have sustained nonsignificant mechanisms of injury and on responsive medical patients. This type of examination is based on the cardinal presentation/chief complaint. For example, in a person reporting a headache, you should carefully and systematically assess the head and/or neurologic system. A person with a laceration on the arm may need to have only the arm evaluated. The focused assessment concentrates on the immediate problem. The most common complaints from a responsive medical patient will involve the head, heart, lungs, or abdomen, individually or in combination.

- *Mental status.* Evaluation of a patient's mental status involves assessing cognitive function (the patient's ability to use reasoning). At a minimum, evaluate the patient's degree of alertness. Use the AVPU mnemonic as described the *Primary Survey* section to help identify the patient's level of consciousness. You can further assess mental status by considering whether the patient is alert and oriented in four areas (A×O): person, place, day of the week, and the event itself. The most reliable and consistent method of assessing mental status and neurologic function is the Glasgow Coma Scale, which assigns a point value (score) for eye opening, verbal response, and motor response; these values are added together for a total score. The GCS score provides much greater insight into the patient's overall neurologic function.

- *Skin, hair, and nails.* The skin, which is the largest organ system in the body, serves three major functions: It regulates the temperature of the body, it transmits information from the environment to the brain, and it protects the body in the environment. Examination of the skin involves both inspection and palpation. Pay careful attention to the skin color, moisture, temperature, texture, turgor, and any significant lesions. Look for evidence of diminished perfusion, evaluate for pallor and cyanosis, and be wary of diaphoresis. Flushed skin is usually apparent in patients with fever, and it may be seen in patients who are experiencing an allergic reaction.

  Examination of the hair is done by inspection and palpation. In this survey, note the quantity, distribution, and texture of the hair. Recent changes in the growth or loss of hair can indicate an underlying endocrine disorder, such as diabetes, or may result from treatment modalities, such as chemotherapy or radiation.

  The examination of the fingernails and toenails can reveal many subtle findings. The color, shape, texture, and presence or absence of lesions should all be assessed. Normal changes to the nails with aging include the development of striation and a change in color (yellowish tint) related to the reduction in body calcium. Overly thick nails or nails that have lines running parallel to the finger often suggest a fungal infection.

- *Head, eyes, ears, nose, and throat.* Physical exam of the head, eyes, ears, nose, and throat consists of a comprehensive evaluation of the head and related structures. It is crucial because the head contains the brain, numerous important sensory organs, and all of the upper airway anatomy. The eyes are a nervous system structure that involves both motor pathways (lids, extraocular muscles, pupillary constrictors, corneal blink reflex) and sensory pathways. The ears provide for both hearing and balance control. The nose is a sensory organ involved with the senses of smell and taste. It also plays an important role in assisting with breathing. The throat consists of the mouth and posterior pharynx and all the structures intrinsic to them. This complicated organ simultaneously coordinates many motor and sensory functions, while also coordinating the initial activities of both the respiratory and digestive systems.

  When you are examining the head, you should both feel it and inspect it visually. This step is important in the management of potential trauma patients and with patients who have altered mental status or are unresponsive. Inspect and feel the entire cranium for signs of deformity or asymmetry, being careful not to palpate any depressions because you do not want to push bone fragments into the cranial vault or the brain. If you find evidence of external bleeding, attempt to separate the hair manually and irrigate the clot. When you are evaluating the face, observe the color and moisture of the skin, as well as expression, symmetry, and contour of the face itself. Asymmetry of the face could suggest an underlying nerve system problem such as a stroke or facial nerve palsy. Take the following steps to examine the head:

1. Visually inspect the head, looking for any obvious deformities, contusions, abrasions, punctures, burns, tenderness, lacerations, and swelling.
2. Palpate the top and back of the head to locate any subtle abnormalities. Use a systematic approach, going from front to back, to ensure that nothing is missed.
3. Part the hair in several places to examine the condition of the scalp. Identify any lesions under the hair.
4. Note any pain or discomfort during the process. This exam should not cause the patient any pain.
5. Palpate the structure of the face, noting any deformities, contusions, abrasions, punctures, burns, tenderness, lacerations, and swelling.

The eyes are a tremendously complex sensory organ. They process light stimuli for the brain, so that the brain is able to decode light impulses presenting to the eyes and form a visual image. The eyes are a critical link to the CNS—they give a useful glimpse into the patient's neurologic status. The eyes are assessed for a conjugate gaze. To do so, shine a penlight into the eye from the side of the face as the patient focuses on a distant object. In an awake and alert patient, the eyes should be open, should face in the same direction, and should move in tandem (**Figure 1-19**).

Adequately perfused pupils are equal, round, and briskly reactive to stimulation with a penlight. Pinpoint pupils suggest opiate abuse or injury to the pons. Pupil dilation indicates toxicity or diminished neurologic function. Shining a light into the patient's eyes should cause the pupils to constrict quickly. Be sure to assess for this response in both eyes, observing whether the muscles of the eyes work synchronously so that the pupils constrict simultaneously. Unilateral dilatation in an unconscious patient may be a sign of brain herniation. Some patients may present with anisocoria, a condition characterized by pupils that are noticeably unequal in size. Pupils that appear unequal in shape and size may also suggest glaucoma. Take the following steps to examine the eyes:

1. Examine the exterior portion of the eye. Look for any obvious trauma or deformity.
2. Ask the patient about any pain, altered vision (blurred or double vision), discharge, or sensitivity to light.
3. Measure visual acuity by having the patient count the number of fingers you are holding up at varying distances from the patient (usually 6 ft, 3 ft, and 1 ft away from the patient). Perform this exam on each eye independently of the other.
4. Examine the pupils for size, shape, and symmetry. They should be equal.

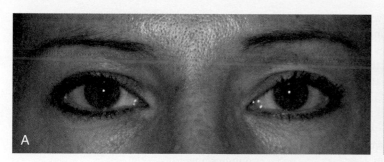
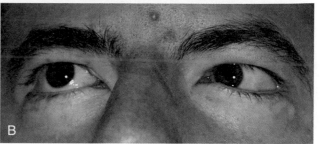
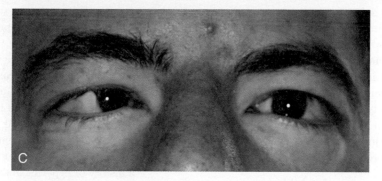

Figure 1-19 A. Baseline eye and lid position in central position. **B.** Right gaze with impaired abduction of the right eye. **C.** Left gaze with impaired abduction of the left eye.

Janet C. Rucker et al. Characterization of ocular motor deficits in congenital facial weakness: Moebius and related syndromes. Brain, April 2014, Vol. 137 (4), 1068–107. By permission of Oxford University Press.

5. Test the pupils for their reaction to light. Both pupils should constrict when exposed to light, and they should be equal in their response.
6. Test the function of the 12 cranial nerves on patients exhibiting altered mentation, syncope, headache, and stroke.
7. Inspect the eyelids, lashes, and tear ducts for evidence of trauma, foreign bodies, or discharge.

Assessing the ears essentially involves checking for new aberrations in hearing perception plus inspecting and palpating for wounds, swelling, or drainage (blood, pus, cerebrospinal fluid). Abnormalities of the external canal and tympanic membrane are visualized by use of an otoscope. Take the following steps to examine the ears:

1. Select an appropriately sized speculum. Dim the lights as much as possible.
2. Ensure that the ear is free of foreign bodies.
3. Place your hand firmly against the patient's head and gently grasp the patient's auricle. Move the ear to best visualize the canal, usually upward and back in the adult patient.
4. Ask the patient not to move during the exam to avoid damaging the ear.
5. Turn on the otoscope and insert the speculum into the ear. Insertion toward the patient's nose usually provides the best view. Do not insert the speculum deeply into the canal.

6. Inspect the canal for any lesions or discharge. A small amount of ear wax is normal.
7. Visualize the tympanic membrane (eardrum), and inspect it for integrity and color. Note any signs of inflammation.

When you are checking the nose, assess it both anteriorly and inferiorly. Look for evidence of asymmetry, deformity, wounds, foreign bodies, discharge or bleeding, and tenderness. Take the following steps to examine the nose:

1. Inspect the exterior of the nose, looking for color changes and structural abnormalities.
2. Examine the column of the nose; it should be midline with the face.
3. Inspect the septum for any deviation from midline.
4. Note gross abnormalities and any drainage or discharge. Small amounts of mucosal discharge are normal, but large amounts of mucus and any blood or cerebrospinal fluid are serious findings.

Assessment of the throat should include an evaluation of the mouth, the pharynx, and sometimes the neck. The throat is a conduit for both respiration and digestion, and it is in close proximity to numerous vital neurovascular structures. As part of the assessment of overall hydration status, pay close attention to the lips, teeth, oral mucosa, and tongue. In patients who present with a markedly altered mental status, you will need to rapidly determine upper airway status. Prompt assessment of the throat and upper airway structures is mandatory. Always be ready to assist with clearing the pharynx using manual techniques and suction. Take the following steps to examine the throat:

1. If trauma is suspected, take precautions to protect the cervical spine.
2. Assess for usage of accessory muscles during respiration.
3. Palpate the neck to find any structural abnormalities or subcutaneous air, and ensure the trachea is midline. Begin at the suprasternal notch and work your way toward the head. Be careful about applying pressure to the area of the carotid arteries because it may stimulate a vagal response.
4. Assess the lymph nodes and note any swelling, which may indicate infection.
5. Assess the jugular veins for distention; it may indicate a problem with blood returning to the heart.

- *Cervical spine.* The cervical spine is the pathway by which the spinal cord makes its way out of the brain and into the torso, enabling the spinal nerves to emanate to and innervate the rest of the body. Cervical injury can present in a variety of ways, and the assessment for such injury must be conducted in a careful manner. Evaluate the patient first for the mechanism of injury and then for the presence of pain.

  When you are examining the cervical spine, inspect and palpate it, looking for evidence of tenderness and deformity. Pain is the single most reliable indicator of a spine injury or spinal cord injury. Any manipulations that result in pain, tenderness, or tingling should prompt you to stop the exam immediately and place the patient in a proper sized collar. Continued assessment of a patient's range of motion should take place only when there is no potential for serious injury.

- *Chest.* Typically, the chest exam proceeds in three phases. The chest wall is checked, a pulmonary evaluation is conducted, and finally the cardiovascular assessment is performed. The chest must be inspected for deformities in wall patency as well as to look for external clues of respiratory distress. Expose the chest and then begin the assessment, using the techniques of inspection, palpation, auscultation, and percussion. The examination of the posterior chest is the same as the examination of the anterior chest. Take the following steps to examine the chest:

1. Ensure the patient's privacy as best you can.
2. Inspect the chest for any obvious deformities, contusions, abrasions, punctures, burns, tenderness, lacerations, and swelling.
3. If you find any open wounds, dress them appropriately.

4. Note the shape of the patient's chest—it can give you clues to many underlying medical conditions, such as emphysema.
5. Look for any surgical scars or catheter ports that indicate previous cardiac surgery and chronic illness.
6. Auscultate the lung fields, noting any abnormal lung sounds.
7. Observe and palpate for subcutaneous emphysema.
8. Auscultate for heart tones.
9. Repeat the appropriate portions of the examination for the posterior aspect of the thorax.

- *Cardiovascular system.* When you are examining a patient's cardiovascular system, pay attention to distal pulses, noting their location, rate, rhythm, and quality. Are the pulses fast or slow? Regular or irregular? Is the quality weak and thready or strong and bounding? Obtain an accurate blood pressure reading and repeat this measurement periodically to assess the patient's hemodynamic stability. Note if the patient has a history of hypertension. Auscultate the carotid arteries with the bell of the stethoscope to assess for any bruits. While inspecting and palpating the chest, listen for heart sounds. Feel the chest wall to locate the point of maximum impulse and appreciate the apical pulse.

  For a suspected heart problem, assess the pulse for regularity and strength, and examine the skin for signs of hypoperfusion (pallor, cool, wet) or oxygen desaturation (cyanosis). If the pulse feels irregular, assess it over 1 minute, rather than 30 seconds, in order to obtain a more accurate rate. Listen to breath sounds—many cardiac problems are associated with respiratory problems. Obtain baseline vital signs. Serious hypotension with sustained or progressive tachycardia is common in cardiogenic shock; stay alert for this condition because its mortality rate is more than 80%. Check for JVD because it can indicate heart failure, cardiac tamponade, or pneumothorax. Examine the extremities for signs of peripheral edema that may result from right-sided heart failure.

- *Abdomen.* One of the most challenging complaints for you to assess in the field setting is that of abdominal pain, because it can result from multiple causes and often presents with few or no external signs. Always proceed with abdominal assessment in a systematic fashion, routinely performing inspection, auscultation, percussion, and palpation, in that order, quadrant by quadrant. Take the following steps to examine the abdomen:

1. Inspect the abdomen for any deformities, contusions, abrasions, punctures, burns, tenderness, lacerations, and swelling.
2. Note any surgical scars because they may be clues to an underlying illness.
3. Look for symmetry and the presence of any distention.
4. Auscultate the abdomen for bowel sounds.

5. Perform percussion.

6. Palpate the four quadrants of the abdomen in a systematic pattern, beginning with the quadrant farthest from the patient's complaint of pain.

7. Note any tenderness or rigidity, and pay special attention to the patient's expressions because they may yield valuable information.

- *Female and male genitalia and anus.* In general, assessment of female genitalia is performed in a limited and discreet fashion. Reasons to examine the genitalia include concern over life-threatening hemorrhage or imminent delivery in childbirth (checking for crowning). Assessment of the female genitalia can be performed while you are assessing the abdomen. Palpate both the bilateral inguinal regions and the hypogastric region. If the decision is made to inspect the genitalia specifically, limit the examination to inspection only. Clinically significant causes of this pain include ectopic pregnancy, complications of third-trimester pregnancy, and nonpregnant ovarian problems or pelvic infections. Note any bleeding. In the case of injury involving intentional trauma, significant bleeding is possible. In general, make note of the amount and quality of any bleeding, as well as any inflammation, discharge, swelling, or lesions of the genitalia.

  When you are examining the male genitalia, make certain that the exam is performed in a limited and discreet fashion. Always assess the entire abdomen and note any pertinent findings, because occasionally lower abdominal problems are referred from the genitalia. Situations of testicular torsion or inguinal hernia sometimes present with a complaint of lower abdominal pain but minimal abdominal tenderness. In the case of a trauma patient, assess for the possibility of significant genital bleeding and injury or underlying fracture.

  The anus is often evaluated at the same time as the genitalia. It is examined in only a limited number of circumstances, and is always done with the patient appropriately draped and your partner present. Examine the sacrococcygeal and perineal areas, noting obvious bleeding trauma, lumps, ulcers, inflammation, rash, abrasions, or evidence of fecal incontinence.

- *Musculoskeletal system.* When you are examining the skeleton and joints, pay attention to their structure and function. Consider how the joint and associated extremity look and how well they work. Does the extremity look normal, and does it move in a normal pattern? In particular, note any limitation of range of motion, pain with range of motion, or bony crepitus. When you are assessing the joints and extremities, look for evidence of inflammation or injury, such as swelling, tenderness, increased heat, redness, ecchymosis, or decreased function. Also evaluate the joint or extremity for obvious deformity, diminished strength, atrophy, or asymmetry from one side to the other. The examination of the musculoskeletal system should not cause the patient any pain. If any pain occurs, it should be considered an abnormal finding. Take the following steps to examine the musculoskeletal system:

  1. Beginning with the upper extremities, inspect the skin overlying the muscles, bones, and joints for soft-tissue damage.

  2. Note any deformities or abnormal structure.

  3. Check for adequate distal pulse, motor, and sensation to each extremity.

  4. Inspect and palpate the hands and the wrists, noting any deformities, contusions, abrasions, punctures, burns, tenderness, lacerations, and swelling.

  5. Ask the patient to flex and extend the joints of the fingers, hands, and wrist, noting any abnormalities in the range of motion. If the patient experiences any discomfort, stop that portion of the exam immediately.

  6. Inspect and palpate the elbows, noting any abnormalities. Ask the patient to flex and extend the elbow to determine the range of motion.

  7. Ask the patient to turn the hand from the palm-down position to the palm-up position and back again, noting any pain or abnormalities.

  8. Inspect and palpate the shoulders. As the patient to shrug the shoulders and raise and extend both arms.

  9. Inspect the skin overlying the lower extremities.

  10. Ask the patient to point and bend the toes to establish the range of motion.

  11. Ask the patient to rotate the ankle, checking for pain or restricted range of motion.

  12. Inspect and palpate the knee joints and patella. Ask the patient to bend and straighten both to establish the range of motion.

  13. Check for structural integrity of the pelvis by applying gentle pressure to the iliac crests and pushing in and then down.

  14. Ask the patient to lift both legs by bending at the hip and then turning the legs inward and outward. Note any abnormalities.

- *Peripheral vascular system.* When you are assessing the peripheral vascular system, pay attention to both the upper and lower extremities. Look for signs indicative of either acute or chronic vascular problems. A wide range of disorders can affect the peripheral vascular system—from chronic venous stasis and lymphedema to intermittent claudication (cramp-like pain in the lower legs due to poor circulation or low potassium levels) and acute arterial occlusion. Peripheral vascular disease can manifest in many forms, depending on the point in the vasculature where the abnormality is located. Carotid artery disease can manifest as a stroke, for example, while arterial embolization involving the mesenteric vessels can result in bowel ischemia and necrosis. Take the following steps to examine the peripheral vascular system:

1. When you are examining the upper extremities, note any abnormalities in the radial pulse, skin color, or condition. Always one extremity to the opposing extremity.
2. If abnormalities are noted in the distal pulse, work your way proximally, checking these pulse points and noting your findings.
3. Palpate the epitrochlear and brachial nodes of the lymphatic system, noting any swelling or tenderness.
4. Examine the lower extremities, noting any abnormalities in the size and symmetry of the legs.
5. Inspect the skin color and condition, noting any abnormal venous patterns or enlargement.
6. Check distal pulses, noting any abnormalities.
7. Palpate the inguinal nodes for swelling and tenderness.
8. Evaluate the temperature of each leg relative to the rest of the body and to each other.
9. Evaluate for pitting edema in the legs and feet.

- *Spine.* Assessment of the cervical spine was introduced after the section on examination of the throat and neck. This section lists the complete assessment steps for the examination of the spine.
  1. Inspect the cervical, thoracic, and lumbar curves for any abnormalities.
  2. Evaluate the heights of the shoulders and the iliac crests. Differences from one side to the other may indicate abnormal curvature of the spine.
  3. Palpate the posterior portion of the cervical spine, noting any point tenderness or structural abnormalities.

4. In the nontrauma patient and in the absence of reported pain, ask the patient to move the head forward, backward, and from side to side.
5. Move down the spine, palpating each vertebra with the thumbs to note any tenderness or instability.
6. In the absence of pain or trauma, ask the patient to bend at the waist in each direction to establish the range of motion.

- *Nervous system.* The nervous system includes two portions: the central nervous system, which consists of the brain and spinal cord, and the peripheral nervous system, which includes the remaining motor and sensory nerves. Motor and sensory function should be evaluated in all patients whether they are conscious or unconscious, or have altered mental status. If the patient is conscious, gently touch the hands and feet to determine the ability to feel light touch, indicating that distal perfusion is adequate and sensory nerve tracts are functioning properly. Withdrawal of an extremity may indicate pain or discomfort. Assessing for sensation will determine the function of the afferent sensory nerve tracts in the posterior spinal column. The check of the nervous system is one of the most time-consuming elements of the physical exam.

  All levels of healthcare providers should be proficient in performing a cranial nerve assessment as part of their physical exam. The cranial nerves play roles in a wide variety of motor and sensory functions that involve both the voluntary and autonomic nervous systems. Findings identify cranial nerve impairment and glean timely information about the patient's neurologic status. The cranial nerves and their functions are summarized in **Table 1-6**.

Table 1-6 Cranial Nerves and Their Functions

Nerve No.	Name	Function	Assessment
I	Olfactory	Sense of smell	Ask the patient to close her eyes. Place spirits of ammonia or an alcohol wipe under her nose. The patient should be able to identify the odor.
II	Optic	Sense of sight	Evaluate visual acuity using a Snellen visual acuity chart or Rosenbaum card. Ask the patient to cover one eye and tell you how many fingers you're holding up. Then evaluate the opposite eye.
III	Oculomotor	Size, symmetry, and shape of pupils Eye movement	Test the pupil response to light for equality, reactivity, and roundness. Pupils should briskly constrict with light and dilate in darkness.
IV	Trochlear	Downward gaze	Hold the patient's chin to prevent movement. Ask the patient to follow a penlight or object in an "H" pattern to track the six visual fields.

(continues)

Table 1-6 Cranial Nerves and Their Functions (*continued*)

Nerve No.	Name	Function	Assessment
V	Trigeminal	Cheek Jaw motion Chewing Facial sensation	Ask the patient to clench his teeth to determine the strength of the jaw and the ability to close the mouth without difficulty. The patient should feel a slight touch bilaterally.
VI	Abducens	Lateral eye movement	Same as for cranial nerve IV.
VII	Facial	Strength of facial muscles Taste Saliva secretion	Assess for weakness or asymmetry by inspecting the face at rest and when speaking. Ask the patient to raise his eyebrows, frown, show his upper and lower teeth, smile, and puff out both cheeks.
VIII	Acoustic	Sense of hearing Balance	Occlude each ear independently to test for hearing and balance.
IX	Glossopharyngeal	Tongue and pharynx sensation Taste Muscles of swallowing	Ask the patient to say "ahhh," and observe the uvula and soft palate response. The soft palate should move up, and the uvula should remain midline.
X	Vagus	Sensation of throat and trachea Taste Muscles for voice production Heart rate	Same as cranial nerve IX
XI	Spinal accessory	Shoulder movement Ability to turn head	Ask the patient to raise and lower her shoulders against the resistance of your hand on her shoulder.
XII	Hypoglossal	Speech articulation Tongue movement	Ask the patient to stick out his tongue and move it in several directions with symmetry.

Motor function in all extremities should be evaluated for bilateral equality and strength. Unequal responses of left and right limbs should be considered a sign of hemiparesis (unilateral paralysis) or hemiplegia (unilateral weakness), which can be caused by stroke, meningitis, brain tumors, or seizure activity. Bilateral upper or lower extremity weakness should raise concern for a spinal cord lesion.

Cerebellar function can be evaluated by how a patient stands and walks. Ataxia (unsteady gait) may indicate damage from toxicity or chronic neurologic dysfunction. A shuffling gait may indicate neurologic damage caused by Huntington's disease or Parkinson's disease. Tremors, muscle rigidity, and repetitive motion may indicate degeneration of the nervous system attributable to Alzheimer's disease or Parkinson's disease.

Patients with a variety of psychological or behavioral disorders may take antipsychotic medications that have spasmodic muscle movement as a side effect. These medications may also induce muscle dystonia, expressed as contortion of the extremities or facial tics.

Reflexes are tested to evaluate symmetry and strength of response. Reflexes are involuntary motor responses to specific sensory stimuli, such as a tap on the knee or stroking the eyelash. Testing may include deep tendon reflexes and superficial reflexes, including superficial abdominal reflexes. Inappropriate responses may indicate damage to neuronal pathways at corresponding spinal segmental levels. All responses should be thoroughly documented.

Deep tendon reflexes are stretch reflexes, requiring the muscles being tested to be relaxed and the tendons gently stretched (Table 1-7). Using a reflex hammer and keeping the wrist relaxed, gently swing the hammer to tap the tendon. Support the joint or extremity being tested with your nondominant hand (Figure 1-20). Upper motor neuron lesions, such as in the brain or spinal cord, typically lead to hyperreflexia, whereas peripheral nerve lesions, such as with Guillain-Barré syndrome, cause hyporeflexia.

The arm drift (see Figure 1-21) is used to evaluate motor and sensory function in a suspected stroke patient. Patients are asked to close their eyes and extend their arms with palms up. Note any downward drift or drop or any inward rotation of either arm.

The Babinski test may be used to check for neurologic function in conscious patients and in patients with altered mental status. To perform this exam, take a pen

Table 1-7 Superficial and Deep Tendon Reflexes

Reflex	Spinal Level Evaluated
Superficial	
Upper abdominal	T7, T8, and T9
Lower abdominal	T10 and T11
Cremasteric	T12, L1, and L2
Plantar	L4, L5, S1, and S2
Deep Tendon	
Biceps	C5 and C6
Brachioradial	C5 and C6
Triceps	C6, C7, and C8
Patellar	L2, L3, and L4
Achilles	S1 and S2
Scoring Deep Tendon Reflexes	
Grade	Deep Tendon Reflex Response
0	No response
1+	Sluggish or diminished
2+	Active or expected response
3+	More brisk than expected, slightly hyperactive
4+	Brisk, hyperactive, with intermittent or transient clonus

Modified from Rudy EB: Advanced Neurological and Neurosurgical Nursing, St. Louis, 1984, Mosby.

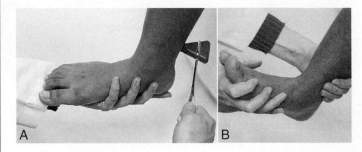

Figure 1-20 Location of tendons for evaluation of deep tendon reflexes. **A.** Patellar. **B.** Achilles.

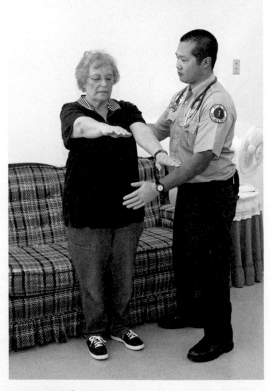

Figure 1-21 Arm drift test (National Institutes of Health Stroke Scale).

From Sanders MJ: *Mosby's paramedic textbook*, revised reprint, ed 3, St. Louis, MO, 2007, Mosby.

or similar dull object and run it along the lateral length of the sole of the foot. Normal reaction to this stimulation is for the toes to move downward, a response known as plantar flexion. This movement indicates a negative test result. A positive Babinski test is indicated by abnormal extension of the great toe and fanning of the remaining toes, a response called dorsiflexion. This movement suggests neurologic dysfunction (**Figure 1-22**). Periodic reevaluation of the patient's response to questions about pain, discomfort, and difficulty breathing is important in gauging the effectiveness of interventions.

The patient's physical exam should also be reevaluated, as appropriate, for diminished pain and discomfort, bleeding, and edema. Capillary refill time, distal pulses, and skin color, temperature, and moisture should also be reevaluated. Central nervous system function should be reassessed for improvement in GCS scores and motor, sensory, and pupil response. Take the following steps to examine the nervous system:

1. Assess the patient's mental status by using the AVPU mnemonic.
2. Note the patient's posture.
3. Evaluate cranial nerve function.
4. Evaluate the patient's neuromuscular status by checking muscle strength against resistance.
5. Evaluate the patient's coordination by performing the finger-to-nose test using alternating hands.
6. If appropriate, check the patient's gait and balance by having the patient walk heel to toe or perform the heel to shin stance.
7. Perform the arm drift test. There should be no difference in movement on either side.
8. Evaluate the patient's sensory function by checking the responses to both gross and light touch.
9. If appropriate, check for deep tendon reflexes.

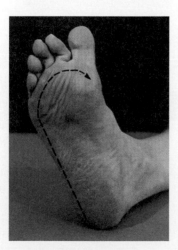

Figure 1-22 Check to determine the presence or absence of the Babinski sign.

Trauma Patients

Any trauma patient who is unresponsive or has altered mentation should be considered a high-risk, priority patient and requires immediate transport to a trauma center. An unresponsive patient may have a traumatic brain injury, stroke, hypoglycemia, or alcohol or drug intoxication. All are serious and potentially lethal events.

Recall that you will perform the rapid exam on trauma patients to obtain a quick 60- to 90-second impression of a patient's injuries before the patient is immobilized. Although there may not always be time for further physical examinations of trauma patients, when time and patient condition do allow for it, perform further physical examinations. The most visible injury you may be looking at (for example, a scalp laceration) or the most painful injury the patient reports (such as a fractured ankle) may not be nearly as serious as the most lethal injury the patient has (for example, a ruptured spleen).

Before you physically examine a trauma patient, make sure that the patient's cervical spine is manually immobilized in the neutral position. Quickly reassess the patient's current mental status, comparing it with the baseline that was established when you first encountered the patient. Last, revisit your transport decision. If you decide that the patient needs immediate transport, perform the rapid exam and do not delay transport in order to perform more thorough examinations.

If additional physical examinations are performed beyond the rapid exam, remember to check your gloves for blood after each area of the body is assessed. This will enable you to note any areas that have active bleeding. If you do not check your gloves frequently, you may be unsure which part of the body the blood came from, and will have to redo the entire process.

Mentally piece together all you know about your patient, including the chief complaint, the history of the present event, the medical history, and any information about the patient's current health status. Combine that knowledge with the other information and insights you have gained from your various assessments, along the information obtained from your diagnostics, and you should have enough information to make appropriate clinical choices for your patient. Keep in mind that a trauma patient may have also experienced a traumatic event and a medical patient may also have an injury. The provider must prioritize the most urgent complaint and condition for treatment. Some cases may involve both medical and trauma considerations.

Diagnostics

Whereas the history taking and secondary survey process are the best methods for determining a differential diagnosis in the patient, the use of certain diagnostic and monitoring devices in addition to performing laboratory tests aids in the assessment process. These devices are designed to assist the provider with diagnostic assessment and monitoring of patients. Keep in mind that while these devices are helpful, they cannot replace a good history and secondary survey. Patient history, physical exam, and diagnostic tools can be targeted to a specific body system. Each body system presents a set of unique assessment options to rule in or rule out differential diagnoses. Using clinical reasoning, the provider can integrate new information pertinent to the current patient with previous assessment and treatment knowledge.

Diagnostic tools can help identify a broad range of medical conditions. Prehospital diagnostic tools can provide valuable information and prompt early, lifesaving intervention.

Laboratory Studies

There are a variety of elements found in the blood that aid you in determining a differential diagnosis. Laboratory studies to obtain values for serum bilirubin, serum albumin, hemoglobin, hematocrit, serum urea nitrogen, and creatinine can be done. Measuring the blood glucose level of every patient who has altered mentation is a must in EMS. Laboratory results are evaluated for blood loss, metabolic acidosis, renal or hepatic disease, dehydration, and malabsorption syndromes. Laboratory and radiographic tests are ordered to identify the presence of kidney stones, ulcers, and obstructions to the GI, GU, and reproductive systems.

Stroke Scales

Research indicates that using a stroke scale can help determine whether a patient has had a stroke. Although other assessment data and physical exam findings are needed to establish such a diagnosis, several consensus guidelines advocate using such a scale to make the rapid determination that a stroke is likely to have occurred. This early identification will prioritize the patient's treatment and transport. Common scales utilized are the Los Angeles Prehospital Stroke Screen and the Cincinnati Prehospital Stroke Scale. Many protocols also specify notification of a designated stroke team early in the assessment process (**Tables 1-8** and **1-9**).

Pulse Oximetry

A pulse oximeter takes advantage of hemoglobin's propensity to absorb light, which results in an indirect measurement of oxygen saturation when a pulse oximetry probe is placed on a finger or toe (without nail polish) or earlobe. Oxygen saturation is an indication of how many hemoglobin-binding sites in the blood are occupied by (saturated with) oxygen molecules relative to the number available. This measurement is expressed as a percentage. Healthy people have an oxygen saturation of 97% to 99%. In a patient with a normal hemoglobin level, a saturation of 90% is minimally acceptable but oxygen should be administered to patients with breathlessness, signs of heart failure, shock or an oxygen saturation less than 94%.

Table 1-8 Los Angeles Prehospital Stroke Screen

Criteria	Yes	Unknown	No
1. Age > 45	❑	❑	❑
2. History of seizures or epilepsy absent	❑	❑	❑
3. Symptoms < 24 hours	❑	❑	❑
4. At baseline, patient is not wheelchair bound or bedridden	❑	❑	❑
5. Blood glucose level between 60 and 400 mg/dL	❑	❑	❑
6. Obvious asymmetry (right vs. left) in any of the following three exam categories (must be unilateral):	❑	❑	❑
	Equal	**Right Weak**	**Left Weak**
Facial smile/grimace	❑	Droop ❑	Droop ❑
Grip	❑	Weak grip ❑ No grip ❑	Weak grip ❑ No grip ❑
Arm strength	❑	Drifts down ❑ Falls rapidly ❑	Drifts down ❑ Falls rapidly ❑

Interpretation: If criteria 1–6 are marked yes, specificity of a stroke is 97%.

Table 1-9 **Cincinnati Prehospital Stroke Scale**		
Assessment	**Normal**	**Abnormal**
Facial Droop		
Ask patient to smile and show his or her teeth.	Both sides of the face move equally.	One side of the face does not move as well as the other side.
Arm Drift		
Ask patient to close eyes and hold arms out for 10 seconds.	Both arms move the same or neither arm moves.	One arm does not move or one arm drifts down compared with the other.
Abnormal Speech		
Ask patient to repeat the phrase "You can't teach an old dog new tricks."	Uses correct words, no slurring.	Slurs words, uses inappropriate words, or is unable to speak.

Interpretation: If any one is abnormal, probability of a stroke is 72%.

The tool is of minimal value in patients with poor perfusion attributable to autoimmune disease, endocrine emergencies, drug toxicity, or blood loss. In addition, pulse oximetry readings may be unreliable in patients with carbon monoxide poisoning, in smokers, and in diabetics with advanced peripheral vascular disease.

A patient whose oxygen saturation is less than 94% should be administered supplemental oxygen by a nasal cannula or nonrebreathing mask. (**Figure 1-23**). The percentage of supplemental oxygen administered will depend on assessment findings. Oxygen saturation findings are helpful to measure if assessed before and after application of supplemental oxygen.

Peak Flow Meter

Peak flow meters measure peak expiratory flow rate, or the rate at which a patient can breathe out. The rate is expressed in liters per minute (L/min). In patients with reactive airway disease, the rate diminishes because of increased resistance during exhalation. To participate in this test, the patient must be able to follow instructions to take deep breaths in and out (maximum inhalation and exhalation; see Figure 1-12A).

Capnography

Capnography is used to monitor carbon dioxide levels in exhaled gases, or end-tidal carbon dioxide ($ETCO_2$). This diagnostic assessment can give you a better understanding of the patient's ventilatory status. Capnography is projected as a waveform and a numerical value. The normal value of $ETCO_2$ in the blood is between 32 and 43 mm Hg.

Digital capnography can measure on a waveform tracing the exact amount of exhaled carbon dioxide. In addition, it can

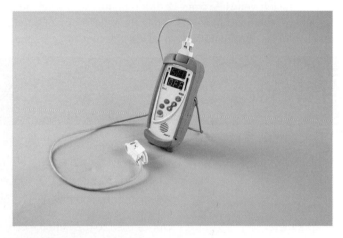

Figure 1-23 A pulse oximeter.
© Jones & Bartlett Learning. Courtesy of MIEMSS.

record air movement during inhalation and exhalation. This device allows continual monitoring of tracings. Abnormalities in inhalation or exhalation will alter the pattern of the waveforms.

Capnometry is the quantitative measurement of CO_2 without the waveform, often referred to as end-tidal CO_2 ($ETCO_2$). A colorimetric capnometer provides semiquantitative information. This is a device with litmus paper that changes color in response to pH. The device can be placed between the airway and ventilating device. Exhaled air that contains no carbon dioxide will not change the paper color. Initially there is a dark purple color, and it turns to yellow/gold when there are near-normal levels of CO_2. If the litmus paper is exposed to stomach contents, it will also turn yellow/gold owing to acidity. The color should go from purple to yellow to purple with each ventilation to indicate the capnometer is accurately detecting CO_2.

Hypoventilation causes retention of CO_2, leading to respiratory acidosis. Increasing the percentage of supplemental oxygen, checking proper tracheal tube placement, and assisting ventilation with a bag-mask device are essential (Table 1-10).

Electrocardiography

An ECG records the electrical activity of the atrial and ventricular cells of the heart and represents this activity as specific waveforms and complexes. The ECG continuously detects and measures electrical flow on the patient's skin. Electrocardiographic testing is used to detect acute myocardial ischemia and to monitor a patient's heart rate, evaluate the effects of disease or injury on heart function, analyze pacemaker function, and assess response to medications. The ECG does not provide information about the heart's contractile (mechanical) function.

Whether using a 3-lead, 12-lead, 15-lead, or 18-lead ECG, reviewing various views of the frontal surface, horizontal axis, and left ventricle of the heart provides key information about ischemia and infarction. The standard 12-lead ECG visualizes the heart in the frontal and horizontal planes and views the surfaces of the left ventricle from 12 different angles. Having multiple views of the heart makes possible the recognition of bundle branch blocks, the identification of ST-segment changes such as ischemia, injury, or infarct, and the analysis of ECG changes associated with medications. Extended lead placement, as in the 15- and 18-lead devices, allows additional anterior and posterior views.

ECG monitoring is typically performed in patients who are having difficulty breathing or who have chest or abdominal discomfort or pain, particularly if the patient has both complaints. ST-segment elevation MI (STEMI) points toward an acute, evolving myocardial necrosis. Non–ST-segment elevation MI (NSTEMI) may show up on an ECG as ST-segment depression and T-wave inversion. When reviewing 12-lead ECGs, several patterns may mimic ST elevation, including left bundle branch block (LBBB) and pericarditis.

▼ Refine the Differential Diagnosis

Throughout the assessment process, the provider will be distinguishing one disease from another based on accumulated data and clinical reasoning. The clues that have been obtained from the patient's symptoms, history, physical examination, and diagnostic testing help narrow down the possible diagnoses. The differential diagnosis, which is the process of the elimination of potential diagnoses, eventually leads to one diagnosis.

Table 1-10 Capnography-Related Terms

Term	Description
Capnography	Continuous analysis and recording of CO_2 concentrations in respiratory gases Output is displayed as a waveform. Graphic display of the CO_2 concentration versus time during a respiratory cycle CO_2 concentration may also be plotted versus expiratory volume.
Capnometer	Device used to measure the concentration of CO_2 at the end of exhalation
Capnometry	A numeric reading of exhaled CO_2 concentrations without a continuous written record or waveform Output is a numerical value. Numeric display of CO_2 on a monitor
Capnograph	A device that provides a numeric reading of exhaled CO_2 concentrations and a waveform (tracing)
Exhaled CO_2 detector	A capnometer that provides a noninvasive estimate of alveolar ventilation, the concentration of exhaled CO_2 from the lungs, and arterial CO_2 content; also called an end-tidal CO_2 detector
Colorimetric ETCO$_2$ detector	A device that provides CO_2 readings by chemical reaction on pH-sensitive litmus paper housed in the detector The presence of CO_2 (evidenced by a color change on the colorimetric device) suggests tracheal placement.
Qualitative ETCO$_2$ monitor	A device that uses a light to indicate the presence of ETCO$_2$

ETCO$_2$, end-tidal carbon dioxide

From Aehlert BJ: *Paramedic practice today: Above and beyond*, St. Louis, MO, 2010, MosbyJems.

The patient's differential diagnosis also helps you decide whether the patient's condition is life threatening, critical, or nonemergent. At any moment your patient's condition may decline from being critical to life threatening, and appropriate management and transport must begin without delay.

▼ Ongoing Management

After the primary survey, reassessment is the single most important assessment process you will perform. When performing reassessment, you must reassess the patient's airway, breathing, and circulation/perfusion (ABCs), make certain you have adequately addressed the chief complaint, obtain another set of vital signs, and close any other patient care loops, such as dressing small wounds and placing ice packs. Reassessment represents a continuous, yet cyclical, process that you perform throughout transport, right up to the time you turn patient care over to the emergency department staff. For patients in stable condition, you should do a reassessment every 15 minutes or so. For patients in unstable condition, you need to make a concerted effort to repeat the reassessment every 5 minutes.

Reassess the Patient

Reassessment combines repetition of the primary survey, reassessment of vital signs and breath sounds, and repetition of the secondary survey. During the reassessment, you continue to evaluate and reevaluate the patient's status and any treatments already administered. Trends in the patient's current condition may give clues about the effectiveness of treatments. Compare vital signs. Have interventions improved the patient's condition?

First, compare the patient's LOC with your baseline assessment. Is the LOC changing? Second, review the patient's airway. Is it patent? Always be prepared to suction, and do not delay if you hear gurgling in the upper airway. Third, reassess breathing. Is the patient breathing adequately? If not, figure out why and correct the problem. Finally, reassess the patient's circulation and perfusion. Assess overall skin color as an initial measure of cardiovascular function and hemodynamic status. Make certain that all bleeding is controlled.

Refine the Differential Diagnosis

As you perform your reassessment, you will continually be able to rule in or rule out certain conditions from your differential diagnosis. Keep an open mind as you gather all your patient information and modify your differential diagnosis based on new findings.

Modify Treatment

After reassessing the patient, think about your present care plan. Have you addressed all life threats? On the basis of what you know now, do you need to revise your priority list? If so, make

the change and continue with patient care. In contrast, if your plan is working well and you have addressed most or all of the patient's complaints, there is no need to revise the care plan.

While you are reevaluating your patient care priorities, you should reassess the transport plan as well. Should routine transport be stepped up to priority? Is the patient's condition worsening to the point that you need to consider diverting to a closer facility? Do you need to set up a rendezvous with an air ambulance and fly the patient to the healthcare facility? If your patient's condition has improved and stabilized, you should step down from priority and transport the patient as a routine case—the clearly safer choice.

Monitor the Therapeutic Response

Continue to monitor the patient's condition. Obtain another complete set of vital signs, and compare them with the expected outcomes from your therapies. For example, if you administered a 500-mL bolus of normal saline to a patient with gastrointestinal bleeding, you usually would expect a rise in blood pressure and a decrease in pulse rate. With any priority patient, you should have a minimum of three sets of vital signs—and that would be if there is a short transport. With most priority patients, you will have four or five sets of vital signs. With several sets of vital signs, you can look for trends or patterns in your patient's condition.

Last, revisit your patient's complaints, as you've recorded during history taking. Have any complaints improved or resolved? Which situations remain unresolved? Situations that are worsening are especially concerning because they could mean an unseen problem or ineffective interventions. If you have not reached the receiving facility, repeat the reassessment process again. Document all of your findings with each reassessment so that your medical record is accurate and complete for handoff at the emergency department.

Special Populations
Older Adult Patients

The American Geriatrics Society has estimated that more than a third of all EMS calls are in response to an older adult patient. Many older adults lead healthy, active lives, but others have chronic health problems. Assessment of the geriatric patient is more challenging than that of a younger adult for a variety of reasons.

Geriatric patients lack appropriate compensatory mechanisms and therefore may not show signs of deterioration as their conditions become unstable. In addition, many of these patients have underlying diseases or take medications that mask the true assessment findings. Orthostatic hypotension attributable to diminished baroreceptor function can be a concern during the physical exam. Take care to have older patients move slowly to better accommodate blood volume changes.

Medications

Most older adults take three to five prescription medications, which is referred to as polypharmacy. **Pharmacokinetics**—the absorption, distribution, metabolism, and excretion of medications—differs in older adults compared to younger patients. As a result, older adults tend to have adverse drug reactions more often, especially when they are also taking OTC medications or dietary supplements such as herbal preparations or nutritional drinks. The most common adverse reactions to medications are confusion, sedation, loss of balance, nausea, and electrolyte abnormalities.

Communication

Communication may be difficult if the patient has a hearing or speech–language impairment. However, many older adults are able to hear normally. If a patient does have hearing aids, make sure they're set at the proper volume.

Patience is vital when taking a history. Older adults sometimes can't recall the names of medications or the conditions for which they've been prescribed. In addition, they may process questions slowly and feel obligated to share information they believe is important before answering the question directly. Such extra information may prove helpful when trying to work through the differential diagnosis.

Pulmonary System Changes

The pulmonary system undergoes changes in the older adult. The kyphosis (curvature) of the thoracic spine that often occurs with advancing age can make expanding the lungs more difficult. The respiratory muscles weaken, causing respiratory fatigue and failure earlier than in younger adults. This decrement is perhaps attributable to lifelong exposure to environmental pollutants or to repeated lung infections over the years. In addition, the elasticity of the lungs and chest wall decreases with age, diminishing tidal volume. Because of these changes, the respiratory rate normally increases to compensate and maintain an adequate minute volume.

If a patient shows signs or symptoms of hypoxia, oxygen must be given in an effort to attain an oxygen saturation of 95% or greater. When you are transporting a patient who has shortness of breath, the patient may ask to sit upright. Follow the patient's lead because patients are usually better able to determine for themselves which position makes breathing easier.

Cardiovascular System Changes

Many changes occur in the cardiovascular system of an older adult patient. Large arteries become less elastic, creating more pressure in the arteriole system during systole. This raises systolic blood pressure, leading in turn to a widened pulse pressure (the difference between systolic and diastolic blood pressure). Peripheral vascular resistance (PVR) may increase, and diastolic blood pressure and mean arterial pressure may rise, resulting in hypertension. Common cardiac problems among older adults include MI, heart failure, dysrhythmias, aneurysms, and hypertension.

When obtaining a history from the older adult patient complaining of chest pain or discomfort, try to ascertain his or her level of cardiovascular fitness. Older people who regularly engage in physical activity are able to maintain more efficient cardiac function.

Assessment of the older adult for cognitive changes can be difficult without family members or friends to whom you can direct questions about the patient's history. If possible, determine the patient's baseline mental status, and then assess for any changes in behavior, thought processes, and mood. Ask family or friends about any recent changes in the patient's hygiene and food preparation habits.

Terminally Ill Patients

Hospice services include supportive social, emotional, and spiritual care for patients and their families at the end of life. Patients who are terminally ill, such as those with advanced cancer or acquired immunodeficiency syndrome (AIDS), often receive palliative care (comfort care). Medical needs vary depending on the disease but typically center on pain management.

The terminally ill patient may have medical and legal documents such as advance directives or do-not-resuscitate (DNR) orders. Some states have specific DNR paperwork, so healthcare providers should be familiar with specific policies, procedures, and regulations in their part of the country. In many states, a provider's scope of practice governs whether a prehospital healthcare provider may honor legal DNR advance directives or living wills.

Bariatric Patients

Obesity is an excessive amount of weight relative to height. Being overweight is defined as a body mass index (BMI) of 25 to 29.9 kg/m^2. The CDC defines obesity in terms of body mass index, a height/weight ratio calculated as follows:

$$\text{BMI} = [\text{Weight (lb)} \div \text{Height (inches)} \times \text{Height (inches)}] \times 703$$

For example, a person who is 5 feet 5 inches tall and weighs 135 lb has a BMI of 22.5, which falls in the normal range for a person of that height and weight. A person of the same height who weighs 180 lb has a BMI of 30 and is thus, by definition, obese. BMI is calculated more precisely for children and teens, factoring in their precise height and weight as well as their age and sex. A BMI of 39 or greater, or being 100 lb or more over recommended weight for height, constitutes morbid obesity, which carries more serious health risks.

Obesity is a chronic disease and is the second leading cause of preventable death in the United States (behind tobacco use).

Obese (bariatric) patients are at increased risk of diabetes, hypertension, coronary heart disease, dyslipidemia, stroke, liver disease, gallbladder disease, sleep apnea, respiratory disorders, osteoarthritis, and certain types of cancer; obese women are also at increased risk of infertility. Morbidly obese persons may develop pulmonary hypertension and right-sided heart failure, known as cor pulmonale.

Moving an Obese Patient

Healthcare personnel must have policies for moving and lifting obese patients because of the additional risk they pose to providers and the extra demands they place on staff and resources. Scene and situational assessment is especially important because a specially equipped bariatric ambulance and additional providers may be necessary (**Figure 1-24**). Ask the patient's weight, and call for lift assistance if necessary.

Both provider and patient are at particularly high risk as the patient is being moved. Providers are subject to heavy-lifting injuries. Patients can be dropped or may roll off surfaces that were not designed to accommodate them, such as standard-sized backboards. High-capacity carrying sheets made of plastic with built-in side handles may be a good alternative to moving the patient on a stretcher.

Providing Specialized Medical Devices and Supplies

All EMS agencies and healthcare institutions must have the proper equipment and supplies needed to care for obese patients, such as extra-large blood pressure cuffs, long-length needles for intramuscular injections or needle decompression, large cervical collars, extra-long straps and taping supplies, and large gowns, sheets, and blankets.

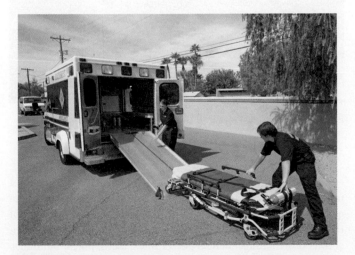

Figure 1-24 Some EMS systems have specialized equipment and vehicles to care for bariatric patients.

Obstetric Patients

Pregnancy-related emergencies include spontaneous abortion, ectopic pregnancy, premature labor, hemorrhage, blood clots, preeclampsia, infection, stroke, amniotic fluid embolism, diabetes, and heart disease. Begin by assessing the patient's skin color, temperature, and moisture. Maternal physiology changes as early as the first trimester of pregnancy. Heart rate quickens by 10 to 15 beats/min. Respiratory rate also increases as the enlarging uterus pushes up on the diaphragm, causing breathing to become more rapid and shallow. Assess the patient's vital signs for evidence of dehydration and shock.

In the early stages of pregnancy, usually the fifth to tenth weeks, abdominal pain, vaginal bleeding, and signs of shock can indicate ectopic pregnancy. Pregnant patients in the fifth to tenth weeks should be assessed for pregnancy-induced hypertension and gestational diabetes.

In later stages of pregnancy, patients who complain of tearing abdominal pain and vaginal bleeding with dark-colored blood may be experiencing an abruption, or separation of the placenta from the uterine wall. Painless vaginal bleeding in the last trimester can indicate a placenta previa, where the placenta is bleeding. Both conditions are life-threatening medical emergencies and require rapid transport.

Postpartum pathology may include hemorrhage, infection, and pulmonary embolism. Fever and severe abdominal pain are symptoms of endometritis (infection of the uterus), which can be very serious. A medical history related to the pregnancy must be obtained, including delivery by cesarean section.

Special Transport Considerations

Air Transport

Depending on the proximity to the hospital and its specialization, some patients will be transported by air. Transfer from one facility to another, such as from a community hospital to a burn center, may also occur by air. Helicopters and fixed-wing aircraft (airplanes; **Figure 1-25**) have been used for patient transport by both civilian and military medical systems almost since the dawn of aviation.

Patients who are critically ill and medically unstable may be considered for helicopter transport, especially when definitive care on the ground will be delayed. Examples of medical conditions that might be considered for air transport are as follows:

- Bleeding or imminent rupture of a dissecting aortic aneurysm
- Intracranial bleeding
- Acute (time-dependent for treatment) ischemic stroke
- Severe hypothermia and hyperthermia
- Cardiac dysfunction requiring immediate intervention
- Status asthmaticus
- Status epilepticus

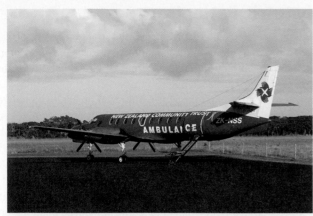

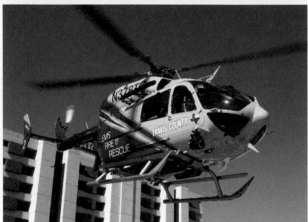

Figure 1-25 A. Air medical fixed-wing aircraft. **B.** AMLS group helicopter.

A © ChameleonsEye/Shutterstock, Inc. B Courtesy of Travis County STARFlight.

Table 1-11 **Advantages and Disadvantages of Air Medical Transport**
Advantages
■ Rapid transportation   ■ Access to remote areas   ■ Access to specialty units such as neonatal intensive care units and burn centers   ■ Access to personnel with specialized skills   ■ Access to specialized equipment and supplies
Disadvantages
■ Weather and environmental restrictions to flight   ■ Limitations on patient weight   ■ Limitations on number of patients who can be transported   ■ Altitude limitations   ■ Airspeed limitations   ■ High cost   ■ Difficulties delivering patient care because of limited access and cabin size   ■ Limitations of the amounts of equipment and supplies that can be carried

From Aehlert BJ: *Paramedic practice today: above and beyond*, St. Louis, MO, 2009, Mosby.

Each EMS provider should be familiar with the ground and air transport options in his or her geographic area. The decision to transport a patient by air has some advantages and some drawbacks (Table 1-11). Air transport allows the patient to be rescued in a remote area if necessary, transported quickly, and transferred rapidly to a specialty unit. In addition, specialized personnel or supplies (e.g., antivenin, blood products) can be delivered in minutes or hours rather than days. However, flying is often restricted in bad weather, and all aircraft have load restrictions that limit the number and weight of patients who can be transported at once or at all. It's not just total passenger weight that counts, but the number of passengers, since the weight in an aircraft must be properly distributed. Each aircraft is different; one may be able to accommodate a tail-heavy load, whereas the same distribution pattern would be unsafe in another aircraft.

In addition, patients with certain conditions cannot easily tolerate high altitude, vibration, and rapid changes in barometric pressure. The altitude at which an aircraft flies depends on the type of aircraft, weather conditions, noise abatement procedures pilots must follow to reduce engine noise in certain areas, geography of the terrain below (for obvious reasons, aircraft fly higher over mountainous terrain and forested areas), altitude restrictions in heavily trafficked urban air corridors, and other factors.

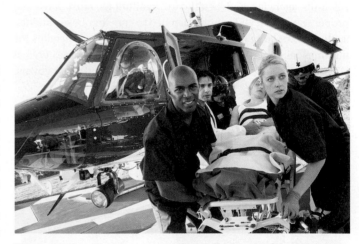

Figure 1-26 Helicopters can provide rapid transport for critical patients.

© Monkey Business Images/Shutterstock, Inc.

Helicopter transport (**Figure 1-26**) requires observance of proper safety procedures, such as finding a landing zone of adequate size (at least 100 × 100 feet) and a location (downwind of the patient care area) that is relatively level, firm, and free of dangerous obstructions such as power lines, trees, poles, buildings, and rocks (Table 1-12). Each EMS provider should be updated annually on local helicopter safety requirements and communication procedures.

Table 1-12 Landing Zone and Scene Operations

Landing Zone

- Ensure the landing zone is a minimum of 100 × 100 feet.
- Identify and mark any obstructions in the immediate area.
- Identify the landing zone by GPS coordinates or a major nearby intersection.
- Inform the flight crew of the landing surface and slope.
- Mark the corners of the landing zone with cones or other easily visible objects in the daytime. Place a fifth marker on the upwind side of the landing zone. Make sure markers are secured or heavy enough that they will not blow away.
- For night operations, mark the corners of the landing zone with ground strobes, secured flares, or vehicles with their lights on. Place a fifth lighted marker on the upwind side of the landing zone.

Scene Operations

- Keep spectators at least 200 feet away.
- Ensure personal equipment is secured.
- Do not approach the helicopter until you are signaled by one of the crew members.
- Always approach from the front of the helicopter, never from the tail.
- Never bend over when approaching the helicopter. The rotors are 10 feet above the ground, and you are more likely to trip and fall if you are looking down.
- Do not hold anything above your head.
- Do not wear a hat.

GPS, global positioning system.

From Aehlert BJ: *Paramedic practice today: above and beyond*, St. Louis, MO, 2009, Mosby.

Flight Physiology

The healthcare provider—in many instances the paramedic—must select the most suitable mode of transportation for patients based on their condition, the specialty care offered at the receiving facility, and the safest, most efficient means available by which to move them. Likewise, in-hospital providers use similar criteria to determine whether to transfer a patient by air or ground.

If air medical transport is thought to be in the best clinical interest of the patient, you must prepare the patient for transport. Although the transport crew is responsible for the patient's safety during the flight, proper preflight preparation is the responsibility of the prehospital or in-hospital provider, who must be aware of factors that affect the patient during flight. For example, you should understand how factors such as vertigo (dizziness), changes in temperature and barometric pressure, gravity, and spatial disorientation might affect the patient.

Barometric Pressure Patients with underlying pulmonary disease such as COPD, asthma, or pulmonary edema are at high risk of hypoxia when barometric pressure drops. Diminished barometric pressure during flight can reduce the PaO_2 in the alveoli, in turn reducing blood oxygen saturation. During flight, the patient may need supplemental oxygen or tracheal intubation to maintain adequate oxygen saturation.

Patients who have sinus infections may experience severe sinus pressure or pain during flight, or epistaxis (nosebleed) can occur during ascent as gases trapped in the sinus cavity expand. In such patients, nasal vasoconstrictors can be administered prophylactically before the flight.

Helicopters rarely fly above 1,000 feet, so changes in barometric pressure are not clinically significant. However, with fixed-wing transport, this must be taken into consideration.

Humidity As altitude increases, the amount of moisture in the aircraft decreases as fresh air from the outside is drawn into the cabin. Therefore, supplemental oxygen should be administered with humidification to prevent dehydration of the patient's mucous membranes and nasal passages.

Temperature The patient should be adequately protected from wind and cold to ensure that he or she remains normothermic. The transport team should be notified of the patient's hydration status and of any medications, such as sedatives, that have been administered. Alterations in cabin temperature with descent and ascent can disrupt a poorly hydrated and sedated patient's ability to maintain core body temperature.

Other Considerations Anxiety is an emotional factor to consider when a patient is being transported by air. If conscious, the patient should be briefed on the types of aircraft vibrations and sounds that might be experienced during flight and on how long the flight is expected to take. Ill or injured patients can have physiologic signs and symptoms attributable to air turbulence or engine vibrations. The patient may have motion sickness or abdominal pain or trouble staying warm.

Patients with a history or risk of seizures should be visually protected from the flashing lights they might see during the aircraft's ascent and descent.

Take basic safety precautions when you are around fixed-wing or rotary aircraft. Navigate carefully around rotating helicopter and propeller blades. Always approach a helicopter from the front or side, in view of the pilot. Whether you are a prehospital or in-hospital provider, you must heed the flight crew's instructions when you are loading or unloading a patient.

Special Environmental Considerations
Wilderness Conditions

EMS providers are often confronted with austere conditions that complicate the assessment process. Care delivery in such conditions is often called wilderness medicine. Loosely defined, wilderness medicine is medical management in situations in which care is limited by environmental considerations, prolonged extrication, or limited resource availability. You may encounter such situations in remote areas like national parks, or in cities or suburbs, such as when caring for a patient who is suffering from hypothermia or has been struck by lightning. Unfamiliar situations occurring in a familiar environment, such as an earthquake in your city, may call upon your wilderness medicine skills. Chapter 9, *Environmental-Related Disorders*, discusses medical conditions you may encounter in patients as a result of environmental exposure.

Wilderness EMS is a subset of EMS operations that requires specialized training. Personnel need training in technical rope rescue, prevention of hypothermia, and the safety precautions to follow when working in an unpredictable, unsafe outdoor environment that poses threats ranging from ravines to rattlesnakes. The National Association of Emergency Medical Technicians (NAEMT) has compiled a list of variables that affect wilderness EMS activities, which include the following:

- Access to the scene
- Weather
- Daylight
- Terrain
- Special transport and handling times
- Access and transport times
- Available personnel
- Communications
- Medical rescue equipment available
- Hazards present

The wilderness EMS scope of practice is often expanded to include cervical spine clearance, administration of medications (e.g., steroids, antibiotics), and additional interventions such as shoulder reductions and sutures. According to the Academy of Wilderness Medicine, many programs in this specialty have been developed, and fellowship and residency programs are available within emergency medicine and paramedic programs. Programs that have been established in the field are offered by the U.S. National Park Service, the National Ski Patrol, the Mountain Rescue Association, the Divers Alert Network, and many other organizations.

Putting It All Together

A systematic, thorough, efficient patient assessment process is the backbone of effectively managing patients with medical or traumatic emergencies. The AMLS assessment pathway is built on the assumption that providers already have a broad understanding of human anatomy, physiology, pathophysiology, and epidemiology to complement the assessment and management processes. Clinical reasoning, therapeutic communication, clinical decision making, and pattern recognition skills all affect your ability to integrate historical information, physical exam findings, and the results of diagnostic assessments to arrive at a working diagnosis. Implementation of appropriate treatment modalities hinges on the accuracy of this assessment information.

Initial patient presentations are often subtle; the dependability of your judgment is the key to timely, effective intervention. Most of the assessment information, especially in patients with emergent presentations, is obtained during history taking. When patients are poor historians, you must use your senses and let your experience guide your decisions.

Initial observations begin with the dispatch information or a prehospital radio report. A scene or situation assessment gives you a preview of the patient's condition even before any direct interaction takes place. All scenes or situations, whether prehospital or in-hospital, should be evaluated for safety. Home environments should be assessed for medical devices, environmental issues, and indications of chronic disease processes. Once the area is deemed safe, providers should note the patient's affect and body position, breath sounds and respiratory pattern, coloring, odor, and other physical characteristics. Any life threats must be addressed immediately. Proceed to the primary survey to identify and manage life threats relevant to airway, breathing, circulation, or perfusion. This assessment, while finished in a matter of seconds, should be systematic and thorough to identify any emergent conditions for which urgent intervention is needed. Determine an initial impression, including how sick the patient is and whether the patient is likely to deteriorate. If deterioration seems imminent, determine which body systems might be affected.

History taking is then performed. Historical information is obtained by soliciting information about the present illness (OPQRST) and past medical history (SAMPLER). During the secondary survey, the provider applies clinical reasoning and pattern recognition to the patient's initial presentation. Diagnostic information is obtained and interpreted from pulse oximetry devices, blood glucose meters, laboratory tests, 3-lead or 12-lead ECG monitoring, and $ETCO_2$ devices to eliminate or confirm diagnoses. Vital signs, pain assessment, and a physical exam help rule in or rule out differential diagnoses to determine a working diagnosis.

Associated symptoms are investigated to determine the acuity of the working diagnoses and to identify underlying conditions that need to be managed. A focused physical exam should be performed on patients with nonemergent presentations. A full-body (head-to-toe) physical exam is performed on patients with minimal LOC if on-scene and transport time allow.

Communication, assessment, and management barriers can be encountered in patients with special challenges, such as bariatric patients, older adults, and obstetric patients. Transport decisions take into consideration the patient's condition but must also yield to exogenous factors such as weather, maximum aircraft load capacity, capabilities of the receiving hospital, and distance of the most appropriate facility.

Healthcare providers at all levels and scopes of practice can work as a team to apply the AMLS pathway to provide comprehensive assessment and management of patients experiencing medical emergencies. The AMLS pathway is a dynamic and ongoing assessment process in which conclusions are continually revised as more information about the patient's history and current status becomes available. The process promotes teamwork for efficient and accurate patient assessment and care from dispatch to delivery at the receiving facility.

SCENARIO SOLUTION

© HunThomas/ShutterStock, Inc.

- Several communication barriers may inhibit an efficient assessment. There may be hearing deficits and a short attention span due to fatigue and feelings of frustration. This requires the providers to use closed-ended questions and actively listen to what the patient and daughter state. Assistive devices may indicate inability to care for self or multiple complaints causing perfusion deficit. This patient may not be an accurate historian, so an efficient and thorough history and physical assessment are necessary to determine if this patient's presentation is life threatening. At this time, the patient's condition appears to be a potential life threat.
- The providers should investigate for congestive heart failure, bowel impaction, stroke, dehydration and nutrition concerns, head injury or bruising from falls or abuse, and STEMI or cardiac rhythm changes.
- Assessment should include a thorough OPQRST and SAMPLER exam to note current status and any changes since last week's complaints, as well as a neurologic exam to include motor/sensory and pupil status. A focused physical exam should evaluate pulmonary or systemic edema. Auscultation of breath, heart, and bowel sounds should be performed.

Diagnostic evaluation of blood glucose, pulse oximetry, ECG, and waveform capnography should be performed.

Reassessment en route to the receiving facility is essential to determine if the patient's condition is stable or deteriorating, despite interventions.

- The providers should be concerned about the patient's condition rapidly deteriorating; therefore an organized, systematic approach to assessment and management is essential. Multiple underlying diagnoses in this patient are a concern that is attributed to the decrease in efficiency of all body systems in the elderly. Changes in metabolic rates, reduction in blood vessel elasticity, osteoarthritis, slowed reflexes, and diminished neurotransmitter activity all contribute to diminished efficiency of body systems in the elderly. Respiratory, cardiovascular, and neurologic assessments are key to determining differential diagnoses and ultimately a working diagnosis. The AMLS assessment pathway, while dynamic and flexible, can provide a tool for systematic and comprehensive assessments in patients with challenging medical presentations.

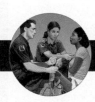

Summary

- The AMLS assessment pathway is a dependable framework allowing for early recognition and management of a variety of medical emergencies, with a goal of improved patient outcome.
- The patient's history, physical exam, risk factors, chief complaint, and cardinal presentation help suggest possible differential diagnoses.
- Therapeutic communication skills, keen clinical reasoning abilities, pattern recognition, and expert clinical decision making are the foundation for the AMLS assessment.
- Patient assessment and management can be hindered by social, language, behavioral, or psychological barriers.
- Effective clinical reasoning requires gathering and organizing relevant historical and diagnostic information, filtering out irrelevant or extraneous information, and reflecting on similar experiences to efficiently determine working diagnoses and management priorities.
- Clinical reasoning is a bridge between historical information and diagnostic test results, allowing the provider to draw inferences about underlying etiologies to formulate differential diagnoses.
- Barriers for efficient assessment and management of patient presentations involve the level of medical knowledge and experience and scope of practice of the healthcare provider.
- Clinical decision making is the ability to integrate diagnostic data and assessment findings with experience and evidence-based recommendations to improve patient outcomes.
- The primary survey consists of identifying and managing life-threatening medical emergencies related to the patient's level of consciousness, as well as his or her airway, breathing, circulatory, and perfusion status.
- An emergent or critical patient is one who is hemodynamically unstable and "sick," with a decreased level of consciousness, signs and symptoms of shock, severe pain, and difficulty breathing.

Summary (CONTINUED)

- The provider's senses can contribute and enhance information obtained from observation of the scene and the initial presentation of the patient.
- The physical exam can be a focused exam related to the chief complaint or initial presentation or a full-body head-to-toe exam.
- All healthcare providers should be familiar with the benefits and risks in transportation options for patients.
- Wilderness medicine is medical management in situations where care is limited by environmental considerations, prolonged extrication, or limited resources.

KEY TERMS

© HunThomas/ShutterStock, Inc.

Advanced Medical Life Support (AMLS) assessment pathway A dependable framework to support the reduction of morbidity and mortality by using an assessment-based approach to determine a differential diagnosis and effectively manage a broad range of medical emergencies.

assessment-based patient management Utilizing the patient's cardinal presentation; historical, diagnostic, and physical exam findings; and one's own critical thinking skills as a healthcare professional to diagnose and treat a patient.

blood pressure The tension exerted by blood on the arterial walls. Blood pressure is calculated using the following equation: Blood pressure = Flow × Resistance.

clinical decision making The ability to integrate assessment findings and test data with experience and evidence-based recommendations to make decisions regarding the most appropriate treatment.

clinical reasoning The second conceptual component underpinning the AMLS assessment pathway, which combines good judgment with clinical experience to make accurate diagnoses and initiate proper treatment. This process assumes the provider has a strong foundation of clinical knowledge.

differential diagnosis The possible causes of the patient's cardinal presentation.

initial patient presentation The patient's primary presenting sign or symptom; often this is the accompanied by the patient's chief complaint, but it may be an objective finding such as unconsciousness or choking.

pattern recognition A process of recognizing and classifying data based on past knowledge and experience.

pharmacokinetics The absorption, distribution, metabolism, and excretion of medications.

primary survey The process of initially assessing the airway, breathing, circulation, and perfusion status to identify and manage life-threatening conditions and establish priorities for further assessment, treatment, and transport.

pulse pressure The difference between the systolic and diastolic blood pressures; normal pulse pressure is 30 to 40 mm Hg.

secondary survey An in-depth systematic evaluation of the patient's history, physical exam, vital signs, and diagnostic information used to identify additional emergent and nonemergent conditions and modify differential diagnoses and management strategies.

signs Objective evidence that a healthcare professional observes, feels, sees, hears, touches, or smells.

symptoms The S in SAMPLER; subjective perceptions by patients indicating what they feel, such as nausea, or have experienced, such as a sensation of seeing flashing lights.

therapeutic communication A communication process in which the healthcare provider uses effective communication skills to obtain information about the patient and his or her condition, including the use of the four Es: engagement, empathy, education, and enlistment.

working diagnosis The presumed cause of the patient's condition, arrived at by evaluating all assessment information thus far obtained while conducting further diagnostic testing to definitively diagnose the illness.

BIBLIOGRAPHY © HunThomas/ShutterStock, Inc.

Aehlert B: *Paramedic practice today: above and beyond*. St. Louis, MO, 2009, Mosby.

American Academy of Orthopaedic Surgeons, American College of Emergency Physicians, University of Maryland, Baltimore County: *Critical care transport*. Burlington, MA, 2011, Jones & Bartlett Learning.

American Academy of Orthopaedic Surgeons: *Emergency care and transportation of the sick and injured*, ed 10. Burlington, MA, 2011, Jones & Bartlett Learning.

American Academy of Orthopaedic Surgeons: *Nancy Caroline's emergency care in the streets*, ed 7. Burlington, MA, 2013, Jones & Bartlett Learning.

Centers for Disease Control and Prevention: *Guide to infection prevention for outpatient settings: minimum expectations for safe care*. www.cdc.gov/HAI/pdfs/guidelines/Outpatient-Care-Guide-withChecklist.pdf

Donohue D: Medical triage for WMD incidents: An adaptation of daily triage. *JEMS*. 33(5), 2008. http://www.jems.com/article/major-incidents/medical-triage-wmd-incidents-i

Edgerly D: *Assessing your assessment*. www.jems.com/news_and_articles/columns/Edgerly/Assessing_Your_Assessment.html, January 23, 2008.

Hamilton G, Sanders A, Strange G, et al: *Emergency medicine: An approach to clinical problem-solving*, ed 2. Philadelphia, PA, 2003, Saunders.

Marx J, Hockberger R, Walls R, Eds: *Rosen's emergency medicine: concepts and clinical practice*, ed 5. St. Louis, MO, 2002, Mosby.

Mock K: Effective clinician–patient communication. *Physician's News Digest*. 2001;1-6.

National Highway Traffic Safety Administration: *Drug and human performance fact sheets*. http://www.nhtsa.gov/people/injury/research/job185drugs/technical-page.htm, 2014.

Occupational Safety and Health Administration: *General description and discussion of the levels of protection and protective gear*, Standard 1910.120, App B. www.osha.gov/pls/oshaweb/owadisp.show_document?p_table=STANDARDS&p_id=9767

Occupational Safety and Health Administration: *Toxic and hazardous substances: Bloodborne pathogens*, Standard 1910.1030. www.osha.gov/pls/oshaweb/owadisp.show_document?p_table=STANDARDS&p_id=10051

Ogden CL, Carroll MD, Kit BK, et al.: Prevalence of childhood and adult obesity in the United States, 2011–2012. *JAMA*. 311(8):806–814, 2014. doi: 10.1001/jama.2014.732.

Pagana K, Pagana T: *Mosby's diagnostic and laboratory test reference*. St. Louis, MO, 1997, Mosby.

Paramedic Association of Canada: *National occupational competency profile for paramedic practitioners*. Ottawa, Canada, 2001, The Association.

Pi Y, Liao W, Liu M, et al.: Pattern recognition techniques, technology and applications. In Sanders M, Ed: *Mosby's paramedic textbook*, revised ed 3. St. Louis, MO, 2007, Mosby, pp. 433–462.

Urden L: *Priorities in critical care nursing*, ed 2. St. Louis, MO, 1996, Mosby.

U.S. Department of Transportation National Highway Traffic Safety Administration: *EMT-paramedic national standard curriculum*. Washington, DC, 1998, The Department.

U.S. Department of Transportation National Highway Traffic Safety Administration: *National EMS education standards*, Draft 3.0. Washington, DC, 2008, The Department.

CHAPTER REVIEW QUESTIONS © HunThomas/ShutterStock, Inc.

1. While performing a comprehensive assessment, the provider recognizes the patient's assessment and diagnostic findings are similar to patient complaints she has treated in the past. Integrating new patient presentation information with past experiences to determine management strategies can be defined as:
   a. Active listening
   b. Clinical reasoning
   c. Therapeutic communication
   d. Clinical decision making

2. When approaching the patient in an apartment that has been secured by law enforcement, the providers find a semiconscious patient who has a needle in her arm. The patient moans with verbal stimulation, pupils are pinpoint, and respirations are noted as shallow at 4 breaths/min. The initial observation indicates the patient's presentation is:
   a. Nonemergent
   b. Emergent
   c. A potential life threat
   d. A life threat

3. An 18-year-old adolescent male has a syncopal episode with tremors in his upper extremities. He is currently alert and oriented and denies any significant medical history. His skin is cool and diaphoretic. His vital signs include a pulse rate of 118 beats/min and regular; respirations, 20 breaths/min and unlabored; and blood pressure, 102/68 mm Hg. Which diagnostic test would most likely narrow your differential diagnoses?
   a. 12-lead ECG
   b. Pulse oximetry
   c. Blood glucose analysis
   d. End-tidal CO_2 measurement

4. Geriatric patients experience a reduction in vessel elasticity. This would likely cause which change in the patient's signs and/or symptoms?
   a. Decrease in respiratory fatigue
   b. Increase in systolic blood pressure
   c. Increase in resting cardiac output
   d. Decrease in tidal volume

5. After ensuring the scene or situation is a safe environment, the provider's highest priority is to:
   a. interpret diagnostic information.
   b. determine a differential diagnosis.
   c. identify and manage life threats.
   d. determine a working diagnosis.

6. When initially approaching the patient, the provider uses which of the following relevant questions to form an initial impression?
   a. Is this patient likely to die now?
   b. Has the patient traveled outside the country?
   c. Is the complaint gradual or sudden in onset?
   d. Has the patient ingested over-the-counter medications?

7. One of the essential components in the initial observation of the AMLS assessment pathway is identification of the:
   a. cardinal presentation/chief complaint.
   b. focused physical exam.
   c. medical history information.
   d. interpretation of diagnostic information.

8. The provider finds an unconscious patient with no gag reflex. Which would be most appropriate device to begin to manage the airway?
   a. Nasopharyngeal airway
   b. Endotracheal tube
   c. Oropharyngeal airway
   d. Needle decompression

9. The provider performs a focused physical exam and observes an implanted vascular access device. This finding is most indicative of:
   a. chronic obstructive pulmonary disease.
   b. chemotherapy regimens.
   c. tension pneumothorax.
   d. gastrointestinal bleeding.

10. The provider is assessing a smoker who presents with dyspnea, chest discomfort, and a productive cough. The patient exhibits pedal edema and coarse, scattered rhonchi. The patient's oxygen saturation is 88% and his respiratory rate is 28 breaths/min. Which working diagnosis would be most likely considered to begin immediate treatment?
   a. Foreign body airway obstruction
   b. Chronic obstructive pulmonary disease
   c. Ludwig's angina
   d. Cardiac tamponade

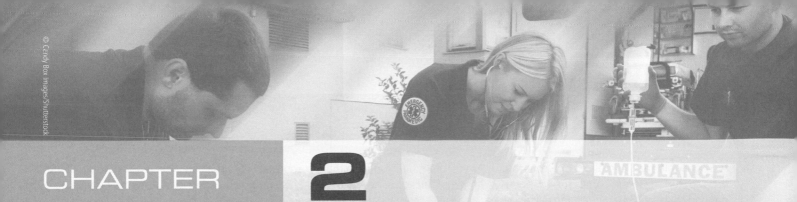

CHAPTER 2

Respiratory Disorders

In this chapter, the anatomy and function of the respiratory system are discussed, and common diseases and conditions that generate respiratory complaints are described. More important, providers will be asked to apply their knowledge to patient assessment, determining whether a pathologic condition is present, identifying the cause of the condition from among several plausible diagnoses, and applying clinical reasoning to select the best treatment plan for the patient. In addition, several critical procedures for monitoring and treating patients with respiratory complaints are reviewed.

LEARNING OBJECTIVES

At the conclusion of this chapter, you will be able to:

- Explain the anatomy, physiology, and pathophysiology of diseases and conditions often accompanied by respiratory complaints and describe their typical clinical presentations.

- Describe how to obtain a thorough history from the patient with a respiratory complaint.

- Carry out a comprehensive physical examination of a patient with a respiratory complaint using the Advanced Medical Life Support pathway.

- Form an initial impression and generate a list of likely differential diagnoses on the basis of a patient's history, signs, and symptoms.

- Order or recommend appropriate diagnostic tests and apply the results to aid in diagnosis.

- Perform critical procedures necessary to stabilize and treat patients with emergent respiratory conditions.

- Follow accepted evidence-based practice guidelines for the overall management of each condition.

- Provide an ongoing assessment of the patient, revising your clinical impression and treatment strategy on the basis of the patient's response to interventions.

A 57-year-old man complains of a sore throat. As you greet him you note that he appears ill. His eyes are infected and he constantly dabs sputum from the corners of his mouth. With a muffled voice, he explains that his symptoms began today. He says he feels achy, has had chills, and is experiencing pain in his ear and lower teeth. His medical history includes type 2 diabetes and hypertension. Initial vital signs include a blood pressure of 104/72 mm Hg; pulse rate, 124 beats/min; respirations, 20 breaths/min; and a temperature, 103°F (39.4°C). As you continue examining the patient, he becomes more anxious and restless. You note a high-pitched noise as he breathes in.

- What differential diagnoses are you considering based on the information you have now?
- What additional information will you need to narrow your differential diagnosis?
- What are your initial treatment priorities as you continue your patient care?

The function of the respiratory system is to bring in oxygen and eliminate carbon dioxide from the body. If this process is interrupted, vital organs of the body will not function properly. Providers must understand the importance of early detection of airway problems, rapid and effective intervention, and continual reassessment of a patient with airway or breathing compromise.

The Respiratory System: Anatomy

The respiratory system consists of all the structures in the body that make up the airway and help people breathe, or ventilate. The respiratory system has two primary functions, ventilation and respiration. Ventilation is the movement of air in and out of the lungs. The process of ventilation is the first step in providing oxygen (O_2) to the cells and removing carbon dioxide (CO_2) and other waste products from the circulation. Delivery of clean, humidified air to the alveoli in sufficient quantities to maintain an appropriate level of oxygen in the blood is the function of the oropharynx, pharynx, trachea, bronchi, and bronchioles. Respiration is the process of **gas exchange**, in which oxygen from the atmosphere is taken up by circulating blood cells and carbon dioxide from the bloodstream is released to the atmosphere. The exchange of gases also helps to control the pH in the blood.

The respiratory system can be divided into the upper and lower airways (**Figure 2-1**). The upper airway comprises all structures above the vocal cords (the nose, mouth, jaw, oral cavity, and pharynx), and the lower airway comprises the structures that fall below that anatomic point (externally, from the fourth cervical vertebra to the xiphoid process; internally, from the glottis to the pulmonary capillary membrane). Most of the respiratory system lies within the thorax, sharing space with the cardiovascular and gastrointestinal systems. The patient who complains of chest pain, cough, shortness of breath, or a choking sensation may be experiencing symptoms from any of these three thoracic systems.

The Upper Airway

The major functions of the upper airway are to warm, filter, and humidify air as it enters the body through the nose and mouth. Humidification is accomplished as the air picks up moisture from the soft tissues of the airway. The pharynx is a muscular tube that extends from the nose and mouth to the level of the esophagus and trachea. Air that passes through the mouth to the posterior pharynx does not become as moist as air that passes through the nasal cavity, but it still contributes to ventilation. Let's take a closer look first at the nasal cavity.

Nasal Cavity

The nasal cavity includes the following structures:

- Nares (nostrils)
- The nasal cavity, which contains the nasal turbinates (curved bony plates, or shelves, that extend from the lateral wall of the nasal cavity; they increase the surface area of the nasal mucosa, thereby improving the processes of warming, filtering, and humidification of inhaled air)
- The nasopharynx, which is formed by the union of the facial bones

The nasal cavity serves several important purposes. It humidifies and warms inhaled air, protecting the lower mucosa. The mucus-producing cells that line the nasopharynx capture large airborne particles, preventing lower respiratory tract infections. In addition, the nasopharynx functions as a resonating chamber, giving the voice its timbre and pitch.

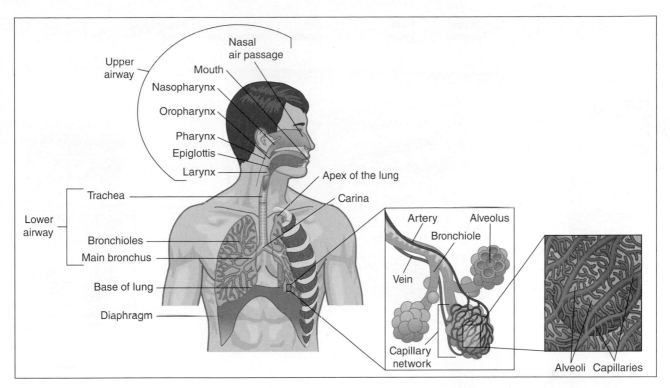

Figure 2-1 The upper and lower airways contain the structures in the body that help us breathe.

Pharynx and Oral Cavity

While not dedicated to ventilation, the structures of the mouth—the lips, teeth, gums, tongue, and salivary glands—function in mastication and speech creation.

Inhaled air that passes through the oral cavity reaches the pharynx and then the hypopharynx, which is immediately behind the base of the tongue (**Figure 2-2**). This area also contains the tonsils, lymph tissue that helps fight infection. Directly below the hypopharynx is the epiglottis, a cartilaginous flap that covers the trachea during swallowing. This flap, which normally remains open, protects the airway from aspiration by closing involuntarily during swallowing when a bolus of liquid or food passes over it. In unconscious patients, this reflex is often absent, putting them at risk of aspirating vomitus. Such aspiration can be life threatening because of the volume and acidity of stomach contents.

Below the epiglottis lie three glottic structures:

1. The thyroid cartilage, which surrounds everything.
2. The arytenoid cartilages, which help support the vocal cords.
3. The false vocal cords and true vocal cords, mobile structures that partially cover the glottis and move back and forth to create basic sounds that are tuned by the oropharynx and nasopharynx. The false vocal cords are made up of fibrous connective tissue and are attached to the true vocal cords. The true vocal cords are composed of fine ligamentous tissues. The space between the two true vocal cords and the narrowest portion of the adult airway is referred to as the glottis.

The Lower Airway

The function of the lower airway is to exchange oxygen and carbon dioxide. When air enters the lower airway (**Figure 2-3**), it passes through the trachea and bronchi to the lungs, where it sweeps through the bronchioles and finally reaches the alveoli, the tiny sacs in which gas exchange takes place.

Trachea

The trachea, or windpipe, is the conduit for air entry into the lungs. The trachea is a membranous tube supported by a series of C-shaped cartilaginous rings. The trachea begins immediately below the cricoid cartilage, the only ring with a circumferential cartilage framework. Below the cricoid cartilage are successive rings connected posteriorly by small muscles that help determine the diameter of the cartilage as they relax and contract. This structure keeps the trachea from collapsing with vigorous coughing or bronchial constriction.

The trachea divides into the right and left mainstem bronchi at the level of the carina. The bronchi are the only source of ventilation for each lung. The right mainstem bronchus is straighter and larger in diameter than the left, making it more susceptible to aspiration and inadvertent intubation. Thus, an endotracheal tube that is inserted too far will often come to lie in the right mainstem bronchus. These bronchi are also composed of C-shaped rings, connected in the back by a small muscle. The trachea and mainstem bronchi are lined with columnar epithelium, providing humidification and secreting mucus to protect the lower airway against harmful particulates. Microscopic hairs called cilia help move the mucus and trapped particles up the respiratory tract to be eventually expelled by coughing and expectoration.

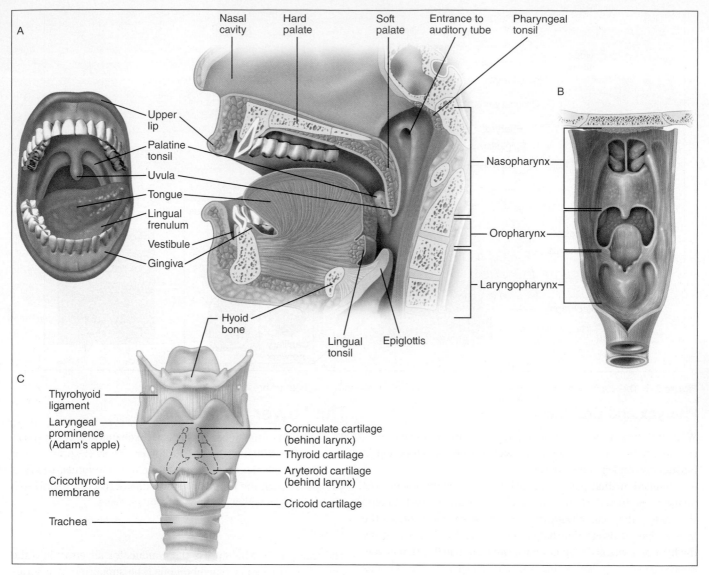

Figure 2-2 **A.** The oral cavity. **B.** The larynx. **C.** The pharynx.

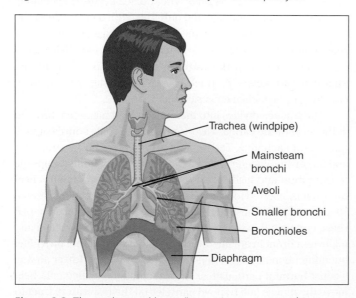

Figure 2-3 The trachea and lungs (lower airway structures).

Lungs

The lungs are the primary organs of breathing. The lungs consist of the entire mass of tissue (parenchyma) that includes the smaller bronchi, bronchioles, and alveoli. The right and left lungs are the next structures in the path of airflow. The right lung has three main lobes: upper, middle, and lower. The left lung shares its side of the intrathoracic space with the heart, so it has only two lobes—the upper and lower. These lobes are covered with a thin, slippery outer membrane called the visceral pleura. The parietal pleura lines the inside of the thoracic cavity. A small amount of fluid is found between the pleurae, which decreases friction during breathing.

On entering the lungs, each bronchus divides into increasingly smaller bronchi, which in turn subdivide into primary, secondary, and tertiary bronchioles. These increasingly smaller bronchioles distribute inhaled air to all areas of the lung for effective ventilation. The bronchioles can dilate or constrict in response to various stimuli. The smaller bronchioles eventually terminate in alveoli, small sacs with walls only a single cell thick, so as to allow gas exchange (respiration) to occur. Millions of alveoli exist in a healthy lung, forming grapelike clusters. Gas exchange takes place across the few layers of cells that separate the alveoli from the pulmonary capillaries. This reciprocal passage of oxygen into the blood and carbon dioxide into the alveoli is called **respiration**. As it leaves the alveoli, gas passes through the single layer of cells that makes up the alveolar wall, through a thin layer of interstitial tissue, and finally through the single layer of cells that makes up the capillary wall. Any increase in the thickness of this cell layer can profoundly jeopardize respiration.

Alveoli are held open and in position by connective tissue in the interstitial tissues that surround the alveoli. A chemical called *surfactant* coats the inner walls of the alveoli, helping keep open these tiny pouches. Surfactant is a chemical that acts much like soap, reducing surface tension and providing an interface between oil and water so the alveoli will not readily collapse on exhalation. Premature infants can have a deficiency of surfactant, which leads to serious respiratory problems. But whatever the patient's age, even normal amounts of surfactant and adequate connective-tissue support can't prevent alveolar collapse or atelectasis. Atelectasis occurs secondary to shallow breathing, infection, trauma, or inflammation, and can be reversed with a sigh or yawn. Atelectasis is a major risk factor for pneumonia.

Musculoskeletal Support of Respiration

The bones, muscles, and connective tissues serve an integral function in ventilation. Without the support of these structures, effective ventilation would be impossible. Structural support ranges from the cartilaginous trachea to the bony vault of the thorax, which maintains the pressure necessary for ventilation.

The main muscle of ventilation is the diaphragm, a thick muscle that separates the thorax from the abdomen. Contraction of the diaphragm, along with that of the chest wall muscles, assists with allowing air to be drawn into the lungs. The diaphragm is under both voluntary and involuntary control. It acts like a voluntary muscle when you take a deep breath, cough, or hold your breath. You control these variations in the way you breathe. However, unlike other skeletal or voluntary muscles, the diaphragm performs an automatic function. Breathing continues during sleep and at all other times. Even though you can hold your breath or temporarily breathe faster or slower, you cannot continue these variations in breathing patterns indefinitely. When the concentration of carbon dioxide becomes too high, automatic regulation of breathing resumes. Therefore, although the diaphragm appears to be a voluntary skeletal muscle that is attached to the skeleton, it behaves, for the most part, like an involuntary muscle. The diaphragm is innervated by the phrenic nerve, which signals the diaphragm to contract and relax. The phrenic nerve originates in the brainstem and exits from the cervical spine at levels C3, C4, and C5. Injury to the cervical spine at these levels, particularly from trauma, may cause fatal apnea.

The thoracic cage is the truss that supports and shelters the structures within the thoracic cavity, including the lungs. Its architecture facilitates the intrathoracic pressure changes necessary for ventilation. The ribs, sternum, and thoracic spine form a protective framework (**Figure 2-4**). In addition to shielding the intrathoracic organs, the ribs help create the pressure necessary for inspiration and expiration. The anatomic structures that support ventilation and respiration share the intrathoracic space with several other important structures, including the heart, venae cavae, aorta, pulmonary trunk, and thoracic duct. These vascular structures circulate oxygenated blood to tissues and return deoxygenated blood to the lungs for lymph exchange and removal of waste materials such as carbon dioxide.

The intercostal muscles are considered accessory muscles to respiration and assist the diaphragm in creating the pressure changes necessary for ventilation. Other accessory muscles include the abdominal and pectoral muscles. The muscles of the chest wall are innervated by the intercostal nerves. When the diaphragm contracts, it moves down slightly, enlarging the thoracic cage from top to bottom. When the external intercostal muscles contract, they move the ribs up and out. These actions combine to enlarge the chest cavity in all dimensions. Pressure in the cavity then falls, making it lower than atmospheric pressure, and air rushes into the lungs. This is referred to as negative-pressure breathing because air is sucked into the lungs. This part of the cycle is active, requiring the muscles to contract.

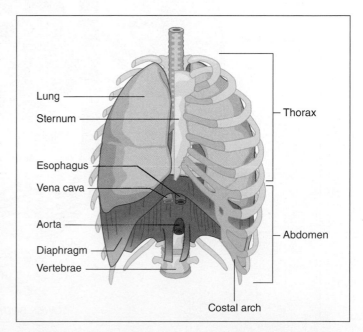

Figure 2-4 The thoracic cage. The dome-shaped diaphragm divides the thorax from the abdomen. It is pierced by the great vessels and the esophagus.

During exhalation or expiration, the diaphragm and the intercostal muscles relax. Unlike inhalation, exhalation does not normally require muscular effort. As these muscles relax, all dimensions of the thorax decrease, and the ribs and muscles assume a normal resting position. When the volume of the chest cavity decreases, air in the lungs is compressed into a smaller space and pressure is greater than atmospheric pressure. Intrapulmonic pressure, which is the pressure within the lungs and airways, is increased, and air is pushed out through the trachea. This phase of the cycle is passive. Exhalation ends when the intrapleural pressure is equal to the atmospheric pressure, at which point air stops flowing from the lungs to the outside.

The esophagus, a muscular tube lined with mucous membrane, lies just behind the trachea and collapses easily with negative pressure. The posterior muscular wall of the trachea lies next to the anterior esophagus. When a person is swallowing large bites of food, the esophagus accommodates the bolus, and the food is propelled down towards the stomach by a wavelike muscular contraction called peristalsis. Esophageal strictures and lesions may create a feeling of burning or fullness in the thorax because of this elasticity.

The process of breathing is typically easy and requires little muscular effort. If you note that a patient is having to use accessory muscles to breathe, respiratory compromise or impending **respiratory failure** should be included in your differential diagnosis.

The heart is the main pump of the circulatory system, and proper functioning is critical to distribution of blood throughout the body (**Figure 2-5**). Deoxygenated blood returns to the heart via the superior and inferior venae cavae. The superior vena cava returns the blood from the head, arms, and shoulders (that is, parts above the heart), and the inferior vena cava returns blood from the lower body (that is, parts below the heart). Deoxygenated blood passes from the venae cavae into the right atrium and is

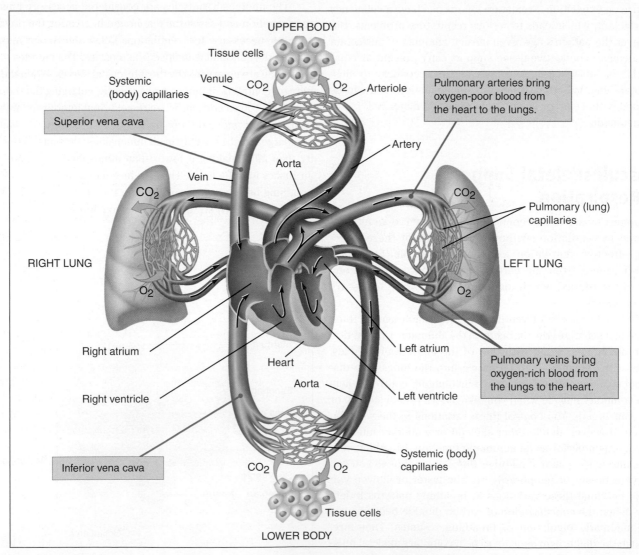

Figure 2-5 The circulatory system includes the heart, arteries, veins, and interconnecting capillaries. The capillaries are the smallest vessels and connect venules and arterioles. At the center of the system, and providing its driving force, is the heart. Blood circulates through the body under pressure generated by the two sides of the heart.

then pumped into the right ventricle, then into the pulmonary trunk. The pulmonary trunk branches into the right and left pulmonary arteries, which flow into the lungs. Oxygenated blood returns to the heart and left atrium through the pulmonary veins. This is the only place in the body where the arteries carry deoxygenated blood and the veins carry oxygenated blood.

From the left atrium, blood is pumped into the left ventricle, the most robust chamber of the heart. The left ventricle is strong enough to counter the force of aortic pressure in order to eject blood into the aorta. Blood is then distributed to the body by successively smaller arteries and arterioles.

The **thoracic duct**, located in the left upper thorax, is the largest lymph vessel in the body. The thoracic duct returns to the venae cavae any excess fluid from the lower extremities and abdomen that is not collected by the veins. The amount of lymph fluid returned is small compared with the blood volume that flows through the veins, but its evacuation is important because the fluid would otherwise pool in the lower extremities.

The Respiratory System: Physiology

The primary function of the respiratory system is to exchange gases at the alveolocapillary membrane or conduct respiration. Respiration and ventilation are regulated by a complex interaction of nerves, sensors, and hormones. The level of carbon dioxide (CO_2) in the body is the primary modulator of respiration. CO_2 is the chief waste product of metabolism. Metabolism is the process of breaking down sugars (dextrose, or glucose) into energy for use by the cells of the body. A high CO_2 level damages the cellular machinery responsible for this metabolism. **Aerobic metabolism**, in which glucose is converted into energy in the presence of oxygen, is the basic process of life. This process is very efficient but relies on a steady supply of both oxygen and glucose, because the cell cannot stockpile either resource.

When denied oxygen, the cells resort to **anaerobic metabolism**, which allows the cells to generate small amounts of energy but releases excessive acids as by-products, especially lactic and carbonic acids. This excess of acid must be removed by the bicarbonate, carbonic acid buffer system or acidosis will result. Often, though, the same problem that impaired oxygen delivery also compromises the circulation, and acids build up, causing cellular injury or tissue death.

When air from the environment enters the respiratory tract, the potential for infection is always present, but the body is quite efficient in responding to this threat. The respiratory system has several strategies for preventing disease-causing organisms (pathogens) from entering from the upper respiratory tract and reaching the alveoli.

If a pathogen bypasses the skin (which acts as a primary barrier against injury and infection) and enters the body through the respiratory tract, the lining of epithelial cells in the trachea acts as a secondary barrier against infection. The epithelium is made up of mucus-secreting goblet cells. The sticky mucus intercepts would-be invaders. Other cells contain microscopic hairs (cilia) that help move the mucus to the upper respiratory tract, where it can be expectorated by coughing. Mucus also contains an immune antibody called immunoglobulin A (IgA). IgA is secreted into bodily fluids and binds to pathogenic organisms, allowing white blood cells to recognize and destroy them.

In the lower respiratory tract, white cells can physically enter the alveoli and bronchioles by squeezing between the cell borders. White cells attack pathogens and engulf any small particles not carried away in the mucus of the upper airway. These white cells are often expectorated in mucus and account for the yellow-green color of sputum in patients with certain kinds of respiratory infections.

Respiration

Each time a person takes a breath, the alveoli receive a supply of oxygen-rich air. The oxygen then passes into a fine network of pulmonary capillaries, which are in close contact with the alveoli. The capillaries in the lungs are located in the walls of the alveoli. The walls of the capillaries and the alveoli are extremely thin. Thus, air in the alveoli and blood in the capillaries are separated by two very thin layers of tissue.

Oxygen and carbon dioxide pass rapidly across these thin tissue layers by diffusion. Diffusion is a passive process in which molecules move from an area with a higher concentration of molecules to an area of lower concentration. There are more oxygen molecules in the alveoli than in the blood. Therefore, the oxygen molecules move from the alveoli into the blood. Because there are more carbon dioxide molecules in the blood than in the inhaled air, carbon dioxide moves from the blood into the alveoli. This process is completely passive. Gas moves naturally from areas of high concentration to areas of low concentration.

The Chemical Control of Breathing

The brain—or more specifically, the respiratory center in the brainstem—controls breathing. This area is in one of the best protected parts of the nervous system—deep within the skull. The nerves in this area act as sensors for the level of carbon dioxide in the blood and subsequently the spinal fluid. The brain automatically controls breathing if the level of carbon dioxide or oxygen in the arterial blood is too high or too low. In fact, adjustments can be made in one breath.

Breathing occurs as the result of a buildup of carbon dioxide, which causes the pH to decrease in the cerebrospinal fluid. The cells are constantly working to eliminate carbon dioxide to regulate the acid–alkaline balance of the body. When the level of carbon dioxide becomes too high, a slight change occurs in the pH (the measure of acidity) of the cerebrospinal fluid. The medulla oblongata (a portion of the brainstem), which is sensitive to pH changes, stimulates the phrenic nerve, sending a signal to the diaphragm that causes a person to breathe.

The person then exhales to reduce the level of carbon dioxide in the body.

Chemical receptors, or **chemoreceptors**, sense changes in the composition of blood and body fluids. The primary chemical changes registered by chemoreceptors include levels of hydrogen (H^+), carbon dioxide (CO_2), and oxygen (O_2):

- H^+. The chemoreceptors sense when an increase in the hydrogen level in the fluid surrounding the cells of the medulla stimulates an increase in the rate of ventilation. The opposite occurs when H^+ levels fall. This change can be detected in the bloodstream by measuring pH. Normal pH in the human body is 7.35 to 7.45.
- CO_2. The CO_2 level in the blood will rise if respiration is too slow or shallow, causing **hypercapnia** or CO_2 retention, or if the blood becomes too acidic. The excess CO_2 spills over into the cerebrospinal fluid, triggering an increase in H^+ and in turn precipitating an increase in the respiratory rate. This level can be measured in the blood by measuring the partial arterial pressure of CO_2 ($Paco_2$). Normal $Paco_2$ is 35 to 45 mm Hg. CO_2 level is the principal regulator of respiration.
- O_2. When peripheral chemoreceptors sense an excessive drop in the oxygen level, the respiratory rate increases. Normal partial arterial pressure of O_2 (Pao_2) is 80 to 100 mm Hg.

Normal respiration is controlled by the hypercarbic (high CO_2 level) drive, whereby respiration increases when CO_2 becomes even slightly elevated. Chemoreceptors undergo a change when chronic lung disease causes a perpetual elevation of the CO_2 level. The body also has a backup system, called the hypoxic drive, to control respiration. When the oxygen level falls, this system will also stimulate breathing. There are areas in the brain, the walls of the aorta, and the carotid arteries that act as oxygen sensors. These sensors are easily satisfied by minimal levels of oxygen in the arterial blood. Therefore, the backup system, the hypoxic drive, is much less sensitive and less powerful than the carbon dioxide sensors in the brainstem. A patient is said to convert to a hypoxic drive, whereby he or she is dependent on a low level of oxygen to stimulate a rise in ventilation rate or depth. This fact explains why patients with chronic lung disease should not be given excessive amounts of oxygen long term. In the initial management of patients with chronic lung disease, if marked hypoxemia is present and a high percentage of oxygen is necessary, oxygen should not be deprived for fear of causing respiratory arrest. The patient has likely run out of energy because inspiration is an active process.

Buffer Systems A buffer is a substance that can absorb or donate hydrogen (H^+). Buffers absorb hydrogen ions when they are in excess and donate hydrogen ions when they are depleted. Therefore, buffer systems act as rapid defenses for acid–base

changes in the hydrogen ion concentration of the extracellular fluid. The respiratory system and the renal system work in conjunction with the bicarbonate buffer to maintain homeostasis. The fastest way the body can get rid of excess acid is through the respiratory system. Excess acid can be expelled as $CO_2 + H_2O$ from the lungs. Conversely, slowing respirations will increase CO_2 in alkalotic states. The renal system regulates pH by filtering out more hydrogen and retaining bicarbonate in an acidotic state and doing just the reverse in alkalotic states. This is a slow process, and it may take days for enough H^+ to be eliminated to achieve acid–base balance.

The kidneys can sense decreased oxygen levels in the blood. Sensors in the renal artery note hypoxia and then release erythropoietin, a hormone that stimulates the creation of red blood cells. When the sensors register chronic low levels of oxygen, more red blood cells are created. Patients who suffer from chronic bronchitis, for example, often have an elevated number of red blood cells, a condition called polycythemia. This disorder increases the risk of forming blood clots. Erythropoietin has been chemically synthesized and is used as an injectable medication in patients who are receiving chemotherapy, in an effort to encourage the body to generate red blood cells.

The Nervous System Control of Breathing

The dorsal respiratory group (DRG) is the main pacemaker for breathing and is responsible for initiating inspiration. It sets the base pattern for respirations. The pons, another area within the brainstem, helps regulate the DRG activities. The pons has two areas. The **pneumotaxic center**, located in the superior portion of the pons, helps shut off the DRG, resulting in shorter, faster respirations. The **apneustic center**, located in the inferior portion of the pons, stimulates the DRG, resulting in longer, slower respirations. Both areas of the pons are used to help augment respirations during emotional or physical stress. The two areas of the medulla and the two areas of the pons work together to help you get the right amount of air when you need it.

Ventilation

A substantial amount of air can be moved within the respiratory system. An adult male has a total lung capacity of 6,000 mL (equivalent to three 2-L bottles of soda). An adult female has about one third less total capacity because the lung size is smaller. The amount of air movement during rest is approximately 500 mL. This is called tidal volume. Tidal volume is the amount of air that is moved into or out of the lungs during a single breath. The precise volume can be affected by many variables, including lung disease, body size, physical fitness, and less obvious factors such as elevation above sea level. Residual volume is the amount of air that remains in the lungs after maximum expiration. This air maintains partial inflation of the lungs and does not move during ventilation. Vital capacity is the total amount of air moved in and out of the lungs with maximum inspiration and expiration.

There are two kinds of reserve capacity: expiratory and inspiratory. Expiratory reserve capacity is the difference between a normal exhalation and an exhalation of the remaining air in the lungs. You can demonstrate this concept by forcing as much air out of the lungs as possible after a normal exhalation—this volume of air is the expiratory reserve capacity. Likewise, inhaling as deeply as possible after a normal inhalation allows you to take in an additional volume of air, the inspiratory reserve capacity. The inspiratory reserve capacity helps keep the alveoli inflated. It is often expelled in yawning.

When you assist a patient's breathing, you move air in and out of the lungs using a bag-mask device. The typical bag-mask device holds approximately 1,000 to 2,000 mL of air. Note that although a person's resting tidal volume is 500 mL, you need to use a bag-mask device that provides more than twice that volume. This is because of dead space.

Dead space is the portion of the respiratory system that has no alveoli, and, therefore, little or no exchange of gas between air and blood occurs. This includes the air in the upper airway and parts of the lower airway to the alveoli and is normally accepted to be about 150 mL. The mouth, trachea, bronchi, and bronchioles are all considered dead space. When a patient is ventilated with any device, more dead space is created. Gas must first fill the device before it can be moved into the patient. The amount of dead space can increase when a disease process like atelectasis occurs.

The depth of each breath is critical information to know when assessing ventilation. There is another measurement called minute volume that provides a more accurate determination of effective ventilation. Minute volume, also referred to as minute ventilation, is the amount of air that moves in and out of the lungs in 1 minute minus the dead space. Dead space is an important factor to consider when determining adequate rates and depths of ventilation as it must be subtracted from the tidal volume.

Minute Volume = Respiratory Rate × Tidal Volume

This calculation helps you to determine how deeply a patient is breathing. Survival requires an adequate amount of minute volume, not just tidal volume alone. Consider the scenario of a patient who is breathing at a normal rate of 20 breaths/min. Yet, when you look at the patient's chest, it is barely moving. When you feel for air movement out of the mouth, you find very little movement. Even though the patient's respiratory rate is normal, the amount of air being moved is inadequate. The minute volume is too low, and the patient needs ventilatory assistance. Always evaluate the amount of air being moved with each breath when assessing a patient's respirations. Analysis of the volume of air involved in ventilation can help you understand the pathology of many respiratory diseases and evaluate how well a patient is responding to treatment (**Figure 2-6**).

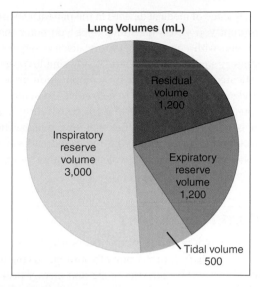

Figure 2-6 Lung volumes.

The AMLS Assessment Pathway

▼ Initial Observations

Dyspnea is both a sign and a symptom. An outward sign of dyspnea, for example, is the use of accessory muscles. The patient may complain of breathlessness or express an uncomfortable awareness of breathing difficulties, using terms such as *shortness of breath* or *chest tightness* or *having trouble breathing*.

When you are responding to an emergency dispatch, the chief complaint of the patient with trouble breathing (sometimes expressed by bystanders when the patient is unable to speak) varies from obvious shortness of breath to weakness or altered mental status. The dispatcher may have obtained additional information from the caller, or your memory of having responded to this patient's residence before may be a clue that the patient has chronic disease.

Scene Safety Considerations

Evaluating the scene for hazards is a key step in the AMLS assessment pathway. Patients with respiratory distress rarely pose a threat to emergency responders, but caution must be exercised when dealing with any hypoxic patient who is restless. You must also consider the potential for violence by family members or bystanders who find it distressing to watch a patient, particularly a loved one, struggle to breathe. Extreme frustration combined with few coping resources is a recipe for aggression. Gaining a command of the scene with tact and empathy can lay the groundwork for good patient care.

The presence of medical devices in the patient's environment should prompt you to ask questions once you enter the home. Some patients with chronic respiratory disease require airway and ventilatory support 24/7, from relatively simple oxygen tanks to sophisticated ventilators. When a complication arises, emergency services are implemented to help solve the acute problem.

A note of caution about settings in which drug overdoses may have occurred: In communities that have a high crime rate, police protection should usually be requested early in the dispatch process. Be alert for loud voices and other red flags that danger may be at hand.

Standard Precautions

Any combination of respiratory complaints with a stated history of fever warrants barrier protection of your mucous membranes, especially while performing suctioning and airway procedures. Putting on a mask, gloves, and gown seems so simple, but it's a precaution that is easy to forget when you view a very sick patient from across the room.

Other Hazards

When patients show evidence of mucous membrane irritation and increased work of breathing, especially when there are isolated groups of victims, special attention to scene safety is warranted. Hazardous materials (hazmat) equipment and teams may have to be dispatched before you enter the scene.

Evaluation of any scene, whether a business or a private home, should be done using all your senses. You should not see particulates suspended in the air, and you should not enter an area where the air is smoky, foggy, or dusty. If your patient is in such an area, respiratory complications are likely. Look for chemical placards or pictograms within business settings. Obtain personal protection equipment and hazmat resources to gain safe entry to such scenes if you are trained to do so. Be sure to smell the air. Chemical odors may alert you to the presence of invisible chemicals in the air. The same protection and resources must be used if you detect this hazard. Within industrial scenes, unusual sounds should alert you to gas leaks or the potential for hazardous situations.

Social, psychological, and physiologic stressors assail the body's immune systems and create an environment conducive to respiratory disorders. Hypothermia, for instance, leads to respiratory compromise and failure. Heat and humidity combined with environmental pollution is also a hazard for chronic respiratory patients. Secondary smoke pollutes the air of everyone in the general vicinity but especially triggers reactive airway difficulties in those with asthma or chronic obstructive pulmonary disease (COPD).

Patient Cardinal Presentation/Chief Complaint

Many patients with chronic respiratory disease have some symptoms all of the time. The pertinent question for them is "What changed that made you call an ambulance or come to the hospital?" Some common respiratory problems include:

- Asthma with fever
- Failure of a metered-dose inhaler
- Travel-related problems after a lengthy journey
- Dyspnea triggers such as pets, perfume, or cigarette smoke
- Seasonal issues with bacteria, molds, and fungi
- Noncompliance with therapy
- Failure of technology, such as an oxygen tank, or running out of medicine

Primary Survey

Level of Consciousness

Whether in an emergency department (ED), a triage area, or the prehospital environment, you assess the patient's level of consciousness and work of breathing from across the room but assess the airway at the patient's side. If the patient is alert, awake, not working hard to breathe, and reaches out to shake your hand when you introduce yourself, the patient is in relatively stable condition and safe from immediate respiratory life threats. Look for the work of breathing. Normal breathing should be peaceful and subtle while at rest. If you are able to note the patient's breathing from across the room, he or she is probably using accessory muscles to breathe, which indicates labored breathing and signals that the patient's condition is probably unstable. The airway must be carefully evaluated. Remember that recognizing and treating life threats are the priority in the primary survey and throughout care. Because many respiratory ailments are life threatening, the respiratory assessment is always an early step in patient assessment.

Airway and Breathing

Immediately open the airway with your gloved hands, using a jaw-thrust or head tilt-chin lift maneuver. Look for signs of upper airway obstruction, such as secretions or blood inside the mouth. Listen to the sounds of the airway. Are there unusual noises that indicate upper airway compromise such as stridor, or lower airway noises such as wheezing, even with the head and jaw in proper position? Suction should always be readily available for your use in the primary exam.

If you need to provide ongoing manual airway management, an immediate plan for positioning or initiation of invasive techniques should be instituted. Preoxygenation/ventilation is always the first step in the plan while you map out a safe, effective means of managing the airway on the basis of your resources, the differential diagnosis, your location, and the patient's anatomy.

If the patient already has an artificial airway in place, evaluate its effectiveness and the patient's tolerance of the device. Confirm proper placement of the device before moving on to assess breathing.

Assessment of breathing begins at your first encounter with the patient. Quickly visualize the chest and observe for obvious movement. As a general rule, any respiratory noises that are audible without a stethoscope are abnormal. Tactile (or vocal) fremitus is a vibration palpable when a person speaks; pneumonia will cause vibration to be more prominent, whereas pneumothorax and pleural effusion lead to a decrease in fremitus. Listen to the patient speak. Is the patient hoarse or does the patient complain of dysphagia? How many words can the patient speak in a sentence before taking a breath? The ability to use six- or seven-word sentences rather than two- to three-word sentences says a great deal about how the patient is breathing.

Assessing the rate and depth of breathing is an obvious component of respiratory assessment, but rate and depth are often not accurately determined. The rate may be a commonly guessed vital sign, but respiratory depth is even more commonly misjudged. A patient with an adequate rate but a low volume will still have an inadequate minute volume. The respiratory rate can vary significantly from minute to minute. Be sure to monitor trends in respiratory rate (whether it is decreasing or increasing) rather than concentrating on the specific rate from the beginning of the assessment.

Distinguishing Respiratory Distress from Respiratory Failure

When a patient reports dyspnea or has an observable increased work of breathing, you must pause and ask yourself a question: Is this patient in respiratory distress, or does he have signs of respiratory failure? If the patient improves with simple resuscitation maneuvers, then respiratory distress is the answer. If, on the other hand, the patient does not improve with basic interventions, or if any patient with respiratory distress has signs of fatigue or altered mental status, respiratory failure is imminent. Immediate resuscitation measures should be implemented to support the patient's airway and ventilation. The following lists some of the indicators of impending respiratory failure.

- Respiratory rate > 30 or < 6 breaths/min
- Oxygen saturation < 90%
- Use of multiple accessory muscle groups
- Inability to lie supine
- Tachycardia with a rate > 140 beats/min
- Mental status changes
- Inability to clear oral secretions/mucus
- Cyanosis of nail beds or lips

After the primary survey, you may have already initiated some basic resuscitation maneuvers if warranted by the patient's condition. You may have supplied oxygen or continuous positive airway pressure (CPAP), or you may have administered positive-pressure ventilation with a bag-mask device. Reevaluate how the patient is tolerating these interventions. Assess whether the patient is feeling better. Have the patient's vital signs improved? Is the patient's chest rising symmetrically with bag-mask ventilation? If these

methods fail, you may need to consider endotracheal intubation and mechanical ventilation or rapid-sequence intubation.

Rapid sequence airway (RSA) is a form of rapid sequence intubation that uses the same pharmacologic approach, but instead of intubation of the trachea, the provider inserts a supraglottic airway device or laryngeal tube device. Studies have shown not only successful airway control but in a shorter time than endotracheal intubation. RSA would appear to work well in patients where endotracheal intubation would be difficult.

Circulation/Perfusion

Assessing skin color is a fast way to begin forming an early impression of the patient's circulation. Although it is important to note the generalized cyanosis of oxygen desaturation or the profound pallor of shock, more subtle information can be gained by assessing the mucous membranes. The tissue inside the mouth, under the eyelids, and even under the nail beds is usually the same pink color in all healthy patients. Note whether the patient's mucous membranes are moist. Dehydration can be seen in the mucous membranes of the mouth and eyes. Dry, cracked lips; a dry, furrowed tongue; and dry, sunken eyes point to obvious dehydration. The skin of an older patient may always look dry with poor turgor, so skin assessment may be of less value in some older people.

▼ First Impression

Your knowledge of anatomy, physiology, and pathophysiology is the first step in being able to perform a thorough physical exam and obtain an appropriate history from the patient to determine the cause of the breathing complaint. Chapter 1 outlined the process of forming that clinical impression, and the Appendix of airway procedures describes rapid-sequence intubation (also referred to as pharmacologically assisted intubation), which is generally used for responsive or combative patients who need to be intubated but who are unable to cooperate.

Initial Presentation

The patient's initial presentation is important. In certain circumstances, the family will bundle up an ill patient having respiratory problems and go to the ED, without calling for the aid of emergency services. Occasionally, emergency care is given in a clinic. Regardless of the setting, assess for overall level of consciousness and work of breathing and do a quick check of perfusion status. You can obtain these assessments while helping the patient out of the car or wheelchair or onto a gurney.

All healthcare providers must be aware of the safety and environmental clues that can be assessed when first encountering the patient. Clues to a variety of pathologic conditions may be evident immediately, but keep in mind that they are only clues. Avoid making a hasty field impression based on minimal information. The patient's presentation may suggest a particular condition, but these suspicions must be confirmed by a thorough assessment.

▼ Detailed Assessment

History Taking

Always ask a patient with a history of a complaint similar to the current one to compare today's symptoms with those experienced previously—are they the same or different from the last time? A patient with a history of heart failure and an acute onset of dyspnea may relate that the symptoms today are the same as the last time pulmonary edema developed. Ask the patient what he or she thinks is wrong. Some patients are so familiar with their disorder, they can relate current symptoms to how they felt on previous occasions and the cause.

OPQRST and SAMPLER

The **history of the present illness (HPI)** is perhaps the most important element of patient assessment. As is often quoted in medical education, "95% of your diagnosis is made by asking the right questions." The primary elements of the HPI are easily remembered by using the OPQRST and SAMPLER mnemonics. Even if the patient does not have pain, those who have had dyspnea before can give you many key pieces of information. For example, a patient with asthma might rate the severity of discomfort of a current episode at 8. It is important to determine how the patient compares this discomfort to that of previous episodes. Identifying if they have ever been intubated when experiencing this type of discomfort can be a key indicator of the need for imminent airway management interventions and the likelihood of respiratory failure. Using these mnemonics, you can systematically obtain a basic HPI.

Also elicit information from the patient about aggravating or alleviating factors—what makes the symptoms worse, and what makes them better? A detailed HPI is decisive in developing an accurate differential diagnosis and formulating an effective treatment plan. Key findings in the patient with dyspnea are listed in Table 2-1. Important elements of a pulmonary history include the following:

- Fever or chills
- Ankle edema
- Calf swelling or tenderness
- Back, chest, or abdominal pain
- Vomiting
- Orthopnea
- Cough
- Dyspnea on exertion
- History of bronchitis
    - Asthma
    - COPD
- Blood in sputum
    - Color of sputum
    - History of sputum production
- Prior respiratory admissions
- History of smoking or passive smoke exposure
- Prior intubations
- Home nebulizer use

Current Health Status

Your history taking should include an exploration of the patient's risk factors to help you narrow the differential diagnosis. For example, the patient may have risk factors for the development of venous thrombosis and pulmonary embolus: use of oral contraceptives, obesity, smoking, and a sedentary lifestyle.

Table 2-1 Key Findings in the Patient with Dyspnea
Duration
• Chronic or progressive dyspnea is usually related to cardiac disease, asthma, chronic obstructive pulmonary disease (COPD), or neuromuscular disease (e.g., multiple sclerosis). • An acute dyspneic spell may be due to exacerbation of asthma, infection, pulmonary embolus, intermittent cardiac dysfunction, a psychogenic cause, or inhalation of a toxic substance, allergen, or foreign body.
Onset
• Sudden onset of dyspnea should raise suspicion of pulmonary embolism or spontaneous pneumothorax. • Dyspnea that develops slowly (hours to days) points toward pneumonia, congestive heart failure, or malignancy.
Patient Position
• Orthopnea can be attributed to congestive heart failure, COPD, or a neuromuscular disorder. • Paroxysmal nocturnal dyspnea is most common in those with left heart failure. • Exertional dyspnea is associated with COPD, myocardial ischemia, and with the abdominal loading that occurs in obesity, ascites, and pregnancy.

Secondary Survey

Vital Signs

Obtain the patient's baseline vital signs—temperature, pulse, respiration, blood pressure, oxygen saturation, and end-tidal CO_2 measurements, and repeat these periodically guided by the severity of the patient's condition. In monitoring vital signs, it's important to keep a close eye on how respiration and perfusion are affecting the patient's mental status. Record your findings in the patient's chart, noting the time they were obtained.

The patient's work of breathing has already been assessed as being quiet (normal) or increased. You've also determined whether the patient is in respiratory distress (obvious from across the room) or has signs of impending respiratory failure (increased work of breathing with altered mental status).

In the primary survey, you were attending to vital functions and addressing life threats. During the secondary survey, however, you should count the patient's breaths per minute to determine the respiratory rate. An extremely high or low respiratory rate may alert you that a secondary organ system is responsible for the respiratory distress. For example, a patient who is breathing without difficulty, using no accessory muscles, but at a fast rate is exhibiting tachypnea. This subtle finding has ominous implications for shock. Tachypnea occurs when the chemoreceptors sense a rise in acidity (metabolic acidosis), stimulating the respiratory system to breathe faster in an attempt to blow off excess CO_2. At the other end of the spectrum, a patient who is breathing slowly, with no accessory muscle use, is exhibiting bradypnea, which can be caused by a central nervous system (CNS) disturbance or by the action of depressant drugs.

In monitoring vital signs, it's especially important to keep a close eye on how respiration and perfusion are affecting the patient's mental status.

Physical Exam

By the time a patient's history has been elicited, some important information should be known about the patient's physical signs, such as level of consciousness, position, and degree of distress. This section presents the components of the focused physical exam in sequence, noting at each step the points of particular relevance to a patient with dyspnea.

Neurologic Exam

Assessing the level of consciousness is imperative in patients with dyspnea. Mental status is a good rough indicator of adequate perfusion and oxygenation of the CNS. The CNS, and the brain in particular, is intolerant of prolonged interruption of its supply of blood, oxygen, or glucose. Mental status can deteriorate rapidly when any of these three components is deficient for as little as a few minutes. Dysfunction of the pulmonary system can lead to hypoxia, hypercapnia, and decline of mental status even in the presence of a functioning circulatory system.

Evaluation of mental status is an important part of patient examination. Assess the patient's orientation to person, place, and time. Assess clarity of speech, verbal coherence, and response time. Slurred speech, poor articulation, mumbling or rambling speech, and aphasia can all be attributable to hypoxia. The combination of new-onset altered mental status and respiratory distress is a hallmark of respiratory failure.

Neck Exam

In the neck, look for jugular venous distention when a patient is in a semisitting position. Jugular venous distention is a condition in which the jugular veins are engorged with blood. It is common in patients who have an obstructive lung disease such as asthma or COPD.

When jugular venous distention is present in patients who are sitting upright, it can provide a rough measure of the pressure in the right atrium of the heart. Distended neck veins may implicate cardiac failure as the source of dyspnea. Jugular venous distention may also indicate high pressure in the thorax, which keeps the blood from draining out of the head and neck. Cardiac tamponade, pneumothorax, heart failure, and COPD can all cause jugular venous distention. Hepatojugular reflux occurs when mild pressure on the patient's liver causes the jugular veins to engorge further. This is a specific sign of right-sided heart failure.

Jugular venous distention must be interpreted in light of the patient's position and other vital signs. Grossly distended jugular veins despite a blood pressure of 80/40 mm Hg in a trauma patient should cause considerable concern; however, jugular vein distention in a healthy 20-year-old person while lying flat (but not while sitting) is of little concern.

While you are looking at the neck, note the trachea. Tracheal deviation is a classic, late sign of a tension pneumothorax. The deviation occurs behind the sternum, so it may not be seen or felt. Consider palpating the trachea at the suprasternal notch.

Chest and Abdominal Exam

Hepatojugular reflux is specific to right-sided heart failure. When the right ventricle is not pumping effectively, blood backs up, making it difficult for the jugular veins and the large reservoir of blood in the liver to drain into the thorax. As a result, the combination of jugular venous distention and a distended liver may present in right-sided heart failure. Pressing gently on the liver will further engorge the jugular veins (hepatojugular reflux). You can elicit this sign of right-sided heart failure when a patient in respiratory distress is sitting up in a semi-Fowler's (45-degree) position.

Feel the chest for vibrations as the patient breathes (tactile fremitus); secretions in the large airways are usually easy to feel and to hear. Some recommend percussion of the chest. With experience, it is possible to distinguish between the sounds of a normal chest and the sounds of a large pneumothorax, but percussion remains a difficult procedure to use in the field because of ambient noise.

One of the key assessments of a patient with respiratory difficulty is auscultation of breath sounds. Evaluate all fields of respiration, both anterior and posterior. Auscultate each of the three lobes of the right lung and the two lobes of the left lung during both inspiration and expiration, paying close attention to ensure that breath sounds are equal bilaterally. Best practices for performing auscultation are outlined as follows:

- Use the diaphragm of the stethoscope; place the diaphragm on the patient's skin if possible.
- To eliminate outside interference, do not allow the stethoscope tubing to touch anything during auscultation.
- To avoid abnormal airway noises, ask the patient to breathe with the mouth open and the head in a neutral position or slightly extended.

- Always move with purpose: superior to inferior, side to side, and site to site.
- If you hear something unusual, stop, move the stethoscope to a new site, and listen again for comparison.

Breath sounds can be categorized simply as normal or abnormal. You might hear normal sounds in one area and abnormal sounds in another. Abnormal sounds, sometimes called adventitious breath sounds, can be heard in any lung area. Sounds associated with particular respiratory disease processes are summarized in **Table 2-2**.

- Wheezing is the classic sound of airway obstruction or a reactive airway. Patients usually do not have trouble drawing air in, but they have difficulty letting air out, which causes expiration to be longer than inspiration. Wheezing is usually heard on expiration and can have a musical quality or a harsh discordant tone. The pitch

Table 2-2 Breath Sounds Associated with Selected Conditions			
Location	**Sound**	**Phase**	**Disease Process**
Upper airway	Stridor	Inspiration	Viral croup Epiglottitis Foreign body aspiration
Lower airway	Rhonchi	Primarily expiration	Frank aspiration Bronchitis Cystic fibrosis
	Wheeze	Primarily expiration	Reactive airway disease Asthma Congestive heart failure Chronic bronchitis Emphysema Endobronchial obstruction
	Crackles	End inspiration	Pneumonia Exacerbation of congestive heart failure Pulmonary edema
	Diminished breath sounds	Either or both	Emphysema Atelectasis Pneumothorax (simple or tension) Flail chest Neuromuscular disease Pleural effusion
Chest wall	Pleural rub	Either	Pleuritis Pleurisy Pleural effusion

varies with the size of the airway. Expiratory wheezes are heard in asthma, bronchitis, and chronic obstructive lung disease. Wheezes associated with other diseases, such as pneumonia and heart failure, signal a reactive airway. The area is inflamed, and bronchi are edematous.

- The auscultation of crackles (also known as rales) on inspiration is associated with accumulated fluid in the alveoli. The sound has a fine, high-pitched, shrill quality and sometimes clears with coughing. If the sound clears after a few deep breaths, the patient probably has atelectasis. Pneumonia, congestive heart failure (CHF), and pulmonary edema are the conditions most often associated with crackles.
- The word *rhonchi* (the plural of rhonchus) derives from the Greek word *rhonkos*, meaning "snoring." Auscultation of rhonchi indicates accumulation of secretions in the larger airways. Rhonchi are often described as bubbly or slurpy sounds heard on expiration. The sounds are generated as air passes through secretions trapped in the airways. Bronchiectasis, cystic fibrosis, and aspiration pneumonitis are often accompanied by rhonchi.
- As noted earlier, fluid between the pleural layers reduces friction, helping the lungs expand and contract during normal respiration. When this fluid buffer is absent, a pleural friction rub can be auscultated. This sign is associated with chest wall pain caused by pneumonia, pleurisy, and lung contusion. The friction rub may be heard in an area adjacent to the site of pain.
- Diminished or distant breath sounds are heard in patients with the following respiratory difficulties:
  - Disorders that lead to increased functional residual capacity—that is, an increase in the resting volume of gas in the lung
  - Diminished air exchange
  - Inappropriate presence of air or fluid
- Auscultation of diminished breath sounds is a classic sign of emphysema. This disease process destroys the alveolar walls, creating greater surface area in the lungs. Gas flow becomes less turbulent, producing a softer sound. Other disorders associated with diminished breath sounds are atelectasis, pneumothorax, pleural effusion, and neuromuscular disorders that limit inspiratory volume.
- Stridor is a sound produced by inflammation or a large obstruction in the upper airway. It is heard only on inspiration and is described as a high-pitched musical sound. While viral croup and epiglottitis are two respiratory disorders accompanied by stridor, a foreign body airway obstruction, laryngitis, stenosis, or tumor of the airway may also be present and may be determined in the history. In the critical care arena, angioedema and trauma are most commonly associated with stridor.

Examination of the Extremities

Does the patient have edema of the ankles or lower back? If so, does it pit when a finger is pushed into the edematous tissue? Is there peripheral cyanosis? Check the patient's pulse. The radial pulse is the point most commonly assessed in a stable patient, but you can gather additional information by evaluating the pulse at alternative arterial sites like the carotid, femoral, and dorsalis pedis. Proximal pulses correspond to larger arteries. The body can shift circulation to these larger vessels during times of stress or hemorrhage. When this occurs, the peripheral pulses may be weak or absent while central circulation is preserved. Does the patient have profound tachycardia (from exertion or hypoxia)? Is there pulsus paradoxus? Also note the patient's skin temperature—whether an obvious fever is present or whether the patient's skin is cool and clammy from shock.

Diagnostics

As appropriate to the patient care plan, apply any monitors that are immediately available. Repeated vital signs, ECG, and pulse oximetry readings are the data most commonly collected. In some situations, depending on available equipment, peak expiratory flow, ETCO$_2$, and transcutaneous carbon monoxide levels might be recorded.

Stethoscope

Practically speaking, the stethoscope is the single most important investment a provider will make. The diaphragm of the stethoscope is for high-pitched sounds (breath sounds); the bell (if present) is for low-pitched sounds (some heart tones). The bell should be placed lightly against the skin to hear the lower pitched sounds.

Pulse Oximeter

Under normal circumstances, a pulse oximeter is a noninvasive device that measures the percentage of a patient's hemoglobin that has oxygen attached to it. For example, an oxygen saturation of 97% indicates that 97% of the patient's hemoglobin has oxygen attached to it. Most healthy people would feel short of breath at a saturation rate of less than 90%. Transcutaneous oxygen saturation monitoring, also known as "pulse ox," "O$_2$ sat," and "sat monitoring," has become an easy, commonplace way to assess blood oxygenation. Transcutaneous oxygen saturation monitors are relatively inexpensive and can quickly approximate the level of oxygen in the blood without the need for an invasive procedure. The technology depends on hemoglobin's ability to absorb infrared light to varying degrees, depending on the number of hemoglobin-binding sites occupied by (i.e., saturated by) oxygen molecules. The monitor calculates the amount of light absorption and translates it into a percentage that represents the level of oxygen saturation. This percentage is displayed on the monitor.

At rest, most healthy individuals have an oxygen saturation of 95% to 100%. More accurate oxygen levels are assessed through invasive arterial blood gas (ABG) monitoring, which requires the puncture of an artery to obtain a sample for testing. This test is valuable for patients experiencing respiratory distress/failure, for ventilated patients, and for the assessment of respiratory and metabolic acidosis. While this test is not typically performed in the prehospital environment, it may prove to be quite helpful in the specialty care transport arena.

The normal partial pressure of oxygen dissolved in arterial blood (Pa_{O_2}), expressed in millimeters of mercury (mm Hg), is 80 to 100. Generally, if oxygen saturation stays above 92%, the Pa_{O_2} is above 60 mm Hg. As the oxygen level drops, the saturation monitor will show a declining reading. There is a slight lag so your patient's oxygen level may be lower before you actually see a change on the saturation monitor. Because of the relationship between the partial pressure of oxygen and the saturation percentage, the latter is not very sensitive to changes in Pa_{O_2} above 90%. When oxygen saturation is 90%, Pa_{O_2} is approximately 60 mm Hg. However, below 90%, the saturation will decrease markedly when decreases in the O_2 partial pressure occur. A minor dip in oxygen saturation at this level can translate to significant hypoxia. As the reading tumbles further, the oxygen level in the blood falls significantly. In some cases, readings below 90% can be used only to evaluate qualitative improvements in ventilation, not absolute improvements in oxygenation. For example, when intubating a severely hypoxic patient, if the patient initially shows 70% saturation, the Pa_{O_2} may be in the 40s. After intubation, the oxygen saturation might improve to 80%, but the Pa_{O_2} may actually have improved only marginally, to about 50 mm Hg.

Other factors can compromise the reliability of oxygen saturation monitoring. Nail polish, paint, or stain on the fingers; cool extremities or a cold environment; shock; poor sensor-to-skin contact, and low batteries can cause inaccurate readings. The saturation monitor needs to sense a pulsatile flow in the digit and indicates this by a pulsating bar or flashing light. Make sure your saturation monitor is picking this up, as without it your readings may be unreliable. Carbon monoxide poisoning can cause falsely high readings; the saturation may be 100%, but the patient may nevertheless be severely hypoxic due to carbon monoxide binding. The bottom line on saturation monitoring is that the value you obtain indicates the hemoglobin you have that is saturated with a gas. It does not verify effective ventilation, it does not determine the amount of hemoglobin you have present so it can be high when in fact if you are anemic you can still be hypoxic, and it does not indicate which gas is attached to the hemoglobin.

Carbon Monoxide Sensor

Relatively new in the healthcare industry, carbon monoxide oximeters have now become reliable indicators of the attachment of carbon monoxide molecules to hemoglobin. Hemoglobin likes carbon monoxide more than oxygen—it's said to have a much higher affinity for carbon monoxide than for oxygen when both are available for attachment, resulting in a higher than normal **carboxyhemoglobin** reading. When a patient has been exposed to a toxic carbon monoxide inhalation, it's clinically useful to have a simple method of detecting the precise amount of carbon monoxide binding that has occurred. The highly accurate sensor attaches to the patient the same way a traditional oximeter device does, but it relies on different wavelengths of light on the spectrum to detect carbon monoxide. Comparing the results of carbon monoxide oximetry and standard carboxyhemoglobin detection using ABG analysis, an invasive laboratory test, the CO-oximetry method comes within 4.3% of the ABG result.

End-Tidal Carbon Dioxide Detector

Analysis of exhaled gases for CO_2, known as **end-tidal carbon dioxide ($ETCO_2$) monitoring**, is a useful method of assessing a patient's ventilatory status. When you are using skin sensors to measure oxygen levels, an accurate reading depends on the patient's distal perfusion. Perfusion strongly influences the accuracy of CO_2 detection as well; CO_2 cannot be detected if there is no perfusion.

Capnometry and Capnography

Capnometry is a reliable method of confirming proper initial placement of an endotracheal tube, because the esophagus normally has a low level of CO_2 or none at all. It is also useful in detecting inadvertent extubation, effectiveness of chest compressions, and return of spontaneous circulation. Capnometry often employs a detector placed between the endotracheal tube and the ventilator or bag-mask device. One type of detector contains a paper indicator that is sensitive to pH changes. Exhaled CO_2 causes the paper to change color, serving as a visual indicator of the presence of CO_2. The degree of color change approximates the amount of CO_2 present, so this type of capnometry is referred to as colorimetric CO_2 detection. These devices provide only semiquantitative measurements. Colorimetric detectors have limited clinical use and a short shelf life. The pH-sensitive paper must remain in sealed packaging until needed, it must be used within 15 minutes of opening, and aspiration of gastric acid into the device will render the device useless, as will administration of acidic drugs through the endotracheal tube. Consumption of carbonated beverages may also give a false-positive result.

Digital capnometry provides a true quantitative reading, with the patient's CO_2 level expressed numerically after each exhalation. Capnography takes carbon dioxide detection a step farther by making the measurement graphic and dynamic, mapping the CO_2 level throughout the respiratory cycle and over time, providing information about the rate of airflow and quality of respiration. The resulting waveform can be broken down into the following several phases that represent metabolism in the body:

- Phase I is the initial exhalation, consisting of dead space air that contains no significant amount of CO_2 and thus does not move the graph.

- Phase II is the active exhalation, which contains escalating amounts of CO_2 owing to the increasing percentage of alveolar air.
- Phase III continues as the alveolar air is exhaled and the CO_2 level eventually reaches a plateau.

Figure 2-7 shows a typical waveform produced by capnography. Point A-B (phase I) shows the waveform at zero, or baseline, on the graph. This baseline occurs at the end of inspiration, just before exhalation. As exhalation begins, an upstroke appears on the waveform, represented by point B-C (phase II). This positive deflection occurs as the device immediately begins to detect CO_2. Point C-D (phase III) indicates a slowing of the velocity of the exhalation, with point D representing the peak of exhaled CO_2 at the end of exhalation. As the plateau of the wave is graphed, a negative deflection (dip), or cleft, may indicate the patient's spontaneous respiratory effort. This can be an early sign that neuromuscular paralysis is wearing off. Point D-E on the waveform reflects rapid inhalation as the next breath begins. This stroke is negatively deflected (moving in a downward direction) because little CO_2 is expelled during this part of the respiratory cycle.

Proper endotracheal tube placement should produce a regular, predictable waveform, as illustrated. Inadvertent placement of the endotracheal tube in the esophagus produces no regular waveform, because there is no significant continuous production of CO_2. Placement of the tip of the endotracheal tube near the glottis may produce some irregular but measurable readings; however, they will not appear as a typical waveform. Any waveform that departs the expected contours should prompt immediate reevaluation of intubation status.

As mentioned earlier along with the waveform in the intubated patient there will also be a number. A normal $ETCO_2$ level is 35–45 mm Hg and is present when ventilation and perfusion are well matched. Conditions such as cardiac arrest, pulmonary embolism, and hypovolemic shock make it difficult to achieve normal $ETCO_2$ levels. In cardiac arrest the $ETCO_2$ level should be able to exceed 10 mm Hg if chest compressions are adequate. If $ETCO_2$ levels above 10 mm Hg cannot be achieved, place a fresh compressor to perform high-quality chest compressions and rotate providers at least every 2 minutes. If $ETCO_2$ levels still do not exceed 10 mm Hg, check the patient's perfusion for possible pulmonary embolus, pleural effusion, or hypovolemia. In an intubated patient, failure to achieve an $ETCO_2$ of greater than 10 mm Hg by waveform capnography after 20 minutes of effectively performed CPR may be considered as one of several pieces of evidence when weighing a decision to discontinue resuscitative efforts. Should spontaneous circulation return, $ETCO_2$ levels will return to or exceed normal measurements, indicating a need to stop chest compressions and assess the patient for a pulse and rhythm. Supraglottic and glottic airways may also produce similar results, and $ETCO_2$ should be measured with these as well.

Sidestream $ETCO_2$ Evaluation in the Nonintubated Patient

Another valuable means of evaluating the patient's CO_2 level at the end of exhalation occurs in the nonintubated patient through sidestream capnography. A CO_2 sampling tube is placed within the patient's nose or mouth, and airway gas samples of the patient's exhalation are sent to a sensor in the machine. Monitoring of nonintubated patients can occur while simultaneously providing supplemental oxygen via bag-mask or cannula. This technique provides breath-to-breath information and will detect problems such as hypercapnia, apnea, respiratory depression, and hypoperfusion. Changes will be seen almost immediately, whereas it may take minutes for oxygen saturation to decrease. Sidestream $ETCO_2$ can be used to assess the severity of COPD or an asthma exacerbation and the effectiveness of interventions. With a mild exacerbation, the patient may initially hyperventilate, and $ETCO_2$ will decrease, but with a severe exacerbation, there will be retention of CO_2 or air trapping that may signal respiratory failure.

Chest Radiography

A chest radiograph is an invaluable evaluation tool for assessing patients with chest pain and dyspnea. A plain radiograph conveys a surprising amount of information about the lungs, heart, chest wall, bones, diaphragm, and soft tissues of the chest. A routine two-view chest radiograph is usually performed with lateral and posteroanterior (PA) views, with the patient's chest against the film.

For more critically ill patients, a chest radiograph may be done at the bedside using a portable machine that yields only one view—the anteroposterior (AP) view. The two-view chest radiograph is better for diagnosing pulmonary disease, but an AP view is sufficient to identify most disorders. An AP film tends to have some image degradation and is subject to more variance in technique than a two-view chest radiograph because the unit

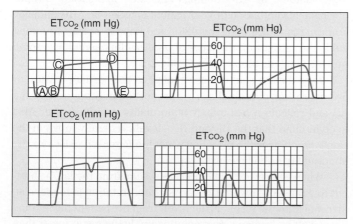

Figure 2-7 Four phases of a normal capnogram. A-B. Carbon dioxide–free portion of the respiratory cycle. B-C. Rapid upstroke of the curve, representing the transition from inspiration to expiration and the mixing of dead space and alveolar gas. C-D. Alveolar plateau, representing alveolar gas rich in carbon dioxide and tending to slope gently upward with uneven emptying of alveoli. D-E. Respiratory downstroke, a nearly vertical drop to baseline. $ETCO_2$, end-tidal carbon dioxide.

is portable. In addition, the AP portable chest unit can somewhat magnify the size of the heart.

Radiographic examination should include the following basics:

- To detect pneumothorax, confirm full expansion of the lungs on both sides.
- Examine the borders of the lungs and margins of the diaphragm to look for fluid collection that suggests pleural effusion, hemothorax, or empyema (pus in the pleural space).
- Explore the interior of each lung to identify pneumonia or any free air that suggests a pneumomediastinum.
- Evaluate the heart's size and position.
- Check both sides for air beneath the diaphragm that might indicate a perforated bowel.
- Confirm that the trachea is in the middle of the mediastinum and any endotracheal tubes are above the carina.

Ultrasonography

Ultrasound examination, also called sonography or diagnostic medical sonography, is an imaging method that uses high-frequency sound waves to produce precise images of structures within your body. The images produced through ultrasound examination often provide information that's valuable in diagnosing and treating a variety of diseases and conditions.

Ultrasound imaging is a valuable tool in emergency settings and has been increasingly used to detect aneurysmal rupture and other life-threatening hemorrhages. Used in its early days primarily for evaluation of pregnancy, new-generation, real-time ultrasound imaging is now used by some emergency care providers to detect ectopic pregnancy, pericardial tamponade, abdominal aneurysm, pleural effusion, pneumothorax, and intra-abdominal hemorrhage. The equipment is relatively expensive, however, and reliable ultrasound evaluation requires training and significant expertise. Such drawbacks tend to limit the availability of this diagnostic tool.

Blood Tests: Arterial Blood Gases and Venous Blood Gases

Arterial blood gases (ABGs) and venous blood gases (VBGs) are used to evaluate both the oxygenation and the acid–base balance of the blood. ABGs are obtained by needle perforation and aspiration of arterial blood into a syringe. The blood is then analyzed rapidly and used to direct clinical management of a patient in respiratory distress. A VBG analysis is an alternative method of estimating systemic carbon dioxide and pH that does not require arterial blood sampling. Performing a VBG rather than an ABG is particularly convenient in the intensive care unit because most patients have a central venous catheter from which venous blood can be quickly and easily obtained.

The pH is a reflection of the acidic or alkalemic condition of the blood. Normal pH in the human body ranges between 7.35

and 7.45. A decreased pH level, such as 7.20, represents acidosis caused by a body malfunction. An elevated pH level, such as 7.55, represents alkalosis.

Acidosis and alkalosis can be further divided into respiratory and metabolic components. Acidosis of a respiratory nature—that is, respiratory failure—can evolve rapidly. Metabolic conditions can also cause acidosis; diabetic ketoacidosis is a primary example, although shock is the most common cause of metabolic acidosis.

Measuring the partial pressure of arterial oxygen (Pao_2) is essential in evaluating the presence and degree of hypoxia. Normal values for patients who are able to breathe room air range from 80 to 100 mm Hg and normally are achieved while breathing 21% oxygen (room air). Patients receiving 100% oxygen with values exceeding 500 mm Hg have been shown to have poorer neurological outcomes. Providers should titrate the fraction of inspired oxygen (Fio_2) to the lowest percentage required to achieve an arterial oxygen saturation between 94% and 99% to avoid potential oxygen toxicity. Hypoxia ranging from 50 to 70 mm Hg is not uncommon in patients with chronic lung disease such as COPD. Patients with decreased levels between 50 and 70 mm Hg may have a more severe clinical presentation because of the tolerance that occurs with chronic hypoxia. The bicarbonate (Hco_3) level reflects the body's acid–base status from a metabolic perspective. A low Hco_3 indicates a metabolic acidosis, and a high Hco_3 level indicates a metabolic alkalosis. The base excess (BE) or base deficit can also be used to evaluate the presence of a metabolic or respiratory condition. The BE normally ranges from –3 to +3. A negative value indicates metabolic acidosis. A positive value indicates metabolic alkalosis.

Arterial Blood Gas Interpretation

As a healthcare provider, it is important that you have a basic understanding of ABG findings and their application. Proper mechanical ventilation of your patient is based on ABG findings. You can't just turn on a ventilator and hope it works. You must guide the settings on the basis of precise clinical findings, some of which include blood gases (Table 2-3).

Note that an acid or base change in the partial pressure of arterial carbon dioxide ($Paco_2$) is proportionately opposite of the pH and reflects a respiratory abnormality or adjustment. Also keep in mind that the BE and Hco_3 levels generally move in the same direction as the pH when a metabolic reason exists for the abnormality or body adjustment.

When you review the blood gas results from the lab, a shortcut to guide you toward the correct interpretation is to place an arrow next to the result. Is the result from the patient higher than normal? If so, use an arrow pointing up. Is the result lower than the normal range? If so, use an arrow pointing down.

For example, your patient's blood gas results read as follows:

Pao_2: 60 mm Hg
pH: 7.20
$Paco_2$: 78 mm Hg
BE: –2
Hco_3: 22 mEq/L

Table 2-3 Key Blood Gas Results

Parameter	Normal Range	Abnormal Findings	
		Acid	Alkali
pH	7.35–7.45	↓	↑
P_{CO_2}, mm Hg	35–45	↑	↓
Base excess	−2 to +2	↓	↑
Bicarbonate, mEq/L	22–26	↓	↑

You note that the P_{O_2} is low, indicating the delivery of oxygen is not sufficient. If the patient is breathing room air you would consider administering high-flow oxygen. The pH is down, the P_{CO_2} is up, and the BE and H_{CO_3} levels are normal. These findings, taken together, indicate acidosis—respiratory acidosis. All laboratory results must be correlated with the patient's clinical condition. In this case, you know that the way to correct the acidosis is to increase the patient's minute volume. If you were providing mechanical ventilation to the patient, you could correct the minute volume by increasing the rate (frequency), the tidal volume, or both.

The body continually tries to recalibrate its balance, or homeostasis. The mechanisms by which the body adjusts for acid or alkali abnormalities come first and most rapidly through the buffer system, second and more slowly through the respiratory system, and third—days later—through the renal system.

The following blood gas results show successful compensation in a patient who is in early hemorrhagic shock:

pH: 7.36
$Paco_2$: 25 mm Hg
BE: −8
HCO_3: 15 mEq/L

Clinically, this patient is demonstrating tachypnea (an early sign of shock) and is blowing off CO_2 to minimize the availability of carbonic acid. In fact, the respiratory system has done so well that the patient's pH remains normal. This is termed *complete compensation*. Alternatively, you could say the metabolic acidosis is fully compensated.

Adjusting positive-pressure ventilation on the basis of blood gas results is standard practice in the critical care arena. One way to do this is from a practical standpoint as follows:

1. $Paco_2$ is largely a function of rate (f) and tidal volume (VT).
   - For increased $Paco_2$: increase f × 2 to 5 or VT × 50 to 100 mL
   - For decreased $Paco_2$: decrease f × 2 to 5 or VT × 50 to 100 mL

2. For acute changes in oxygen saturation as measured by pulse oximetry (Spo_2), changes in F_{IO_2} and positive end-expiratory pressure (PEEP) should occur. Changes in PEEP must be undertaken with caution, especially where PEEP levels are greater than 7 to 10 cm H_2O.
   - For increases in Spo_2 greater than 95%: decrease F_{IO_2} in increments of 5% to maintain Spo_2 above 94%.

Venous Blood Gas Interpretation

Some EDs are beginning to rely on VBG values in certain clinical circumstances. This practice has obvious clinical advantages: it reduces the number of high-risk arterial punctures required to obtain laboratory samples, it provides enough data for physicians to determine the presence of some metabolic disorders, and it eliminates a painful experience for the patient. VBG values, except for Po_2, serve as predictors of arterial values.

One disadvantage to VBG testing is the necessity of drawing ABGs in the event that clinical correlation cannot be made with venous values. Another is the obvious gap in reliable Po_2. Pulse oximetry may be used as an adjunct to VBG sampling. Table 2-4 demonstrates the differences in normal venous and arterial blood gas values.

Pulmonary Function Tests

Pulmonary function tests (PFTs) are a group of tests often ordered by pulmonologists for a patient with breathing difficulties in order to better characterize the nature and severity of the illness. PFTs measure how well the lungs take in and release air and how well they move gases such as oxygen from the atmosphere into the body's circulation.

In the field or ED, you may measure a peak expiratory flow rate, or peak flow, in patients with bronchospasm. This rate is a measure of airflow and is evaluated against an expected norm

Table 2-4 Comparison of Arterial and Venous Blood Gas Values in Healthy Volunteers		
	Arterial Blood Gas Values	**Venous Blood Gas Values**
pH	7.38–7.42	7.35–7.38
P_{CO_2} mm Hg	38–42	44–48
P_{aO_2} mm Hg	80–100	40
H_{CO_3} mEq/L	24	22–26

Reproduced from Sherman and Schindlbeck: Arterial and venous blood gas values. *Emerg Med*. 38(12):44–48, 2006. Copyrighted 2015. IMNG. 119131:0815BN

based on age, height, and sex or against the patient's known baseline. Measurements can determine the effectiveness of your therapies or direct you to another cause of the patient's shortness of breath.

▼ Refine the Differential Diagnosis

You should perform certain diagnostics, ask questions, and select assessments on the basis of the patient's chief complaint, such as dyspnea, weakness, fever, altered mental status, syncope, or chest pain. The following tables will help you formulate a set of differential diagnoses associated with common complaints. Differential diagnosis of dyspnea by body system is summarized in **Table 2-5**. Differential diagnosis by sign or symptom is outlined in **Table 2-6**.

Table 2-5 Differential Diagnosis of Dyspnea by Body System		
Critical	**Emergent**	**Nonemergent**
Pulmonary Diagnoses		
Airway obstruction	Spontaneous pneumothorax	Pleural effusion
Pulmonary embolus	Asthma	Neoplasm
Noncardiogenic edema	Cor pulmonale	Pneumonia
Anaphylaxis	Aspiration pneumonia	COPD
Cardiac Diagnoses		
Pulmonary edema	Pericarditis	Congenital heart disease
Myocardial infarction		Valvular heart disease
Cardiac tamponade		Cardiomyopathy
Abdominal Diagnoses		
Abdominal dissection	Ischemic bowel	Ascites
Bowel perforation	Pancreatitis	Ileus
Perforated diverticula	Cholecystitis	Obesity
Gangrenous gallbladder	Bowel obstruction	
Perforated esophagus	Herniated diaphragm	

(continues)

Table 2-5 Differential Diagnosis of Dyspnea by Body System (*continued*)		
Critical	**Emergent**	**Nonemergent**
Metabolic Diagnoses		
Diabetic ketoacidosis	Hyperglycemia	
Thyroid storm	Hyperthyroidism	
Infectious Diagnoses		
Sepsis	Pneumonia, viral	Influenza
Pneumonia	Pneumonia, bacterial	Bronchitis
Epiglottitis	Pneumonia, fungal	Human immunodeficiency virus (HIV) infection
Bacterial tracheitis	Pneumonitis	Tuberculosis
Retropharyngeal abscess	Aspiration pneumonitis	
Foreign object aspiration	Lung abscess	
Meningitis	Empyema	
Hematologic Diagnoses		
Severe anemia	Anemia	Chronic anemia
Hemorrhage, gastrointestinal	Leukemia	
	Lymphoma	
Neuromuscular Diagnoses		
Intracerebral hemorrhage	Encephalopathies	Neuromuscular degenerative disease (amyotrophic lateral sclerosis [ALS])
Cerebrovascular accident	Alcohol intoxication	Myasthenia gravis
Transient ischemic attack	Basilar artery syndrome	Multiple sclerosis

Table 2-6 Differential Diagnosis of Dyspnea by Sign or Symptom

Critical	Emergent	Nonemergent
Weakness		
Sepsis	Electrolyte abnormality	Dehydration
Intracerebral hemorrhage	Pneumonia	Heat exhaustion
Myocardial infarction	Basilar artery syndrome	
Pulmonary embolus		
Pneumothorax		
Drug overdose		
Fever		
Sepsis	Pneumonia	Bronchitis
Heat stroke	Empyema	Urinary tract infection
Epiglottitis		
Bacterial tracheitis		
Retropharyngeal abscess		
Syncope		
Sepsis	Congestive heart failure	Dehydration
Pulmonary embolus	Myocarditis	Vertigo
Myocardial infarction		Vasovagal stimulation
Myocardial ischemia		
Cardiac arrhythmia		
Chest Pain		
Acute myocardial infarction	Pericarditis	Bronchitis
NSTEMI	Myocarditis	Chest wall pain
Pericardial tamponade	Pericardial effusion	Costochondritis
Aortic dissection	Pneumonia	Hiccough
Status asthmaticus	Dressler's syndrome	Tietze's syndrome

(continues)

Table 2-6 Differential Diagnosis of Dyspnea by Sign or Symptom (*continued*)

Critical	Emergent	Nonemergent
Arrhythmia	Cholecystitis	
	Hepatitis	
	Superior vena cava embolus	
Altered Mental Status		
Hypoglycemia	Drug intoxication	Alcohol intoxication
	Acute coronary syndrome	
Stroke/TIA	Hypercalcemia	
Sepsis	Hyperkalemia	
Respiratory failure	Hyponatremia	
Aortic dissection	Pneumonia	
Intracerebral hemorrhage		
Status epilepticus		

NSTEMI, Non–ST-segment elevation myocardial infarction; TIA, transient ischemic attack.

▼ Ongoing Management

Before administering the treatment discussed in the following sections, a variety of other standard interventions should have already been implemented. Oxygen to keep the saturation above 94% and an intravenous line are typical interventions for any patient who needs advanced life support. Psychological support is also an important consideration for a patient with dyspnea. Your efforts to reduce that patient's anxiety with a calm, professional, and caring demeanor can help reduce the patient's heart rate and blood pressure and allow the patient to maximize breathing effectiveness.

Initial and Basic Management Techniques

Supplemental Oxygen

Supplemental oxygen is the easiest, quickest, and most efficient way to improve oxygenation in a breathing patient. Oxygen is usually delivered by nasal cannula, which can effectively provide 24% to 40% oxygen. Higher flow rates greater than 6 L/min can cause patient discomfort, especially when given long term.

Oxygen may be administered with humidification, reducing the drying effect of the inspired air.

Use of a face mask can increase the concentration of oxygen administered up to 60% when 15 L/min of oxygen is given. The Venturi (air entrainment) mask is a specialized face mask that gives the provider more precise control over the amount of inspired oxygen, from 28% to 40%. The Venturi mask and the standard face mask have one problem in common: placing a device over both the nose and mouth of a dyspneic patient will almost certainly increase the patient's anxiety and often results in the patient removing the mask.

The nonrebreathing face mask adds an oxygen reservoir to the standard face mask, increasing the inspired oxygen level to 100% at 15 L/min of oxygen flow. The nonrebreathing mask often functions as a bridging device to another modality, because a patient who needs 100% oxygen typically requires some other type of ventilatory support such as bilevel positive airway pressure (BiPAP) or intubation. If aggressive care is successful, the patient can be weaned down to a lower FIO$_2$ instead of being intubated.

Achieving oxygen saturations of 100% indicates hyperoxemia (excessive acidity in the blood) and has been associated with poorer neurologic outcomes. In a patient with a normal hemoglobin level, a saturation of 90% is minimally acceptable, but oxygen should be administered to patients with breathlessness, signs of heart failure, shock or an oxygen saturation less than 94%.

Positive-Pressure Ventilation

Patients with respiratory failure need positive-pressure ventilation to improve gas exchange, relieve respiratory distress, and allow for uncomplicated lung healing. Criteria to establish ventilation are as follows:

- $Pao_2 < 55$ mm Hg
- $Paco_2 > 50$ mm Hg
- pH < 7.32

You can provide this ventilatory support noninvasively through a bag-mask device, CPAP, or BiPAP.

Bag-Mask Device

The bag-mask device has become a standard respiratory resuscitation tool for patients of all ages. Certain considerations are typical regardless of which manual resuscitator system you purchase and use. You must stock and select the correct size bag and masks for all patients.

The manual resuscitator should have PEEP valve capability, especially in the hospital and interfacility transport setting. If you need to administer temporary manual ventilation with a bag-mask to a patient who just came off a bedside intensive care unit (ICU) ventilator equipped with PEEP, that parameter must be maintained. In addition, oxygenation is improved when a reservoir bag or tube is added, *and* you administer ventilation slowly with just enough tidal volume to raise the chest.

Another misconception about manual (self-inflating) bag-mask systems is that they all deliver 100% oxygen if you add 12 to 15 L of oxygen to the reservoir. *If* you administer ventilation slowly, with moderate tidal volume, you can approach 100% oxygen using those devices, but it is difficult to do so. A more realistic estimate is 65% to 80% oxygenation. Non–self-inflating devices or anesthesia bags do deliver 100% oxygen to the patient. Providers in many critical care areas prefer these bags because they are sensitive to the patient's lung compliance while administering ventilation, although they are not easy to use in practice. The flow-control valve on an anesthesia bag gives it built-in PEEP capability.

Continuous Positive Airway Pressure

Continuous positive airway pressure (CPAP) is a ventilatory technique used to apply a modest amount of continuous pressure in the airway to an alert patient to keep smaller airways open, reduce the work of breathing, and improve alveolar oxygenation. CPAP devices can be beneficial for patients who are having moderate to severe respiratory difficulty, such as those with asthma, emphysema, and CHF. The technique reduces left ventricular preload and afterload in patients with CHF. For the device to be effective, the patient must keep a seal between the mask and his or her face.

Bilevel Positive Airway Pressure

BiPAP (**Figure 2-8**) is a modality being used more frequently in the emergency setting. This noninvasive technique can ease the work of breathing, improve ventilation, and greatly reduce the morbidity of intubation and possible subsequent ventilator dependence. BiPAP holds great promise for avoiding at least some intubations.

In BiPAP, one pressure can be delivered during inspiration (inspiratory positive airway pressure) and a different pressure can be delivered during exhalation (expiratory positive airway pressure). BiPAP is a form of CPAP, but it has two different levels of pressure support. One level is higher and supports inspiration (IPAP). The second, lower level assists expiration (EPAP) and helps keep the airway open. Ventilation is delivered through a mask that covers either the nose only or both the face and nose. The mask is often secured to the face with adjustable straps, allowing the patient to relax rather than worry about holding the mask in place.

Both CPAP and BiPAP are valuable noninvasive tools for supporting a patient's respiratory effort, but they are not without drawbacks. Some patients, especially those prone to claustrophobia, cannot tolerate having their nose and mouth covered. The continuous positive pressure can impede venous return and thus reduce blood pressure; it may also contribute to gastric distention and raise the risk of aspiration. Finally, increased positive airway pressure carries the risk of barotrauma, specifically pneumothorax or tension pneumothorax (discussed later).

Invasive Airway Ventilation

Emergent ventilatory management is always or almost always performed in response to a clinical presentation of respiratory distress and a declining level of consciousness. The initial goal of invasive airway ventilation is to ensure the airway is secure and protected and ventilation and oxygenation are adequate.

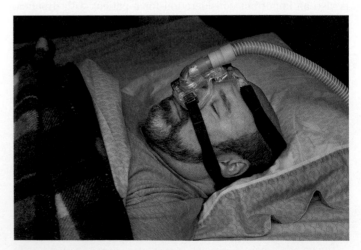

Figure 2-8 Patient with a bilevel positive airway pressure (BiPAP) mask applied.
© Howard Sandler/ShutterStock, Inc.

The secondary goal is to successfully wean the patient from the support without complications. The selection of the mode of ventilation should take into consideration the patient's level of consciousness, pulmonary function, degree of respiratory distress, prior intubation history, coexisting medical conditions, and degree of hypoxia.

Invasive techniques for intubated patients include pressure-cycled and volume-cycled ventilators. With the ultimate goal of successful extubation, you should select the mode that will allow the patient to exercise as much control as possible over his or her own breathing.

Pressure-Cycled Ventilation

In pressure-cycled ventilation, a breath is delivered until a preset airway pressure has been reached. This predetermined level is called the peak inspiratory pressure, and the ventilator carefully maintains ventilation within this parameter. Higher pressure allows air to move from the ventilator until the peak inspiratory pressure has been achieved and inspiration occurs. Passive exhalation follows inspiration, because the pressure is higher in the chest than in the ventilator.

Pressure-cycled ventilation is most beneficial in the ICU, where patients often have reduced compliance of the lungs or chest wall (as in acute respiratory distress syndrome [ARDS]) or increased lung pressure (as in asthma). In treating such patients, the ability to control peak pressure dictates the selection of pressure-cycled ventilation.

Volume-Cycled Ventilation

In volume-cycled ventilation, a preset tidal volume is programmed into the device. Inhalation is terminated when the limit has been reached. A major advantage of this type of ventilator is that it delivers the tidal volume regardless of changes in lung compliance. Assist/control and intermittent mandatory ventilation are types of volume-cycled ventilators.

Modes of Ventilatory Support

The following four principal methods of ventilation are used to deliver volume-cycled and pressure-cycled ventilation:

1. *Controlled mechanical ventilation (CMV).* The ventilator delivers breaths at a preset interval, regardless of the patient's respiratory effort. This mode is appropriate only for apneic patients and for those who have been pharmacologically paralyzed.
2. *Assist/controlled (A/C) ventilation.* If the patient takes a breath, an assisted breath is given simultaneously and the ventilator monitor resets to watch for a breath in the next 5 seconds. If no breath is taken within 5 seconds, the machine delivers one, and the clock starts again. This is a common ventilator setting during the early phase of ventilatory support.

3. *Intermittent mandatory ventilation (IMV).* This combines CMV with the patient's spontaneous ventilation. The background CMV breathes for the patient regardless of his or her own respiratory effort. If the patient puts forth a respiratory effort, the ventilator does not support it with positive pressure. Instead, it supplies only warm, humidified oxygen. IMV in an alert patient requires less sedation and no paralysis, and it allows the patient to preserve muscle tone in the muscles of ventilation, which makes it easier to wean the patient from mechanical ventilation.
4. *Synchronous intermittent mandatory ventilation.* This supports the patient's spontaneous breaths with A/C ventilation. Synchronous delivery prevents stacking of breaths (a mechanical breath being delivered at the same time as a spontaneous breath—a drawback of IMV), which may cause barotrauma from hyperinflation.

Determine how the ventilator should respond to a patient's spontaneous respiration. Consider the patient's mental status, and take into account whether the patient will be aware of the activity of the ventilator. Attempting to breathe and receiving no response from the ventilator can make even the calmest patient extremely anxious. Conscious patients can be placed on synchronous intermittent mandatory ventilation, and totally awake patients who are being prepared for extubation may be placed on pressure-support ventilation.

A heavily sedated patient or one with severe brain injury, on the other hand, may put forth no respiratory effort. Such patients require near-total mechanical control and are candidates for A/C ventilation.

Mechanical Ventilator Settings

When initiating mechanical ventilation, you must select a ventilatory mode, tidal volume, respiratory rate, and initial oxygenation concentration. Supplemental choices include PEEP. The parameters can be altered to meet clinical requirements, such as an anxious patient with respiratory failure and COPD who prefers to breathe at a rate of 20 breaths/min but whose tidal volume is less than that predicted on the basis of body weight. Table 2-7 summarizes typical ventilator settings.

Minute Volume Minute volume is the amount of air inspired per minute. Minute volume combines tidal volume with rate to ensure that enough air is inspired to support adequate ventilation.

Tidal Volume Tidal volume (ventilation volume) and respiratory rate should approximate the patient's own normal rate of respiration. Most adults draw a tidal volume of between 5 and 10 milliliters per kilogram (mL/kg) of body weight. Typical settings for an adult who is not in distress are a volume of 6 to 8 mL/kg of body weight and a respiratory rate of 12 breaths/min. Several calculations used to determine tidal volume on the basis of weight are shown in Table 2-8.

Table 2-7 Common Ventilator Settings

Setting	Description	Common Settings	Comments
Rate or frequency (f)	Number of breaths delivered per minute	6–20/min	
Tidal volume (TV)	Volume of gas delivered to the patient	6–8 mL/kg	
Oxygen (F_{IO_2})	Fraction of inspired oxygen delivered	21%–100%	Blender required if < 100%
PEEP	Positive pressure delivered at the end of exhalation	5–20 cm H_2O	This mode improves oxygenation.
Pressure support (PS)	Pressure support to augment inspiratory effort	5–20 cm H_2O	
Inspiratory flow rate/time	Speed with which VT is delivered	40–80 L/min Time: 0.8–1.2 seconds	
Inspiration/expiration (I/E) ratio	Duration of inspiration to expiration	1:2	
Sensitivity	Determines the amount of effort the patient must generate to initiate a breath	0.5–1.5 cm H_2O below baseline pressure	
High pressure limit	The maximum pressure with which the ventilator can deliver the tidal volume	10–20 cm H_2O above peak inspiratory pressure	The ventilator will stop the breath and release the rest to the atmosphere when the limit is reached.

If the patient is a man who is 6 feet tall and weighs 225 lb and you convert his weight to kilograms, you might set his tidal volume at 800 mL if you calculate 8 mL/kg. Instead, you should calculate that his ideal body weight is 177 lb, or about 81 kg. Your setting, then, should be closer to 650 mL.

The fraction, or concentration, of oxygen in the inspired air (F_{IO_2}) is also chosen as an initial ventilator setting. Choices range from 100% down to 21%. A severely dyspneic patient who has low P_{O_2} may benefit from an initial setting of 100% until his or her condition has stabilized. Few patients who require emergent or urgent intubation will tolerate 21% oxygen, which is the same as room air. Virtually all patients requiring aggressive airway management will need some oxygen supplementation, but the precise degree will vary from patient to patient. Settings typically fall between 40% and 80%.

Pressure Support Initially, choose the ventilatory mode on the basis of the patient's spontaneous respiratory effort and sedation level. Pressure-support ventilation is a mode used in patients who have retained a spontaneous respiratory drive. It allows the operator to set minimum parameters for breaths per minute, tidal volume, and minute volume. Pressure support can be used to hold a constant positive pressure in the airways, much like BiPAP.

Positive End-Expiratory Pressure Most ventilators accommodate PEEP, a small amount of positive pressure that remains even at the peak of expiration. This pressure opens alveoli clogged with mucus, vomitus, infiltrate (in patients with pneumonia), and edema (in patients with CHF), and it helps keep them open. PEEP can help patients who have alveolar collapse, as is seen in pneumonia and pulmonary edema, but larger tidal volumes and high-pressure support increase the risk of pneumothorax.

Table 2-8 Weight-Based Formulas for Calculating Tidal Volume*

Devine Formula

For women: 45.5 kg + 2.3 kg for every inch more than 5 feet of height

For men: 50 kg + 2.3 kg for every inch more than 5 feet of height

Broca's Formula

Women: 100 lb for the first 5 feet + 5 lb for every inch above that

Men: 110 lb for the first 5 feet + 5 lb for every inch above that

Hamwi Formula

Women: 45.5 kg for the first 5 feet, then 2.2 kg for every inch above that

Men: 48 kg for the first 5 feet, then 2.7 kg for every inch above that

Generic Height-Weight Formula

Women: 105 lb + 5 × (Height in inches − 60)

Men: 105 lb + 6 × (Height in inches − 60)

*When choosing an appropriate tidal volume for your patient, you must consider what the patient's ideal weight is—not his or her actual weight. Many formulas have been devised to calculate ideal body weight. Most rely on the patient's height and sex.

Complications of Mechanical Ventilation

A number of serious risks are associated with invasive mechanical ventilation. Volutrauma (also known as barotrauma) is lung injury or alveolar rupture from overdistention of the alveoli. Pneumothorax and tension pneumothorax are the primary concerns in ventilator-induced barotrauma; pneumomediastinum and pneumoperitoneum are less frequent complications. Prolonged administration of high-concentration oxygen can damage cells with resultant atelectasis. Persistent high intrathoracic pressure can cause decreased cardiac return and low systolic blood pressure.

Another complication can occur while providing positive-pressure ventilation. You already know from earlier discussions that applying PEEP can help keep distal alveoli open and improve oxygenation. Using too much ventilation or administering ventilation to patients who have air-trapping diseases such as asthma or COPD, however, may cause a complication called auto-PEEP. In this condition, too little time for exhalation leads to progressively increased air trapping. This phenomenon can compromise gas exchange and allow intrathoracic pressure to become so high that hemodynamic compromise occurs as a result of decreased cardiac output, placing a squeeze on the heart itself.

Special Circumstances with Mechanical Ventilation

Closely monitoring the patient during intubation and subsequent mechanical ventilation is imperative, because adequate sedation to allow mechanical ventilation can prevent the patient from communicating symptoms of an evolving complication. Immediately investigate and address any unexplained tachycardia, bradycardia, hypotension, or hypertension. Use capnographic and oxygen saturation monitoring—including periodic measurement of ABGs—to direct your selection of ventilator settings. Reduce the F_{IO_2} as soon as possible, consistent with maintaining an adequate P_{O_2}.

Patients with asthma or COPD may require a high inspiratory pressure and increased pressure support. These patients tend to retain air volume and have high airway pressure, putting them at markedly increased risk of barotrauma. The use of BiPAP in patients with COPD has been shown to reduce the need for intubation by 59%. Should intubation become necessary, adding PEEP may help reduce the air retention that puts these patients at higher risk.

Intubation

Ultimately, patients who are in respiratory failure may need to be intubated and ventilated. Intubation can be lifesaving, and many patients can be extubated within a day or two and have an excellent outcome. However, when you are deciding whether to intubate a patient, the following issues must be weighed along with the protocols, medical direction, and any expression of the patient's wishes:

- Intubation should be the last option for patients who have severe asthma. Patients with asthma are extremely difficult to ventilate and are prone to pneumothoraces.
- Be proactive; ventilate patients before cardiac arrest occurs. When is doubt, attempt to ventilate. A patient who is combative may not be ready for intubation. If a patient allows intubation, it was probably necessary. Patients who are conscious, yet still in respiratory distress will require sedation and neuromuscular blocking medications (through rapid-sequence intubation) to facilitate intubation.

- Patients who have had a stroke or who are severely intoxicated may have little or no gag reflex, the lack of which poses a grave danger if the patient vomits. Consider intubating patients in these situations to protect the airway even if ventilation is adequate.
- Some patients who have diabetes or have overdosed present with an obvious need for intubation. However, if an ampule of 50% dextrose or naloxone (Narcan) is likely to completely change that picture, it might be better to use bag-mask ventilation for a few minutes to monitor the effect of the initial therapy, assuming ventilation can be done without causing gastric distention and vomiting. Ventilate slowly (over 1 second), and use only enough ventilation to produce visible chest rise.

Upper Airway Conditions

The upper respiratory tract is vulnerable to many conditions that can obstruct the airway and consequently impair ventilation. Infection is the most common cause of such conditions, but allergic reactions and foreign bodies can also obstruct airflow. Patients with airway obstructions may have no obvious outward signs of illness (e.g., swelling and positional breathing) but may have difficulty swallowing (dysphagia) to the point of drooling. Abnormal sounds may be generated when they breathe or speak. The most common sound associated with upper airway obstruction is stridor, which typically is heard on inspiration. Some of these airway diseases like epiglottitis can become life threatening, and you must have a safe and smart plan for airway management that includes proper positioning of the patient.

Aspiration

The inhalation of anything other than breathable gases is called aspiration. Patients can aspirate fresh or salt water, blood, vomitus, or food. Patients who receive tube feedings are at particular risk for aspiration if they are placed supine immediately after receiving a large feeding. A large percentage of geriatric patients have impaired swallowing from strokes or other neurologic impairments. Unresponsive patients are at risk for the aspiration of vomitus. The aspiration of stomach contents carries the additional risk of aspiration pneumonitis, in which the gastric acid irritates the lung tissue. This risk is in addition to the risk of pneumonia from any bacteria in the aspirated material.

Pathophysiology

Aspiration of stomach contents into the lungs has a significantly high mortality rate. It is a common but profoundly dangerous complication in patients who have had trauma or who have overdosed. Aspiration of foreign bodies, such as nuts or broken teeth, may also occur. Most adults choke only when they are intoxicated or traumatized or have a reduced gag reflex from a stroke or aging. Chronic aspiration of food is also a common cause of pneumonia in older patients.

Signs and Symptoms

What is the scenario surrounding your patient's sudden onset of dyspnea? Did it occur immediately after eating? Does the patient have a gastric feeding tube, and if so, when was the last feeding and how large was it? Is the material suctioned from the patient's airway the same color as the tube feeding? Is there particulate matter in the suctioned material? A fever and cough may present several hours after an aspiration-prone event, such as a seizure or episode of unresponsiveness. Some patients aspirate chronically and may have a history of aspiration pneumonia.

Treatment

Use the following guidelines when treating patients at risk for aspiration or who have aspirated:

- Aggressively reduce the risk of aspiration by avoiding gastric distention when ventilating and by decompressing the stomach with a nasogastric tube whenever appropriate.
- Aggressively monitor the patient's ability to protect his or her own airway, and protect the patient's airway with an advanced airway when needed.
- Aggressively treat aspiration with suction and airway control if the other steps described fail.

If basic life support maneuvers fail to clear an obstructed airway, use laryngoscopy and Magill forceps, and, if necessary, perform a needle or surgical cricothyrotomy if allowed by local protocol.

Airway and Foreign Body Obstruction

The most common cause of upper airway obstruction in a semiconscious or an unconscious patient is the tongue. Every year, obstruction caused by the tongue results in results in the death of some trauma patients, patients in insulin shock, patients who have had a seizure, or patients who are intoxicated.

Aspiration of foreign objects can be a source of significant anxiety for patients and their caregivers. With a peak incidence among infants and toddlers, aspiration of foreign bodies is perhaps a predictable result of young children's tendency to mouth everything they handle. Older children and adults are not seized by this temptation so frequently; aspiration of a foreign object by an adult should prompt assessment for intoxication and mental impairment. According to the American Academy of Pediatrics, food, coins, and toys are the most frequently aspirated items by children.

Signs and Symptoms

Sudden onset of coughing, dyspnea, and signs of choking are the hallmarks of aspiration of a foreign object. Depending on the size and position of the object and the diameter of the airway, the patient may have total or partial obstruction. Partial obstruction of the lower airway may cause air trapping, with a sudden change in thoracic pressure leading to pneumothorax or pneumomediastinum. Sudden onset of wheezing, especially in an infant or child and particularly in one lung, should raise suspicion that a foreign object has been aspirated.

In some cases, aspirated foreign objects may remain trapped in the airway for several days, weeks, or even months. Chronic blockage of a bronchus can cause bronchial collapse and obstructive pneumonia. Even those in the esophagus can be responsible for airway compromise.

Treatment

Management of an aspirated foreign object should be dictated by the patient's ability to breathe or cough effectively. Supplemental oxygen may alleviate symptoms sufficiently to allow transport to the ED. Patients who exhibit severe stridor, low oxygen saturation, cyanosis, or signs of impending respiratory failure must receive immediate intervention. Management of such scenarios is challenging for even the most experienced provider—not just the physical act of removing a foreign object from an anxious, dyspneic patient, but calming the distressed parents or other family members.

For conscious patients with partial obstruction who cannot clear the obstruction on their own, abdominal thrusts may simulate a deep cough. If the patient loses consciousness, initiation of chest compressions has been found to be the best method of helping the patient clear the airway obstruction. Preoxygenate the patient if possible to ensure you can ventilate the patient, prepare the necessary medications for RSI, and prepare an alternative rescue airway. Ready the equipment necessary for endotracheal intubation, and have forceps handy. Preparing the family with a brief, simple description of the procedure before you attempt removal can alleviate some anxiety. After sufficient sedation and/or paralyzation has occurred, you may see well enough using direct laryngoscopy to grasp and remove the offending object. Suction should be nearby to prevent aspiration in case the patient vomits. Assist ventilations with a bag-mask device and, if needed, prepare for intubation.

An object visualized below the glottis may be difficult to grasp and not easily removed. Blindly passing an endotracheal tube into the trachea in an effort to move the object to a less obstructive position has been known to

be successful, but this is a maneuver that should only be attempted if you're a skilled, experienced provider faced with a complete obstruction.

After removal of a foreign object, intubation may still be indicated if the patient has a decreased level of consciousness, is intoxicated or bleeding, or requires oxygenation and respiratory support. Retain the object so it can be inspected at the receiving facility. The patient's posttransport condition or suspicion that portions of the aspirated object have been retained may warrant bronchoscopy. Bronchoscopy is performed under general anesthesia in the ICU or operating room.

Anaphylactic Reactions

Anaphylaxis is an extreme systemic form of an allergic reaction involving two or more body systems. Although the immune system is essential to life and health, sometimes it becomes overzealous in defending the body. The resulting problems may range in severity from hay fever to anaphylaxis and exist along the spectrum from a simple annoyance to a life-threatening crisis. During anaphylactic reactions, the immune system becomes hypersensitive to one or more substances. The body often has these reactions to substances that should not be identified as harmful by the immune system—substances such as ragweed, strawberries, and penicillin. The immune cells of the allergic person are more sensitive than the immune cells of a person without allergies. Although these cells are able to recognize and react to dangerous invaders such as bacteria and viruses, they also identify harmless substances as posing a threat.

Pathophysiology

When an invading substance enters the body, the mast cells recognize it as potentially harmful and begin releasing chemical mediators. Histamine, one of the primary chemical weapons, causes the blood vessels in the local area to dilate and the capillaries to leak. Leukotrienes, which are even more powerful, are released and cause additional dilation and leaking. White blood cells are called to the area to help engulf and destroy the enemy, and platelets begin to collect and clump together. In most cases, this overreaction to harmless invaders is usually restricted to the local area being invaded. The runny, itchy nose and swollen eyes associated with hay fever are examples of a local allergic reaction.

In the case of anaphylaxis, however, chemical mediators are released, and the effect involves more than one system throughout the body. The initial effect may be seen from the histamine release, causing skin symptoms (hives) and hypotension. Later responses from the much more powerful leukotrienes compound the effects of histamine. The patient's respiratory status will deteriorate as the highly potent bronchoconstrictors are released.

Signs and Symptoms

Patients may present with CNS symptoms in response to decreased cerebral perfusion and hypoxia. These symptoms include headache, dizziness, confusion, and anxiety. The most common complaints are usually respiratory symptoms, which often present as shortness of breath or dyspnea and tightness in the throat and chest. Stridor and/or hoarseness may also be noted. These signs and symptoms are often due to upper airway swelling in the laryngeal and epiglottic areas. Affected patients may report a lump in the throat. The lower airway is often involved as well. Bronchoconstriction and increased secretions may result in wheezes and crackles. It is not uncommon for the patient to cough or sneeze as the body tries to clear the airway. These symptoms may progress slowly or alarmingly fast. You may have only 1 to 3 minutes to halt this rapid, life-threatening process. Table 2-9 lists the signs and symptoms of anaphylaxis.

Differential Diagnosis

Determining a differential diagnosis in a patient having an anaphylactic reaction can be very challenging. You may have to simultaneously assess the patient, identify the problem, and intervene within seconds of arriving on the scene to save the patient's life. Index of suspicion for anaphylaxis must be high on your list if any of the symptoms previously discussed are present.

Treatment

Patients having allergic reactions are divided into two groups for management. The first group includes patients who have signs of an allergic reaction—for example, hives—but no respiratory distress of dyspnea. The drug of choice is diphenhydramine (Benadryl). Continue to monitor for changes in the patient's condition, but most patients in this group will recover with no further problems.

The second group includes patients with signs of an allergic reaction and dyspnea. These patients require oxygen, epinephrine, and antihistamines (usually Benadryl). Whenever dyspnea is present with signs of an allergic reaction, you should administer epinephrine and monitor the patient for development of anaphylaxis.

Psychological support is a crucial component of treatment. Anaphylaxis can progress rapidly and has the potential to be a life-threatening event. Patients and their families will need reassurance as you perform the necessary interventions. Many of the patients have experienced similar events and may recognize how serious their condition has become. For others, this may be a first-time event. You need to be professional and reassuring and focus on early intervention and transport.

Table 2-9 Signs and Symptoms of Anaphylaxis*

System	Signs and Symptoms
Skin	<ul><li>Warm</li><li>Flushed</li><li>Itching (pruritus)</li><li>Swollen, red eyes</li><li>Swelling of the face and tongue</li><li>Swelling of the hands and feet</li><li>Hives (urticaria)</li></ul>
Respiratory	<ul><li>**Dyspnea**</li><li>Tightness in the throat and chest</li><li>Stridor</li><li>Hoarseness</li><li>Lump in throat</li><li>Wheezes</li><li>Crackles</li><li>Coughing</li><li>Sneezing</li></ul>
Cardiovascular	<ul><li>Dysrhythmias</li><li>**Hypotension**</li><li>**Tachycardia**</li></ul>
Gastrointestinal	<ul><li>Abdominal cramping</li><li>Nausea</li><li>Bloating</li><li>Vomiting</li><li>Abdominal distention</li><li>Profuse, watery diarrhea</li></ul>
Central nervous	<ul><li>Headache</li><li>Dizziness</li><li>Confusion</li><li>Anxiety and restlessness</li><li>Sense of impending doom</li><li>Altered mental status</li></ul>

*Key indicators are represented by bold type.

Pharyngitis and Tonsillitis

Pharyngitis and tonsillitis are both infections of the posterior pharynx. While sharing many of the same causes, *tonsillitis* specifically refers to infection of the tonsils, whereas *pharyngitis* refers to infection of the pharynx, which often includes some degree of tonsillitis.

Pathophysiology

The etiology of pharyngitis and tonsillitis is usually either viral or bacterial; about 40% to 60% of infections are viral, and 5% to 40% are bacterial. Most bacterial infections are caused by group A streptococcus. A very small percentage of cases are due to trauma, cancer, allergy, or a toxic exposure.

Bacterial and viral infections cause inflammation of the local pharyngeal tissues. In addition, streptococcal infections release local toxins and proteins that may trigger additional inflammation. This inflammation and infection are usually self-limiting, but streptococcal infections have two important side effects. First, the bacterial surface carries antigens that are similar to proteins found normally in the heart. In the process of fighting off a streptococcal infection, the body can inadvertently attack the heart and heart valves, causing rheumatic fever. Second, the glomeruli in the kidneys can become damaged by the antibody-antigen combination, causing acute glomerulonephritis.

Signs and Symptoms

Signs and symptoms of pharyngitis and tonsillitis may include the following:

- Sore throat
- Fever
- Chills
- Muscle aches (myalgia)
- Abdominal pain
- Rhinorrhea
- Headache
- Earache

Physical exam will reveal a red and swollen posterior pharynx, enlarged and tender anterior cervical lymph nodes, and sometimes a fine red rash that feels like sandpaper. This rough-feeling rash, called scarlatina, begins on the torso and spreads to the entire body and is caused by streptococcal infection. In addition, whitish exudates (pockets of pus) on the tonsils may be seen. These exudates are more common with streptococcal infection, although their presence does not confirm a bacterial infection. Viral infections are more often associated with the presence of other upper respiratory infection (URI) signs and symptoms such as cough and nasal congestion. A particular viral infection, mononucleosis, is associated with anterior and posterior cervical lymph node swelling and tenderness and should be identified because of potential complications such as splenic rupture.

Treatment

Viral pharyngitis and tonsillitis are best treated symptomatically with fluids, antipyretic medications, and anti-inflammatory agents. Bacterial infections require antibiotics, usually penicillin or amoxicillin. Alternative treatments such as ceftriaxone, vancomycin, clindamycin, and erythromycin are often used as an alternative in patients who are allergic to penicillin.

Peritonsillar Abscess

In **peritonsillar abscess**, a superficial soft-tissue infection progresses to create pockets of purulence in the submucosal space adjacent to the tonsils. This abscess and its accompanying inflammation cause the uvula to deviate to the opposing side (**Figure 2-9**).

Pathophysiology

Peritonsillar abscess is the most common infection of the peritonsillar region. The incidence of peritonsillar abscess in the United States is about 3 in 10,000 people annually. *Streptococcus* is often isolated in cultures of peritonsillar abscess, along with other bacteria such as *Peptostreptococcus*.

Signs and Symptoms

Signs and symptoms of peritonsillar abscess may include the following:

- Sore throat (especially unilaterally)
- Dysphagia
- Fever
- Chills
- Muscle aches
- Neck and anterior throat pain
- Hoarseness

Additional signs of peritonsillar abscess include tachycardia, dehydration, "hot potato" or thickened voice, cervical lymph nodes, difficulty swallowing, asymmetric bulging of the tonsils in the posterior pharynx, which often causes the uvula to deviate to the other side of the mouth, and exudates on the tonsils.

Differential Diagnosis

The differential diagnosis of peritonsillar abscess includes other serious illnesses such as retropharyngeal and prevertebral abscess, epiglottitis, bacterial tracheitis, mononucleosis, herpes pharyngitis, carotid artery aneurysm, and cancer.

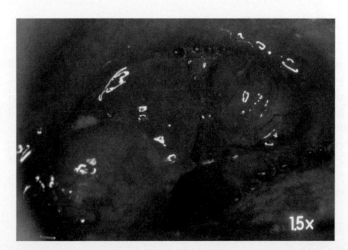

Figure 2-9 Peritonsillar abscess. Note extensive swelling of left tonsil and deviation of uvula.
© Dr. P. Marazzi/Science Source.

Treatment

Treatment includes hydration with intravenous (IV) fluids and administration of anti-inflammatory agents and antibiotics. If an abscess is present, surgical drainage is often indicated and can be performed in the operating room. Occasionally, needle drainage is performed in the ED.

Epiglottitis

Epiglottitis is a life-threatening infection that causes inflammation of the epiglottis and often the supraglottic region. This swelling can obstruct the trachea, inducing hypoxia or anoxia.

Once considered a disease of toddlers, the incidence of epiglottitis has changed dramatically since the United States began immunizing against *Haemophilus influenzae*. Adults are more likely to present with this illness in the emergency setting; men develop epiglottitis about three times more often than women. The infection remains most common in children 2 to 4 years of age. Mortality is estimated at 7% in adults and 1% in children.

Pathophysiology

Before a vaccine to *H. influenzae* type b (Hib) became available, epiglottitis occurred 2.6 times more often in children than in adults. *Streptococcus* spp. have now edged out *H. influenzae* as the pathogen most often responsible for causing epiglottitis.

Signs and Symptoms

Epiglottitis often begins with a sore throat and progresses to pain on swallowing and a muffled voice. Physical exam may reveal a patient in moderate or severe distress assuming a tripod position, with fever, heavy drooling, stridor, respiratory distress, notable pain when the larynx is palpated, tachycardia, and perhaps a low oxygen saturation. The stridor may be of a softer, lower pitch than that caused by croup.

Differential Diagnosis

The differential diagnosis should include bacterial tracheitis, retropharyngeal or prevertebral abscess, Ludwig's angina, and peritonsillar abscess. A diagnosis of epiglottitis should be suspected on the basis of clinical presentation and history, but it can be confirmed with plain-film lateral neck radiographs. Computed tomographic (CT) imaging may be performed but is often unnecessary because plain-film radiographs are usually sufficient. Fiber-optic laryngoscopy may provide direct information about the extent of airway edema and can assist in placement of an endotracheal tube.

Treatment

Emergency treatment should be limited to maintaining adequate oxygenation and ventilation. Humidified oxygen can be of some relief to the patient, but the severity of this condition cannot be overstated. Avoid sticking anything in the patient's mouth. Limit suction to only those situations where secretions are obstructing the airway. If the patient is drooling heavily, have the patient sit up and lean forward to allow drooling. Intubation should be performed in the field only if absolutely necessary. Manipulating the epiglottis with a laryngoscope blade while the tissue is inflamed may irritate the airway and make further intubation attempts extremely difficult. Endotracheal intubation in this setting is best achieved in the surgical suite with an ear, nose, and throat (ENT) surgeon nearby. Antibiotics are indicated, often amoxicillin/sulbactam (Unasyn) or clindamycin, as well as corticosteroids, inhaled beta-agonists, and nebulized epinephrine. If respiratory failure occurs with this condition, it is comforting to note that positive-pressure ventilation is usually successful, even without endotracheal intubation.

Ludwig's Angina

Named for the physician who first described it in the early 19th century, **Ludwig's angina** refers not to chest pain but to a deep-space infection of the anterior neck just below the mandible. Sensations of choking and suffocation are reported by most patients with this condition.

Pathophysiology

Swelling, redness, and warm tissue (induration) between the hyoid bone and the mandible may be the most notable sign on clinical exam. This inflammation is caused by bacteria in the oral cavity. *Streptococcus* spp. are often cultured, but such infections are rarely due to a single organism and may contain anaerobic organisms.

Submental (beneath the chin) infection often migrates from dental caries in the incisors. Sublingual infection can usually be attributed to infection in the anterior mandibular teeth and can manifest as tongue elevation caused by swelling. Submandibular infection, which usually originates in the molars, is characterized by swelling in the angle of the jaw.

Since fluoridation of public drinking water became widespread in the 1970s, the prevalence of dental caries has decreased in developed countries. However, dental caries remains the most common chronic disease in the world.

Signs and Symptoms

Because it often arises from dental decay and subsequent infection, Ludwig's angina is characterized by:

- Severe gingivitis and cellulitis, with firm swelling and rapidly spreading infection in the submandibular, sublingual, and submental spaces (**Figure 2-10**)
- Swelling of the sublingual area and tongue
- Drooling
- Airway obstruction
- Elevation and posterior displacement of the tongue as a result of edema

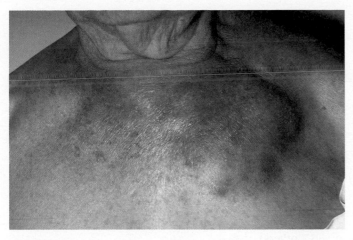

Figure 2-10 Ludwig's angina. Rapid progression may compromise a patient's airway in a few hours.
© Mediscan/Visuals Unlimited, Inc.

Symptoms of Ludwig's angina include sore throat, dysphagia, fever, chills, dental pain, and dyspnea. The patient tends to look anxious and toxic, with poor dentition and a firm, red, pronounced swelling in the anterior throat area. The location of caries may suggest which primary spaces are affected. The patient's tongue may be elevated, portending a difficult intubation should a mechanical airway become necessary.

Differential Diagnosis

Your differential diagnosis should include retropharyngeal and prevertebral abscess, bacterial tracheitis, and epiglottitis. Patients who have recently had chemotherapy or an organ transplant with immunosuppression are at increased risk of having this infection develop, including abscess.

Treatment

A patient suspected of having Ludwig's angina should be considered to have a life-threatening illness, perhaps accompanied by a compromised airway. Maintaining a patent airway is of paramount importance. In a rapidly progressing infection, prophylactic intubation may be performed electively in the ED or operating room. Stridor, dysphagia with difficulty controlling secretions, and dyspnea may prompt intubation. In the prehospital environment, supplemental humidified oxygen can make the patient more comfortable. Electrocardiographic monitoring and IV placement should be initiated. Antibiotics are initiated in the ED, and an ENT surgeon may be consulted.

Bacterial Tracheitis

Bacterial tracheitis is a rare infection of the subglottic trachea. Since *H. influenzae* vaccination became widespread, bacterial tracheitis may rival epiglottitis as the least common obstructive airway infection. One study showed that of 500 children hospitalized for croup over a 3-year period, 2% had bacterial tracheitis. While it may occur in any age group, tracheitis is more common in children because of their smaller airways and the narrow diameter of the subglottic tissues. Twice as many male patients as female patients contract the infection.

Pathophysiology

Tracheitis is caused by multiple organisms, such as *Staphylococcus aureus* (including community-associated methicillin-resistant *S. aureus* [CA-MRSA] and healthcare-associated [HA-MRSA]), *Streptococcus* spp., *H. influenzae*, *Klebsiella* spp., and *Pseudomonas* spp.

Signs and Symptoms

Bacterial tracheitis begins as a URI and progresses to become a life-threatening infection of the subglottic tracheal lining. Symptoms include productive cough, voice changes, high fever, chills, and dyspnea. Signs include rapid progression to a toxic state during as few as 8 to 10 hours, stridor, a brassy cough, and occasionally neck or upper chest pain. Unlike epiglottitis, drooling is uncommon, and the patient may be able to lie supine.

Differential Diagnosis

Bacterial tracheitis is sometimes difficult to differentiate from epiglottitis and retropharyngeal abscess.

Treatment

As with any airway infection, maintaining a patent airway is of primary importance. Provide supplemental oxygen, initiate electrocardiographic monitoring, and obtain IV access. Many patients with bacterial tracheitis will require intubation, but the procedure is best performed under controlled circumstances unless the patient is in acute respiratory failure. If intubation is absolutely necessary in the field, you should be ready to implement a backup airway if necessary. If intubation is successful, be alert for tracheal exudates and mucus clogging the tube, and provide appropriate suction. These patients may have features of sepsis, so initiate an appropriate fluid challenge and if necessary a pressor drug to aid in maintaining blood pressure.

Retropharyngeal and Prevertebral Abscess

Retropharyngeal and prevertebral abscesses are both infections that develop behind the esophagus and in front of the cervical vertebrae. As noted earlier, an abscess is a localized collection of pus in a tissue or other confined space in the body. A retropharyngeal abscess may originate in the sinuses, teeth, or middle ear. Up to 67% of patients with such an abscess report having had a recent ENT infection. Retropharyngeal infections can be life threatening if they begin to cause airway obstruction. Infection that spreads to the mediastinum, called mediastinitis, is a grave complication that carries a startlingly high mortality rate of nearly 50%.

Pathophysiology

Common causal organisms in retropharyngeal abscess are *Staphylococcus* spp., *Streptococcus* spp., and *H. influenzae*, although the infection can be attributed to other organisms, especially anaerobes from the mouth. Retropharyngeal lesions can be seen in adults as well as in children but usually affect those 3 to 4 years old or younger.

Signs and Symptoms

Signs of retropharyngeal abscess include the following:

- Pharyngitis
- Dysphagia
- Dyspnea
- Fever
- Chills
- Neck pain, stiffness, swelling, or erythema
- Drooling

The following are worrisome signs of possible airway compromise:

- Difficulty opening the mouth (trismus)
- Vocal changes
- Inspiratory stridor

Differential Diagnosis

Early retropharyngeal abscess may be misdiagnosed as unspecified or streptococcal pharyngitis. If the patient's condition rapidly declines, you should consider more threatening illnesses such as epiglottitis, bacterial tracheitis, and meningitis.

Treatment

Treatment includes ensuring a patent airway and providing supplemental oxygen. Be careful not to puncture the abscess during intubation, because aspiration of the purulent contents may be fatal. Initiate electrocardiographic monitoring and obtain IV access. Initiate appropriate fluid replenishment if the patient is dehydrated from decreased oral intake.

Definitive care often involves intubation in the operating suite (or under other controlled circumstances), surgical drainage of the lesion, and antibiotics. With aggressive management of retropharyngeal abscess before it progresses to mediastinitis, many patients recover promptly and can be extubated immediately following or a few days after the procedure.

Angioedema

Angioedema is a sudden swelling, usually of a head or neck structure such as the lip (especially the lower lip), earlobes, tongue, or uvula, but it has been described in other tissues including the bowel. While not fully understood, angioedema is considered to be an allergic reaction and is treated as such. Sometimes the cause is idiopathic (of unknown cause). A few cases are hereditary, referred to as hereditary angioedema.

Up to 15% of the general population has episodic idiopathic angioedema. No racial predominance exists. Women are more likely to have angioedema than men, and the condition is most often seen in adults. Exposure to certain agents increases the risk of angioedema. Common triggers are listed as follows:

- ACE inhibitors (captopril, enalapril, and others)
- Radiologic dyes
- Aspirin
- NSAIDs (ibuprofen, naproxen, and others)
- Hymenoptera insect stings (wasps, yellow jackets, and others)
- Food allergies
- Animal hair or dander (shed skin cells)
- Sunlight exposure
- Stress

Pathophysiology

In angioedema, some insult triggers leakage from the small-vessel circulation, prompting interstitial tissues to swell. Edema can originate in the epidermal and dermal tissues, in the subcutaneous tissues, or both. This inflammation is a response to the actions of circulating hormones and histamines, serotonin, and bradykinins.

Signs and Symptoms

Signs of angioedema include clearly demarcated swelling with or without a rash and occasionally with dyspnea or anxiety. Stridor, wheezing on chest auscultation, or history of intubation should prompt careful observation for deterioration. Angioedema of the bowel may cause bowel obstruction with consequent nausea, vomiting, and abdominal pain.

Differential Diagnosis

Carefully assess the patient for other life-threatening illnesses, such as cellulitis/abscess, retropharyngeal abscess, and Ludwig's angina. If the patient has hives, consider the possibility of anaphylaxis.

Treatment

Although extensive angioedema may threaten the airway, many cases are self-limiting or require only minimal treatment. Allow the patient to assume a comfortable position. If there are no signs of respiratory failure, the patient will maintain his or her own airway with simple positioning.

Emergent intubation can be extremely difficult in severe cases of angioedema because the swollen tissue may prevent adequate visualization of the vocal cords. In addition to normal intubation equipment, prepare rescue airway equipment before you attempt intubation. If time permits, intubation should be performed under controlled circumstances, where the services of an anesthetist and an ENT surgeon or general surgeon are available. In nonemergent patients, it is prudent to initiate electrocardiographic monitoring, obtain IV access, and transport the patient to a nearby emergency facility.

Lower Airway Conditions

Obstructive lower airway diseases are characterized by diffuse obstruction to airflow within the lungs. The most common obstructive airway diseases are emphysema, chronic bronchitis, and asthma; these three conditions collectively affect as many as 20% of adults in the United States.

Obstructive disease occurs when the positive pressure of exhalation causes the small airways to pinch shut, trapping gas in the alveoli. The harder the patient tries to push air out, the more it is trapped in the alveoli. Patients with obstructive disease have large amounts of gas trapped in their lungs that they cannot effectively expel. Patients with obstructive disease learn that exhaling slowly at a low pressure is more effective than exhaling rapidly at high pressure.

Asthma

Asthma is a common disease, prompting millions of ED visits a year and accounting for 20% to 30% of hospital admissions. Patients have a high relapse rate, with 10% to 20% returning within 2 weeks of treatment. In the United States, asthma prevalence increased from 7.3% in 2001 to 8.4% in 2010, when 25.7 million persons had asthma. For the period 2008–2010, asthma prevalence was higher among children than adults, and among multiple-race, black, and American Indian or Alaska Native persons than white persons.

Children who have wheezing that begins before age 5 years and persists into adulthood have a greater likelihood of compromised lung function. Children who begin to wheeze after age 5 have a lower incidence of pulmonary disease even if the wheezing persists into adulthood. As many as 90% of patients with asthma have their first symptoms before age 6. Some children present with nocturnal coughing as a symptom, without the typical wheezing.

Pathophysiology

Asthma is a chronic inflammation of the bronchi with contraction of the bronchial smooth muscle, resulting in narrowed bronchi and the associated wheezing. The airways become overly sensitive to inhaled allergens, viruses, and other environmental irritants—even strong odors can precipitate an episode. This oversensitivity is responsible for the reactive airway component of the disease.

Inflammation is at the center of asthma symptoms such as dyspnea, wheezing, and coughing. The body may respond to persistent bronchospasm with bronchial edema and tenacious mucous secretions that can cause bronchial plugging and atelectasis.

Signs and Symptoms

Patients with asthma are usually acutely aware of their symptoms, even if the symptoms are considered clinically mild. Early symptoms of asthma include some combination of the following:

- Wheezing
- Dyspnea
- Chest tightness
- Cough
- Signs of a recent URI, such as rhinorrhea, congestion, headache, pharyngitis, and myalgia
- Signs of exposure to allergens, such as rhinorrhea, pharyngitis, hoarseness, and cough
- Chest tightness, discomfort, or pain

The patient initially hyperventilates, causing a decrease in CO_2 levels (respiratory alkalosis). As the airways continue to narrow, complete exhalation becomes more and more difficult, and air trapping results and CO_2 levels begin to increase. The lungs become overinflated and stiff, increasing the work of breathing. Tachypnea, tachycardia, and pulsus paradoxus may occur, with accompanying agitation. Few retractions should be seen. Oxygen saturation should be near normal, even on room air.

Patients with moderate exacerbations may show increased tachycardia and tachypnea, with increased wheezing and decreased air movement. Oxygen saturation may dip, but it should be easily restored with supplemental oxygen. Retractions may be seen, and the degree and types will increase with the severity of the episode. Recruitment of more muscle sets (e.g., intercostal, subcostal) indicates a worsening condition.

Certain factors in a carefully taken patient history may help predict the severity of an asthma episode: respiratory illness, exposure to potential allergens, compliance with home inhaled medications, and the frequency of ED visits, hospital admissions, and corticosteroid use.

Allergens such as animal material and airborne ragweed and pollen particles are common precipitants of asthma episodes. Inhalation of smoke or cold, dry air may also touch off a flare-up. The following factors indicate it is likely a patient is having a severe asthma exacerbation:

- Presenting oxygen saturation < 92%
- Tachypnea
- Recent ED visit or hospitalization
- Frequent hospitalizations
- Any history of intubation for asthma
- Peak flows < 60% of predicted values
- Accessory muscle use and retraction

- Duration of symptoms > 2 days
- History of frequent corticosteroid use
- Currently taking theophylline

Differential Diagnosis

When you are gathering a history, new-onset wheezing is not enough to make a diagnosis of asthma. Repeated bouts of this disease are usually necessary for a clinician to make a definitive diagnosis because many other conditions are characterized by wheezing. Bacterial pneumonia, such as that caused by *Streptococcus* spp., can cause wheezing, as can atypical infections from *Mycoplasma* and *Chlamydia*. Viral infections are also potential causes of wheezing, especially respiratory syncytial virus (RSV), a common infection among infants during the winter and early spring months.

What other diseases present with wheezing? The differential diagnosis should include both primary pulmonary and systemic disease. COPD often has at least some component of asthma, but it can also have features of bronchitis and emphysema. What distinguishes asthma from COPD? The reactive airway process in asthma, unlike in COPD, is largely reversible. Consider upper airway obstruction, such as that caused by croup, epiglottitis, bacterial tracheitis, or retropharyngeal infection, especially if stridor is present. Congestive heart failure may present with new-onset wheezing, as can aspiration of a foreign object (see earlier discussion). Chest pain may prompt evaluation for cardiac ischemia, especially if the quality of the pain is different from that of previous asthma episodes.

Treatment

Therapy should be scaled to the severity of the exacerbation. First-line treatment for actively wheezing patients includes inhaled beta-agonists such as albuterol and levalbuterol (Xopenex). Beta$_2$-agonists used early and aggressively in the course of disease can reduce the likelihood of hospitalization. Albuterol 2.5 to 5 mg is given every 20 minutes for three doses, or it can be given continuously, followed by 2.5 to 10 mg every 1 to 4 hours as needed. The pediatric dose is 0.15 mg/kg (with a minimum dose of 2.5 mg) every 20 minutes, followed by 0.15 mg to 0.3 mg/kg every 1 to 4 hours as indicated by the patient's clinical condition, up to 10 mg.

Parenteral beta$_2$-agonists may be a useful supplement for severe asthma episodes. Terbutaline, 0.25 mg, or 0.3 mg of 1:1,000 epinephrine administered intramuscularly or subcutaneously, can assist inhaled beta$_2$-agonists. Because of their tendency to cause hypertension and increase myocardial workload and oxygen demand, however, they should be used with caution, especially in patients who have coexisting ischemic disease. IV or intraosseous (IO) administration of terbutaline or epinephrine may also be indicated, but you should seek medical consultation first.

Ipratropium, 0.5 mg, is occasionally given and has the greatest effect on patients with coexisting COPD or a history of tobacco use. Ipratropium can be given every 20 minutes for three doses and then as indicated.

IV corticosteroids help slow down the inflammatory response, thereby reducing the edema that narrows bronchial passageways. In adults, 40 to 125 mg of methylprednisolone (Solu-Medrol) is given, or 2 mg/kg IV in pediatric patients. In adults, 60 mg of triamcinolone (Aristocort) IM can be given. In children older than age 6, use 0.03 to 0.3 mg/kg IM. Remember that corticosteroids may take hours to work. EMS providers may initiate corticosteroid treatment rather than wait until the patient reaches the ED so that the agent can begin to take effect as quickly as possible.

Magnesium sulfate given intravenously has shown promise in controlling severe exacerbations of asthma. It is typically given as a 2-g dose over 30 to 60 minutes to help relax smooth bronchial muscles.

While not widely used, Heliox, a gaseous mixture of helium and oxygen, is another inhaled agent that has shown promise for severe exacerbations. Given either in an 80:20 or a 70:30 mixture, helium acts as a lighter-than-air carrier to help distribute oxygen and nebulized agents and decrease the work of breathing. Albuterol given with Heliox uses twice the normal dose of albuterol at a flow rate of 8 to 10 L/min.

Despite aggressive pharmacologic therapy, some patients still face severe respiratory distress or respiratory failure.

Chronic Obstructive Pulmonary Disease

COPD is an airflow obstruction caused by chronic bronchitis or loss of alveolar surface area associated with emphysema. It is characterized by some degree of wheezing and airway edema, and even though the mechanism is slightly different from that of asthma, both are air-trapping diseases of the lungs. COPD is a chronic, devastating disease ranked as the fourth-leading cause of death in the United States. About 14 million people have COPD. Of those, 12.5 million have chronic bronchitis and 1.7 million have emphysema. The number of patients diagnosed with COPD has increased by 41.5% since 1982. The incidence of this disease in the United States is between 6.6% and 6.9% for mild and moderate COPD. It is more prevalent in men than women and in Caucasians than in African-Americans. According to the National Health and Nutrition Examination Survey (NHANES), the rate of COPD climbs with age, especially in those who smoke.

The primary cause of COPD is cigarette smoking. Most patients with clinically significant COPD have smoked at least 1 pack a day for 20 years. An estimated 15% of all smokers develop clinically significant COPD. Many factors affect the rate at which COPD evolves, including the age at which the person began smoking, the number of packs per day, the existence of other illnesses, the person's level of physical fitness, and his or her current tobacco abuse. Secondhand smoke contributes to reduced pulmonary function, asthma exacerbations, and increased risk of upper respiratory tract infections. The only genetic risk factor known to cause COPD in nonsmokers is a deficiency of alpha$_1$-antitrypsin, a protein that inhibits neutrophil elastase, a lung enzyme.

Pathophysiology

Chronic inflammation from exposure to inhaled particles injures the airways. The body tries to repair this injury by remodeling the airways, which causes scarring and narrowing. Changes in the alveolar walls and connective tissue permanently enlarge the alveoli. On the other side of those alveoli, the important connection to the capillary membrane is remodeled with a thickened vessel wall, which impedes gas exchange. Mucus-secreting glands and goblet cells multiply, increasing mucus production. Cilia are destroyed, limiting the elevation and clearing of this abundant mucus.

External changes in the body, such as a barrel-shaped chest, occur in response to the remodeled airways and chronic air trapping. Chronic shortness of breath and chronic cough are also manifestations of this remodeling. Because of chronic hypoxia, chemoreceptors fail to react to fluctuations in the blood's oxygen level. Unfortunately, these changes reflect a permanent adjustment of the body in response to chronic inhalation of irritants.

Lung function gradually declines, and body remodeling slackens. Sputum production increases, and the patient has retained secretions with a chronic cough. The classic air trapping is caused by the limited ability of the lungs to move air out of enlarged distal airways. The lungs become hyperinflated, and only limited gas exchange occurs, which leads to hypoxia and high CO_2 levels, a condition known as hypercarbia or hypercapnia. Chronic hypercarbia blunts the body's normal chemoreceptor sensitivity, and hypoxia becomes the primary mechanism for ventilation control. At this stage, the patient is vulnerable to infection and intolerant of exercise. Any condition that increases the work of breathing may quickly lead to respiratory failure. To compensate for the CO_2 retention, the body must maintain a slightly alkalotic state, which affects the pH.

Signs and Symptoms

Signs and symptoms of acute exacerbation of COPD may include:

- Dyspnea
- Cough
- Intolerance of exertion
- Wheezing
- Productive cough
- Chest pain or discomfort
- Diaphoresis
- Orthopnea

You may note the following clinical signs of COPD:

- Wheezing
- Increased respiratory rate

- Decreased oxygen saturation
- Use of accessory muscles
- Elevated jugular pulse
- Peripheral edema
- Hyperinflated lungs
- Hyperresonance on percussion
- Coarse, scattered rhonchi

Critical episodes are indicated by:

- Saturation below 90%
- Tachypnea (about 30 breaths per minute)
- Peripheral or central cyanosis
- Mental status changes caused by hypercapnia

A patient with COPD can have single or multiple triggers of acute exacerbations. As noted, cigarette smoking is the primary cause of COPD, and continued tobacco abuse can be a seminal trigger of a critical episode. Exposure to environmental allergens can precipitate an episode or exacerbate an existing flare-up. Air pollution can contribute to a COPD exacerbation but by itself usually does not touch off a critical episode.

Differential Diagnosis

The presentation of COPD should prompt you to consider other serious diseases, particularly because the chief complaint of dyspnea may be associated with chest pain. The differential diagnosis of COPD should include asthma, bronchitis, emphysema, pneumonia, pneumonitis, pulmonary fibrosis, respiratory failure, pneumothorax, and cardiac causes of dyspnea such as acute myocardial infarction, angina, CHF, pulmonary embolus, and pulmonary hypertension.

Treatment

Management of a COPD exacerbation hinges on maintaining oxygenation and ventilation. Emergency management includes supplemental oxygen delivered by either nasal cannula or venturi mask and sufficient to maintain a saturation of at least 94%. If the patient remains hypoxic with low-flow oxygen, apply a nonrebreathing mask with high-flow oxygen, and prepare for aggressive airway and ventilation management. Poor peak flow performance, an oxygen saturation that falls into the 80s, and pale or cyanotic extremities also indicate a need for aggressive intervention. Small studies have shown a trial of mask CPAP may be warranted before intubation attempts in an alert, acutely hypercapnic patient with COPD. Using CPAP has shown to decrease the work of breathing, improve oxygenation, and decrease the likelihood of needing to intubate. Endotracheal intubation, either rapid sequence or nasotracheal, may be indicated in severe cases. Patients with COPD may require extended periods of intubation, so nasotracheal intubation may have some advantages because it requires less sedation and may allow for earlier extubation.

Never withhold oxygen from a hypoxic patient. It is a common misconception that giving oxygen to COPD patients with dyspnea will eliminate the drive to breathe. Although elevated oxygen levels may marginally decrease the drive to breathe, permissive hypoxia is a poor management plan.

Once you have secured the airway, administer $beta_2$-agonists early and often. Even though these agents are not as effective in COPD as in asthma, they are a mainstay of treatment. Three nebulized doses can be administered 20 minutes apart for stabilization of the patient's condition. In emergent cases, these doses can be administered back to back. Anticholinergic agents such as ipratropium bromide are beneficial, particularly in concert with $beta_2$-agonists. Although they do not act as quickly as the $beta_2$-agonists, the anticholinergics can provide an additional 20% to 40% bronchodilation when combined with $beta_2$-agonists.

Systemic corticosteroids, usually in the form of injectable Solu-Medrol, are considered routine treatment in moderate to severe episodes. Although oral corticosteroids, notably prednisone, are useful in mild exacerbations, they are not used in moderate to severe episodes.

Patients with COPD in acute respiratory failure require positive-pressure ventilation in the form of **noninvasive positive-pressure ventilation (NPPV)** or endotracheal intubation with invasive ventilation through a ventilator. Patients with COPD may benefit from NPPV if they are hemodynamically stable, have a patent airway, have minimal secretions, and are alert and oriented. If tolerated, NPPV is usually better for short-term ventilatory support because it tends to have fewer side effects. A bag-mask device with a PEEP valve or CPAP/BiPAP may be used.

Conversely, the patient with COPD who must be placed on invasive mechanical ventilation may be difficult to wean from that therapy and is vulnerable to ventilator-associated pneumonia. Mechanical ventilation is indicated when, despite aggressive therapy, the patient has mental status changes, acidosis, respiratory fatigue, and hypoxia. The patient may have discussed the use of long-term ventilatory support with his or her family. Be sure to ask the family whether the patient has an advance directive and what the patient's wishes are in regard to long-term mechanical ventilation.

Atelectasis

Atelectasis is the collapse of the alveolar air spaces of the lungs.

Pathophysiology

The alveoli are vulnerable to a number of disorders. They may collapse from obstruction somewhere in the proximal airways or from external pressures produced, for example, by pneumothorax or hemothorax. They may fill with pus in pneumonia, with blood in pulmonary contusion, or with fluid in near-drowning or congestive heart failure. In addition, smoke or toxic gases may displace the fresh air that should be present in the alveoli.

The human body has billions of alveoli, and it is common for some of them to collapse from time to time. Humans periodically, sigh, cough, sneeze, and change positions—all actions that are thought to help open closed alveoli and avoid decreased ventilation any one part of the lung. When people do not use these actions, for example, because they are sedated or in a coma or deep breathing or moving causes pain, increasing numbers of alveoli in sections of the lung may collapse and not reopen. Like balloons, alveoli are more difficult to flow open once they have completely collapsed. Eventually entire lung segments collapse. This condition describes atelectasis, and it increases the chance of pneumonia developing in the affected areas.

Signs and Symptoms

Although atelectasis can be a significant disease by itself, the larger concern is that the affected areas become breeding grounds for pathogens, resulting in pneumonia. This is a concern in any patient who has a fever in the days following chest or abdominal surgery, particularly if breath sounds are decreased or abnormally colored sputum is coughed up.

Treatment

Postsurgical patients are encouraged to cough, deep breathe, and get out of bed, even though it is painful. People who cannot get out of bed may experience atelectasis, which can lead to hypoxia or predispose a patient to lung infections and pneumonia. EMS providers can reinforce deep breathing in patients who would benefit from it and can be watchful for atelectasis in patients who are sedentary or who take medications with sedative effects, including some analgesics.

Pneumonia

Lung infection that causes fluid to collect in the alveoli is referred to as pneumonia. The resulting inflammation can cause dyspnea, fever, chills, chest pain, chest wall pain, and a productive cough. There are three broad types of pneumonia: community acquired, hospital acquired (nosocomial; begins 48 or more hours after hospital admission), and ventilator associated. The cause may be viral, bacterial, fungal, or chemical (aspiration of gastric contents).

More than 3 million cases of pneumonia are diagnosed annually in the United States. Untreated pneumonia has a mortality rate approaching 30%. Even with appropriate and timely treatment, coexisting medical conditions (comorbidities) can drastically increase the likelihood of mortality. Advanced age increases susceptibility to pneumonia. In a 20-year study, overall mortality in pneumonia caused by *Staphylococcus pneumoniae* was 20%, but in patients older than 80 years, mortality exceeded 37%.

Recovery may be complicated by comorbid conditions such as human immunodeficiency virus (HIV) infection, CHF, diabetes, leukemia, and pulmonary diseases such as asthma, COPD, and bronchitis. Development of pneumonia in an already compromised patient can touch off a downward spiral of dyspnea, destruction of lung tissue by infection, further infection, more dyspnea, and a worsening condition. Ravaged alveoli can be replaced by pus-filled saccules. This inflammatory material perpetuates the cycle, resulting in empyema or lung abscess, which can be difficult to treat without surgical intervention. Even in patients who recover, scarring from the infection can compromise respiratory gas exchange, reducing pulmonary reserve capacity and increasing susceptibility to another infection.

Pathophysiology

Pathogens that can cause community-acquired pneumonia include *Streptococcus pneumoniae*, *Legionella* spp., *H. influenzae*, *S. aureus*, respiratory viruses, *Chlamydia*, and *Pseudomonas*. Hospital-acquired pneumonia can be caused by the same pathogens, along with *Klebsiella* and *Enterococcus* spp. The two pathogens most commonly associated with ventilator-assisted pneumonia are *S. aureus* and *Pseudomonas aeruginosa*. Pneumonia most commonly develops because of a defect in the host's immune system or an overwhelming burden of strong pathogens.

Signs and Symptoms

Patients with pneumonia usually have the classic symptoms of cough and fever, but they may also have more subtle signs, such as abdominal pain, low-grade fever, and weakness with accompanying tachycardia. An acute onset of symptoms and a rapid progression are more suggestive of a bacterial cause than a viral cause. Clinical signs and symptoms of pneumonia may include any of the following:

- Fever
- Chills
- Cough
- Malaise
- Nausea and vomiting
- Diarrhea
- Myalgia
- Pleuritic chest pain
- Abdominal pain
- Anorexia
- Dyspnea
- Tachypnea
- Tachycardia
- Hypoxia
- Abnormal breath sounds, including rales, rhonchi, and even wheezing

Differential Diagnosis

While you are auscultating the lungs over an area with decreased breath sounds, ask the patient to make an *e* sound and hold it. The tone transmitted may more closely resemble an *a* than an *e*. This phenomenon is known as *egophony*, derived from the Greek words for *goat* and *sound*, because the pitch is said to mimic a goat's bleating. There may also be dullness to percussion over the affected lobe and increased tactile fremitus. Altered mental status and cyanosis are signs of severe illness.

Diagnosis can be made on the basis of clinical presentation, a careful HPI, and a thorough physical exam. Radiologic evaluation, including anteroposterior and lateral chest radiographs, shows fair to good sensitivity to infiltrate, although normal findings do not rule out pneumonia. CT is sensitive to pneumonia but exposes the patient to higher radiation than plain films.

The differential diagnosis of pneumonia should include asthma, bronchitis, COPD exacerbation, tracheal or supraglottic foreign objects, epiglottitis, empyema, pulmonary abscess, CHF, angina, and myocardial infarction.

Treatment

Supplemental oxygen is helpful for any patient with a clinically significant pneumonia. It should be provided by nasal cannula, with the goal of maintaining saturation above 94%. Consider more aggressive airway maneuvers for patients who require more intensive oxygenation. Use of a CPAP mask may alleviate the need for intubation in patients who are able to tolerate having the mask covering the face (see earlier discussion).

Blood cultures are often obtained, but antibiotics are administered empirically as soon as possible, before the results of such cultures become available. Studies have shown that administration of antibiotics within 6 hours of arriving in the ED decreases morbidity and mortality in patients with pneumonia. Sudden inflammatory response syndrome (SIRS) may accompany the infection. SIRS is an abnormal, generalized inflammatory reaction remote from the initial insult, and clinically, it is the presence of two or more of the following:

- Temperature less than 96.8°F (36°C) or greater than 100.4°F (38°C)
- Heart rate greater than 90 beats/min
- Respiratory rate greater than 20 breaths/min or a $Paco_2$ less than 32 mm Hg
- White blood cell count less than 4,500 or greater than 10,000 L/mm³

The identification of SIRS does not confirm a diagnosis of sepsis, or even an infection; other etiologies of SIRS exist, including trauma, burns, and pancreatitis. Sepsis is said to occur when there is an identifiable infection plus clinical criteria for SIRS. Hydration may also be effective, especially if the patient is bordering on septic shock. In such patients, vigorous fluid resuscitation and possibly vasopressor therapy may be needed. Fluid resuscitation in dehydrated patients may make the pneumonia visible on plain radiograph by making enough fluid available to cause an infiltrate. In such cases, a decrease in oxygenation may be seen as alveoli labor to carry out gas exchange under an increasing burden of collected fluid. Chest physical therapy and regular ambulation can loosen such infiltrates and collections of mucus.

Acute Lung Injury/Acute Respiratory Distress Syndrome

Acute lung injury/acute respiratory distress syndrome (ALI/ARDS) is a systemic disease that causes lung failure. Typically, ARDS is not seen in the field, but providers might be asked to transport a patient with ARDS between facilities.

When the lungs fail in ALI/ARDS, a noncardiogenic pulmonary edema develops, in which fluid from the blood plasma migrates into the lung parenchyma and fills the lung tissue and air spaces, accompanied by respiratory distress, pulmonary edema, and respiratory failure. Ventilatory support may be required to treat the associated severe hypoxemia.

Pathophysiology

ARDS is seldom seen in the field, but EMS providers may have a vital role in preventing this devastating pathologic condition. This syndrome is caused by diffuse damage to the alveoli, perhaps as a result of shock, aspiration of gastric contents, pulmonary edema, or a hypoxic event. It seems to be worse when there is some direct damage to the lungs, as in trauma patients who have severe pulmonary contusions. The onset of ALI/ARDS begins with a breakdown of the alveolar-capillary border that allows fluid to seep into the alveoli, decreasing gas exchange in the lungs. In severe cases, high levels of oxygen are required to maintain adequate oxygenation.

Signs and Symptoms

Development of progressive dyspnea and hypoxemia within hours to days after an acute traumatic or medical event characterizes ALI/ARDS; ARDS is most often seen in hospitalized patients, usually in the ICU. A typical patient has recently undergone major surgery, seems to recover and is in a non-ICU bed, and then phase 1 ALI/ARDS develops and the patient must be readmitted to the ICU. Physical signs of ALI/ARDS include the following:

- Dyspnea
- Hypoxemia, sometimes accompanied by cyanosis of the mucous membranes
- Tachypnea
- Tachycardia
- Increasing demand for supplemental oxygen to maintain adequate saturation
- Fever and hypotension in patients with sepsis
- Rales/crackles (may or may not be heard on auscultation)

Treatment

Supporting oxygenation and assisting respiration are the cornerstones of ALI/ARDS treatment. Document oxygen saturation, breath sounds, and any sudden changes in condition. Patients with ARDS typically have "stiff" lungs (that is, low compliance). No specific remedy exists other than aggressively managing the inciting medical or traumatic event. Intubation and mechanical ventilation, along with pressure support and suctioning as needed, are indicated. Once ventilatory support has been instituted, ventilation pressures should be monitored and care taken to not overventilate the lungs and cause further damage.

Severe Acute Respiratory Syndrome

Severe acute respiratory syndrome (SARS) is a disease that arose from the merger of two viruses, one from mammals and one from birds. The source of the virus has been identified as bats found in Hong Kong. SARS was first reported in Asia in February 2003. Within a few months, the disease had spread to Canada, South America, and Europe. In the United States, there were eight confirmed cases (all mild) and no deaths; all of the cases involved people who had traveled to areas where SARS cases had been reported. In the United States, no healthcare providers have contracted SARS.

Pathophysiology

Transmission of SARS is by close personal contact—that is, living with and caring for a person with the disease or having direct contact with respiratory secretions or body fluids of an infected person. The incubation period is about 10 days from the date of exposure; the communicable period has not been well defined.

Signs and Symptoms

Signs and symptoms of SARS include a temperature of greater than 100.4°F (38°C), headache, overall feeling of discomfort, and body aches. Initially, SARS resembles any general flulike illness; however, after 2 to 7 days, a dry cough appears, and severe cases may progress to pneumonia; patients may need respiratory support.

Treatment

Caring for a person suspected of having SARS includes using adequate personal protective equipment (an N95 or P100 respirator), notifying the infection control practitioner, completing an exposure form, and a possible 10-day quarantine.

Respiratory Syncytial Virus

Respiratory syncytial virus (RSV) is a major cause of illness in young children, creating an infection in the lungs and breathing passages. The more serious infections found in premature infants and children with depressed immune systems can lead to other serious illnesses that affect the lungs or heart. An RSV infection can cause respiratory illnesses such as bronchiolitis and pneumonia.

Pathophysiology

The RSV is highly contagious and spread through droplets when the patient coughs or sneezes. The virus can also survive on surfaces, including hands and clothing. The infection tends to spread rapidly through schools and in child care centers.

Signs and Symptoms

When you are assessing a child, look for signs of dehydration. Infants with RSV often refuse liquids, so look for signs and symptoms of dehydration. The RSV can also cause severe upper respiratory infections and typical asthma symptoms in adults and geriatric patients.

Treatment

Treat airway and breathing problems with supplemental oxygen. Humidified oxygen is helpful if available.

Pneumothorax

Pneumothorax is best defined as a partial or complete accumulation of air in the pleural space. As discussed earlier, normally the pleural space is occupied by only a small amount of fluid that lubricates the pleura to minimize friction. Pneumothorax is most often caused by trauma, but it can be caused by some medical conditions.

Normally, the "vacuum" pressure in the pleural space keeps the lung inflated. When the surface of the lung is disrupted, however, air escapes into the pleural cavity, and the negative vacuum pressure is lost. The natural elasticity of the lung tissue causes the lung to collapse. The accumulation of air in the space may be mild or severe.

Pathophysiology

Primary spontaneous pneumothorax can occur without an obvious cause. Nearly all patients who experience primary spontaneous pneumothorax have bullae, or air pockets, that rupture to cause the pneumothorax (**Figure 2-11**).

Primary spontaneous pneumothorax is seen predominantly in patients without a prior diagnosis of lung disease. However, more than 90% of persons who experience primary spontaneous pneumothorax are smokers. The condition is also more common in tall, thin, young men. Developing evidence suggests that certain genetic factors may predispose patients to spontaneous pneumothorax. Use of inhaled or injected cocaine is also a known risk factor for spontaneous pneumothorax.

Secondary spontaneous pneumothorax can be caused by a variety of lung diseases but occurs primarily in patients with

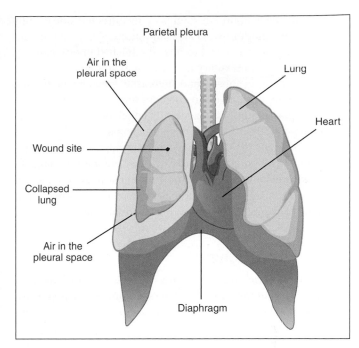

Figure 2-11 A pneumothorax occurs when air leaks into the pleural space from an opening in the chest wall or the surface of the lung. The lung collapses as air fills the pleural space and the two pleural surfaces are no longer in contact.
© Jones & Bartlett Learning.

COPD and is most often due to tobacco abuse. Pulmonary fibrosis, sarcoidosis, tuberculosis, and infection with *Pneumocystis jiroveci* (almost exclusively in patients with acquired immunodeficiency syndrome [AIDS]) are other reported causative factors. Secondary spontaneous pneumothorax occurs more frequently in patients aged 60 to 65, and patients with COPD who experience secondary spontaneous pneumothorax are 3.5 times more likely to die of the condition than patients without COPD as a cofactor.

Signs and Symptoms

The cardinal signs of primary and secondary spontaneous pneumothorax are chest pain and dyspnea. The chest pain is often described as sudden, sharp, or stabbing and made worse by breathing or other chest wall motion. Decreased lung reserve capacity, as in COPD, may make dyspnea more pronounced in patients with secondary spontaneous pneumothorax. Additional symptoms of pneumothorax may include diaphoresis, anxiety, back pain, cough, and malaise.

Look for the following clinical signs of spontaneous pneumothorax:

- Tachypnea
- Tachycardia
- Pulsus paradoxus
- Decreased breath sounds
- Hyperresonance on percussion
- Hypoxia and altered mental status (in some patients)

The presence of breath sounds on the affected side cannot rule out a pneumothorax because an estimated 25% of the lung would need to be collapsed to hear diminished breath sounds. Auscultating the midaxillary line may help you pick up on this earlier. Hypoxia, cyanosis, and increased jugular venous distention should prompt you to consider tension pneumothorax. A tension pneumothorax is generally considered to be present when a pneumothorax (primary spontaneous, secondary spontaneous, or traumatic) leads to significant impairment of respiration and/or blood circulation. The most common findings in people with tension pneumothorax are chest pain and respiratory distress, often with an increased heart rate (tachycardia) and rapid breathing (tachypnea) in the initial stages.

Differential Diagnosis

Other pneumothoraces may occur as a result of volume or barotrauma from high intrathoracic pressure during positive-pressure ventilation. If you are administering positive-pressure

Assessing Causes of Acute Deterioration in the Intubated Patient

When you are evaluating an intubated patient for acute deterioration, begin by taking the patient off of the ventilator and performing ventilation with a bag-mask device during the assessment. Use the DOPE acronym to guide you.

D Displaced tube. Has the tube been accidentally displaced? Auscultate for bilateral breath sounds and absence of epigastric sounds. Use capnography/capnometry.

O Obstructed tube. Does the patient have thick secretions that have plugged the distal tube? Perform sterile suctioning. Is the patient biting on the tube to obstruct it? Insert a bite block.

P Pneumothorax. Has pneumothorax occurred during positive-pressure ventilation? Listen for breath sounds. Sense lung compliance while ventilating. Is it hard to squeeze the bag because of high intrathoracic pressure? If a tension pneumothorax is present, perform needle decompression until a chest tube can be inserted.

E Equipment failure. Has the ventilator run out of oxygen to drive the ventilatory pressure? Check the oxygen tank and ventilator for correct function.

ventilation and your patient exhibits acute status changes, barotrauma with pneumothorax must be immediately ruled out. In fact, in the intubated patient, a rapidly declining condition usually warrants a quick assessment of the most common causes of acute deterioration in the intubated patient, using the DOPE mnemonic shown in the Rapid Recall box.

Although a diagnosis can be made on the basis of clinical exam findings, a chest radiograph can confirm the degree of pneumothorax. Performing a chest radiograph while the patient is exhaling will allow the practitioner to see the severity of the pneumothorax, although a regular chest radiograph is also acceptable. CT can also demonstrate a pneumothorax and can be especially useful when the pneumothorax is small and the patient has a comorbidity. Bedside ultrasound is also helpful in diagnosing pneumothorax. When the patient is in severe respiratory distress, diagnosis of a tension pneumothorax must be clinical, not radiographic, and cared for immediately as time dies not allow for radiological studies.

The differential diagnosis of primary and secondary spontaneous pneumothorax includes tension pneumothorax, pleurisy, pulmonary embolism, pneumonia, myocardial infarction, angina, pericarditis, esophageal spasm, and cholecystitis.

A distinction should be made when differentiating pneumothorax from tension pneumothorax (**Figure 2-12**). Accumulation of air in the pleural space on the affected side eventually forces the mediastinum to shift against the "good" lung and the vena cava. These changes cause worsening dyspnea, increased work of breathing, and a drop in cardiac output, leading to obstructive shock. The patient with unilateral diminished breath sounds who is clinically deteriorating and slipping into shock should be diagnosed with tension pneumothorax. Immediate lifesaving chest decompression must occur. Tension pneumothorax is best diagnosed by clinical exam. Waiting for radiologic confirmation can prove a fatal delay.

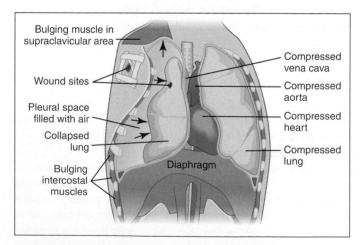

Figure 2-12 A tension pneumothorax can develop if a penetrating chest wound is bandaged tightly and air from a damaged lung cannot escape. The air then accumulates in the pleural space, eventually causing compression of the heart and great vessels.
© Jones & Bartlett Learning.

Treatment

The goal of treating pneumothoraces is to restore an air-free pleural space. The treatment you select should be guided by the patient's medical history, comorbid conditions and clinical status, the likelihood of resolution, and follow-up avenues. Most patients will not require acute intervention, such as needle chest decompression, but they must at least receive oxygen and have their respiratory status closely monitored en route to the hospital.

The least invasive management strategy is simple observation; this approach is ideal for stable patients with no comorbid conditions who have good oxygenation and reserve capacity and a small pneumothorax. These patients may be observed in the ED for a period of 6 hours. If a repeat chest radiograph shows no increase in the size of the pneumothorax, they can be discharged in 24 to 96 hours, provided they receive close follow-up.

Simple aspiration may be performed on certain patients whose condition is unlikely to resolve without intervention. Candidates include symptomatic but stable patients and those who have a small pneumothorax but comorbid conditions such as COPD. To perform this procedure, a needle is introduced into the chest under local anesthesia, and air is aspirated to induce reexpansion of the lung. The patient is then observed, usually as an inpatient. Needle aspiration, or **thoracentesis**, is the treatment of choice if possible for patients with AIDS, because placement of a chest tube in a patient with AIDS often leads to a protracted hospital stay.

Patients who are significantly symptomatic often warrant tube **thoracostomy**. If time permits, local anesthesia and conscious sedation are provided. The tube may be connected to a Heimlich valve, a one-way valve that lets air escape but not enter the pleural space. Alternatively, the tube may be connected to continuous wall suction. Patients in whom a Heimlich apparatus has been placed may be eligible for discharge sooner than those who require continuous suction. Surgical intervention may be necessary in severe or prolonged cases, or in cases in which tube thoracostomy does not rectify the pneumothorax.

EMS responders and members of the resuscitation team should have a working knowledge of chest tube insertion. Even if you never perform the procedure yourself, knowing how the procedure is accomplished will help you assist and anticipate the needs of the provider who does so.

Pleural Effusion

Pleural effusion is a collection of fluid outside the lung on one or both sides of the chest. It compresses the lung or lungs and causes dyspnea. This fluid may collect in large volumes in response to any irritation, infection, congestive heart failure, or cancer. Though it can build up gradually, over days or even weeks, patients often report that their dyspnea came on suddenly. Pleural effusions should be considered as a contributing diagnosis in any patient with lung cancer and shortness of breath (**Figure 2-13**).

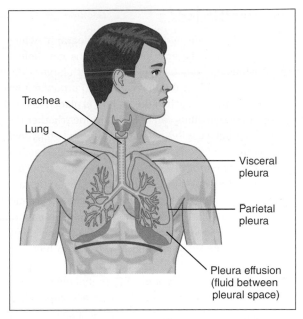

Figure 2-13 With a pleural effusion, fluid may accumulate in large volumes on one or both sides, compressing the lungs and causing dyspnea.
© Jones & Bartlett Learning.

Pathophysiology

When fluid collects between the visceral and parietal pleura, it produces a pleural effusion. The sac of fluid formed is similar to a blister, in which repeated trauma to the tissues causes more fluid to collect. Effusions can be caused by infections, tumors, or trauma.

To visualize how this condition arises, imagine a blister forming at the base of the lung. The tissues rub against each other breath after breath, causing inflammation and fluid to accumulate in the space. Some pleural effusions can contain several liters of fluid. A large effusion decreases lung capacity and causes dyspnea.

Signs and Symptoms

The most common symptom of patients with effusion is dyspnea. Chest pain (particularly pleuritic), cough, dyspnea on exertion, or orthopnea may also be present. The absence of a pleuritic component of chest pain does not rule out effusion. Certain etiologies of effusion may carry additional symptoms (e.g., pneumonia causing fever and productive cough), and systemic effects such as hypotension and hypoxia may suggest sepsis.

When you listen with a stethoscope to the chest of a patient with dyspnea resulting from pleural effusion, you will hear decreased breath sounds over the regions of the chest where fluid has moved the lung away from the chest wall. The patients frequently feel better if they are sitting upright. Nothing will really relieve their symptoms, however, except removal of the fluid, which must be done by a physician in the hospital.

Differential Diagnosis

Effusions can be confirmed on chest radiograph, which can help guide treatment. Lateral decubitus films can help image smaller effusions but may be unnecessary with larger effusions. Approximately 200 mL of fluid is required to produce a layer of fluid throughout the lung when the patient is placed in the decubitus position. Supine films can help determine whether the fluid is loculated (within a cavity), which may suggest empyema.

Pneumonia, pulmonary abscess, empyema, pulmonary embolism, and hemothorax can have symptoms and physical findings similar to pleural effusion. Of these, hemothorax often has a traumatic etiology, whereas the other causes are medical. Consider malignancy in patients who present with new pulmonary effusion. Consider tuberculosis in patients known to have been exposed to the infection and in those who have a newly converted purified protein derivative (PPD) test.

CHF should also be part of the differential diagnosis, as well as myocardial infarction and ischemia with accompanying heart failure. Collection of fluid in the pericardial space or in both the pericardial and pleural spaces after a recent myocardial infarction should prompt you to consider Dressler's syndrome.

Treatment

Shifting positions may cause significantly more dyspnea, and patients usually will resist being placed into anything other than the Fowler's position. Supportive care, including proper position and aggressive supplemental oxygen administration, should be used until the patient can be transported to a facility at which the effusion can be definitively treated.

Fluid from significant effusions can be extracted by needle thoracentesis for both diagnostic purposes and symptomatic relief. Chemical and microscopic examination of the aspirated fluid can determine its etiology. In rare cases, tube thoracostomy or surgery may be required to relieve very large effusions or to treat the cause of the effusion, as in the case of certain aggressive cancers. Imaging with CT may be performed in patients who have a new-onset effusion; this study can help diagnose lung cancer and tuberculosis that may be associated with the effusion.

Pulmonary Embolism

Pulmonary embolus (*pl.*, emboli) is the sudden blockage of an artery in the lung with a blood clot, an air bubble, a fatty plaque, or even a group of tumor cells. Deep venous thrombosis (DVT), a blood clot that has traveled to the lung from a deep vein in the leg, is one of the most common causes of pulmonary embolism.

Pathophysiology

The pulmonary circulation may be compromised by a blood clot (embolism), a fat embolism from a broken bone, an amniotic fluid embolism from leakage of amniotic fluid during pregnancy, or an air embolism resulting from air entering the circulation

from a laceration in the neck or an IV administration set that was improperly flushed or not flushed. A large embolism, of whatever type, will usually lodge in a major branch of the pulmonary artery and prevent blood flow through that branch. Adequate gas exchange in the lungs requires functional alveoli to provide oxygen and take up carbon dioxide and intact pulmonary vessels to convey oxygen-poor blood to the alveoli. Normal alveoli will be of little use if the venous blood cannot reach them, as is the situation in pulmonary embolism.

Signs and Symptoms

Because this vascular event tends to generate only vague, nonspecific symptoms, it is one of the most challenging diagnoses to make in the ED. Patients at risk of pulmonary embolism include those who have recently had surgery or major trauma and those with indwelling catheters. Signs and symptoms suggesting pulmonary embolism include the following:

- Chest pain
- Chest wall tenderness
- Dyspnea
- Tachycardia
- Syncope
- Hemoptysis (blood-tinged sputum)
- New-onset wheezing
- New cardiac arrhythmia
- Thoracic pain

The classic triad of chest pain, hemoptysis, and dyspnea is seen in fewer than 20% of patients. Early symptoms of pulmonary embolism may be minimal, but massive pulmonary embolism evolves quickly and may rapidly become symptomatic, leading to cardiac arrest with pulseless electrical activity as the presenting rhythm.

Differential Diagnosis

Pulmonary embolism is one of the most frequently misdiagnosed conditions in emergency medicine because of its confusing presentation. The early presentation may reveal normal breath sounds with good peripheral aeration, diverting attention away from a pulmonary pathology. The classic presentation is sudden dyspnea and cyanosis and, perhaps, a sharp pain the chest. A hallmark of pulmonary embolism is that the cyanosis does not resolve with oxygen therapy.

On physical exam, massive pulmonary embolism can cause hypotension secondary to cor pulmonale. More subtle pulmonary embolism can evolve into atelectasis that appears much like pneumonia over the course of a few days. New wheezing may be noted and can be deceptive, especially in COPD and asthma patients. Chest radiograph is typically normal, and the classic triad seen infrequently as an S wave in lead I, Q wave in lead III, and inverted T waves in lead III cannot be used to rule in or out pulmonary embolism. If present, SI QIII TIII should draw suspicion. Tachycardia is often seen due to the hypoxia but is a nonspecific finding. Lung sounds are often clear as there is nothing preventing the air from moving in and out of the chest; the circulation is obstructed by the pulmonary embolism leading to ventilation–perfusion mismatch. Oxygen saturations show little improvement with oxygen administration.

Treatment

Bedridden patients are often prescribed anticoagulants or wear special stockings or other devices to reduce the formation of blood clots in the legs. Especially for patients with a history of deep venous thrombosis, a Greenfield filter may be inserted by a physician. This device, which opens like a mesh umbrella in the main vein that returns blood to the heart, is intended to catch clots that break loose and travel from the legs.

Cardiac arrest caused by a large pulmonary embolus is a perilous situation that few patients survive. Patients who do not respond to oxygen or who complain of chest pain must be transported to the nearest facility.

Pulmonary Artery Hypertension

Pulmonary hypertension is a rare chronic disease characterized by elevated pulmonary artery pressure. The high pressure in the pulmonary artery makes it difficult for the heart to pump enough blood to the lungs, eventually affecting both the heart and the lungs.

Affecting only 1 to 3 people per million in the U.S. population, the disease can have a genetic component. Side effects from drugs such as cocaine, methamphetamine, and fenfluramine/phentermine/dexfenfluramine (known as *fen/phen* and withdrawn from the market in 1997 because of safety concerns) have also been implicated. The disease is most common among women of childbearing age and women in their 50s and 60s. Severe chronic lung disease is another cause.

Pathophysiology

Pulmonary hypertension begins with inflammation and changes in the cells that line the pulmonary arteries. Other factors also can affect the pulmonary arteries and cause pulmonary hypertension. For example, the condition may develop if:

- The walls of the arteries tighten.
- The walls of the arteries are stiff at birth or become stiff from an overgrowth of cells.
- Blood clots form in the arteries.

These changes make it hard for your heart to push blood through your pulmonary arteries and into your lungs. Thus, the pressure in the arteries rises, causing pulmonary hypertension.

Many factors can contribute to the process that leads to the different types of pulmonary hypertension.

Pulmonary arterial hypertension (PAH) may have no known cause, or the condition may be inherited. Some diseases and conditions also can cause PAH. Examples include HIV infection, congenital heart disease, and sickle cell disease. Also, the use of street drugs (such as cocaine) and certain diet medicines can lead to PAH.

Many diseases and conditions can cause a different type of pulmonary hypertension (often called secondary PH), including:

- Mitral valve disease
- Lung diseases, such as COPD
- Sleep apnea
- Sarcoidosis

Signs and Symptoms

Signs and symptoms of pulmonary hypertension include the following:

- Dyspnea (cardinal symptom)
- Weakness
- Fatigue
- Syncope
- Increased second heart sound (S_2)
- Tricuspid murmur
- Jugular venous pulsations
- Pitting edema

Lung sounds are often normal.

Differential Diagnosis

Echocardiography and blood tests can be performed to help confirm the diagnosis.

Treatment

Administering oxygen to dilate pulmonary vessels is an important part of treatment. A pulmonary vessel dilator or an anti-inflammatory agent may be prescribed, along with medications that hinder the growth of endothelial layers that can narrow the pulmonary artery.

Other Conditions That Affect Respiratory Function
CNS Dysfunction

A wide range of CNS diseases can impair respiratory tract function, as shown in Table 2-10. CNS disorders can be divided into the following three categories:

1. *Acute.* Illnesses lasting less than 1 week
2. *Subacute.* Diseases and disorders lasting between 1 week and 2 months
3. *Chronic.* Conditions lasting 2 months or longer

Table 2-10 CNS Conditions That Can Impair Respiration		
Acute	**Subacute**	**Chronic**
Intoxication	Guillain-Barré syndrome	HIV/AIDS
Overdose	Encephalopathy	Neuromuscular degenerative disease (ALS)
Stroke/TIA	Meningitis	Dementia
Tick paralysis	Delirium	Myasthenia gravis paralysis
Myasthenia gravis paralysis	Myasthenia gravis paralysis	
Guillain-Barré syndrome		
Meningitis		
Encephalopathy		
Delirium		
Psychiatric illness		
Seizure		
Epidural abscess		

ALS, Amyotrophic lateral sclerosis; HIV/AIDS, human immunodeficiency virus/acquired immunodeficiency syndrome; TIA, transient ischemic attack.

Acute CNS Dysfunction

Acute CNS dysfunction can have numerous medical and traumatic causes. The focus here is on acute medical illnesses of the CNS that impair respiratory function. The primary concern in such cases is maintaining a patent airway. An occluded airway may lead to rapid deterioration and cerebral anoxia. Stroke, seizure, CNS infection, and other acute neuromuscular disorders may cause a decreased level of consciousness and place the patient at great risk for poor airway and ventilation control.

General changes in respiration such as hyperpnea, tachypnea, or both often accompany CNS dysfunction. Abnormal respiratory patterns, given in Table 2-11, sometimes suggest the etiology of the problem (Figure 2-14).

Subacute CNS Dysfunction

Subacute CNS dysfunction can be responsible for prolonged respiratory compromise, including respiratory failure, atelectasis, pneumonia, lobar collapse, or infiltrate. An extended period of immobility can impair the ability to expel mucus, increase the

risk of mucous plugging of bronchi, and raise the risk of pneumonia as the alveoli lose their ability to expand. Persistent immobility can increase the threat of deep venous thrombosis and pulmonary embolus.

Chronic CNS Dysfunction

Chronic CNS dysfunction carries many of the same risks as subacute CNS dysfunction, such as an increased chance of deep venous thrombosis and pulmonary embolism. Prolonged respiratory compromise may necessitate a tracheostomy to maintain a secure airway. Inspired air thereby skirts the defenses of the upper airway, increasing the risk of a lower airway infection.

Furthermore, long-term care of CNS dysfunction is associated with exposure to hospitals and healthcare facilities, where serious infection with *Pseudomonas* spp., HA-MRSA, and vancomycin-resistant *Enterococcus* (VRE) is more likely.

Generalized Neurologic Disorders

Neuromuscular diseases such as myasthenia gravis and neuromuscular degenerative disease, often called amyotrophic lateral

Table 2-11 Abnormal Breathing Patterns

Pattern	Description
Kussmaul's respiration	Hypertachypneic, hyperpneic respiration that points to metabolic acidosis, particularly diabetic ketoacidosis.
Cheyne-Stokes respiration	Apnea alternating with tachypnea in a crescendo-decrescendo sequence, suggesting injury to the respiratory centers in the brainstem.
Biot's respiration	Characterized by groups of quick, shallow inspirations followed by regular or irregular periods of apnea. This rhythm, which may be caused by opioid overdose, indicates injury to the medulla oblongata in the brainstem.
Apneustic respiration	Deep, gasping breaths with a pause at full inspiration, followed by an incomplete release that suggests injury to or infection of the pons or upper medulla section of the midbrain. It may also be caused by ketamine sedation.
Ataxic respiration	Characterized by a disorganized pattern and depth of respiration that often progresses to apnea. Damage to the medulla oblongata is responsible for this chaotic pattern.

sclerosis (ALS), or Lou Gehrig's disease, are chronic diseases that have profound effects on the respiratory tract. Respiratory muscle weakness or ineffective nervous system control can cause hypoventilation, resulting in atelectasis. Subsequent pneumonia can be life threatening in patients who are already debilitated by disease. Acute respiratory failure can be superimposed on pneumonia or, conversely, pneumonia may precipitate respiratory failure.

A few chronic neuromuscular diseases bear mention individually. Guillain-Barré syndrome is an ascending paralysis believed to represent an overzealous immune system response to a viral infection. Patients with this disease may report having had a recent upper respiratory infection and may have an ascending paralysis develop over a few days. Respiratory compromise may be seen if the disorder progresses to involve the chest muscles and muscles of breathing.

Neuromuscular degenerative disease (ALS/Lou Gehrig's disease) is a chronic muscle-wasting disease that affects the muscles of the extremities, some skeletal muscles, and the respiratory muscles. Respiratory muscle paralysis can be partial or complete and may make the patient permanently dependent on a ventilator.

A few final tips and cautions are in order:

- Do not use depolarizing neuromuscular blocking agents (i.e., succinylcholine) for medication-assisted intubation in patients with chronic neuromuscular diseases.
- Follow standard precautions because many nontraumatic respiratory complaints of CNS origin are infectious.
- Consider suctioning for any patient who is producing sputum. Suctioning may induce coughing, which helps clear the plugs of mucus.
- Provide supplemental oxygen and initiate endotracheal intubation with any necessary sedation if you have any concern about the patient's ability to protect the airway.

Remember, all situations—acute, subacute, and chronic CNS dysfunction—should prompt meticulous attention to airway maintenance.

Medication Side Effects

Many medications have pulmonary side effects. Narcotics are among the most commonly abused categories of drugs. Narcotics induce sleep as well as respiratory depression. Both illicit and prescription narcotics are prone to abuse. In a well patient, small to moderate doses of narcotics induce pain relief and mild sedation. In larger doses, narcotics induce respiratory depression and eventually respiratory arrest, to which almost all fatal narcotics overdoses can be attributed. Both naloxone (Narcan) and naltrexone (Revia) are effective in reversing opioid toxicity, although naloxone is more frequently given emergently because it is available in IV form. Naloxone is administered to an adult as 0.4 to 2 mg IV push or 2 mg intranasally, and its effects are both naloxone-dose and opioid-dose dependent. Alcohol has a synergistic effect with opioids, and acute intoxication with both substances increases the risk of respiratory depression.

Benzodiazepines such as diazepam (Valium), lorazepam (Ativan), alprazolam (Xanax), and midazolam (Versed) may also cause respiratory depression or, in significant quantities, respiratory failure. Among the most commonly prescribed medications, agents in this class of drugs also have significant potential for abuse. Nevertheless, benzodiazepines have a relatively low toxicity, with less than 1% resulting in death. Like opioids, benzodiazepines have synergistic effects with alcohol, and combined ingestions increase the likelihood of an adverse outcome. Hypoventilation, respiratory depression, and respiratory failure can accompany major toxicity. Flumazenil (Romazicon) can be administered as a reversal agent, given

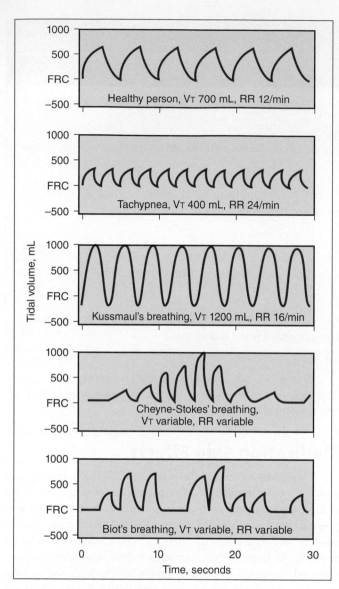

Figure 2-14 Abnormal respiratory patterns.

intravenously in a 0.1- to 0.2-mg dose, up to a total of 1 mg. If the patient has not responded after 5 minutes or a total dose of 5 mg, consider other causes.

Use caution with any reversal agent in the setting of chronic use or abuse. Naloxone use may precipitate opioid withdrawal, which is rarely life threatening but almost always unwelcome. Benzodiazepine withdrawal may precipitate seizures in severe cases. Treatment with flumazenil may make treating withdrawal seizures problematic. Both medications have variable duration, so monitor the patient carefully if airway compromise is suspected.

Cancer

Lung cancer is one of the most common forms of cancer, especially among people who smoke cigarettes and people exposed to occupational lung hazards, such as asbestos, coal dust, and secondhand smoke. Although lung cancer was traditionally considered predominantly a disease of men, today 45% of new cases of lung cancer occur in women, most likely because of the increase in smoking among women.

Signs and Symptoms

Lung cancer often is identified when tumors in the large airways bleed, causing hemoptysis (coughing up blood in the sputum) and uncontrollable coughing. It is frequently accompanied by COPD and impaired lung function. The lung is also a common site for the metastasis of cancer from other body sites.

Other cancer may invade the lymph nodes in the neck, producing tumors that threaten to occlude the upper airway. Patients with various types of cancer may have pulmonary complication from chemotherapy or radiation therapy. Lung irradiation, for example, may be associated with some degree of pulmonary edema. Tumors or treatment may also cause pleural effusion, which can present rapidly progressing dyspnea.

Clinical symptoms mirror the extent of disease and metastasis but may include the following:

- Cough
- Dyspnea
- Dyspnea on exertion
- Wheezing
- Hemoptysis
- Chest wall pain from pleural irritation or pleural effusion (decreased breath sounds may not be noted until a significant pleural effusion develops)

Regional spread of the cancer can compress structures or destroy tissue, generating a broad range of symptoms. For example, superior vena cava obstruction can cause extensive central thrombus and emboli formation, paralysis of the recurrent laryngeal nerve can cause hoarseness, pressure on the esophagus can cause swallowing difficulties, and so on. The cancer may cause markedly elevated calcium, which may be responsible for muscle pain, renal problems, kidney stones, and mental status changes. A chest radiograph will often demonstrate the malignancy as well as any associated effusion.

Treatment

Treatment involves administering supplemental oxygen, assisting respiration, ensuring a patent airway, and providing appropriate suctioning. Pneumothoraces are extremely rare with lung cancer, but consider this condition if the patient has had a recent lung biopsy. Pleural effusions, if present, are rarely drained emergently (see earlier discussion).

Toxic Inhalations

Many potentially toxic substances can be inhaled into the lungs. The type of damage depends largely on the water solubility of the toxic gas.

Signs and Symptoms

Highly water-soluble gases like ammonia will react with the moist mucous membranes of the upper airway and cause swelling and irritation. If the substance gets in the patient's eyes, they will also burn and feel inflamed and irritated.

Less water-soluble gases may get deep into the lower airway, where they may do damage over time. Such toxic gases have been used in war to disable the enemy because they do not cause immediate distress, but rather cause pulmonary edema up to 24 hours later. The gases phosgene and nitrogen dioxide behave in this manner.

Some common gases, for example chlorine, are moderately water soluble and cause problems somewhere between the extremes of irritation and pulmonary edema. Severe exposure may present with upper airway swelling, whereas lower level exposure may present with the classic delayed onset, lower airway damage. A common household error is pouring drain cleaner and chlorine bleach into a drain in an attempt to clear a clog, which may produce an irritant chlorine gas that can sicken the person and everyone in the home or building. Industrial settings often use irritant gas-forming chemicals in large quantities and in higher concentration than available for home use, creating the possibility for incidents that expose a larger number of people or a more toxic gas. EMS providers should note industrial settings in their area that are high risk for this type of incident.

Toxic gases can also affect people outside the industrial setting. One common type of exposure is carbon monoxide. Natural gas has an odor because of a chemical additive, but carbon monoxide is odorless and tasteless, and you cannot see it. Carbon dioxide is the leading cause of accidental poisoning deaths in the United States. People who survive carbon monoxide poisoning can have permanent brain damage.

Carbon monoxide is produced by household appliances such as gas water heaters, space heaters, grills, and generators, and it is even present in cigarette smoke. A common cause of carbon monoxide poisoning occurs at the onset of cold weather when people turn heaters on for the first time of the season. The combined effects of incomplete combustion and generally poor or no ventilation in a cold weather-sealed building result in the perfect setting for the production of carbon monoxide. Other common sources of carbon monoxide poisoning are smoke from fires and motor vehicle exhaust. Some people will attempt suicide by closing the car in the garage, turning the vehicle on, and inhaling the exhaust. The signs and symptoms associated with CO poisoning are listed in Table 2-12.

Differential Diagnosis

People who are exposed to carbon monoxide may think they have the flu. They initially complain of headache, dizziness, fatigue, and nausea and vomiting. They may complain of dyspnea on exertion and chest pain and display nervous system symptoms such as impaired judgment, confusion, or even hallucinations. The worst exposures may result in syncope of seizure.

Treatment

A patient who has been exposed to a toxic gas must be removed from contact with the toxic gas immediately and provided with 100% supplemental oxygen or assisted ventilation if breathing is impaired (if there is reduced tidal volume). If the upper airway is compromised, aggressive airway management (such as intubation or a cricothyrotomy) may be required.

Patients who have been exposed to slightly water-soluble gases may feel fine initially but have acute dyspnea many hours later. When such an exposure is suspected, patients should strongly consider transport to the closest emergency department for observation and further assessment.

Special Populations
Older Adult Patients

Aging patients undergo multiple changes in the respiratory system, all of which ultimately impair the body's ability to oxygenate the blood. A wide range of physiologic changes can occur both within the respiratory tract and in the body structures that

Table 2-12 Signs and Symptoms of Carbon Monoxide Poisoning		
Severity	**CO-Hb Level**	**Signs and Symptoms**
Mild	< 15–20%	Headache, nausea, vomiting, dizziness, blurred vision
Moderate	21–40%	Confusion, syncope, chest pain, dyspnea, weakness, tachycardia, tachypnea, rhabdomyolysis
Severe	41–59%	Palpitations, dysrhythmias, hypotension, myocardial ischemia, cardiac arrest, respiratory arrest, pulmonary edema, seizures, coma
Fatal	> 60%	Death

support ventilation. A summary of physiologic changes associated with advancing age follows.

- Thinning of the epithelial linings
- Decreased mucus production
- Flagging activity of respiratory cilia
- Reduced lung compliance due to calcification of cartilage in the trachea and bronchioles and calcification of interstitial tissues
- Decreasing respiratory surface area as the number of alveoli reduces
- Reduced intrathoracic volume secondary to fractures, slumping, or bone changes
- Less vigorous immune response, including fewer immunoglobulins and leukocytes
- Weakened muscles of respiration, including diaphragm, intercostal muscles, and accessory muscles

Because these changes occur gradually, often over a period of years or even decades, the body has time to adapt to a significant decrease in function. If these same changes were to happen over a compressed period of days or weeks, the sudden loss of function could be fatal. A good example is the decrease in respiratory surface area that occurs as a person ages. The blood oxygen level (called the partial pressure) in a young adult normally averages 95 mm Hg. In the older adult, a value as low as 60 mm Hg is not uncommon. If the partial pressure of oxygen was noted to be 60 mm Hg in a young, seemingly healthy individual, you would be quite concerned.

The likelihood of pathologic changes in the respiratory system and supporting structures increases as a patient ages. Some intrapleural diseases impair the ability of the lungs to inspire and expire air. Others inhibit diffusion of oxygen into the blood and carbon dioxide out of the blood. In addition, tumors can occupy lung space, decreasing the area available for ventilation. Chronic smoking can damage alveoli, narrow bronchi and choke them with mucus, and displace functioning alveoli with large blebs, or air pockets. Circulatory changes can result in delivery of less or thinner blood to the lung capillaries, impairing oxygenation. Decreased hemoglobin levels can reduce the oxygen-carrying capacity of red blood cells.

All these changes can combine to make it more difficult for an individual to perform normal activities of daily living. In the elderly, a relatively minor respiratory infection can pose a life threat. Pneumonia may cause an already marginally hypoxic elderly patient to become severely hypoxic, requiring respiratory support and mechanical ventilation.

Obstetric Patients

Pulmonary physiology changes in pregnancy. Upper airway mucosal edema, mucus secretion, nasal congestion, and rhinitis can create difficulties with bag-mask ventilation and endotracheal intubation. A pregnant patient has reduced respiratory reserve because of the elevated oxygen demand on her system. In a critical illness, rapid and severe respiratory decompensation may occur. A pregnant patient is also at greater risk of gastric aspiration.

The following conditions may cause respiratory disorders in a pregnant patient:

- Preeclampsia (hypertension and proteinuria occurring after the twentieth week of gestation)
- Pulmonary embolism (may occur throughout pregnancy, but the highest incidence is in the immediate postpartum period)
- Respiratory infection (such as pneumonia and influenza)
- Asthma
- ARDS

Bariatric Patients

Increased body mass can impede or complicate many functions of the respiratory system in the following ways:

- The larger body mass increases the need for energy for routine activities, with a consequent increase in the need for delivery of oxygen and removal of carbon dioxide and other waste products.
- The body's sheer physical mass limits the range of motion of the chest, reducing contraction of the diaphragm and subsequent expansion of the lungs. Obstructive sleep apnea is common, as are other respiratory conditions such as pulmonary embolus, COPD, CHF, and pneumonia.
- When a person is lying supine, excessive weight in the anterior abdomen can shift to the upper abdomen, limiting expansion of the chest and perhaps decreasing tidal volume, leading to hypercapnia and subsequent respiratory acidosis.

The lungs can expand somewhat in response to increased demand, but their size is limited by the abdomen and its contents. The chest can increase in diameter, a response often seen in patients who chronically abuse tobacco (an indicator of chronic bronchitis), but the size of the chest is also limited. The heart can become more efficient by pumping faster and harder, but these adjustments may have long-term cardiovascular side effects including heart failure.

Putting It All Together

Disorders that result in respiratory compromise are common to all ages of patients and are seen by all levels of healthcare providers. Respiratory complaints can result in significant ventilation, perfusion, and diffusion compromise. A thorough patient history, physical exam, and evaluation of diagnostic findings will aid your early recognition of the underlying etiologies of respiratory distress and respiratory failure.

As a healthcare provider, your understanding of the anatomy, physiology, and pathophysiology of the respiratory system and the diseases that contribute to inadequate ventilation, perfusion, and diffusion can be critical in evaluating your patient's level of distress and initiating proper care.

Ineffective work of breathing may be due to a variety of dysfunctional processes. Be familiar with the differences and similarities of reactive airway diseases, bacterial versus viral infections, and the causes of airway occlusion—accidental, traumatic, and idiopathic. Maintain your skill levels at peak performance, and be ready to initiate prompt basic life support (BLS) and advanced life support (ALS) airway adjunct interventions. The expertise you bring to the work of responding to and attending patients with respiratory disorders can save lives.

SCENARIO SOLUTION

© HunThomas/ShutterStock, Inc.

- Differential diagnoses may include pharyngitis, tonsillitis, peritonsillar abscess, epiglottitis, Ludwig's angina, bacterial tracheitis, retropharyngeal abscess, and prevertebral abscess.
- To narrow your differential diagnosis, you will need to complete the history of prior and present illness. Perform a physical examination of the patient's mouth and throat. Do not insert anything into the mouth to examine the throat. This could worsen airway swelling. Assess his oxygen saturation. Palpate his submental area and his neck. This examination should not delay transport or transfer to an area where advanced airway management is possible.

- The patient has signs of impending airway obstruction. Airway management in patients with airway obstruction is best provided by anesthesia or ENT physicians when immediately available. Administer humidified oxygen. Prepare to suction his oropharynx (provide him with an emesis basin to spit secretions if he prefers). Establish vascular access, and deliver IV fluids. Prepare to intubate. Select several tube sizes. Prepare equipment for cricothyrotomy if the airway cannot be secured by oral endotracheal intubation. Consider medication for fever, antibiotics, and pain once the airway is managed.

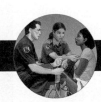

Summary

- Upper and lower airways conduct air (ventilation) to the alveoli, the site of gas exchange (respiration).
- Sensors tell the respiratory system when and how to adjust the respiratory cycle to meet the body's needs for oxygen and carbon dioxide (CO_2) and maintain its acid–base balance.
- The interdependence of respiratory anatomy on other thoracic structures helps it provide oxygen to all tissues and eliminate CO_2.
- Diseases of the cardiovascular system, which shares intrathoracic space with the respiratory system, should be included in the differential diagnosis when the patient complains of respiratory distress or failure, weakness, airway compromise, chest pain, altered mental status, cough, or fever.
- Specific disease processes that may compromise the upper airway include anatomic obstruction, aspiration, allergic reactions, and inflammation caused by infection.
- Specific disease processes characterized by lower airway dysfunction include asthma, COPD, pulmonary infections, pneumothorax, pleural effusion, pulmonary embolism, and pulmonary artery hypertension.
- Other conditions that affect respiratory function include CNS dysfunction, generalized neurologic disorders, medication side effects, cancer, and toxic inhalations.
- Your assessment of the patient with respiratory complaints should include a standard emergency approach. Special monitoring and diagnostic clues can help you narrow the differential diagnoses.
- Patient management includes airway and ventilatory support, with ongoing assessment that reassures the patient that the treatment plan is being reassessed and carried out on the basis of your findings.
- The recognition of a potential or actual life threat is essential by EMTs. Early recognition will prompt an immediate request for ALS backup and support timely and effective BLS and ALS treatment interventions, ensuring quality patient care.

KEY TERMS

© HunThomas/ShutterStock, Inc.

abscess (peritonsillar) An abscess in which a superficial soft-tissue infection progresses to create pockets of purulence in the submucosal space adjacent to the tonsils. This abscess and its accompanying inflammation cause the uvula to deviate to the opposing side.

acute lung injury/acute respiratory distress syndrome (ALI/ARDS) A systemic disease that causes lung failure.

aerobic metabolism Metabolism that can proceed only in the presence of oxygen.

anaerobic metabolism The metabolism that takes place in the absence of oxygen; the principal byproduct is lactic acid.

angioedema A vascular reaction that may have an allergic cause and may result in profound swelling of the tongue and lips.

apneustic center A portion of the pons that assists in creating longer, slower respirations.

atelectasis The collapse of the alveolar air spaces of the lungs.

carboxyhemoglobin Hemoglobin loaded with carbon monoxide.

chemoreceptors Chemical receptors that sense changes in the composition of blood and body fluids. The primary chemical changes registered by chemoreceptors are those involving levels of hydrogen (H^+), carbon dioxide (CO_2), and oxygen (O_2).

end-tidal carbon dioxide ($ETCO_2$) monitoring Analysis of exhaled gases for CO_2, a useful method of assessing a patient's ventilatory status or lung perfusion. In cardiac arrest it may indicate the effectiveness of chest compressions or return of spontaneous circulation.

gas exchange The process in which oxygen from the atmosphere is taken up by circulating blood cells and carbon dioxide from the bloodstream is released to the atmosphere.

history of the present illness (HPI) The most important element of patient assessment. The primary elements of the HPI can be obtained by using the OPQRST and SAMPLER mnemonics.

hypercapnia A condition of abnormally elevated carbon dioxide (CO_2) levels in the blood, caused by hypoventilation, lung disease, or diminished consciousness. It may also be caused by exposure to environments containing abnormally high concentrations of carbon dioxide, or by rebreathing exhaled carbon dioxide. Usually defined as a carbon dioxide level over 45 mm Hg.

Ludwig's angina A deep-space infection of the anterior neck just below the mandible. The name derives from the sensation of choking and suffocation reported by most patients with this condition.

noninvasive positive-pressure ventilation (NPPV) A procedure in which positive pressure is provided through the upper airway by some type of mask or other noninvasive device.

peritonsillar abscess *See* abscess (peritonsillar).

pneumotaxic center Located in the pons, this center generally controls the rate and pattern of respiration.

respiration The reciprocal passage of oxygen into the blood and carbon dioxide into the alveoli.

respiratory failure A disorder in which the lungs become unable to perform their basic task of gas exchange, the transfer of oxygen from inhaled air into the blood and the transfer of carbon dioxide from the blood into exhaled air.

thoracentesis A procedure to remove fluid or air from the pleural space.

thoracic duct Located in the left upper thorax; the thoracic duct is the largest lymph vessel in the body. It returns the excess fluid that is not collected by the veins from the lower extremities and abdomen to the venae cavae.

thoracostomy A procedure in which a tube may be connected to a Heimlich valve, a one-way valve that lets air escape but not enter the pleural space.

ultrasound Also called *sonography* or *diagnostic medical sonography,* this imaging method uses high-frequency sound waves to produce precise images of structures within the body.

BIBLIOGRAPHY

© HunThomas/ShutterStock, Inc.

Acerra JR: *Pharyngitis.* http://emedicine.medscape.com/article/764304-overview, updated February 5, 2015.

Aceves SS, Wasserman SI: Evaluating and treating asthma, *Emerg Med.* 37:20–29, 2005.

American Academy of Orthopaedic Surgeons: *Emergency care and transportation of the sick and injured,* ed 10, Burlington, MA, 2011, Jones & Bartlett Learning.

American Academy of Orthopaedic Surgeons: *Nancy Caroline's emergency care in the streets,* ed 7, Burlington, MA, Jones & Bartlett Learning, 2013.

American Academy of Pediatrics: Prevention of choking among children. *Pediatrics.* 125:601–607, 2010.

Amitai A: *Ventilator management.* http://emedicine.medscape.com/article/810126-overview, updated December 17, 2013.

Asmussen J, Gellett S, Pilegaard H, et al: Conjunctival oxygen tension measurements for assessment of tissue oxygen tension during pulmonary surgery, *Eur Surg Res.* 26:372–379, 1994.

Centers for Disease Control and Prevention: *National health and nutrition examination survey.* http://www.cdc.gov/nchs/nhanes.htm

Daley BJ: *Pneumothorax.* http://emedicine.medscape.com/article/424547-overview, updated April 28, 2014.

Dumitru I: *Heart failure.* http://emedicine.medscape.com/article/757999-overview, updated June 9, 2014.

Fink S, Abraham E, Ehrlich H: Postoperative monitoring of conjunctival oxygen tension and temperature, *Int J Clin Monit Comput.* 5:37–43, 1988.

Flores J: *Peritonsillar abscess in emergency medicine.* http://emedicine.medscape.com/article/764188-overview, updated February 4, 2015.

Gompf SG: *Epiglottitis.* http://emedicine.medscape.com/article/763612-overview, updated August 8, 2014.

Goswami VJ: *Dilated cardiomyopathy.* http://emedicine.medscape.com/article/757668-overview, updated October 6, 2014.

Green TE: *Acute angioedema: Overview of angioedema treatment.* http://emedicine.medscape.com/article/756261-overview, updated January 14, 2015.

Gresham C: *Benzodiazepine toxicity.* http://emedicine.medscape.com/article/813255-overview, updated January 15, 2015.

Harman EM: *Acute respiratory distress syndrome.* http://emedicine.medscape.com/article/165139-overview, updated February 18, 2014.

Howes DS: *Encephalitis.* http://emedicine.medscape.com/article/791896-overview, updated April 11, 2014.

Jenkins W, Verdile VP, Paris PM: The syringe aspiration technique to verify endotracheal tube position, *Am J Emerg Med.* 12(4):413–416, 1994.

Kamangar N: *Bacterial pneumonia.* http://emedicine.medscape.com/article/807707-overview, updated October 8, 2014.

Kaplan J: *Barotrauma.* http://emedicine.medscape.com/article/768618-overview, updated October 2, 2013.

Khan JH: *Retropharyngeal abscess.* http://emedicine.medscape.com/article/764421-overview, updated February 6, 2015.

Link MS, Berkow LC, Kudenchuk, PJ, et al. Part 7: Adult Advanced Cardiovascular Life Support: 2015 American Heart Association Guidelines Update for Cardiopulmonary Resuscitation and Emergency Cardiovascular Care. *Circulation,* 132(18 Suppl 2), S444–64. http://doi.org/10.1161/CIR.0000000000000261

Maloney M, Meakin GH: *Acute stridor in children.* http://www.medscape.com/viewarticle/566588, March 27, 2015.

Marx J, Walls R, Hockberger R: *Rosen's emergency medicine: concepts and clinical practice,* ed 5, St. Louis, MO, 2002, Mosby.

Memon MA: *Panic disorder.* http://emedicine.medscape.com/article/806402-overview, updated January 5, 2015.

Morris MJ: *Asthma.* http://emedicine.medscape.com/article/806890-overview, updated September 30, 2014.

Mosenafir Z: *Chronic obstructive pulmonary disease.* http://emedicine.medscape.com/article/297664-overview, updated September 25, 2014.

Murray AD: *Deep neck infections.* http://emedicine.medscape.com/article/837048-overview, updated March 28, 2014.

Nadel JA, Murray JF, Mason RJ: *Murray & Nadel's textbook of respiratory medicine,* ed 4, Philadelphia, PA, 2005, Elsevier Saunders.

National Highway Traffic Safety Administration: *National EMS education standards (NEMSES).* http://www.ems.gov/pdf/811077a.pdf. March 27, 2015.

Oudiz RJ: *Primary pulmonary hypertension.* http://emedicine.medscape.com/article/301450-overview, updated September 16, 2014.

Ouellette DR: *Pulmonary embolism.* http://emedicine.medscape.com/article/759765-overview, updated January 30, 2015.

Pappas DE, Hendley JO: Retropharyngeal abscess, lateral pharyngeal abscess and peritonsillar abscess. In Kleigman RM, et al, Eds: *Nelson textbook of pediatrics,* ed 18, Philadelphia, PA, 2007, Saunders.

Paramedic Association of Canada: *National occupational competency profile for paramedic practitioners.* http://www.paramedic.ca/nocp/. March 27, 2015.

Paul M, Dueck M, Kampe S, et al: Intracranial placement of a nasotracheal tube after transnasal trans-sphenoidal surgery, *Br J Anaesth.* 91:601–604, 2003.

Peng LF: *Dental infections in emergency medicine.* http://emedicine.medscape.com/article/763538-overview, updated February 27, 2015.

Petrache I: *Pleurodynia.* http://emedicine.medscape.com/article/300049-overview, updated November 20, 2013.

Rackow E, O'Neil P, Astiz M, et al: Sublingual capnometry and indexes of tissue perfusion in patients with circulatory failure, *Chest.* 120:1633–1638, 2001.

Rajan S, Emery KC: *Bacterial tracheitis.* http://emedicine.medscape.com/article/961647-overview, updated September 25, 2014.

Ren X: *Aortic stenosis.* http://emedicine.medscape.com/article/757200-overview, updated November 10, 2014.

Rubins J: *Pleural effusion.* http://emedicine.medscape.com/article/299959-overview, updated September 5, 2014.

Shah SN: *Hypertrophic cardiomyopathy.* http://emedicine.medscape.com/article/152913-overview, updated April 21, 2014.

Shapiro JM: Critical care of the obstetric patient. *J Intensive Care Med.* 21:278–286, 2006.

Shores C: Infections and disorders of the neck and upper airway. In Tintinalli J, Ed: *Emergency medicine: A comprehensive study guide,* New York, NY, 2004, McGraw-Hill Professional Publishing, pp. 1494–1501.

Stephens E: *Opioid toxicity.* http://emedicine.medscape.com/article/815784-overview, updated April 4, 2014.

Tan WW: *Non-small cell lung cancer.* http://emedicine.medscape.com/article/279960-overview, updated December 22, 2014.

Tanigawa K, Takeda T, Goto E, et al: The efficacy of esophageal detector devices in verifying tracheal tube placement: A randomized cross-over study of out-of-hospital cardiac arrest patients, *Anesth Analg.* 92:375–378, 2001.

Tatevossian RG, Wo CC, Velmahos GC, et al: Transcutaneous oxygen and CO_2 as early warning of tissue hypoxia and hemodynamic shock in critically ill emergency patients, *Crit Care Med.* 28(7):2248–2253, 2000.

Urden L, Stacy K, Lough M: *Thelan's critical care nursing: Diagnosis and management,* ed 5, St. Louis, MO, 2006, Elsevier.

Wilson Tang WH: *Myocarditis.* http://emedicine.medscape.com/article/759212-overview, updated September 5, 2014.

CHAPTER REVIEW QUESTIONS

1. Which of the following is most likely to impair ventilation?
   a. Anaphylaxis
   b. Carbon monoxide poisoning
   c. Congestive heart failure
   d. Pneumonia

2. Which sign or symptom indicates impending respiratory failure in a patient who is having an asthma attack?
   a. End-tidal CO_2 of 32 mm Hg
   b. Increased respiratory rate
   c. S_3 heart sounds
   d. Sleepiness

3. A 65-year-old woman has progressive onset of dyspnea over several days. The patient's temperature is 102.2°F (39°C). Her prescription medications include Accupril (quinapril), spironolactone, Lanoxin (digoxin), ipratropium, and salbutamol. Which of the following would be included in your differential diagnosis?
   a. Pneumonia
   b. Pulmonary edema
   c. Spontaneous pneumothorax
   d. Status asthmaticus

4. Which diagnostic test will quickly detect poor ventilation?
   a. Capnography
   b. Carbon monoxide sensors
   c. Chest radiograph
   d. Transcutaneous oxygen saturation

5. A patient presents with fever, sore throat, and swollen lower jaw. Which should be included in your differential diagnosis?
   a. Foreign-body airway obstruction
   b. Laryngotracheobronchitis
   c. Ludwig's angina
   d. Tonsillitis

6. A 62-year-old man has a sudden onset of dyspnea after a bout of coughing. Lung sounds are diminished on the right side. Which element of the past medical history would help confirm the diagnosis of spontaneous pneumothorax?
   a. Heroin abuse
   b. Pneumonia within 5 years
   c. Tobacco smoker
   d. Treatment with warfarin

7. Which sign or symptom may develop as a result of pulmonary embolism, COPD, or pulmonary hypertension?
   a. Bradycardia
   b. Jugular venous distention
   c. Rhonchi
   d. Right-sided heart strain or right axis deviation

8. You have administered albuterol and parenteral epinephrine to a 21-year-old woman who is having an asthma attack. The patient's P_{CO_2} level is now 55 mm Hg. What additional treatment is indicated?
   a. Apply oxygen and allow the patient's body to reverse the bronchospasm and hypercarbia.
   b. Coach the patient to slow her respiratory rate.
   c. No immediate treatment is indicated except to monitor the patient.
   d. Place the patient on a continuous positive-pressure airway mask.

9. A 24-year-old man was diagnosed with Guillain-Barré syndrome 1 week ago. Which complication should you anticipate?
   a. Hypertension
   b. Metabolic alkalosis
   c. Pneumonia
   d. Spontaneous pneumothorax

10. The risk of barotrauma for a patient with asthma who is receiving mechanical ventilation increases if you decrease the:
    a. Expiratory time
    b. Positive end-expiratory pressure
    c. Respiratory rate
    d. Tidal volume

© Candy_Box_Image-/Shutterstock

CHAPTER 3

Cardiovascular Disorders

Cardiac disorders are a common reason for adults to seek medical attention each year. Chest pain is not only the most common presenting medical complaint, but it can also be a symptom of a life-threatening medical emergency. This chapter describes how to quickly assess the causes of chest pain, from life-threatening to nonemergent, by categorizing this common symptom into the three possible systems affected: cardiovascular, pulmonary, and gastrointestinal. Additional descriptions will help you make an accurate field diagnosis, develop a treatment plan, and monitor the patient in order to adapt treatment as necessary.

LEARNING OBJECTIVES

At the conclusion of this chapter, you will be able to:

- Apply knowledge of anatomy, physiology, and pathophysiology to patients presenting with chest discomfort.

- Employ history collection and physical exam skills to direct the assessment for patients with chest discomfort.

- Apply knowledge of disease processes and the information obtained from the patient presentation, history, and physical to form a list of diagnoses based on the degree of life threat (life-threatening, critical, emergent, and nonemergent diagnoses) using the AMLS assessment pathway.

- Manage patients with chest discomfort by making clinical decisions, performing diagnostic tests, and using the results to modify care as indicated. Decision making includes routing the patient to the correct resources and following accepted practice guidelines.

- Provide an ongoing assessment of the chest discomfort patient to confirm or rule out potential diagnoses and adapt treatment and management based on patient response and findings.

A 37-year-old woman complains of dyspnea and chest pain. She has been feeling ill for about a week and vomited twice today. Her skin is flushed, and her heart rate is increased. She reports smoking two packs of cigarettes a day. Her only medications are birth control pills and insulin.

- Which differential diagnoses are you considering based on the information you have now?
- Which additional information will you need to narrow your differential diagnosis?
- What are your initial treatment priorities as you continue your patient care?

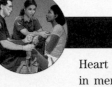

Heart disease is the leading cause of death in men and women. It was for the purpose of providing early, definitive treatment for patients with **acute myocardial infarction (AMI)** that the job of paramedic first came into being more than 40 years ago. Even with paramedic availability, more than 600,000 Americans die of heart disease every year; approximately half die in an emergency department or before reaching a hospital, during the first minutes and hours after the onset of symptoms. It is easy to see why recognition and management of cardiovascular emergencies continue to receive strong emphasis in the education of every level of provider.

Anatomy and Physiology

Several organs and structures within the chest can cause discomfort or pain if affected by disease or injury, including the chest wall, which contains the ribs, vertebrae, muscles, the pleurae and lungs; the heart and great vessels; the esophagus; and the diaphragm (**Figure 3-1**).

The Heart

The heart is a four-chambered, electrically driven, muscular pump located beneath the sternum, slightly offset to the left of midline, and roughly the size of a closed fist. It beats from birth to death and is the body's most exercised muscle, requiring a healthy blood supply of its own. It is estimated that 81 million adult Americans suffer from one or more types of heart disease. The heart and its connection to the great vessels are surrounded by a tough fibrous membrane known as the "pericardial sac" or "pericardium." This sac protects the heart against trauma from surrounding structures, invasion of foreign organisms, and friction from the constant movement. A small amount of pericardial fluid is normally in the pericardium and acts as a lubricant to allow normal heart movement within the chest. The pericardium

provides support in terms of anchoring the heart and prevents overdistention.

The Great Vessels

The great vessels include the aorta, superior and inferior venae cavae, pulmonary arteries, and pulmonary veins (**Figure 3-2**). The section of the aorta that runs through the chest is called the *thoracic aorta* and, as the aorta moves down through the abdomen, it is called the *abdominal aorta*. Serious, life-threatening illness occurs when the aorta becomes diseased and the layers begin to separate.

The Lungs and Pleurae

Chapter 2 covers respiratory disorders in depth, but a brief review the anatomy and physiology is given here. The lungs are the large organs made of spongy lobes of elastic tissue that stretch and constrict as you inhale and exhale. The trachea and bronchi are made of smooth muscle and cartilage, allowing the airways to

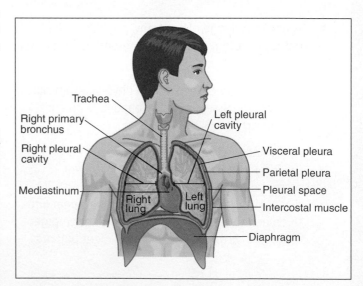

Figure 3-1 Thoracic cavity, including ribs, intercostal muscles, diaphragm, mediastinum, lungs, heart, great vessels, bronchi, trachea, and esophagus.

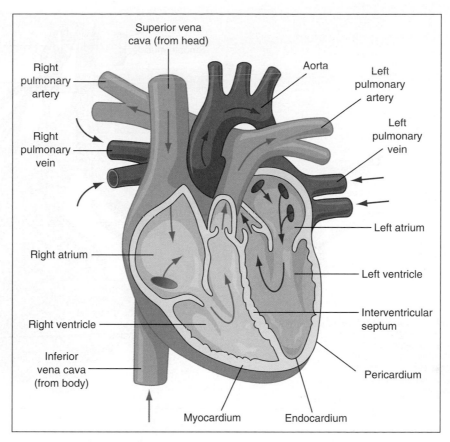

Figure 3-2 Pericardial reflections near the origins of the great vessels, shown after removal of the heart. Note that portions of the caval vessels are within the pericardial space.

constrict and expand. The lungs and airways bring in fresh, oxygen-enriched air and get rid of carbon dioxide, which is a product of metabolism. When you inhale, the diaphragm and intercostal muscles contract and expand the chest. This expansion lowers the pressure in the chest below that of the outside air pressure. Air then flows in through the airways from an area of high pressure to low pressure and inflates the lungs. When you exhale, the diaphragm and intercostal muscles relax, and the weight of the chest wall along with the elasticity of the diaphragm forces the air out.

The lungs are also surrounded by the chest wall, which is lined with **pleura** (**Figure 3-3**). The visceral pleurae surround the lungs, and the parietal pleurae line the chest wall. A small amount of visceral fluid acts as a lubricant to allow normal lung movement within the chest, and a small amount of parietal fluid causes the visceral and parietal pleurae to adhere together. This adherence keeps the lungs expanded and stretches the spongy tissue when the chest cavity expands during inhalation. (To illustrate how fluid can act as an adhesive, take two glass slides. If you place them together, you can easily separate them, but if you place just one small drop of water between them, it is very difficult to pull them apart.)

Oxygenation occurs in the alveoli, the terminal sacs of the lungs (**Figure 3-4**). The alveoli are covered by single-cell capillaries, where the exchange of gases (oxygen and carbon dioxide) takes place. Anything that causes disruption of diffusion between

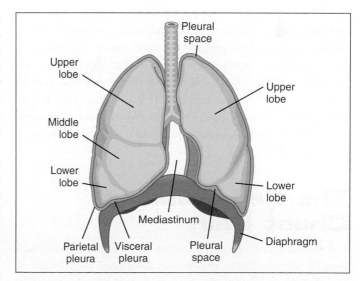

Figure 3-3 The pleura lining the chest wall and covering the lungs is an essential part of the breathing mechanism.

the alveoli and capillaries can interfere with oxygenation, leading to hypoxia. An example of this is a patient with pulmonary edema. In pulmonary edema, fluid accumulates in the interstitial space and alveoli, decreasing the ability of oxygen to cross from the alveoli to the capillaries and contributing to hypoxia.

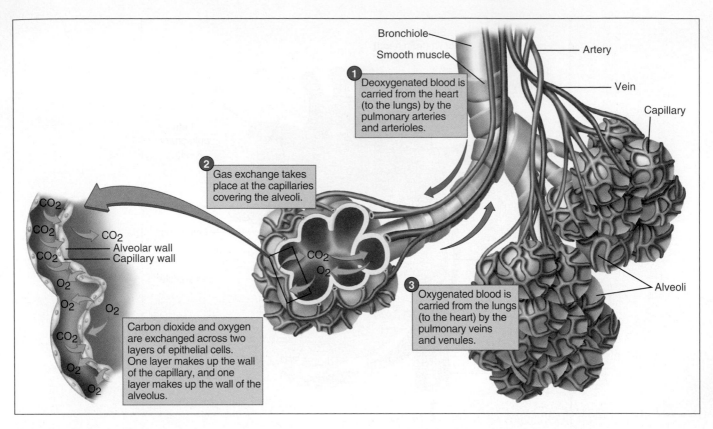

Figure 3-4 Exchange of gases in the lungs.

The Esophagus

When food is swallowed, it passes from the pharynx into the esophagus, initiating rhythmic contractions (peristalsis) of the esophageal wall. This propels the food toward the stomach. Any alteration in these processes can lead to chest discomfort. Esophageal reflux often causes chest discomfort and may be confused with the discomfort caused by a cardiac event. In gastroesophageal reflux disease, or GERD, the contents of the stomach flow back up the esophagus, causing a burning sensation or local discomfort.

The Sensation of Chest Pain

The scientific and clinical definition of *pain* is an unpleasant sensory and emotional experience associated with actual or potential tissue damage. For the purpose of this chapter, *chest discomfort* includes not only pain, but any feeling of discomfort to include burning, crushing, stabbing, or squeezing sensations. Chest pain or discomfort, then, is the direct result of the stimulation of nerve fibers from potentially damaged tissues within the chest. This potential damage may be caused by mechanical obstruction, inflammation, infection, or **ischemia**. For example, with an AMI, ischemic tissues send the brain sensory information that is interpreted as chest pain or discomfort.

Many cardiovascular disorders cause chest pain or discomfort. All complaints of chest discomfort should be taken seriously until potential life threats can be ruled out. At times, it may be difficult to distinguish chest discomfort from pain or discomfort caused by organs or structures outside of the chest cavity (**Figure 3-5**). Although the boundaries of the chest cavity are well defined, organs or structures lying close to those boundaries may be served by similar nerve roots. A patient with gallbladder disease, for example, may complain of discomfort in the upper right side of the chest and shoulder because even though the gallbladder is located in the abdominal cavity, pain can be "referred" to the chest and shoulder. The converse may also be true: pathophysiology inside the chest can be interpreted by the patient as symptoms outside the chest, such as in the abdomen, neck, and back. AMI commonly presents with feelings of epigastric pain, nausea, and vomiting.

To locate the cause of the discomfort, an understanding of somatic pain and visceral pain is important. Patients will often describe the pain or discomfort in terms of how it feels to them, using terms such as "sharp," "burning," "tearing," or "squeezing." These are descriptions of different types of pain. Somatic pain is well localized and described as sharp. Visceral pain, however, results from activation of nociceptors (sensory receptors that respond to pain) within the organs of the chest and abdomen and is often described as heaviness, pressure, aching, or burning that is not easy to pinpoint. Visceral pain may also radiate to other areas of the body and be accompanied by symptoms such as nausea and vomiting.

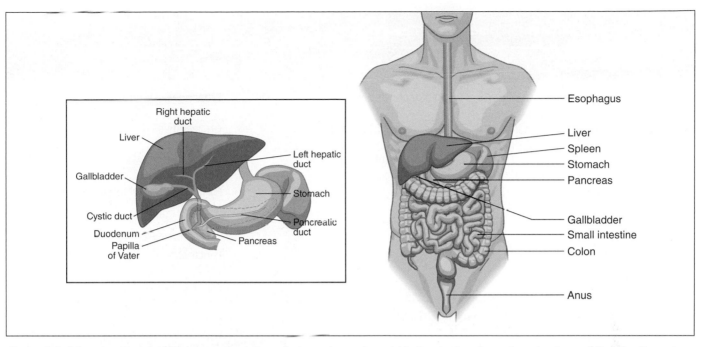

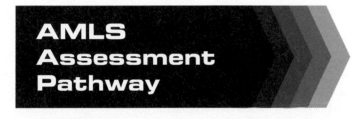

Figure 3-5 Other structures that may cause chest discomfort or pain may be outside the chest cavity, such as structures of the digestive system.

AMLS Assessment Pathway

▼ Initial Observations

Scene Safety Considerations

Ensure that the situation is safe for you to approach. Look for clues in the environment that may give you insight and direct you toward what might have brought on the problem. Which risk factors, medications, medical equipment, and sights or smells support the cause of the complaint? Do you have all the necessary resources to manage this patient right now? Which resources do you need to request to help you manage this patient appropriately? If you are functioning within a basic life support system of EMS, should you request the additional resources of an advanced life support or critical care team? If you are functioning within a small hospital without interventional catheterization lab resources, should you initiate an advanced life support or critical care transport as soon as possible?

Patient Cardinal Presentation/Chief Complaint

Patients experience a wide range of symptoms when they have a cardiovascular problem. The most common complaints include chest pain, dyspnea, fainting, palpitations, and fatigue. If the patient is pulseless or breathless, basic life support measures may be used. In some cases, advanced life support may be needed. Table 3-1 lists the different causes of chest pain. When you are responding to a chief complaint of palpitations, the patient may report a feeling of "skipping a beat." In such a case, inquire about the onset, frequency, and duration of this symptom and any previous episodes. Also ask about the presence of associated symptoms such as chest pain, dizziness, and dyspnea.

Primary Survey

When first assessing the patient, the top priority is looking for any life-threatening causes of chest discomfort. Early recognition of the patient with a critical medical condition should be your initial focus. Should your primary survey reveal life-threatening signs, triage decisions have to be made in both the prehospital and in-hospital settings, with a goal of moving the patient quickly toward a definitive intervention. If the patient's condition is not life threatening, conduct a primary survey assessing the patient's level of consciousness, airway, breathing, and circulation.

Level of Consciousness

The patient's level of consciousness is an excellent indicator of the adequacy of cerebral perfusion. If the patient is alert and oriented, you know that the brain is receiving enough oxygen, which in turn means the heart is functioning well as a pump. Conversely, stupor or confusion may indicate poor cardiac output, which may indicate a myocardial damage or dysfunction. The color and temperature of the patient's skin can provide you with valuable information about circulation—cold, sweaty skin suggests peripheral vasoconstriction.

Table 3-1 Critical Differential Diagnosis of Chest Pain		
Cardiovascular Causes	**Pulmonary Causes**	**Gastrointestinal Causes**
Acute coronary syndrome	Pulmonary embolism	Esophageal rupture
Congestive heart failure	Tension pneumothorax	Cholecystitis
Aortic dissection	Respiratory infections	Dyspepsia
Cardiac tamponade	Pleurisy	Gastroesophageal reflux disease
Arrhythmia		Hiatal hernia
		Pancreatitis
		Peptic ulcer disease

Data from Marx JA, Hockberger RS, Walls RM: *Rosen's emergency medicine*, ed 6, St Louis, Mosby, 2009.

Airway and Breathing

If the patient is able to talk, the airway is patent. The patient may be able to maintain an open airway, or, depending on the patient's level of consciousness, you may need to clear an obstruction (debris, blood, or teeth) by properly positioning the head and/or placing an airway adjunct. Note the rate, quality, and effort of breathing. You may need to use a stethoscope if breathing is in question. Consider using oxygen therapy at this time. Respiratory distress in a cardiac patient suggests the possibility of congestive heart failure, with fluid in the lungs.

Circulation/Perfusion

If the patient is conscious, check the radial pulse; if the patient is unconscious, check the carotid pulse. Note the overall quality of the pulse and whether it is regular or irregular. Continue to assess the skin color and condition. Note any edema, poor turgor, or skin tenting.

▼ First Impression

When you respond to a call for a patient with a complaint of chest pain, your knowledge of anatomy, physiology, and pathophysiology will help guide you toward the common causes of chest pain. The most serious and common life threat is an acute myocardial infarction, or AMI. (However, fewer than half of all patients suffering an AMI call 9-1-1.) Considering the wide range of possible causes, providers must have a high index of suspicion when treating patients with a potential cardiovascular disorder.

What can you discern from across the room? Is the patient awake? What position is the patient in? Is the patient in a tripod position indicating trouble breathing, or lying flat with minimal response to your presence? Is there increased work of breathing?

Does the patient appear anxious? Is there an appearance of shock or poor perfusion? The patient's affect can provide clues as to the etiology or severity of the patient's condition. Your first impression of the patient may tell you whether the patient is sick or not.

Early during the assessment of the patient with suspected ACS, a physical exam should be performed, focusing on the area of the body associated with the chief complaints. Lung sounds should be assessed for the presence of crackles or rhonchi. Wet lungs may be the result of left heart failure and acute pulmonary edema (APE), indicating cardiogenic shock. The presence of a cough with frothy pink sputum may also be evidence of APE.

Jugular vein distention and pedal edema may be present if right-sided heart failure has occurred secondary to left-sided heart failure. Examining the chest for previous scars indicating the presence of a pacemaker or past heart surgery would be important findings as well and would support your diagnosis of acute coronary syndrome (ACS). Having completed your assessment, the diagnosis of ACS can be made and treatment specific to the type of ACS instituted. The information you obtain from a detailed assessment will help you generate an initial diagnosis.

▼ Detailed Assessment
History Taking

Obtain the patient's history by inquiring into the patient's medical history based the patient's cardinal presentation/chief complaint. If the patient has a cough, does he normally have a cough? If so, why? Does he have a past medical history of chronic obstructive pulmonary disease (COPD)? If he normally coughs, is it productive? Is what he is coughing up typical in amount and color? A patient with COPD or pneumonia may have a productive cough, so noting if this is different may help you determine whether or not the patient is experiencing something new.

OPQRST and SAMPLER

The OPQRST and SAMPLER mnemonics can be used to elaborate on the patient's chief complaint. In a patient with chest pain, suspect an acute myocardial infarction. Get the patient's narrative description. Note the exact words the patient uses to describe the pain, and observe the patient's body language during your dialogue. Try not to lead your patient's description unless the patient is clearly unable to describe the pain.

What was the patient doing when the chest discomfort started? Remember, you don't have to be working hard for an AMI to occur. In fact, most happen at rest. If the discomfort began suddenly with activity or during a stressful situation, assess further to determine a past medical history of angina. Gradual onset may suggest pericarditis. An onset a day after heavy lifting or forceful coughing may suggest a chest wall muscle involvement (diagnosis of exclusion only).

What makes the discomfort better or worse? The pain from an AMI is usually constant and is worsened by exertion, but not normally worsened with a deep breath or with palpation on the area where the pain is being felt. It is not made better by a particular position or by splinting the chest with a pillow. If the discomfort is relieved by rest and/or nitroglycerin, then the ACS may be angina. If not, then the pain or discomfort could be the result of **unstable angina (UA)** or an AMI. If the pain increases with palpation or inspiration, pneumonia, pneumothorax, pericarditis, or pulmonary embolism may be the reason for the pain or discomfort. At that time, further assessment for those signs and symptoms should occur.

Have the patient describe the discomfort in his or her own words. Do not coach the patient, which can limit the patient's response and may not accurately describe how the patient feels. Heart-related pain is often accompanied by a sensation of pressure or squeezing. It can be described as indigestion. A tearing pain is associated with dissection of an aneurysm.

Does the discomfort radiate? With acute coronary syndrome, the discomfort radiates to the neck or jaw or down the arms. However, it may also radiate to the back, into the abdomen, or down the legs. Discomfort felt in the shoulder may be referred and associated with gallbladder disease or spleen involvement. The discomfort of an aortic dissection classically radiates straight through to the back and may settle in the flank. Further assessment of those types of discomfort is warranted.

Ask the patient to rate the pain on a scale of 0 to 10, with 1 being the least amount of discomfort and 10 being the worst pain ever felt. If the treatment you provide is effective, that number should go down. If the number goes up, it should signal to you that your patient is not responding to treatment and the condition is probably getting worse. At times the treatment for chest pain in men is taken more seriously because of how they describe its intensity. Women may have little or no complaints of pain, but instead may report a sudden onset of weakness with the associated signs and symptoms of AMI such as nausea, dizziness, malaise, and anxiety.

Ask how long the patient has had the discomfort. If a clot is the cause, the patient may need fibrinolytic or "clot buster" treatment to dissolve a clot in the coronary artery. The decision to administer fibrinolytic therapy will depend on how close the patient is to a definitive therapy or chest pain center capable of cardiac catheterization. The maximum benefit of therapy occurs when fibrinolytics are administered promptly.

Signs and symptoms include sudden onset of weakness; dizziness; pale, cool, clammy skin; or the feeling of impending doom. Ventricular assistive devices can cause skin breakdown at the cannulation site, disturbances in sleep/wake cycles, alterations in mentation and behavior and depression due to the lifestyle changes that occur with end-stage heart failure. Pertinent negatives such as discomfort not being relieved by rest or nitroglycerin would be important to note and suggest unstable angina or AMI.

Knowledge of the patient's allergies to any medications is important because the patient may be given aspirin and other medications. All medications—prescription, herbal, and over-the-counter—are important to note. They may indicate a past medical history of coronary artery disease (CAD) or a previous heart condition. Medications such as nitroglycerin, aspirin, cholesterol-lowering medications, high blood pressure medications such as angiotensin-converting enzyme (ACE) inhibitors, beta-blockers, calcium channel blockers, and oral hypoglycemics would all be pertinent for the possibility of CAD. If the patient has taken any medications in the last 24 to 36 hours for erectile dysfunction (such as Viagra [sildenafil], Cialis [tadalafil], or Levitra [vardenafil]), nitrates should be avoided; they may drastically lower blood pressure.

Does the patient have heart disease? Is there a family history of heart disease? Has the patient had an AMI? Has she ever had a coronary artery bypass graft (CABG) or a percutaneous transluminal coronary angioplasty (PTCA) with a stent to open a coronary vessel? Is there evidence of risk factors? These are all pertinent medical history questions you should attempt to answer.

You should also make note of a surgically implanted left ventricular assistive device (**Figure 3-6**). This implanted mechanical device is used in patients with end-stage heart failure and those waiting for heart transplantation. Patients may also have devices that are right ventricular assistive devices and biventricular assistive devices. Such devices are a "bridge" to transplantation or aids for those who have had heart surgery and experience severe heart failure. Trials of these devices as permanent alternatives to transplantation are taking place.

The patient's last oral intake is important information. This may indicate the presence of a full stomach and an increased risk of vomiting should the patient become nauseated.

Find out the events that led up to the call for 9-1-1. Was the patient engaged in physical activity or a high-stress situation, or did the patient wake up from a sleep with discomfort? Has there been any use of cocaine or methamphetamines? Has there

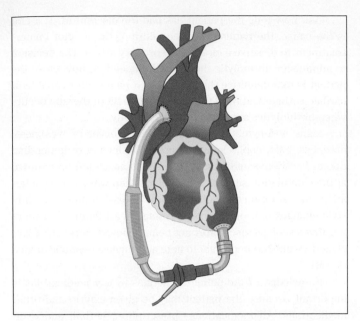

Figure 3-6 Left ventricular assistive device. This device is a small continuous-flow pump. The inflow cannula is connected to the cardiac apex, and the outflow graft is connected to the ascending aorta.

been a long period of inactivity such as an international flight or cross-country road trip (suggesting a pulmonary embolism)?

Risk factors for the development of disease have been described as modifiable and nonmodifiable. If the patient has had previous episodes, have them compare this event with past presentations.

In cases of dyspnea, explore the possibility of left-sided heart failure. When did the dyspnea start? Did it awaken the patient from sleep? Paroxysmal nocturnal dyspnea is an acute episode of shortness of breath in which the patient suddenly awakens from sleep with a feeling of suffocation. It is one of the classic signs of left-sided heart failure.

Fainting (syncope) occurs when cardiac output suddenly declines. Cardiac causes of syncope include dysrhythmias, increased vagal tone, and heart lesions. There are also numerous noncardiac causes of syncope (see Chapter 5, *Neurologic Disorders*). As part of the history taking from someone who has fainted, try to sort out whether the patient fainted from cardiac or noncardiac causes. Find out the circumstances under which the person fainted. A 25-year-old person who faints at the sight of blood is unlikely to have significant underlying heart disease. A 65-year-old person who faints after feeling some fluttering in the chest may have a dangerous cardiac dysrhythmia. Also, losing consciousness while sitting or lying down has more ominous implications than fainting while standing up.

Secondary Survey

Although the secondary survey for medical patients is often similar, when a patient presents with a cardiac problem, certain aspects warrant greater emphasis.

Vital Signs

The patient's pulse should be carefully examined. Although a rapid pulse may indicate anxiety, it may also occur secondary to severe pain, congestive heart failure, or a cardiac dysrhythmia. If the pulse is weak and thready, cardiac output is compromised.

Abnormal pulse findings include the following:

- A *pulse deficit*. This occurs when the palpated radial pulse rate is less than the apical pulse rate; it is reported as the difference between the two. To assess for a pulse deficit, check the peripheral radial pulse while listening to an apical pulse.
- *Pulsus paradoxus*. This is an excessive drop in systolic blood pressure with each inspired breath. The finding is easiest to detect when the rhythm is regular. The affected pulse beats feel weaker than the others. If the variation is slight, it can be detected only by use of a blood pressure cuff and stethoscope.
- *Pulsus alternans*. This occurs when the pulse alternates between strong and weak beats and typically is representative of left ventricular systolic damage.

In patients older than 50 years, a systolic blood pressure of more than 140 mm Hg is a much more important risk factor for cardiovascular disease than the diastolic pressure. It may be beneficial to obtain the patient's blood pressure in both arms and compare the readings. Some conditions, such as stroke or aortic aneurysm, may cause a variation in blood pressure from the right to the left side.

Physical Exam

The physical exam starts with inspection, auscultation, and palpation of the patient's respirations. Inspect the neck and tracheal position. Press down with your finger in the patient's suprasternal notch to verify that the trachea is midline.

Also inspect the adjacent structures such as the neck veins. The external jugular veins reflect the pressure within the patient's systemic circulation. Normally they are collapsed when a person is sitting or standing. If the function of the right side of the heart is compromised, however, blood will back up into the systemic veins behind the right side of the heart and distend those veins.

Continue the assessment by inspecting and palpating the chest. Surgical scars may indicate previous cardiac surgery. A bulge under the patient's skin may indicate a pacemaker or an automated implanted cardioverter-defibrillator. These devices are implanted just below the right or left clavicle and are about the size of a half dollar. A barrel-chested patient indicates chronic obstructive pulmonary disease. On palpation, look for signs of crepitus.

Using your stethoscope, listen for crackles or wheezes, which suggest left-sided heart failure with pulmonary edema. Examine the extremities for pedal edema and examine the back for sacral edema; these are signs of failure of the right side of the heart.

Above all, listen to the patient's heart sounds during your exam. The following lists other abnormal heart sounds:

- *An opening snap.* This sound indicates a noncompliant valve, such as the mitral valve.
- *An ejection click.* This high-pitched sound occurs just after the S[1] sound, which is near the beginning of the ventricular contraction (systole); it may indicate a dilated pulmonary artery or septal defect.
- *A pericardial friction rub.* When the pericardial surfaces rub together and are inflamed, such as in pericarditis, a to-and-fro sound can be heard in systole and diastole.
- *A murmur.* An ambiguous sound associated with turbulent blood flow through the heart valves.
- *A pericardial knock.* A high-pitched sound during the diastole phase. It indicates a thickened pericardium that is limiting how far the ventricle can expand during the diastole phase.

Diagnostics

Prehospital Setting

In the prehospital setting, one of the most widely used diagnostic tools is the ECG monitor-defibrillator. The ECG machine enables healthcare providers to monitor and record 3-lead and 12-lead tracings and to transmit tracings obtained in the field to the receiving facility. The ECG monitor enables prehospital providers to quickly identify suspected AMI, transmit the finding electronically, and make sound transport decisions based on the ECG findings. The monitor also provides rescuers with the ability to defibrillate, cardiovert, and perform transcutaneous pacing in the prehospital setting.

When you are obtaining the patient's vital signs, attach the cardiac monitor, waveform capnography, or pulse oximeter if you have not already done so. Use the ECG and oxygen saturation measurement to guide your assessment and treatment. If multiple healthcare providers are available, essential monitoring equipment, diagnostics, and some early treatment can be initiated while you look for symptoms of those critical diagnoses.

In-Hospital Setting

Cardiac Enzymes

In the hospital setting, the most sensitive and specific enzymes to detect cardiac damage are the cardiac-specific troponins. This test is usually elevated within 6 hours of onset of the infarct, and elevation persists for 5 to 7 days. Besides signaling AMI, these enzymes may also be elevated in the case of unstable angina, myocarditis, and congestive heart failure (CHF). It would also be appropriate to obtain a 15- or 18-lead ECG to obtain a more comprehensive view of the entire myocardium as a 12-lead ECG only views about 50%.

Damaged myocardial tissue cells also release the cardiac enzyme creatine kinase (CK); specifically, a subtype called *CK-MB* is released from heart muscle tissue. CK elevation is seen 4 to 8 hours after MI and returns to normal within 48 hours.

Muscle damage, such as from bruising or rhabdomyolysis, renal failure, low thyroid hormones (triiodothyronine [T_3], thyroxine [T_4], thyroid-stimulating hormone [TSH]), and alcohol and cocaine abuse can increase values unrelated to an MI.

Other hematologic studies frequently ordered include erythrocyte (red blood cell) counts, leukocyte (white blood cell [WBC]) counts, hemoglobin, hematocrit, erythrocyte sedimentation rate, prothrombin time (PT), international normalized ratio (INR), and partial thromboplastin time (PTT). These values are important in patients suspected of having a thrombus or embolus.

Cardiac Stress Testing

Cardiac stress testing can demonstrate the presence of functional ischemia. Stress on the heart may be induced by exercise such as walking on a treadmill or pedaling on a bicycle while the patient is undergoing continuous cardiac monitoring in multiple leads. The ECG is then observed for signs of ischemia during exercise. Cardiac stress can also be induced by administration of vasodilating medications such as adenosine.

Stress testing can be combined with nuclear imaging before and after the cardiac stress portion of the test. The imaging studies can then allow visualization of areas of the heart that show compromised blood flow during exertion. Such compromise is usually caused by stenosis in the coronary arteries.

Cardiac Catheterization

Cardiac catheterization may be warranted in patients with suspected cardiovascular abnormalities who have unstable angina, heart failure with a history that suggests coronary artery disease, or myocardial ischemia. Emergency cardiac catheterization is the treatment of choice for patients with acute **ST-segment elevation myocardial infarction (STEMI)**, one of the two common forms of acute myocardial infarction.

Catheterization can be used to visualize either the right or left side of the heart as well as the coronary arteries. Stenosis, regurgitation, coronary artery occlusion, and ventricular ejection fractions can be identified. The information conveyed by a cardiac catheterization study can be critical in guiding clinical decision making.

▼ Refine the Differential Diagnosis

The history, physical exam, and 12-lead ECG will identify 80% to 90% of the diagnoses with the presentation of chest pain. So far, you have identified those life-threatening causes of chest pain that are initially suggested in the primary survey when the patient is complaining of pain with obvious shortness of breath and/or signs of shock.

For those patients whose conditions are more stable, or for those conditions that cause fewer cardinal signs and symptoms, a more detailed history with the secondary exam will aid you.

When you are obtaining the patient's history, the following key findings may help narrow down the list of possible diagnoses:

- *Character of the pain.* Crushing or pressure-like versus tearing should lead you to think ACS versus thoracic aortic aneurysm. Those with sharp pain can be suffering from a pulmonary embolism, pneumothorax, or a musculoskeletal cause. The complaint of burning or indigestion may lead you to think of gastrointestinal (GI) complaints.
- *Activity with pain.* Pain with exertion is usually indicative of ACS. If at rest, MI is suggested. A sudden onset of pain usually points to aortic dissection, pulmonary embolism, or pneumothorax. Pain after meals may indicate GI problems.
- *The 0-to-10 pain scale.* Now universal. Obtain this information from your patient early in the course of assessment and management. Onset and peak of pain should also be noted, along with an ongoing assessment related to management.
- *Pain location.* Localized pain in a small area is usually somatic (the patient can point to it with one finger, and there's no radiation). Visceral pain, by comparison, is more difficult to localize (the patient circles the chest with his or her hand and talks about referral of pain). Peripheral chest wall pain is usually not cardiac in nature.
- *Radiation of pain.* Radiation into the back may guide you toward aortic dissection or GI causes. Pain located near the scapular area of the back and radiating into the neck suggests aortic dissection as well. Inferior MI may present as thoracic back pain. Any radiation of pain to the jaw, arms, or neck usually points toward cardiac ischemia.
- *Duration of pain.* Very short-lived (measured in seconds) pain is rarely cardiac in nature. Pain that begins suddenly and is described as being worst at the onset is many times aortic dissection. Pain that may begin with exertion but goes away with rest may be cardiac ischemia. Pain that is constant and lasts for days is less commonly life threatening. Pain that is intermittent and fluctuates is more likely serious.
- *Aggravation/alleviation.* Pain that worsens with exertion and improves with rest is usually coronary ischemia. Pain related to meals is associated with GI problems. Pain that worsens with deep breath or cough is generally tied to pulmonary, pericardial, or musculoskeletal problems.

Associated symptoms with chest pain include the following:

- *Diaphoresis*: serious or visceral causes
- *Hemoptysis*: pulmonary embolism
- *Syncope or syncopal feeling*: cardiovascular cause or pulmonary embolism
- *Dyspnea*: cardiovascular or pulmonary causes
- *Nausea and vomiting*: cardiovascular or GI causes

▼ Ongoing Management

Ongoing management of the patient's condition is accomplished en route to the hospital. Repeat the primary assessment. Vital signs should be obtained every 5 minutes for critical patients or every 15 minutes for those patients who are determined to be in stable condition. The physical exam should be repeated to note any changes that have occurred or if any conditions were missed in the initial exam. Assess the effectiveness of your interventions.

Choosing the appropriate method of transport for a patient with ACS should be directed at the needs of the patient. First you must decide whether the patient is critically ill and determine which modes of transportation the patient can tolerate and which facility is best suited for the patient. A chest pain center should be a consideration for patients with ACS. Altitude changes and the stress of flight can increase myocardial demand, so the patient should be closely monitored and supported. Decreasing the transport time to the appropriate facility can serve as a benefit to air transport. Patients with support devices may need additional space and teams for transport. This should be prepared for prior to transport to eliminate delays.

Initial Life-Threatening Causes of Chest Pain

Life-threatening conditions associated with chest discomfort that require immediate treatment include tension pneumothorax, pulmonary embolism, esophageal rupture, aortic dissection, cardiac tamponade, arrhythmia, and acute coronary syndromes (including CHF/APE). Some of these conditions are seen in the primary survey as chest discomfort with respiratory distress, chest discomfort with altered vital signs, or a combination of those three chief complaints/cardinal signs and symptoms.

Tension Pneumothorax

Tension pneumothorax is a life-threatening condition that results from a progressive deterioration and worsening of a simple pneumothorax (the accumulation of air in the pleural space). If allowed to continue, a tension pneumothorax can cause a mediastinal shift, putting pressure on the heart and great vessels and disrupting blood flow. Increased intrathoracic pressure will impede venous return, decreasing preload and leading to a drop in systemic blood pressure.

Pathophysiology

A tension pneumothorax is the most serious type of pneumothorax; it occurs when the pressure in the pleural space is greater than the atmospheric pressure. The increased pressure arises due to trapped air in the pleural space or entering air from a positive-pressure mechanical ventilator. The force of the air can cause the affected lung to collapse completely and shift the heart toward the uncollapsed lung (mediastinal shift), compressing the unaffected lung and heart.

Signs and Symptoms

In the patient with increased work of breathing, unilateral absence or decreased breath sounds suggest a pneumothorax. If shock is also present, a tension pneumothorax has to be immediately recognized and treated. Assessment of a tension pneumothorax will reveal chest discomfort, severe respiratory distress, decreased or absent breath sounds on the affected side, and obstructive shock. Jugular venous distention (JVD) and tracheal deviation can be seen as well but are sometimes difficult to find and are late signs.

Differential Diagnosis

The differential diagnosis should include the following:

- Acute coronary syndrome
- Acute respiratory distress syndrome
- Aortic dissection
- Congestive heart failure and pulmonary edema
- Esophageal rupture and tears
- Myocardial infarction
- Pericarditis and cardiac tamponade
- Pulmonary embolism
- Rib fracture

Treatment

Treatment is aimed at relieving the pressure inside the chest by decompressing the affected side. For most cases, that would mean a needle decompression, accomplished by placing a large-bore (12- to 14-gauge), long (3-inch) needle (for adolescents and adults) in the second intercostal space in the midclavicular line. An alternative location for needle thoracostomy is the fourth or fifth intercostal space in the midaxillary line. However, this site is more difficult to access in immobile and obese patients. In addition, if prehospital decompression can be accomplished via the anterior chest wall, the subaxillary area remains intact for location of landmarks and insertion of a chest tube. Some experts recommend this location because there is less risk for injury to the great vessels in the chest. This will provide a temporizing measure until a chest tube can be placed. See Chapter 2 for more information on pneumothoraces and treatment.

Pulmonary Embolism

Pulmonary embolism (PE) falls into the general category of venous thromboembolism, which includes both deep venous thrombosis (DVT) and pulmonary embolism. A thrombus can form when the fine balance between clot development and clot breakdown is affected. Many factors can create an imbalance toward clot formation, such as malignancy, immobility, and medications such as oral contraceptive pills. In this condition, a vessel injury or sluggish blood flow in large vessels causes a fibrin formation or clot; when this clot forms in a deep vein, a DVT is present.

Pathophysiology

Pulmonary embolism occurs when a clot that has formed in those deeper veins (even weeks earlier) is dislodged and travels through the venous system (embolism), goes through the heart, and lodges in the pulmonary arteries. In the United States, 200,000 to 300,000 persons are hospitalized each year with PE. Up to one-third of these individuals will die. Pulmonary embolism is almost always associated with the presence of risk factors. Strong risk factors include hip or leg fracture, hip or knee replacement, major general surgery, and trauma and spinal cord injury. Moderate risk factors include arthroscopic knee surgery, chemotherapy (which may cause hypercoagulation), CHF or respiratory failure, use of oral contraceptives, and prior venous thromboembolism.

One European study reported that more than one-third of PEs may go undiagnosed in the emergency department. Delayed or missed diagnoses are more common in patients with complex clinical presentations and/or history including coronary artery disease, COPD, asthma, or heart failure relative to the patient's exhibiting signs and symptoms and the more typical risk factor of prior immobilization or recent surgery.

Signs and Symptoms

The initial symptoms of DVT may be quite subtle and may be limited to pain or discomfort only, without outward signs of inflammation. Patients will typically present with unexplained sudden onset of dyspnea or chest pain in the absence of trauma. At times, local inflammation is obvious, and you can act quickly to help prevent the movement of the clot into the central circulation.

The most frequent symptoms of PE include dyspnea, pleuritic chest pain, cough, palpitations, anxiety, and hemoptysis accompanied by tachycardia, tachypnea, and/or swelling of the legs. Nonpleuritic chest pain is also possible. Patients with PE will normally have clear lungs on exam. If the clot occupies a large portion of the vessel, and blood flow to that portion of the lung is compromised, an infarction will occur, and symptoms will be evident. There may be sharp, localized pain that increases with a deep breath or cough (pleuritic) and leads to subsequent "splinting" of the patient's breathing.

Ninety percent of all patients with PE (noninfarcting and infarcting) will have dyspnea, sometimes intermittently. This occurs when there is air going in and out, but blood flow to certain areas of the lung is redirected so the air is not being used. This is called a *ventilation-perfusion ($\dot{V}/\dot{Q}$) mismatch* or *dead space ventilation*. If there is hypoxia and no apparent physiological explanation, PE must be considered.

About half of all patients with PE will have tachycardia. This can be driven by a response to hypoxia or to hypotension from poor left ventricular filling. Computed tomography

(CT), echocardiogram, or electrocardiogram (ECG—classically $S_1Q_3T_3$) may show a strain pattern due to increased pulmonary artery pressures. About 10% of PE patients present with hypotension, which suggests a poor prognosis. The patient will be hemodynamically unstable if one of the main branches of the pulmonary artery is occluded with a saddle embolus, and cardiac arrest will usually present with pulseless electrical activity.

Elements of patient history that suggest PE include an acute onset of shortness of breath, light-headedness or syncope, chest pain, dry cough, and unexplained tachycardia. Pulmonary infarction presents similarly to pneumonia, but high fever is usually found only in pneumonia. An acute onset of chest pain and hemoptysis in the same day suggest the possibility of a PE. There may be unilateral swelling of the leg and risk factors for DVT. Careful history taking and consideration of risk factors are especially important for patients with suspected PE because assessing clinical probability prior to advanced diagnostic testing is an essential element in establishing a diagnosis of PE. A recent study suggests that patients with prior histories of COPD or asthma are more likely to be misdiagnosed when presenting with a PE. An increased index of suspicion by the provider and enhanced readiness for sudden deterioration of the patient might be useful in this context.

Differential Diagnosis

There are many differential diagnoses for PE, and they should be considered carefully with any patient thought to have a PE. These patients also should have an alternative diagnosis confirmed, or PE should be excluded, before you conclude your evaluation. Additional problems to be considered include the following:

- Musculoskeletal pain
- Pleuritis
- Pericarditis
- Hyperventilation

The following procedures should be done to confirm a diagnosis of PE:

1. A 12-lead ECG should be completed as soon as feasible. In patients with chest pain or shortness of breath, this is critical to evaluate for alternative diagnoses. The most common ECG finding in PE is sinus tachycardia. Other findings suggestive for PE, which are seen in the minority of cases, are related to pulmonary hypertension and RV strain. These include a prominence of S wave in lead I, Q wave in lead III, and T-wave inversion in lead III ($S_1Q_3T_3$; **Figure 3-7**).

A constellation of symptoms along with ECG findings is called the *McGinn-White sign*. This sign includes the following:

- A Q wave and late inversion of the T wave in lead III
- Short ST intervals and T waves in lead II
- Inverted T waves in chest leads V_2 and V_3, the electrocardiographic evidence of right ventricular dilatation due to massive pulmonary embolism
- Clinical signs and/or history suggesting acute cor pulmonale
  One study and several case reports suggest that ECG changes in right-sided chest leads occur frequently in PE. These changes include ST elevation and a qr or qs pattern (prominent q waves) in one or more of leads V_4R, V_5R, and V_6R. However, while ECG findings are suggestive of PE, they are not sufficient to confirm a diagnosis of PE.

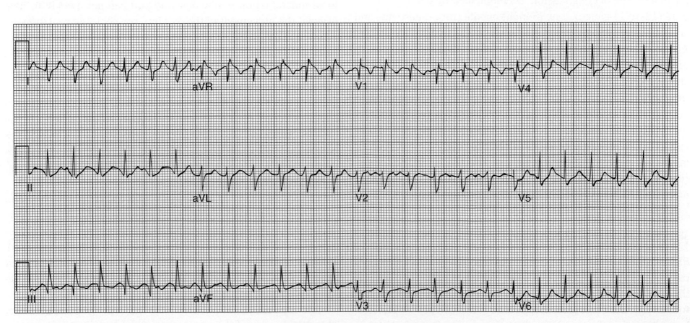

Figure 3-7 A 12-lead electrocardiogram with $S_1Q_3T_3$ pattern.

This article was published in *Rosen's emergency medicine: concepts and clinical practice*, ed 6, Marx JA, Hockberger RS, Walls RM. Copyright Mosby 2006.

2. Although a chest radiograph is unable to show a PE in the hospital setting, it is a necessary diagnostic tool to evaluate for other diagnoses that cause chest pain or shortness of breath. Findings on chest radiographs that are specific but not sensitive for PE include Hampton's hump (wedge-shaped, pleural-based triangular opacity that represents pulmonary infarction) and Westermark's sign (clearing of normal radiologic shadow of pulmonary tissue distal to a PE).

3. Other imaging procedures of value in diagnosing PE include echocardiography, computed tomography angiography (CTA), and V̇/Q̇ scans. An ultrasound of the heart that shows right ventricular strain is common in the case of a large PE. CTA may be used in some hospitals and is fast and about 90% sensitive. Ventilation/perfusion scans may also be employed where the patient inhales radionuclide while an injectable form is used to compare V̇/Q̇ mismatch.

4. Laboratory testing, like the standard chest radiograph in the hospital setting, is usually done to try to differentiate the many causes of chest pain and/or dyspnea. There is no one definitive blood test sensitive enough to diagnose PE. Clotting function tests are usually within normal limits; D-dimer is reasonably sensitive but nonspecific so not diagnostic if positive. While helpful in low-risk patients, D-dimer cannot be relied on for patients who are clinically at high risk for DVT or PE. Blood gas analyses can be done, but PE often fails to produce obvious abnormalities of pulmonary gas exchange.

Treatment

Prehospital Setting

In the prehospital setting, the patient with acute chest pain, dyspnea, and/or alteration in vital signs should have oxygen, vascular access, electronic monitoring, and a 12-lead ECG. Beginning standard therapy for acute coronary syndromes with aspirin is appropriate if the diagnosis is unclear. If the patient has been identified as having respiratory failure, airway control and ventilatory assistance are also required. Stabilization of vital signs may include administration of crystalloids and use of vasopressor infusion to combat obstructive shock.

In-Hospital Setting

Once the patient enters the hospital, appropriate diagnostic tests should be performed. Anticoagulation therapy may include low-molecular-weight heparin, which will reduce the possibility of new clot formation. Placement of a filter in the inferior vena cava will help trap any traveling emboli from moving superiorly. Persistent hypotension and tachycardia usually indicate a more difficult course of treatment and poor outcome. For a hemodynamically significant pulmonary embolism, thrombolytic therapy is a treatment option. In some patients, this therapy can achieve faster results than anticoagulation therapy, but

it must be balanced with the increased risk for bleeding. Surgical embolectomy requires a cardiothoracic surgeon and placing the patient on cardiopulmonary bypass. Catheter thrombectomy can be conducted in the interventional radiology suite of high-resource hospitals.

Esophageal Rupture

Spontaneous rupture or perforation of the esophagus results from a sudden increase in intraesophageal pressure combined with negative intrathoracic pressure, such as in severe straining or vomiting.

Pathophysiology

Chest pain with dyspnea may indicate esophageal rupture. When the esophagus is torn, gastric contents enter into the mediastinum, where an inflammatory infectious process ensues. The most common causes of esophageal perforation include iatrogenic injury from endoscopy or instrumentation, foreign bodies from poorly chewed food or sharp objects, caustic burns, blunt or penetrating trauma, spontaneous rupture (Boerhaave's syndrome from forceful vomiting), or postoperative complications.

Signs and Symptoms

Early clinical signs of esophageal rupture are vague. The patient may complain of pleuritic pain in the anterior part of the chest, and the pain may be worse with swallowing when the head and neck are flexed. Dyspnea and fever often accompany the chest pain as the infectious process worsens.

As air and GI contents enter the mediastinum, subcutaneous air will gather around the patient's chest and neck. Pneumomediastinum and pneumopericardium may be apparent on the chest radiograph. Auscultation of heart sounds may pick up Hamman's sign, in which a crunching sound is heard during systole. As the inflammatory process begins because of mediastinal contamination, sepsis, fever, and distributive shock will ensue. If the diagnosis is delayed for more than 24 hours, the patient's condition may deteriorate rapidly.

Differential Diagnosis

This is a rare condition, but you should consider an esophageal rupture in any patient initially seen with atypical chest or abdominal pain. The differential diagnosis may include, among other conditions, an abdominal aneurysm, ACS, pneumonia, and pulmonary embolism.

Treatment

Management of this life-threatening condition begins with your ability to recognize its signs and symptoms, including them in your differential diagnosis, and conducting a thorough history and physical exam. The patient will present with the previously described symptoms and have one of the common causes in his recent history. Routine treatment includes oxygen, vascular ccess, application of monitors, and obtaining a 12-lead ECG, chest radiograph, and laboratory analysis. Quickly initiating antibiotics, volume replacement, and airway maintenance are other important elements of prehospital treatment. A surgery consult should be obtained as soon as possible.

Acute Pulmonary Edema/Congestive Heart Failure

Pulmonary edema, an accumulation of fluid in the lungs, is often a consequence of congestive heart failure. Heart failure is a complication of nearly all forms of heart disease, both structural and functional; the ventricles are unable to fill or eject blood in adequate amounts to meet the body's needs.

Pathophysiology

Coronary artery disease is the most common underlying cause of CHF. Poor ventricular pumping function leads to an overall decrease in cardiac output (CO), and as more blood is left in the ventricle, pressure builds in the left or right heart circulatory pathways. If the left ventricle fails, the pressure in the pulmonary veins increases, and blood backs up into the lungs, leading to pulmonary edema with poor gas exchange. In the patient with chronic CHF, compensatory mechanisms work to redistribute blood to critical organs and adapt the body to diseased heart function. If the right side of the heart is also involved, blood backs up into the venae cavae, causing congestion of the venous system, which may present as pedal edema, JVD, or sacral edema.

Signs and Symptoms

The signs and symptoms of pulmonary edema/congestive heart failure include dyspnea, fatigue, exercise intolerance, and fluid retention that can lead to pulmonary and peripheral edema. A patient with this condition typically has a combination of chest pain and increased work of breathing. In your primary survey, you may note crackles in the lung fields, often starting in the bases and moving progressively upward with increased severity. A quick assessment of circulation can help you pinpoint the problem, especially if cardiogenic shock is also present.

When you arrive on scene, the patient may be having an MI and have signs of shock with pulmonary edema due to acute systolic dysfunction. Note whether the patient is sitting upright (due to orthopnea), working hard to breathe, and reports chest tightness or discomfort. Look for signs of poor perfusion (weak distal pulses, cool skin, delayed capillary refill, poor urinary output, and acidosis). Systemic and pulmonary congestion will also be present—tachypnea, labored breathing, bilateral crackles (possibly with wheezing ["cardiac asthma"]), pale or cyanotic skin, hypoxemia, and sometimes frothy, blood-tinged sputum.

Differential Diagnosis

A differential diagnosis may include congestive heart failure due to high blood pressure, aortic or mitral valve disease, or cardiomyopathy. Pulmonary edema may be caused by an MI, lung infections, extensive burns, or liver or kidney disease.

Treatment

Prehospital Setting

In the prehospital setting, standard protocols for acute coronary syndromes should be followed if they appear to be the cause of the CHF and pulmonary edema. Care should focus on lowering the patient's blood pressure. Oxygen, vascular access, and monitors should be applied, and a 12-lead ECG should be acquired to evaluate for evidence of an AMI.

Management of heart failure focuses on improving gas exchange and CO. If the patient's blood pressure is adequate (systolic blood pressure > 100 mm Hg), help the patient get into a comfortable position. Many times this can be done with the patient sitting with legs dependent (dangling). Supplemental oxygen should be provided as tolerated. Oxygen saturations above 90% are desired, so you should evaluate the patient for possible ventilatory assistance. If there are signs of respiratory failure along with altered mental status, intubation and invasive pulmonary ventilation will be necessary. If the patient is alert enough, noninvasive positive-pressure ventilation (NIPPV) can be therapeutic in the following two ways: (1) by decreasing venous return and preload, thereby reducing pulmonary edema, and (2) by improving gas exchange. The use of positive end-expiratory pressure, NIPPV, continuous positive airway pressure (CPAP), and bilevel positive airway pressure is explained in Chapter 2. One study regarding the use of CPAP in the treatment of heart failure concluded that prehospital use of CPAP in this context decreases the need for endotracheal intubation, improves vital signs during transport to the hospital, and reduces short-term mortality. Furthermore, another study noted that an Fio_2 of only 28% to 30% improves outcomes of patients in acute pulmonary edema from congestive heart failure.

Along with positive-pressure ventilation, nitroglycerin has emerged as the primary treatment of pulmonary edema if the systolic blood pressure is above 100 mm Hg. This drug acts to decrease preload through peripheral vasodilation. Caution must be exercised when employing these strategies simultaneously; systemic blood pressure can drop quickly. Patients with subacute CHF who also experience volume overload may be given furosemide to initiate diuresis. Diuretics, however, have fallen out of favor for use in the prehospital setting because many patients with crackles on exam are later found to have pneumonia. Diuresis in this group of patients can be detrimental. In addition, many of those who do have CHF are not experiencing total body fluid overload; the fluid is not distributed correctly. Diuresis can be detrimental in these patients because many have existing poor renal function.

Although not typically used in the prehospital setting, angiotensinconverting enzyme inhibitors and beta-blockers are recommended for all levels of the New York Heart Association/ American College of Cardiology classification scale for congestive heart failure. An aldosterone antagonist is added when a patient's ejection fraction remains below 35% despite treatment with ACE inhibitors and beta-blockers.

If your patient's chest pain is complicated by low blood pressure, cardiogenic shock, and dyspnea, vasoactive medications to improve the blood pressure will also be necessary. Dobutamine and norepinephrine (in the field) and milrinone (in hospital settings) may be given to help increase blood pressure and inotropy/chronotropy. Studies suggest that greater longer-term mortality is associated with longer regimens of pressors. Some patients with APE may be found to have abnormal heart sounds indicating mitral regurgitation due to a ruptured papillary muscle or chorda. These patients are in immediate need of a cardiothoracic surgeon.

In-Hospital Setting

In the in-hospital setting, patients require aggressive treatment while a history, physical exam, chest radiograph, and laboratory assessment are completed. If not already performed, a 12-lead ECG should also be done. Arterial and/or venous blood sampling will help evaluate the patient's ability to oxygenate and ventilate. Besides a routine laboratory analysis, brain natriuretic peptide elevation can be useful to help diagnose CHF in unclear cases. These peptides are released when there is stretch in the ventricular muscle. Cardiac enzymes should also be ordered to help evaluate for myocardial injury.

In the intensive care setting, left- and right-sided hemodynamic monitoring can help evaluate the various pressures throughout the heart, along with treatment effectiveness. This type of monitoring can inform decision making as to whether pharmacologic intervention will likely be sufficient or whether some combination of pharmacologic and mechanical intervention might be necessary. Aquapheresis may help remove fluid overload without major derangements in electrolytes. Morphine has historically been used to treat acute CHF but has become controversial owing to studies that show increased mortality in the group of patients with CHF receiving morphine, possibly as a result of depression of the respiratory drive and hypotension.

In conjunction with the medical management discussed, an intra-aortic balloon pump will help reduce afterload and may improve overall perfusion. Patients with ejection fractions of less than 30% and a life expectancy of greater than 6 months may receive implanted intracardiac devices including left ventricular assist devices and biventricular assist devices. Less invasive biventricular pacemakers have been shown to improve quality of life, functional status, and exercise capacity, but they do not affect mortality or morbidity.

Cardiac Arrhythmia

Noting an arrhythmia, or lack of cardiac rhythm, early may help diagnose and speed up treatment of a major cause of chest pain. An arrhythmia may cause chest discomfort and can be life threatening if cardiac output is too low.

Pathophysiology

If the heart rate becomes too slow, cardiac output (known as "Q," or the measure of cardiac output in 1 minute) will decrease. Depending on the effectiveness of the body's compensatory mechanisms, blood pressure may also drop, causing a decrease in coronary artery perfusion. If the heart rate is too fast, Q may decrease as the chambers of the heart are not allowed adequate time to fill. This decreases Q, dropping blood pressure and impairing cardiac function. If the coronary arteries are diseased, the increased workload on the heart may precipitate angina. The cardiogenic shock caused in either case may lead to acute pulmonary edema, causing shortness of breath. Treatment is aimed at control of the heart rate, which will lead to improved pump function. Improving pump function will increase Q and raise blood pressure.

Signs and Symptoms

A patient who is experiencing an arrhythmia may have the following signs and symptoms:

- Chest pain
- Shortness of breath
- Syncope
- Dizziness of light-headedness
- Rapid or irregular heartbeat

Differential Diagnosis

A 12-lead ECG may confirm your suspicion of a cardiac arrhythmia.

Treatment

As the primary survey is being conducted, monitors should be applied by your team to obtain continuous vital signs and evaluate for arrhythmia or acute myocardial injury. For treatment of bradycardia and tachycardia, follow current ACLS guidelines and/or your protocols. The patient may also be experiencing an acute coronary syndrome. A 12-lead ECG and laboratory samples should be acquired early—as the oxygen is applied and vascular access is obtained. If bradycardia is causing the patient to become clinically unstable (chest pain, dyspnea, acute pulmonary edema, shock), measures should be implemented to increase the heart rate. This usually involves the use of medications such as atropine and/or vasoactive agents (epinephrine, dopamine) and/or application of a transcutaneous pacemaker. Care should be taken not to increase the rate excessively, however. Challenging the heart by causing a heart rate that is too high while the patient is experiencing ischemia could lead to myocardial injury.

For the patient with chest pain who is having tachycardia (150 or more beats/min) with a normal blood pressure (> 100 mm Hg systolic), treatment is based on the source of the pacemaker (supraventricular versus ventricular) and the type of arrhythmia present. If the rhythm is tachycardic and very irregular, poor valve function and stagnant blood flow may be present, creating an increased risk of clot formation. Caution must be exercised when encountering new-onset atrial fibrillation or multifocal atrial tachycardia. Medications are prescribed to regulate the heart rate, restore a normal rhythm, and prevent blood clot formation. Such medications help avoid a major change in rhythm that could cause a release of multiple clots into the circulation, with subsequent stroke or other related complications. When applicable, antidysrhythmic agents may also be administered appropriate to the potential pacemaker site. If the tachycardic patient has signs of alterations in mentation and evidence of cardiogenic shock, synchronized cardioversion may be necessary to immediately change the life-threatening rhythm.

Aortic Aneurysm and Dissection

The aorta is suspended from a fixed ligament, the ligamentum arteriosum, near the bifurcations or branches of the left subclavian artery. It has three layers—the intima, media, and adventitia. The middle or medial layer is made up of smooth muscle and some elastic tissue. Normal aging causes this layer to lose its elasticity and the intimal layer to weaken. If chronic hypertension is present, the deterioration is intensified. Some patients have congenital changes in their aorta that also decrease wall strength and hasten the degeneration of the aortic wall. Marfan and Ehlers-Danlos syndromes cause such changes.

Pathophysiology

If the aortic intima layer finally tears, high-pressure blood flow enters the medial layer. The amount of dissection depends on where this tear occurs, the degree of disease in the media layer, and blood pressure. This injury may move up or down the aorta and may extend back into the coronary arteries (usually right), pericardial sac, or pleural cavity. Control of blood pressure is a major factor in controlling the extension of the hematoma. The management approach depends on the location of the dissection—that is, whether it is in the ascending or descending aorta. Dissections in the ascending aorta are much more lethal.

Signs and Symptoms

Chest pain is the most common complaint, with patient descriptions such as "excruciating," "sharp," "tearing," or "ripping." If the patient indicates that the pain is located in the anterior part of the chest, the ascending aorta may be involved. Neck and jaw pain may be associated with injury to the aortic arch, and pain near the scapula may indicate dissection in the descending aorta. Auscultation of heart sounds may yield aortic regurgitation. Congestive heart failure and acute pulmonary edema may quickly develop. It is essential to look for the development of pericardial tamponade.

Tearing pain is usually associated with nausea, vomiting, a feeling of light-headedness, anxiety, and diaphoresis. Syncopal episodes are not common but may be the only presentation in some patients. A change in mental status may also occur.

Blood pressure may present in the following two ways:

1. Hypotension may indicate movement of the dissection into the pericardium, with tamponade or hypovolemia from rupture of the aorta.
2. Hypertension may indicate the catecholamine release associated with the event or, if hypertension continues despite therapy, extension of the dissection into the renal arteries.

Comparison of blood pressure in the right and left arms can indicate aortic branch (usually subclavian) injury. A significant decrease in blood pressure in one of the arms suggests aortic dissection. Neurologic symptoms may indicate injury to proximal aortic branches, which causes signs of stroke, or distal injury, which causes spinal cord signs and symptoms.

Differential Diagnosis

Suspicion of aortic dissection may result from your history taking and physical exam, but diagnostic studies are needed to confirm the differential diagnosis.

Diagnostic Studies

Recent American Heart Association (AHA) guidelines for thoracic aortic disease do not identify 12-lead ECG as a specific diagnostic modality for aortic aneurysm, but all patients with chest pain should receive a 12-lead ECG. Suspicion of a thoracic aortic event occurring simultaneously with new ST-segment elevation should not delay referral of a patient to a facility capable of providing percutaneous coronary intervention and reperfusion therapy. The following diagnostic procedures contribute to the establishment of a diagnosis of aortic aneurysm:

1. *Chest radiography.* A chest radiograph is usually completed on all patients presenting with chest pain. Of the radiographs obtained, 12% are normal, even with aortic dissections. A widened mediastinum may be seen, along with other subtleties that may or may not point the provider to this diagnosis.
2. *Echocardiography.* An echocardiogram can be obtained from two views—transthoracic (where aortic regurgitation may be seen) or transesophageal, which allows a good view of the thoracic aorta.
3. *Computed tomography angiography (CTA).* CTA is the primary diagnostic test chosen to find aortic dissection; the test uses iodinated IV contrast.
4. *Magnetic resonance imaging.* This is good at capturing the true image of an aortic dissection. However, it requires nonferrous equipment around the patient, and because of the prolonged time required for obtaining images, it is not helpful when the patient's condition is unstable.
5. *Angiography.* An angiogram can also be used for diagnosing and evaluating this condition.

Treatment

In general, follow your protocol for chest pain, even when you suspect an aortic dissection. Oxygen, vascular access, and application of monitors are routine. The use of antiplatelet therapy like aspirin in the aortic dissection that requires surgery is problematic but not contraindicated. Transporting the patient to a hospital with emergency cardiac capabilities is of high priority. Suspecting an aortic dissection and passing those signs and symptoms on to the in-hospital team may facilitate more rapid identification.

The most critical presentation of aortic dissection is the patient who presents with hypotension due to aortic rupture and/or pericardial tamponade. The patient needs to be resuscitated with IV crystalloids while preparing for surgery. Pericardiocentesis may afford the patient more time with slight improvements in CO until the definitive repair can be done in surgery.

In the patient who presents with hypertension, beta-blocker administration to decrease rate and strength of contractions is the most common management choice and may be combined with nitroprusside to decrease afterload and preload. Administration of labetalol is advantageous as it a dual alpha- and beta-receptor antagonist. AHA guidelines also emphasize the importance of pain control to blunt sympathomimetic increases in heart rate and blood pressure.

Pericardial Tamponade

The focus of the previous conditions described has been on the patient who presents with chest pain and increased work of breathing and/or chest pain and altered vital signs. One rare event that may present with chest pain, cough, or dyspnea is pericardial tamponade (also called *cardiac tamponade*).

Pathophysiology

Cardiac tamponade occurs when fluid accumulates inside the layered pericardial sac surrounding the heart itself. This causes compression forces around the heart, restricting its movement and causing subsequent obstructive shock. Although you may think of cardiac tamponade as a traumatic injury, many medical causes for this condition also exist (Table 3-2). The fluid that accumulates can come from cancerous lesions and exudate, pus, gas, blood, or a combination of factors. Rapidly accumulating fluid in a confining space usually brings on signs and symptoms very quickly with a minimal amount of fluid. The body space does not have time to compensate or adapt to the change in the environment. Slower-accumulating fluid in a body space allows for adaptation, with slower onset of signs and symptoms and a much larger amount of fluid within the space.

Signs and Symptoms

Generally three factors affect the presentation of cardiac tamponade—how quickly the fluid accumulated, the amount of fluid, and the health of the heart. When symptoms develop, the increased pericardial pressure has squeezed the heart and kept it from filling adequately, decreasing CO.

The signs and symptoms reflecting this squeezing are usually described as a series of three (triad), including hypotension (low CO), distended neck veins (high right-sided heart pressures), and muffled heart tones (fluid outside the heart). In a more subtle

Table 3-2 Most Common Causes of Cardiac Tamponade	
Infectious	Viral: very rare Bacterial: tuberculous, *Coxiella burnetii*, other (rare) Fungal: very rare Parasitic: very rare
Inflammatory and autoimmune	Systemic lupus erythematosus Behçet's syndrome Systemic vasculitides Pericardial injury syndromes: postmyocardial infarction, postpericardiotomy, posttraumatic
Neoplastic	Secondary metastatic tumors: lung cancer, breast cancer, lymphoma Primary tumors: very rare
Metabolic	Uremia (complication of kidney failure), myxedema
Hemopericardium	Postoperative (following sternotomy) Interventional cardiology: flutter ablation, pacemaker insertion Acute aortic dissection Traumatic: blunt or open thoracic injury

Reproduced from: Rodson L, Bouferrache K, Vieillard-Baron A. Cardiac tamponade, *Curr Opin Crit Care*. 17(5):416–424, 2011.

way (with slow accumulation), the patient may present with chest pain, cough, and dyspnea. Your evaluation may note jugular venous distention and muffled heart sounds, although these presentations are rare.

Other classic signs and symptoms that may indicate cardiac tamponade include the following:

- *Pulsus paradoxus, or paradoxical pulse.* Normally the systolic blood pressure decreases slightly with each inhalation. When the heart is being squeezed in tamponade, this decrease is exaggerated. **Pulsus paradoxus** is found when the pulse decreases in size or is nonpalpable during inhalation. Kussmaul's sign, an increase in jugular venous distention during inspiration, may be present as well. Kussmaul's sign is also a paradox. Listening to the heart sounds during inspiration, the pulse weakens or may not be palpable with certain heartbeats, while S_1 is heard with all heartbeats.
- *Dysphoria.* Restless body movements will be observed with unusual facial expressions, restlessness, or a sense of impending death, which has been reported to be present in as many as 26% of all patients with pericardial tamponade.

Differential Diagnosis

The differential diagnosis for cardiac tamponade is a challenge and may include tension pneumothorax or acute heart failure. The patient with cardiac tamponade will be presenting with a complaint of chest pain and dyspnea, possibly with a cough.

A high index of suspicion must guide you toward this diagnosis while reviewing the patient's risk factors for development of a medical cardiac tamponade. To narrow down the possible diagnoses, the following tests need to be performed:

1. *Chest radiography.* A chest radiograph will show a large heart if the fluid accumulated is 200 to 250 mL.
2. *ECG.* An ECG will show low amplitude (decreased voltage). Another diagnostic sign involving the ECG is called *electrical alternans*. This marker is highly specific for chronic pericardial tamponade and is rare in acute accumulation of pericardial fluid. The morphologic features and amplitude of the P waves, QRS complex, and ST-T waves in all leads will alternate in every other beat because of "swinging heart phenomenon," during which the normal heart swings back and forth with each contraction but returns to normal position before the next contraction. In pericardial tamponade, the heart is too heavy to swing back to a normal position in time, and the continuous ECG "sees" the heart out of position for one contraction (**Figure 3-8**).
3. *Echocardiography.* An echocardiogram shows pericardial effusion with RV collapse.
4. *Hemodynamic monitoring.* This monitoring will show that the right and left ventricular pressures are equal.

Treatment

The application of oxygen, gaining vascular access, and applying monitors are routine. Obtaining a 12-lead ECG is also necessary.

Electrical Alternans in Pericardial Tamponade

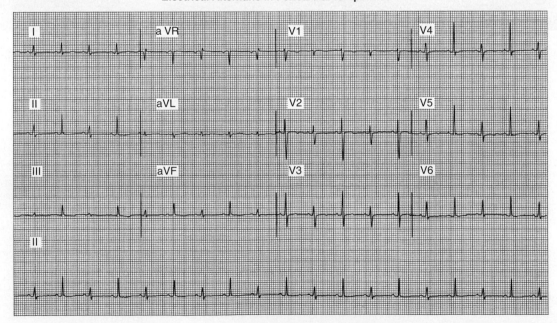

Figure 3-8 Cardiac tamponade. Electrical alternans may develop in patients with pericardial effusion and cardiac tamponade. Notice the beat-to-beat alternation in the P-QRS-T axis; this is caused by the periodic swinging motion of the heart in a large pericardial effusion. Relatively low QRS voltage and sinus tachycardia are also present.

From Goldberger A: *Clinical electrocardiography: a simplified approach,* ed 7, St. Louis, MO, 2006, Mosby.

Standard chest pain protocols in the prehospital setting are warranted, but signs of shock may prevent administration of morphine and nitrates.

If hypotension is present, fluid resuscitation with crystalloids for the obstructive shock state may initially help fill the right side of the heart and improve CO. Fluid administration to the normotensive patient can negatively impact patient hemodynamics and should be avoided. Isoproterenol is the preferred sympathomimetic for circulatory failure due to cardiac tamponade. These interventions serve as temporizing measures until the patient can undergo pericardiocentesis or rarely surgical pericardiotomy.

Figure 3-9 shows pericardiocentesis being used to remove blood from the pericardial sac. Enough fluid should be removed to improve the patient's condition. If tamponade recurs, the procedure may be repeated, and a catheter may be left in with a three-way stopcock. Surgical consultation is warranted if further drainage is required.

Acute Coronary Syndrome

Acute coronary syndrome (ACS) is a group of conditions that involve decreased blood flow to the heart muscle. These conditions often share the common underlying pathology of atherosclerosis. Atherosclerosis comes from the Greek words *athero* (meaning "gruel" or "paste") and *sclerosis* (meaning "hardness"). The "gruel" or "paste" in this case is made up of calcium, lipids, and fats, and is called *plaque*. As plaque clings to the walls of coronary arteries, it narrows the lumen, reducing the amount of blood (carrying nutrients and oxygen) reaching the heart muscle (**Figure 3-10**). The plaque may harden or remain soft.

Pathophysiology

When atherosclerosis occurs within the coronary arteries, it is referred to as *coronary artery disease (CAD)*. Patients with CAD are at increased risk for ACS. Certain risk factors place the patient at a greater risk for developing an ACS. More risk factors mean greater chance of developing ACS.

The risk factors that cannot be modified include age, sex, and heredity. The older you are, the more likely your chance of experiencing CAD. Men have CAD at an earlier age and are more likely to die of ACS. However, heart disease remains the leading cause of death in women, particularly after menopause. Estrogen in younger women is thought to have a cardioprotective effect, but after menopause, the incidence of ACS in men and women is similar. A family history of CAD increases your risk of developing ACS and may be directly linked to lifestyle. If your parents led a lifestyle of high risk for CAD, chances are you will as well.

Those risk factors that can be modified include hypertension, smoking, high cholesterol, diabetes, obesity, stress, and lack of physical activity. Hypertension is defined by the AHA as a blood pressure greater than 140/90 mm Hg, is easily diagnosed, and can usually be successfully managed with diet, exercise, and medications. Hypertension causes the heart to work harder than it should and, over time, causes it to enlarge and weaken. Smoking increases the risk of developing ACS. Smoking is the single most preventable cause of death in the United States. The risk of heart attack in smokers is more than twice that of nonsmokers. The nicotine and carbon monoxide in tobacco smoke reduce the amount of oxygen in the

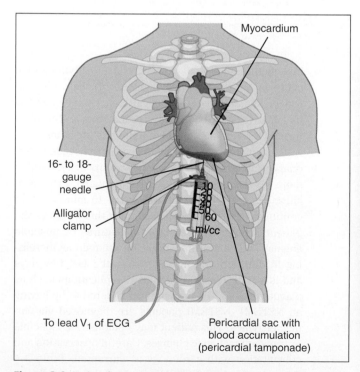

Figure 3-9 Pericardiocentesis to remove blood from the pericardial sac during tamponade.

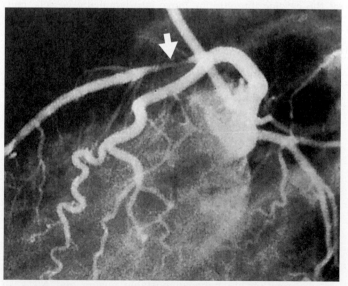

Figure 3-10 Coronary angiography shows stenosis (arrow) of left anterior descending coronary artery.

From Braunwald E: *Heart disease: a textbook of cardiovascular medicine*, ed 4, Philadelphia, PA, 1992, Saunders.

blood and damage blood vessel walls, causing plaque to build up. Tobacco smoke may trigger blood clots to form as well. Smoking promotes heart disease by reducing high-density lipoprotein ("good") cholesterol. Quitting smoking reduces your risk of having ACS even if you have smoked for years. High cholesterol is another easily diagnosed problem that can be managed with diet, exercise, and medications. A heart-healthy diet high in fruits and vegetables and low in fats and carbohydrates reduces low-density lipoprotein ("bad") cholesterol. Diabetes greatly increases the risk of heart disease. In fact, most people with diabetes die of some form of cardiovascular disease because diabetes is usually linked with low high-density lipoprotein ("good") cholesterol and high low-density lipoprotein ("bad") cholesterol levels. Diabetes also affects the blood vessels themselves, accelerating atherosclerosis. Many people with diabetes also have high blood pressure, increasing their risk even more. Obesity, stress, and lack of exercise accelerate the atherosclerotic process, increasing the chances of having ACS.

Current American Heart Association (AHA) guidelines define acute coronary syndrome as a continuum of angina, unstable angina/**non–ST-elevation myocardial infraction** (UA/**NSTEMI**) and STEMI.

Myocardial Infarction

Myocardial infarction is caused by a clot or thrombus that forms in a narrowed coronary artery where the plaque has ruptured, causing platelets to aggregate and a clot to form. If the coronary artery becomes completely obstructed, the ischemic cells in the heart muscle will begin to die. This can cause permanent damage to the heart muscle and is often referred to as a *heart attack.* As heart muscle dies, cardiomyocytes lose their cellular membrane integrity. Biomarkers of this necrosis transit the cardiac interstitium, move into lymphatic vessels, and subsequently move to small vessels of the cardiac circulation. As levels of these products build, they are measurable in the peripheral circulation.

Angina Pectoris

Angina pectoris literally means "chest pain" and is caused by an inadequate blood supply from a narrowed coronary artery filled with plaque. **Stable angina** pain usually comes on with exercise or stress and lasts 3 to 5 minutes, sometimes up to 15 minutes. Angina pain is relieved by rest and/or nitroglycerin. In and of itself, angina is a sign of serious heart disease and may lead to an AMI if it becomes unstable. If left untreated, unstable angina can lead to an AMI. The Canadian Cardiovascular Society (CCS) grading scale for angina is shown in Table 3-3.

- *UA/NSTEMI.* The AHA has formally identified the close relationship between unstable angina and NSTEMI in terms of identifying at-risk patients and delineating their care. Patients presenting with UA/NSTEMI exhibit ST-segment depression or prominent T-wave

Table 3-3 Grading of Angina Pectoris According to CCS Classification

Class	Description of Stage
I	"Ordinary physical activity does not cause . . . angina," such as walking or climbing stairs. Angina occurs with strenuous, rapid, or prolonged exertion at work or recreation.
II	"Slight limitation of ordinary activity." Angina occurs on walking or climbing stairs rapidly; walking uphill; walking or stair climbing after meals; in cold, in wind, or under emotional stress; or only during the few hours after awakening. Angina occurs on walking more than 2 blocks on the level and climbing more than 1 flight of ordinary stairs at a normal pace and under normal conditions.
III	"Marked limitations of ordinary physical activity." Angina occurs on walking 1 to 2 blocks on the level and climbing 1 flight of stairs under normal conditions and at a normal pace.
IV	"Inability to carry on any physical activity without discomfort—anginal symptoms may be present at rest."

CCS = Canadian Cardiovascular Society.

Reproduced from: Anderson JL, Adams CD, Antman EM, et al. 2012 ACCF/AHA focused update incorporated into the ACCF/AHA 2007 guidelines for the management of patients with unstable angina/non-ST-elevation myocardial infarction: A report of the American College of Cardiology Foundation/American Heart Association Task Force on Practice Guidelines, *Circulation.* 127(23) e663–e828, 2013.

inversion and/or the presence of positive cardiac necrosis biomarkers in a context of chest discomfort or anginal equivalent symptoms. Studies suggest that UA/NSTEMI commonly results from a thrombus formed through disruption of a preexisting atherosclerotic plaque and the consequences of subsequent coronary ischemia. Unstable angina occurs at rest and is more severe than prior episodes of angina. Prolonged chest discomfort (lasting more than 15 minutes) that continues at rest or chest discomfort that awakens the patient at night (nocturnal) are features of unstable angina. The patient may describe the pain as increasing in duration and intensity over the last few days and is at risk for more serious complications such as plaque rupture. The patient is considered to be having an NSTEMI. NSTEMI patients are diagnosed via cardiac enzymes. This patient may demonstrate ischemia or transient ischemic changes. Careful observation and consultation with cardiology is warranted. Table 3-4 lists causes of UA/NSTEMI. Each of these conditions ultimately results in a greater coronary oxygen demand

Table 3-4 Causes of UA/NSTEMI

Thrombus or thromboembolism, usually arising on disrupted or eroded plaque
- Occlusive thrombus, usually with collateral vessels
- Subtotally occlusive thrombus on preexisting plaque
- Distal microvascular thromboembolism from plaque-associated thrombus

Thromboembolism from plaque erosion
- Non–plaque-associated coronary thromboembolism

Dynamic obstruction (coronary spasm or vasoconstriction) of epicardial and/or microvascular vessels

Progressive coronary obstruction

Coronary arterial inflammation

Secondary UA

Coronary artery dissection

NOTE: Some patients have two or more causes of UA/NSTEMI.

Modified from Braunwald E. Unstable angina: an etiologic approach to management. Circulation 1998;98:2219–2222.

that can be provided by the patient's obstructed coronary vasculature. Consistent with your local protocol and medical direction, the patient should be transported to a facility capable of monitoring patients for ischemia via serial 12-lead EKG and serial cardiac biomarker studies.

- *STEMI.* ST-elevation myocardial infarction is diagnosed on the basis of symptoms characteristic of myocardial ischemia accompanied by persistent ST elevation and release of cardiac biomarkers confirmed by laboratory tests. In addition, new or presumably new left bundle-branch block in association with a patient presentation consistent with myocardial ischemia is considered a STEMI equivalent, but prior 12-lead electrocardiograms for comparison are frequently unavailable in the field setting. ST-segment depression in the precordial leads (V_1–V_4) may be indicative of a posterior wall MI, but direct assessment of posterior wall MI is possible utilizing leads V_7–V_9. Furthermore, right ventricular infarct (RVI), known to accompany inferior wall MI, can be assessed with right precordial leads, minimally V_4R. Right ventricular infarction or ischemia occurs in 30% to 50% of patients who present with an inferior wall AMI and usually results in right-sided heart failure and hypotension. These conditions can be exacerbated if nitrates or morphine are administered for the complaint of chest pain.

Signs and Symptoms

Healthcare providers receive frequent calls for the most common symptom associated with ACS—chest discomfort. Effective treatment for ACS is time sensitive, so it becomes important to recognize it quickly and provide essential treatment within the first hours of onset. Early intervention can reduce the likelihood of sudden cardiac death and/or myocardial damage. Quick recognition and diagnosis of an ACS starts with readily recognizing the signs and symptoms and obtaining a thorough history and physical exam.

The classic signs and symptoms of ACS include a sudden onset of chest pain or pressure located in the center of the chest beneath the sternum. This pain or pressure may feel like it is radiating to the neck or jaw and down the left arm. It is described as constant, usually lasting longer than 15 minutes. The patient may also complain of shortness of breath, as if the chest is in a vise or an elephant is sitting on the chest, making it difficult to breathe. Associated signs and symptoms include diaphoresis; pale, mottled, cool skin; and weakness or light-headedness. The patient may complain of feeling nauseated, may vomit, and may have a feeling of impending doom. The presence of crackles and rhonchi, with or without JVD, may be present with large infarcts, indicating the presence of CHF.

These classic signs and symptoms of ACS may all be present, or only a few may be present. Elderly persons, patients with diabetes, and postmenopausal women over 55 may present with no pain or discomfort, but instead present as though they are having a sudden onset of weakness. Women may also present with shortness of breath with or without chest discomfort. Nausea, vomiting, and back or jaw pain are also more common in women. Failure to recognize weakness as ACS may lead to the development of serious and life-threatening consequences. These alternate presentations are termed *anginal equivalent symptoms.*

You can organize your approach to the patient with chest discomfort using a SAMPLER history and the OPQRST mnemonic, as discussed in the AMLS assessment pathway.

After completion of the OPQRST and SAMPLER, you will be able to narrow down the differential diagnosis and determine whether your patient is experiencing an ACS and whether the cause is angina, unstable angina, or an AMI. For example, suppose a patient states that he was shoveling heavy snow and suddenly developed chest discomfort. The pain is substernal, constant, radiates to the neck, jaw, and down the arms. He is having difficulty breathing because he feels pressure like an elephant is sitting on his chest. When asked to rate his pain, he describes it as above a 10. The pain has lasted for about an hour and has not been relieved by rest or nitroglycerin. Chances are that he is having an AMI. You may not have completed a 12-lead ECG or have the ability to look at cardiac markers, but you can with some certainty develop the field impression of an AMI.

Differential Diagnosis

Importantly, the absence of a classic presentation should not falsely reassure you. For example, the presence of tenderness to palpation of the chest, a pleuritic component, or presence of a cough does not rule out a cardiac etiology to the pain. Patients with these symptoms should be taken seriously and evaluated for possible ACS depending on age and risk factors. Alternative diagnoses such as GERD and musculoskeletal pain are diagnoses of exclusion.

Pulse Oximetry

Pulse oximetry should be monitored for the presence of hypoxia as defined by the complaint of shortness of breath, increased work of breathing, tachypnea, and oxygen saturations of less than 95%. Administering oxygen in ACS is a high priority and is one of the few interventions that is known to improve the patient's outcome. Oxygen administration should not be delayed to obtain a pulse oximeter reading. Because a pulse oximeter reading is not real time, applying oxygen will not have an instantaneous effect on the number you see on the oximeter. Delaying oxygen administration in a hypoxic patient in need of oxygen is strongly discouraged.

12-Lead ECG

A heart monitor with 12-lead ECG capabilities should be placed on all patients with suspected ACS prior to giving medications for suspected ischemia (e.g., nitroglycerin, morphine). A 12-lead ECG should be immediately acquired on all patients with ischemic chest discomfort In fact, early prehospital recording of a 12-lead ECG and subsequent alerting of the receiving facility has been classified as a Class I intervention in the new 2015 AHA Guidelines. If STEMI is present, a STEMI alert should be called and the patient transported following local or internal guidelines. For patients with STEMI, the AHA advocates primary percutaneous coronary intervention (PPCI) within 90 minutes of first medical contact (FMC), but in any case, no greater than an interval of 120 minutes between FMC and reperfusion. The recommendations regarding fibrinolysis in the absence of a readily available PCI (<120 minutes) have grown complex, and providers should follow local guidelines. More detail is available in Chapter 9 of the 2015 ILCOR/AHA Guidelines. In general, in-hospital fibrinolysis is an acceptable alternative under some circumstances, but the estimated time of symptom onset and expected delay to PPCI drive decision-making. Medications may be administered en route to shorten on-scene times. Extended on-scene times do little more than increase the time to definitive therapy and reperfusion. In some circumstances, field evacuation by helicopter transport of a patient to a PCI-capable center should be considered.

Treatment

Knowing the location where the ischemia or injury is occurring in the heart and the expected complications associated with standard treatments will enhance your ability to provide the most appropriate treatments. As an example, you should suspect right ventricular infarction in patients with inferior wall infarction evidenced by elevated ST segments in leads II, III, and aVF. In patients with inferior wall infarction, the provider should obtain a right-sided ECG by placing the V leads on the left side of the chest to the right side of the chest. ST-segment elevation greater than 1 mm in lead V_4R is suggestive of right ventricular infarction (**Figure 3-11**). The RVI triad of hypotension, elevated jugular venous pressure, and clear lung fields may assist in the field diagnosis of RVI. Patients with acute right ventricular infarction are dependent on maintaining right ventricular filling pressure to maintain CO. Any medication that decreases preload—nitrates, diuretics, or other vasodilators (morphine,

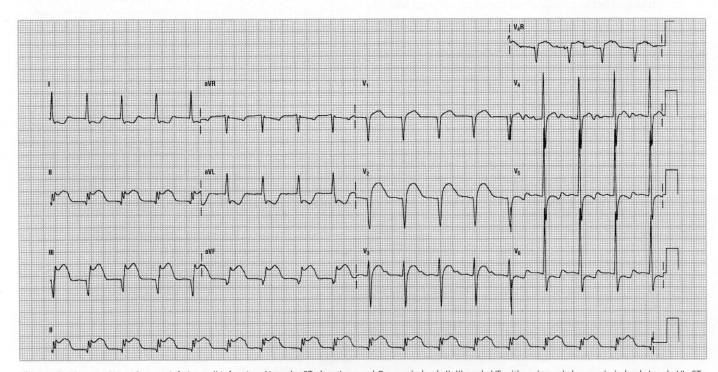

Figure 3-11 Acute RVI with acute inferior wall infarction. Note the ST elevations and Q wave in leads II, III, and aVF with reciprocal changes in in leads I and aVL. ST elevation in lead III exceeds that of lead II and is also seen in V_1–V_3 as a consequence of the RVI.

From *Introduction to 12-lead ECG: the art of interpretation*, ed 2, Courtesy of Tomas B. Garcia, MD.

ACE inhibitors)—should be avoided because it may cause severe hypotension. If your patient with suspected RVI is hypotensive, cautious fluid administration consistent with your local protocols and medical director guidance is appropriate.

Prehospital Setting

As a prehospital provider, you should be able to provide the following care for suspected ACS. Until you have the 12-lead ECG interpretation and determine the patient's level of risk, your initial management of ACS follows standard protocol. The common mnemonic *MONA* is often used to remember the interventions needed once the field impression of ACS has been determined. *MONA* stands for *morphine, oxygen, nitroglycerin,* and *aspirin.* It does not suggest a particular order of administering treatment or a particular importance of one over the other. Oxygen and aspirin are the only prehospital medications known to improve survival from ACS. Nitroglycerin is generally accepted to be a beneficial treatment for ACS, provided there is no RV involvement as described earlier. The use of morphine has been called into question in the context of UA/NSTEMI. Cautious administration of morphine sulfate remains a Class IIa recommendation for UA/NSTEMI and is the drug of choice for pain relief for patients with STEMI. Check with your medical director and review regional protocols for the medications preferred in your area. The following protocol is typical:

- Aspirin, 162 to 325 mg (2 to 4 baby aspirin), nonenterically coated, should be chewed and/or swallowed at the earliest sign of ACS. Make sure the patient is not allergic to acetylsalicylic acid, has no history of recent bleeding ulcers, and is not having an asthma attack. Patients with asthma may develop a condition known as "aspirin-induced asthma." When given aspirin, they may experience an asthma attack that occurs gradually but is more intense and difficult to break. Aspirin administration prior to PCI is a Class I AHA recommendation. All patients complaining of chest pain should receive aspirin unless they are allergic. The AHA is advocating that dispatchers give prearrival instructions to chew 162 to 325 mg of aspirin while awaiting arrival of prehospital EMS providers. Aspirin suppositories (300 mg) are safe and can be considered for patients with severe nausea, vomiting, or disorders of the upper GI tract.
- Oxygen should be administered to patients with breathlessness, signs of heart failure, shock, or an oxygen saturation less than 94%. If there are signs of hypoxia, oxygen should be administered at 10 to 15 L/min via nonrebreathing mask. If shortness of breath is severe or in the presence of acute pulmonary edema secondary to left-sided heart failure, oxygen should be administered with NIPPV/NPPV (CPAP or bilevel positive airway pressure), or at least using a bag-mask device to provide positive pressure. But, in the absence of these conditions, the recent ILCOR/AHA 2015 review fails to identify any benefit of oxygen administration to normoxic patients with suspected or confirmed acute coronary syndrome.

- Establish an IV of crystalloid prior to administration of nitroglycerin, though the IV can be deferred until after nitroglycerin administration if your patient has been administered the drug in the past without complications.

It is in the educational guidelines and the ACLS course to establish an IV for ACS, especially prior to giving nitroglycerin. Should the patient be suffering from a right ventricular MI or have taken an erectile dysfunction drug within 24 to 48 hours, the patient's blood pressure may bottom out and an immediate fluid bolus could be needed, or if the patient would arrest, starting an IV would be difficult.

- Nitroglycerin may be administered sublingually as a 0.4-mg tablet or metered-dose spray. It may be repeated every 3 to 5 minutes three times as long as systolic blood pressure remains above 90 mm Hg. AHA guidelines support 9-1-1 dispatchers advising patients who tolerate nitroglycerin to repeat nitroglycerin every 5 minutes, to a maximum of three doses, while awaiting arrival of EMS personnel. Administering nitroglycerin more than three times may be appropriate with medical direction as long as the blood pressure remains above 90 mm Hg. Nitroglycerin decreases the pain of ischemia by decreasing preload and cardiac oxygen consumption, and it dilates coronary arteries, increasing cardiac collateral flow. Nitroglycerin should be given in patients with ACS, ST-segment elevation or depression, and for the consequences associated with AMI, to include left ventricular failure (APE or CHF). Use with extreme caution in patients with right ventricular infarct, because these patients require adequate preload. Nitroglycerin should not be given to patients with hypotension, extreme bradycardias, or tachycardias. Do not administer nitroglycerin to patients who have taken a phosphodiesterase inhibitor (Viagra [sildenafil], Cialis [tadalafil], Levitra [vardenafil]) for erectile dysfunction within the last 24 to 36 hours. Nitroglycerin may lower the blood pressure in a patient whose vascular system is already dilated. Watch for headache, a drop in blood pressure, syncope, and tachycardia when nitroglycerin is given. The patient should sit or lie down during administration. An infusion of nitroglycerin may be started for more finite control of pain and blood pressure at 10 mcg/min. Titrate to relieve the pain by increasing the dose by 10 mcg every 3 to 5 minutes. Keep a close eye on the blood pressure; if not closely monitored, nitroglycerin infusion can lead to a dangerous drop in blood pressure.
- Consider morphine, 2 to 8 mg IV, titrated for discomfort not relieved by nitroglycerin in patients with STEMI. Morphine may be given once at 1 to 5 mg in a patient with STEMI whose discomfort is not relieved by oxygen and nitroglycerin. Be alert for a drop in blood pressure, especially in patients with volume depletion or if right ventricular infarction is apparent. Respiratory depression may occur, so Narcan (naloxone) should be available.

If the patient is allergic to morphine, other analgesics may be an option. Fentanyl is an option as a short-acting opioid with less effect on blood pressure than morphine. Check with your medical director and the scope of practice within your state for use of these medications.

- Prehospital administration of oral adenosine diphosphate (ADP) inhibitors to STEMI patients has been recognized as potentially valuable for STEMI patients as they are being transported to a receiving facility for PPCI. Studies have identified improved clinical outcomes after PPCI associated with early ADP inhibition. The prehospital setting has been identified as a reasonable setting for ADP inhibition, especially in the case of relatively short first medical contact to PPCI time intervals.

Prehospital administration of fibrinolytics is relatively uncommon in the United States, but out-of-hospital administration of fibrinolytics to patients with STEMI has been shown to be effective in the United States, Europe, and elsewhere. A series of studies suggest that prehospital fibrinolysis may lower mortality rates relative to PCI. Services offering out-of-hospital fibrinolytics require a strict adherence to protocols, 12-lead ECG acquisition and interpretation, experience in ACLS, the ability to communicate with the receiving institution, and a medical director with experience in management of STEMI. A continuous quality improvement process to evaluate all calls where fibrinolytics are used is required. Most EMS services have short enough transport times that they focus on early diagnosis with 12-lead ECG, completing a fibrinolytic checklist, administering first-line medications, and advance notification of the receiving facility to prepare for cardiac catheterization. Selecting the proper fibrinolytic requires a thorough understanding of their properties and complications. The inability to obtain a chest radiograph in the field to determine the presence of a widened mediastinum indicating an aneurysm is another reason for not considering prehospital fibrinolytics. However, in systems where prehospital fibrinolysis is a standard component of the system of care for a STEMI patient, and the alternative is hospital administration of fibrinolytic agents due to delayed or nonavailability of PPCI, prehospital administration of fibrinolytics is reasonable when the transport time exceeds 30 minutes.

In-Hospital Setting

After initial field stabilization of patients diagnosed with STEMI, administration of one or more of the following medications is not uncommon:

- *Unfractionated heparin.* When used as adjunctive therapy with fibrin-specific lytic agents in STEMI, current recommendations call for a bolus dose of 50–70 units/kg followed by infusion at a rate of 12 units/kg/h. While most ground services will not be infusing heparin drips, some are giving a bolus in STEMI confirmed by history and 12-lead ECG. Local protocol, physician medical director involvement, and scope of practice within your state will determine if such treatment is appropriate for your service.

- *Beta-receptor antagonist administration.* These ç which include metoprolol and carvedilol, are indicated for all patients without relative or absolute contraindications of heart failure or reduced cardiac output, prolonged first-degree or high-grade AV block, and/or reactive airway disease. A meta-analysis encompassing over 73,000 patients has confirmed that beta-blocker administration within the first 12 hours of presentation of ACS is associated with significant reduction in ventricular tachyarrhythmias, reinfarction and stroke, as well as an overall decrease in mortality. Contraindications to beta-blockers are moderate to severe left ventricular failure and pulmonary edema, bradycardia, hypotension, signs of poor peripheral perfusion, second-degree or third-degree heart block, and asthma. Some jurisdictions may utilize metoprolol, atenolol, propranolol, esmolol, and labetalol in the field critical care setting. Paramedics should follow their local protocol. Vital signs should be taken between doses to ensure heart rate and blood pressure remain adequate. Sometimes once discomfort is relieved, the catecholamine release stops. If IV beta-blockers are in the patient's system, the patient then becomes hypotensive, and the condition may worsen. Be prepared to treat this reaction with an IV fluid bolus. Local protocol, physician medical director involvement, and scope of practice within your state will determine if such treatment is appropriate for your service.

- *ACE inhibitors, including lisinopril and captopril.* These medications are indicated for oral administration to all patients with STEMI without the contraindications of hypotension, renal failure, and hyperkalemia. In addition to their known effects of lowering blood pressure, ACE inhibitors are thought to minimize destructive changes associated with left ventricular remodeling after MI and thwart plaque disruption by minimizing vessel endothelium apoptosis. A large-scale registry study determined that ACE inhibitors are significantly associated with reduced 6-month mortality in patients with both obstructive and nonobstructive CAD.

Non–Life-Threatening (Emergent) Causes of Chest Pain

All complaints of chest discomfort or those patients presenting atypically with the associated signs and symptoms of an ACS should be assessed first for the presence of an ACS. After initial evaluation, if ACS appears less likely, other differential diagnoses must be investigated (Table 3-5).

Some emergent diagnoses include unstable angina, coronary spasm or Prinzmetal's angina, cocaine-induced chest pain, infection (myocarditis, pericarditis), simple pneumothorax (see Chapter 2), and GI causes such as esophageal tear, cholecystitis, and pancreatitis (see Chapter 6).

Table 3-5 Causes of Chest Discomfort: Differential Diagnoses

- Acute coronary artery occlusion
- Pulmonary embolism
- Coronary artery dissection (often in association with thoracic aortic dissection)
- Uncontrolled hypertension
- Coronary artery spasm
- Coronary artery embolism (secondary to atrial myxoma, platelet thrombi, valvular vegetation, etc.)
- Gastrointestinal diseases
  - Acute gastritis
  - Acute pancreatitis
  - Acid reflux, esophagitis
  - Peptic ulcer disease
  - Boerhaave's syndrome
- Pneumonia, pleuritic
- Viral myocarditis/pericarditis
- Systemic vasculitis with coronary artery involvement
- Toxic exposure (cyanide or carbon monoxide, for example)
- Anemia or red blood cell dysfunction (sickle cell, for example)
- Shock (hypovolemic or septic)
- Cardiac arrhythmias
- Structural abnormalities of the heart (congenital or acquired)

Coronary Spasm or Prinzmetal's Angina

A coronary spasm is a sudden narrowing of a coronary artery that deprives the heart muscle of blood and oxygen. A coronary spasm is also known as "variant angina" or "Prinzmetal's angina."

Pathophysiology

Prinzmetal's angina results in chest pain at rest and is caused by coronary artery vasospasm. Although both men and women can experience Prinzmetal's angina, it is more common in women in their 50s. People with Prinzmetal's angina have an increased risk of experiencing ventricular dysrhythmias, myocardial infarction, heart block, or sudden death.

Signs and Symptoms

Patients with this condition may show little adjustment in their vital signs. Some patients will have significant CAD, whereas others will not. Severe pain usually occurs while the person is resting at night or during the morning hours. The spasms may occur in cycles, with periods of no pain following an episode of pain.

Differential Diagnosis

Because this condition is difficult at times to differentiate from STEMI and AMI, typical categorization, triage, and management should occur.

Treatment

This chest pain may be relieved with rest or nitrates. ECG changes are noted, with ST-segment elevation that looks similar to an AMI.

Cocaine Use

Cocaine or crack cocaine can be taken into the body in various forms. The dangerous consequences to the heart are well documented.

Pathophysiology

Cardiac toxicity occurs because of the direct effect on the heart with an increase in heart rate, blood pressure, and ventricular contractility (beta effect), resulting in increased myocardial oxygen demand. Additionally, there is a decrease in coronary artery blood flow, and a high risk for coronary vasospasm ensues (alpha effect). In fact, coronary vasospasm is thought to be the primary cause of cocaine-induced MI.

Signs and Symptoms

Patients who are abusing cocaine will show signs of agitation and have dilated pupils. Although crack cocaine is smoked, the patient will exhibit many of the same signs and symptoms as a person who has taken the powdered form—aggressiveness, paranoia, and antisocial behavior.

Differential Diagnosis

Diagnoses may include toxicity from other drugs (e.g., barbiturates, benzodiazepines, or alcohol), anxiety disorders (e.g., a panic attack), and depression.

Treatment

First-line treatment for cocaine-induced arrhythmias and hypertensive episodes is usually benzodiazepine administration, which tempers the effects of cocaine on the central nervous system and cardiovascular system. A recently published registry study of over 900 cocaine-positive patients showed them to be younger, male, and as a group exhibiting higher rates of STEMI and cardiogenic shock. Cocaine-positive patients with ACS were also less likely to exhibit multivessel coronary artery disease. Benzodiazepines should be added to the standard ACS management protocols. Because of the risk associated with cocaine, use of fibrinolytics is considered high risk. Beta-blockers are contraindicated, as the resultant unopposed alpha effect can precipitate dangerous hypertensive states and/or coronary vasospasm. Keep in mind also that chronic cocaine/crack use accelerates atherosclerotic disease, so patients at younger ages than normal may be at risk for ACS.

Pericarditis

Pericarditis is an inflammation of the pericardium or pericardial sac. It may be acute—with a 48-hour duration—or chronic, lasting longer and returning frequently.

Pathophysiology

Pericarditis is usually caused by a virus but may be caused by rheumatic heart disease, tuberculosis, leukemia, acquired immunodeficiency syndrome (AIDS), or cancer. Often the cause is unknown. The discomfort of pericarditis differs from ACS. It is often described as a dull ache that increases in intensity gradually over several days.

Signs and Symptoms

Patients with pericarditis may find it difficult to lie flat and may lean forward or be propped up on pillows to make breathing easier (nocturnal dyspnea) while sleeping. Pain may increase on inspiration. Lungs will be clear, with no JVD or pedal edema early. Additional symptoms may include fever, weakness, fatigue, malaise, and pericardial friction rub. If a pericardial effusion is developing as a result of the pericarditis, you might hear the friction rub or pulsus paradoxus. A chest radiograph may show an enlarged cardiac silhouette due to pericardial effusion, and the 12-lead ECG will demonstrate global ST-segment elevation in almost every lead (**Figure 3-12**). Lab studies may show an elevated erythrocyte sedimentation rate, a test that indirectly measures inflammation in the body, and an elevated white blood cell count (WBC), which may indicate the presence of an infection.

Differential Diagnosis

It is difficult to distinguish pericarditis from an acute myocardial infarction. The patient's history and physical exam will help you narrow down the possible diagnoses.

Treatment

Management is aimed at relieving discomfort with analgesics and nonsteroidal antiinflammatory drugs (NSAIDs). Corticosteroids and antimicrobials may be prescribed as well, but they are not initially given in the prehospital or emergency department setting until the definitive cause is known. The patient with pericarditis requires continued monitoring, as more serious cases may develop pericardial tamponade.

Myocarditis

Myocarditis is defined as inflammation of the myocardial layer of the heart.

Pathophysiology

Often undiagnosed clinically, this inflammation is usually caused by a virus (Coxsackie B enterovirus, adenovirus) in the summer months. The 1/3 rule applies to the prognosis of this disease: 1/3 recover without consequences, 1/3 have chronic cardiac dysfunction, and 1/3 progress to have chronic heart failure and need a heart transplant, or they die.

Signs and Symptoms

The patient may present with an influenza-like illness including fever, fatigue, myalgia, vomiting, and diarrhea. Then signs of myocarditis ensue—fever, tachycardia, and tachypnea, with 12% of patients complaining of chest pain. The ECG may show low voltage with a prolonged QT interval, AV block, or AMI patterns.

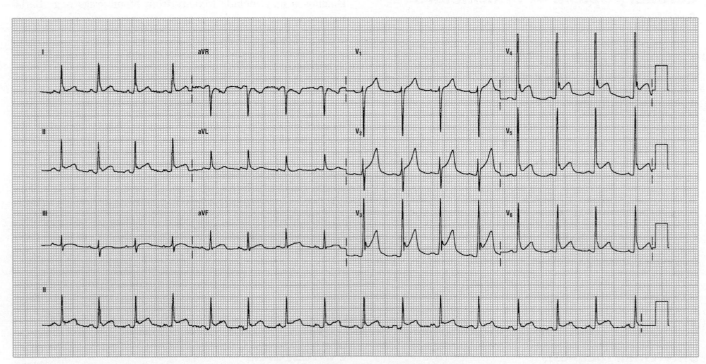

Figure 3-12 A 12-lead ECG showing pericarditis. ST elevation is present in leads I, II, aVF, and V_1–V_6. The QRS complexes are notched, indicating benign ST elevation.

From *Introduction to 12-lead ECG: the art of interpretation*, ed 2, Courtesy of Tomas B. Garcia, MD.

Cardiac enzymes are usually elevated, along with the erythrocyte sedimentation rate.

Differential Diagnosis

Myocarditis can present like an AMI with CHF, but the patient is usually young (< 35 years) and may not have risk factors for heart disease. No coronary obstruction is noted on cardiac catheterization. Other differential diagnoses may include cardiomyopathy, cardiac tamponade, and atherosclerosis.

Treatment

Management is supportive, and severe cases require a heart transplant.

Simple Pneumothorax

Pneumothorax refers to air in the pleural cavity. A small pneumothorax causes mild symptoms and may heal on its own. A larger pneumothorax generally requires aggressive treatment to remove the air and reestablish pulmonary negative pressure.

Pathophysiology

A pneumothorax occurs as the result of a bleb (a small air blister) rupturing on the lung, causing air to leave the lung and collect in the space between the visceral and parietal pleurae. With each ensuing breath, more air is trapped in that space, causing the affected lung to collapse. A simple pneumothorax may occur spontaneously in patients with connective tissue diseases such as Marfan syndrome or in tall, slim males. They can occur as the result of barotrauma or other injuries to the chest. COPD, cystic fibrosis, cancers, and acute lung infections, such as pneumonia, or chronic lung infections, such as tuberculosis, may also cause a pneumothorax. The greatest threat of a pneumothorax is the development of a tension pneumothorax, which may require immediate intervention.

Signs and Symptoms

In addition to histories associated with the causes listed, the patient may feel a sudden tearing as the lung separates from the chest wall. This is often followed with sudden shortness of breath and a sharp pain that increases when a breath is taken. Dry cough with lung sounds diminished on the affected side occur if the pneumothorax is significant in size. Low oxygen saturations may accompany the simple pneumothorax.

Differential Diagnosis

A chest radiograph should be obtained to confirm a diagnosis of a simple pneumothorax. If the radiograph does not show a pneumothorax, a CT scan may be required.

Treatment

Treatment is aimed at maintaining near-normal oxygen saturations by administering oxygen by nasal cannula or mask. Assisting ventilations is usually not required and may worsen the situation, increasing the likelihood of a tension pneumothorax. Some smaller simple pneumothoraces may seal on their own and require only conservative monitoring. Significant pneumothoraces may require insertion of a chest tube to resolve the problem.

Cholecystitis

Because of the close proximity to the thorax, GI problems may also cause chest discomfort and pain. Cholecystitis can be an emergent condition needing immediate attention by healthcare providers.

Pathophysiology

Cholecystitis is inflammation of the gallbladder often caused by bile duct obstruction that leads to infection and inflammation of the walls of the gallbladder. The pain associated with cholecystitis is usually localized to the right upper quadrant, but it may radiate to the shoulders.

Signs and Symptoms

In cholecystitis, the pain is sharp and colicky and often follows ingestion of a greasy meal. Because it may come on suddenly, it is often referred to as an *attack*. Fever may or may not be present, depending on whether the attack is acute (no fever) or chronic (fever). Nausea and vomiting are commonly associated signs and symptoms. Lab studies may show elevated liver function and an elevated WBC count.

Differential Diagnosis

Other possible diagnoses that need to be ruled out include appendicitis and cholelithiasis (gallstones). Imaging studies are required to confirm a diagnosis.

Treatment

Treatment requires removal of the gallbladder, with supportive measures until that can occur. Relief of nausea and pain is a priority, as is ensuring the patient remains hydrated. Broad-spectrum antibiotics may be infused prior to going to surgery.

Additional information on this condition and other GI causes of chest pain, including esophageal spasm, esophageal reflux, peptic ulcer, and biliary colic, is found in Chapter 6.

Pancreatitis

Pancreatitis is an acute inflammation of the pancreas and is often caused by gallstones or excessive alcohol use. Some common medications may also cause pancreatitis, including certain AIDS drugs, diuretics (furosemide and hydrochlorothiazide), and some chemotherapy medications (L-asparaginase and azathioprine). Estrogen replacement therapy may also cause pancreatitis because of its effect of raising blood triglyceride levels.

Pathophysiology

When the pancreas is injured or its function is disrupted, pancreatic enzymes leak into the pancreatic tissue and initiate autodigestion. Pancreatic tissue is replaced by fibrosis, which causes exocrine and endocrine changes and dysfunction of the islets of Langerhans.

Signs and Symptoms

Pancreatitis may be present with lower-left quadrant abdominal pain, serum amylase or lipase more than three times the normal range, and an abnormal CT scan. Early complications of pancreatitis include shock from third spacing, leading to dehydration, hypocalcemia, and hyperglycemia. Frequently, respiratory compromise also occurs with pancreatitis in the form of atelectasis from shallow breathing due to pain. Some degree of pleural effusion or pneumonitis may occur if pancreatic enzymes directly damage the lungs or from third spacing.

Differential Diagnosis

The patient's history and physical examination findings will help narrow down the diagnoses. A prehospital diagnosis is difficult because lab testing and imaging studies (abdominal radiograph, abdominal CT, abdominal magnetic resonance imaging) are helpful in determining the diagnosis.

Treatment

Treatment of pancreatitis will depend on the severity of the disease. General principles include relieving pain with opiates, nausea control, and hydrating the patient. A nasogastric tube for feedings may help avoid pancreatic stimulation. If the patient shows signs of infection, an IV antibiotic may be started as well.

Esophageal Tear

A Mallory-Weiss tear in the esophagus usually follows forceful vomiting. The tear is usually about 1 to 4 cm in length at either the junction of the esophagus and stomach or in the stomach itself. Some GI bleeding will occur, but it is usually not severe. For a full explanation of this condition, see Chapter 6.

Nonemergent Causes of Chest Pain

Several causes of chest discomfort and pain are not emergencies or life threats. Neurologic causes of chest discomfort include thoracic outlet syndrome, herpes zoster, and postherpetic neuralgia. The many respiratory causes of chest discomfort include pneumonitis, pleurisy, lung tumor, and pneumomediastinum, to name a few. Most conditions can be differentiated by the cause and description of the pain. Treatment is supportive, and finding the cause of the pain requires testing not routinely done in an ambulance. Diagnostic testing is often done as a follow-up to discharge from an emergency department after serious life threats have been ruled out.

Thoracic Outlet Syndrome

Thoracic outlet syndrome involves a compression of the brachial plexus (nerves that pass into the arms from the neck) and/or the subclavian vein or artery by muscle groups in the chest, back, or neck. When compressed, these nerves will cause chest discomfort that differs from ACS in that it is often associated with changes in position.

Pathophysiology

In thoracic outlet syndrome, the C8 and T1 nerve roots are usually affected, producing pain and tingling in the ulnar nerve distribution area (lower arm) or the C5, C6, and C7 nerve roots, with pain that refers to the neck, ear, upper part of the chest and upper part of the back, and the outer arm. The people most likely to experience thoracic outlet syndrome are those with neck injuries from motor vehicle collisions and those who use computers in nonergonomic postures for extended periods of time. Young athletes (such as swimmers, volleyball players, and baseball pitchers) and musicians may also experience thoracic outlet syndrome, but significantly less frequently.

Signs and Symptoms

Signs as symptoms may include the following:

- Numbness and tingling in the hands, arms, or fingers
- Discoloration of the extremities due to poor circulation
- Pain in the neck, shoulder, or arms
- Weakness in the hands or arms

Differential Diagnosis

One physical test that may lead you toward this diagnosis is called the *elevated arm stress test*, or *EAST*. Direct the patient to raise the arms to 90 degrees while seated, with elbows flexed 90 degrees. With shoulders back, ask the patient to open and close both fists slowly for about 3 minutes and describe his or her symptoms. A test that indicates thoracic outlet syndrome produces complaints of heaviness of the involved arm, gradual numbness of that hand, and progressive aching through the arm and top of shoulder. It is not unusual to see the patient drop the hand because of increasing pain. The involved arm and hand may have circulatory changes as well.

Treatment

Often, stretching, practicing proper posture, and treatments such as physiotherapy, massage therapy, and chiropractic care will resolve the pain of thoracic outlet syndrome. Cortisone and Botox (onabotulinumtoxinA) injections will lessen the symptoms during a course of treatment. The recovery process, however, is long term, and a few days of poor posture can often lead to setbacks. About 10% to 15% of patients undergo surgical decompression if 6 to 12 months of therapy fails to relieve the pain.

Herpes Zoster

Varicella-zoster virus is the primary agent of both chickenpox and herpes zoster, otherwise known as "shingles" (see Chapter 8 for further information on this condition).

Pathophysiology

Herpes zoster results from the varicella-zoster virus, left dormant in the body following a case of the chickenpox and later reactivated in a cranial nerve or spinal nerve dermatome. Herpes zoster can cause chest discomfort or pain before, during, or after the signature rash develops. Patients who are immunocompromised from human immunodeficiency virus (HIV) or receiving chemotherapy are at a greater risk for herpes zoster outbreaks.

Signs and Symptoms

Unlike the pain of a heart attack, herpes zoster pain is described as burning that typically precedes a rash by several days. The pain can persist for several months after the rash disappears, as in the case of postherpetic neuralgia. The pain and rash most commonly occur on the torso but can appear on the face, eyes, or other parts of the body. At first, the rash appears similar to hives, but unlike hives, it is has a tendency to follow dermatomes on one side of the body, appearing in a beltlike pattern and not crossing the midline. Later, the rash forms small fluid-filled blisters. The patient may develop a fever and general malaise. The painful blisters eventually become cloudy or darkened as they fill with blood, crust over within 7 to 10 days, and usually then fall off. Direct contact with the rash can spread the virus to a person who has never had chickenpox. Until the rash has developed crusts, a person is considered contagious. A person is not infectious before blisters appear or during postherpetic neuralgia (pain after the rash is gone). The pain may persist well after resolution of the rash and can be severe enough to require medications for relief.

Differential Diagnosis

Diagnosis is easy if the rash is present: herpes zoster is the only rash that follows a dermatome and is limited to one side of the body. If no rash is present, as in the case of postherpetic neuralgia, blood tests may be needed for definitive diagnosis.

Treatment

Herpes zoster is usually treated with oral antivirals, which are most effective when started within 72 hours after the onset of the rash. The addition of an orally administered corticosteroid can provide modest benefits in reducing the pain of herpes zoster and the incidence of postherpetic neuralgia. Patients with postherpetic neuralgia may require narcotics for adequate pain control.

Other Pulmonary Causes of Chest Pain

The many respiratory causes of chest discomfort include pneumonitis, pleurisy, lung tumor, and pneumomediastinum, to name a few. See Chapter 2 for an in-depth review of these and other respiratory conditions responsible for chest discomfort.

Pneumonitis

Pneumonitis refers to any inflammation of lung tissue and may be caused by a variety of conditions to include pneumonia, bronchitis, and aspiration. Productive cough and difficulty breathing are the most common symptoms of pneumonitis. Fever may occur with infection, and the cough may burn. Fatigue and malaise may also accompany pneumonitis. Treatment is generally supportive and is aimed at finding the cause. Treatment may be the avoidance of the trigger or may include medications such as IV antibiotics. If the patient is complaining of shortness of breath, administer oxygen to maintain saturations above 94%. An IV should be established and a heart monitor applied. Place the patient in the position of greatest comfort. Obtain a complete blood count, chemistry panel, and chest radiograph to confirm or rule out pneumonia.

Pleurisy

Pleurisy is the term most used to refer to painful respiration and should alert you to conduct a thorough assessment to find the cause of the pain. Pleuritic pain usually increases with respiration and is the result of inflammation of the parietal and visceral pleurae lining the chest wall and lungs, a pathologic process described earlier in this chapter and discussed in detail in Chapter 2. As the patient breathes, the inflamed pleurae rub against each other, causing a sharp pain that increases with inspiration. Fever and cough may be present and can be difficult to distinguish from pneumonia. A possible distinguishing sign includes the rough, scratchy sound heard with a stethoscope when the pleurae rub against each other, known as a "pleural friction rub." It often sounds like leather stretching when the patient inhales deeply.

A chest radiograph may show air or fluid in the pleural space. It also may show the cause of the pleurisy (e.g., pneumonia, a fractured rib, a lung tumor). If significant fluid is present, it may have to be removed with thoracentesis in the inpatient setting. Collected fluid will be tested to determine its origin; fluid may accumulate from lung tissue disease or cancers.

Acetaminophen or NSAIDs may be used for pain, and a codeine-based cough syrup to suppress the cough may also be given. Treatment is generally supportive and aimed at finding the cause. As discussed earlier, life-threatening causes of heart-related chest pain have been ruled out by this point.

Other Heart-Related Causes of Chest Pain

Other causes of chest discomfort may include structural changes in the heart such as valvular heart disease, aortic stenosis, mitral valve prolapse, and hypertrophic cardiomyopathy. All of these conditions may cause chest discomfort and pain similar to that in ACS.

Aortic Stenosis

As people age, the protein collagen of the heart's valve leaflets are damaged, and calcium is deposited. Turbulence from blood flowing across the valve increases scarring, thickening, and stenosis or narrowing of the valve. Why this aging process progresses to cause significant aortic stenosis in some patients but not in others is unknown. The progressive disease causing aortic calcification and stenosis has nothing to do with healthy lifestyle choices, unlike the calcium that can deposit in the coronary artery to cause heart attack.

Pathophysiology

Rheumatic fever is a condition resulting from untreated infection by group A streptococcal bacteria. Damage to valve leaflets from rheumatic fever causes increased turbulence across the valve and similar damage. The narrowing from rheumatic fever occurs from the fusion of the edges of the valve leaflets. Rheumatic aortic stenosis usually occurs with some degree of aortic regurgitation. Under normal circumstances, the aortic valve closes to prevent blood in the aorta from flowing back into the left ventricle. In aortic regurgitation, the diseased valve allows leakage of blood back into the left ventricle as the ventricular muscles relax after pumping. Patients with rheumatic fever also have some degree of rheumatic damage to the mitral valve. Rheumatic heart disease is uncommon in the United States, except in people who have emigrated from underdeveloped countries.

Signs and Symptoms

Chest pain may be the first symptom in patients with aortic stenosis. Chest pain in patients with aortic stenosis resembles the chest pain experienced by patients with angina. In both of these conditions, pain is described as pressure below the breast bone brought on by exertion and relieved by rest. In patients with coronary artery disease, chest pain is due to inadequate blood supply to the heart muscles because of narrowed coronary arteries. In patients with aortic stenosis, chest pain occurs without any underlying narrowing of the coronary arteries. The thickened heart muscle must pump against high pressure to push blood through the narrowed aortic valve. This increases heart muscle oxygen demand in excess of the supply delivered in the blood, causing angina.

Syncope related to aortic stenosis is usually caused by exertion or excitement. Any time a patient's blood pressure drops suddenly, the heart is unable to increase output to compensate for the drop in blood pressure. Therefore, blood flow to the brain is decreased, causing syncope. Syncope can also occur when CO is decreased by an irregular heartbeat. Without effective treatment, the average life expectancy is less than 3 years after the onset of chest pain or syncope symptoms from aortic stenosis.

Shortness of breath from left heart failure is the most ominous sign and is caused by increased capillary permeability in the lungs due to the increased pressure required to fill the left ventricle. Initially, shortness of breath occurs only during activity, but as the disease progresses, shortness of breath occurs at rest. Patients can find it difficult to lie flat without becoming short of breath. Strenuous activities should be avoided and may trigger syncope or angina, causing the patient to seek medical attention.

Differential Diagnosis

A thorough history and the presence of murmur are key to identification.

Treatment

Care is similar to the therapy for the patient with angina, which is usually rest and oxygen. Use extreme caution with medications such as nitroglycerin, which decrease preload. Lack of sufficient preload in patients with syncope may lead to a significant drop in systolic blood pressure and worsening of their condition.

Because valve infection is a serious complication of aortic stenosis, patients are given antibiotics prior to any procedure in which bacteria may be introduced into the bloodstream. This includes routine dental work and minor surgery. When symptoms of chest pain, syncope, or shortness of breath appear, the prognosis for patients with aortic stenosis without valve replacement surgery is poor.

Mitral Valve Prolapse

Mitral valve prolapse is the most common heart valve abnormality, affecting 5% to 10% of the world population. A normal mitral valve consists of two thin leaflets located between the left atrium and the left ventricle of the heart. Mitral valve leaflets, shaped like parachutes, are attached to the inner wall of the left ventricle by a series of strings called *chordae*. When the ventricles contract, the mitral valve leaflets close snugly and prevent the backflow of blood from the left ventricle into the left atrium. When the ventricles relax, the valves open to allow oxygenated blood from the lungs to fill the left ventricle.

Pathophysiology

In patients with mitral valve prolapse, the mitral valve leaflets and chordae degenerate, becoming thick and enlarged. When the ventricles contract, the leaflets prolapse (flop backward) into the left atrium, sometimes allowing leakage or regurgitation of blood through the valve opening.

Signs and Symptoms

Severe mitral regurgitation can lead to CHF and abnormal heart rhythms. Most patients are unaware of the prolapsing of the mitral valve, but others may experience a number of symptoms such as palpitations, chest pain, anxiety, and fatigue. Sharp chest pain that does not respond to nitroglycerin may be reported by the patient. Auscultation of heart sounds with a stethoscope might reveal a clicking sound that reflects the tightening of the abnormal valve leaflets against the pressure load of the left ventricle. If there is associated regurgitation of blood through the abnormal valve opening, a whooshing sound can be heard immediately following the clicking sound.

Differential Diagnosis

Generally, the only physical finding is a clicking sound during cardiac auscultation.

Treatment

Mitral regurgitation usually can be treated with medication, but some people need surgery to repair or replace the defective valve.

Cardiomyopathy

Cardiomyopathy generally refers to a group of conditions that weaken and enlarge the myocardium.

Pathophysiology

Most cardiomyopathies are classified into three groups—dilated, hypertrophic, and restrictive. Cardiomyopathy occurs when heart muscle myocytes are injured by various causes, and the heart remodels itself to accommodate with hypertrophy or thickening of the muscle (**Figure 3-13**). There are genetic and immunologic causes of this debilitating disease process.

Signs and Symptoms

A common patient presentation includes chest pain, weakness, and dyspnea. Left-sided heart failure may be the first presentation, along with exertional chest pain. The ECG may be nonspecific, with intraventricular conduction delay or left bundle-branch block. A chest radiograph will usually show a large heart, and a brain natriuretic peptide test result may be mildly elevated if the patient is asymptomatic and very elevated if symptomatic.

Differential Diagnosis

The differential diagnosis is one of exclusion.

Treatment

Management is supportive and similar to that of CHF and APE. ACE inhibitors are the treatment of choice, along with other techniques to decrease the heart's afterload. This disease is the

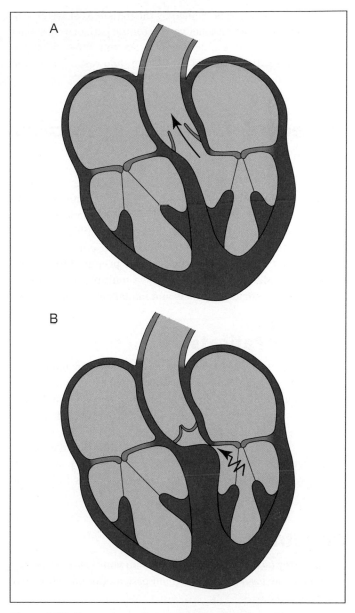

Figure 3-13 Comparison of normal cardiac function with malfunction characteristic of hypertrophic cardiomyopathy. A. Normal heart, illustrating unobstructed flow of blood from the left ventricle into the aorta during ventricular systole. B. Hypertrophic cardiomyopathy, illustrating obstruction to the outflow of blood from the left ventricle by the hypertrophied septum, which impinges on the anterior leaflet of the mitral valve.

leading indication for heart transplantation. As discussed earlier, ventricular assistive devices can be used as bridge therapy to transplantation or as sustained therapy.

Musculoskeletal Causes of Chest Pain

As described in the assessment section, the thoracic cage is made up of musculoskeletal structures and can be a somatic cause for chest pain. Muscle strain, costochondritis, and nonspecific chest wall pain are usually well defined by the patient as sharp or aching. You must rule out all other causes for the patient's chest pain before deciding on this as a diagnosis. As with most inflammation, use of NSAIDs, heat or cold therapy, and rest are the most common tactics for management.

Special Considerations
Older Adult Patients

The older patient may present with ACS, but the symptoms may not be apparent. Weakness or a silent MI (no signs and symptoms) are common, so a high index of suspicion must be maintained. Elderly persons may be taking medications (e.g., beta-blockers) that decrease their ability to compensate for hemodynamic compromise. You must be prepared to address these issues. Many older patients have multiple medical conditions that can make diagnosis and management challenging.

Bariatric Patients

Owing to the decrease in mobility in obese persons, blood clots in the legs may contribute to pulmonary emboli. The complaint of chest pain may be altered because of nerve distribution in the tissues due to torso mass. The increase in myocardial workload obese patients at high risk for ACS. In addition, diabetes is more common and may contribute to cardiovascular issues. Electrolyte imbalance may follow bariatric surgery and result in dysrhythmias as the cause of chest discomfort in bariatric patients.

Obstetric Patients

A pulmonary embolism should be high on your list of suspected diagnoses when assessing a pregnant patient; this condition may be due to the state of hypercoagulation and potential for developing blood clots. Pregnancy also places increased demands on the cardiovascular system and may exacerbate a previous diagnosed or undiagnosed condition. GERD is also common during pregnancy and may contribute to chest discomfort. Consider transport to a facility that cares for high-risk obstetric patients.

Putting It All Together

Caring for a patient with chest pain begins with your initial observation. Your immediate goal is to determine whether the patient is sick or not. Your first impression should tell you whether you have time to continue the assessment or if you should intercede immediately. Evaluate the patient for critical or emergent diagnoses first. Life-threatening diagnoses require immediate narrowing down for management. Include breath sounds to rule out a tension pneumothorax and APE/CHF, then rule out possible ACS (consider a 12-lead ECG as the patient's condition allows, but do not delay treatment with aspirin, oxygen, or nitroglycerin), and check the patient's blood pressures and pulses in both upper extremities and compare them to the lower extremities as you consider an aortic aneurysm. Often the clue to an esophageal rupture, pulmonary embolism, or other life threat is revealed during history taking, so obtain a history to rule these diagnoses out as time allows.

At the receiving facility, chest radiographs, lab analyses, and CT scans are performed as time allows. To confirm or rule out conditions that make up your differential diagnosis, use tools such as SAMPLER, OPQRST, physical examination findings, and lab results. If your patient's condition is unstable or deteriorates, support the ABCs as you work through the AMLS patient assessment process. Immediate life threats take precedence over all else. Once these are ruled out, progress to the other causes of chest pain, but realize initial complaints of chest discomfort may be vague; ongoing reassessment is essential so that that life threats are detected.

SCENARIO SOLUTION

© HunThomas/ShutterStock, Inc.

- Differential diagnoses may include myocarditis, pneumonia, pulmonary embolism, acute coronary syndrome, cholecystitis, and pericarditis.
- To narrow your differential diagnosis, you will need to complete the patient's history of past and present illness. Obtain a more thorough history of her present illness. Perform a physical examination that includes vital sign assessment and evaluation of heart and breath sounds, jugular vein assessment, ECG monitoring and 12-lead ECG, Sao$_2$, capnography, and blood glucose analysis.
- The patient has signs that may indicate acute coronary syndrome, infection, or heart failure. Administer oxygen.

Establish vascular access. Monitor the ECG, and obtain a 12-lead ECG. Further treatment will depend on the rest of your assessment findings. If you suspect acute coronary syndrome, treat the patient with aspirin, nitroglycerin, and morphine. If the patient has signs of congestive heart failure without shock, treat with continuous positive airway pressure and nitroglycerin. If the patient's examination points to cholecystitis, treat for pain. If the patient has diabetic ketoacidosis, administer a large volume of IV fluids. Transport the patient to the closest appropriate healthcare facility.

Summary

- Your standard assessment practice for the patient with chest pain should include looking for life-threatening causes and managing them appropriately—even within the primary survey. In the patient with a patent airway, assessing for breath sounds and looking for shock are key.
- Life-threatening causes of chest pain usually include diseases that produce both chest pain and increased work of breathing, or chest pain and alteration in vital signs (or a combination thereof).
- Standard protocols for chest pain include use of oxygen, vascular access, application of monitors, an ECG, chest radiography, and laboratory studies. Healthcare providers need to triage the patient for additional resources (cardiac catheterization at a specialized heart center) and move the patient toward those specialties early in the process.
- Non–life-threatening causes of chest pain can arise from several body systems, including the cardiovascular, respiratory, gastrointestinal, immunologic, structural cardiac, neurologic, and musculoskeletal systems.

KEY TERMS

© HunThomas/ShutterStock, Inc.

acute coronary syndrome (ACS) An umbrella term that covers any group of clinical symptoms consistent with acute myocardial ischemia (chest pain due to insufficient blood supply to the heart muscle that results from coronary artery disease). ACS covers clinical conditions including angina, unstable angina, ST-segment elevation myocardial infarction (STEMI), and non–ST-segment elevation myocardial infarction (NSTEMI).

acute myocardial infarction (AMI) Commonly known as a "heart attack," AMI occurs when the blood supply to part of the heart is interrupted, causing heart cells to die. This is most commonly due to blockage of a coronary artery following the rupture of plaque within the wall of an artery. The resulting ischemia and decreased supply of oxygen, if left untreated, can cause damage and/or death of heart muscle tissue.

cardiac tamponade Also known as "pericardial tamponade," this is an emergency condition in which fluid accumulates in the pericardium (the sac that surrounds the heart). If the amount of fluid increases slowly (such as in hypothyroidism), the pericardial sac can expand to contain a liter or more of fluid prior to tamponade occurring. If the fluid increases rapidly (as may occur after trauma or myocardial rupture), as little as 100 mL can cause tamponade.

ischemia A restriction in oxygen and nutrient delivery to muscle caused by physical obstruction to blood flow,

increased demand by the tissues, or hypoxia, which leads to damage or dysfunction of tissue.

non–ST-segment elevation myocardial infarction (NSTEMI) A type of MI caused by a blocked blood supply that causes nontransmural infarction in an area of the heart. There is no ST-segment elevation on electrocardiogram (ECG) recordings, but other clinical signs of MI are present. NSTEMI is diagnosed on the basis of positive laboratory tests for cardiac enzymes and other products of myocardium damage and death.

pericarditis A condition in which the tissue surrounding the heart (pericardium) becomes inflamed. This can be caused by several factors but is often related to a viral infection. Accompaniment by cardiac dysfunction or signs of congestive heart failure (CHF) suggests a more serious myocarditis or involvement of the heart muscle.

pleura A thin membrane that surrounds and protects the lungs (visceral pleura) and lines the chest cavity (parietal pleura)

pulmonary embolism (PE) The sudden blockage of a pulmonary artery by a blood clot, often originating from a deep vein in the legs or pelvis, that embolizes and travels to the lung artery, where it becomes lodged. Symptoms include tachycardia, hypoxia, and hypotension.

pulsus paradoxus An exaggeration of the normal inspiratory decrease in systolic blood pressure, defined

KEY TERMS (CONTINUED)

© HunThomas/ShutterStock, Inc.

by an inspiratory fall of systolic blood pressure of greater than 10 mm Hg.

ST-segment elevation myocardial infarction (STEMI) Anginal symptoms at rest that result in myocardial necrosis as identified by elevated cardiac biomarkers with ST-segment elevation on the 12-lead electrocardiogram. These attacks carry a substantial risk of death and disability and call for a quick response by a STEMI system geared for reperfusion therapy.

stable angina Symptoms of chest pain, shortness of breath, or other equivalent symptoms that occur predictably with exertion, then resolve with rest, suggesting the presence of a fixed coronary lesion that prevents adequate perfusion with increased demand.

tension pneumothorax A life-threatening condition that results from progressive worsening of a simple pneumothorax, the accumulation of air under pressure in the pleural space. This can lead to progressive restriction of venous return, which leads to decreased preload, then systemic hypotension.

unstable angina (UA) Angina of increased frequency, severity, or occurring with less intensive exertion than the baseline. This suggests the narrowing of a static lesion, causing further limitation of coronary blood flow with increased demand.

BIBLIOGRAPHY

© HunThomas/ShutterStock, Inc.

Adam A, Dixon AK, Grainger RG, et al: *Grainger and Allison's diagnostic radiology*, ed 5. Philadelphia, PA, 2008, Churchill Livingstone.

Aehlert B: *Paramedic practice today: above and beyond*. Burlington, MA, 2011, Jones & Bartlett Learning.

Aghababian R: *Essentials of emergency medicine*, ed 2. Sudbury, MA, 2011, Jones & Bartlett Learning.

Akula R, Hasan SP, Alhassen M, et al.: Right-sided EKG in pulmonary embolism. *J Natl Med Assoc*. 95:714–717, 2003.

American Academy of Orthopaedic Surgeons: *Nancy Caroline's emergency care in the streets*, ed 7. Burlington, MA, 2013, Jones & Bartlett Learning.

American Heart Association: *2010 AHA guidelines for CPR and ECC*, Dallas, TX, 2010, American Heart Association.

American Heart Association: *ACLS for experienced providers*. Dallas, TX, 2013, American Heart Association.

American Heart Association: *Atherosclerosis*. 2014. http://www.heart.org/HEARTORG/Conditions/Cholesterol/WhyCholesterolMatters/Atherosclerosis_UCM_305564_Article.jsp

American Heart Association: *Classes of heart failure*. http://www.heart.org/HEARTORG/Conditions/HeartFailure/AboutHeartFailure/Classes-of-Heart-Failure_UCM_306328_Article.jsp, reviewed April 6, 2015.

Anderson JL, Adams CD, Antman EM, et al.: 2012 ACCF/AHA focused update incorporated into the ACCF/AHA 2007 guidelines for the management of patients with unstable angina/non-ST-elevation myocardial infarction: A report of the American College of Cardiology Foundation/American Heart Association Task Force on Practice Guidelines. *Circulation*. 127(23): e663–e828, 2013.

Black JM, Hokanson Hawks J: *Medical-surgical nursing*, ed 8. Philadelphia, PA, 2009, Saunders.

Bledsoe BE, Anderson E, Hodnick R, et al.: Low-fractional oxygen concentration continuous positive airway pressure is effective in the prehospital setting. *Prehospital Emergency Care*. 16(2):217–221, 2012.

Bodson L, Bouferrache K, Vieillard-Baron A: Cardiac tamponade. *Curr Opin Crit Care*. 17(5):416–424, 2011.

Braunwald E: *Heart disease: A textbook of cardiovascular medicine*, ed 4. Philadelphia, PA, 1992, WB Saunders.

Damodaran S: Cocaine and beta-blockers: The paradigm. *Eur J Intern Med*. 21(2):84–86, 2010.

Dorland's illustrated medical dictionary. Philadelphia, PA, 2007, Saunders.

Ferrari R, Guardigli G, Ceconi C: Secondary prevention of CAD with ACE inhibitors: A struggle between life and death of the endothelium. *Cardiovasc Drugs Ther*. 24(4):331–339, 2010.

Field J: *Advanced cardiac life support provider manual*. Dallas, TX, 2006, American Heart Association.

Field J, Hazinski M, Gilmore D: *Handbook of ECC for healthcare providers*. Dallas, TX, 2008, American Heart Association.

Frownfelter D, Dean E: *Cardiovascular and pulmonary physical therapy*, ed 4. St. Louis, MO, 2006, Mosby.

Go AS, Mozaffarian D, Roger VL, et al.: Heart disease and stroke statistics—2013 update: A report from the American Heart Association. *Circulation*. 127(1):e6–e245, 2013.

Goldman L, Ausiello D: *Cecil medicine*, ed 23. Philadelphia, PA, 2007, Saunders.

Haji SA, Movahed A: Right ventricular infarction: Diagnosis and treatment. *Clin Cardiol (Hoboken)*. 23(7):473–482, 2000.

Herlitz J, Bång A, Omerovic E, et al.: Is pre-hospital treatment of chest pain optimal in acute coronary syndrome? The relief of both pain and anxiety is needed. *Int J Cardiol*. 149(2):147–151, 2011.

BIBLIOGRAPHY (CONTINUED)

© HunThomas/ShutterStock, Inc.

Hiratzka LF, Bakris GL, Beckman JA, et al.: 2010 ACCF/AHA/AATS/ACR/ASA/SCA/SCAI/SIR/STS/SVM guidelines for the diagnosis and management of patients with thoracic aortic disease: A report of the American College of Cardiology Foundation/American Heart Association Task Force on Practice Guidelines, American Association for Thoracic Surgery, American College of Radiology, American Stroke Association, Society of Cardiovascular Anesthesiologists, Society for Cardiovascular Angiography and Interventions, Society of Interventional Radiology, Society of Thoracic Surgeons, and Society for Vascular Medicine. *Circulation.* 121(13):e266–e369, 2010.

Ikematsu Y: Incidence and characteristics of dysphoria in patients with cardiac tamponade. *Heart Lung: J Crit Care.* 36(6):440–449, 2007.

Johnson D, Ed: The pericardium. In Standring S, et al., Eds: *Gray's anatomy.* St. Louis, MO, 2005, Mosby.

Lange RA, Cigarroa RG, Yancy CW Jr, et al.: Cocaine-induced coronary-artery vasoconstriction. *N Engl J Med.* 321.1557–1562, 1989.

Manfrini O, Morrell C, Das R, et al.: Management of acute coronary events study: Effects of angiotensin-converting enzyme inhibitors and beta blockers on clinical outcomes in patients with and without coronary artery obstructions at angiography (from a register-based cohort study on acute coronary syndromes), *Am J Cardiol.* 113(10):1628–1633, 2014.

Marx JA, Hockberger RS, Walls RM, et al.: *Rosen's emergency medicine: Concepts and clinical practice,* ed 6. St. Louis, MO, 2006, Mosby.

O'Connor RE, Ali Al AS, Brady WJ, et al. Part 9: Acute Coronary Syndromes: 2015 American Heart Association Guidelines Update for Cardiopulmonary Resuscitation and Emergency Cardiovascular Care. *Circulation.* 132 (18 Suppl 2), S483–S500, 2015.

O'Gara PT, Kushner FG, Ascheim DD, et al.: ACCF/AHA guideline: 2013 ACCF/AHA guideline for the management of ST-elevation myocardial infarction. *Circulation.* 127:e362–e422, 2013.

Parikh R, Kadowitz PJ: A review of current therapies used in the treatment of congestive heart failure. *Expert Rev Cardiovasc Ther.* 11(9):1171–1178, 2013.

PHTLS: *Prehospital trauma life support,* ed 8. St. Louis, MO, 2014, MosbyJems.

Story L: *Pathophysiology: A practical approach,* ed 2. Burlington, MA, 2015, Jones & Bartlett Learning.

Torres-Macho J, Mancebo-Plaza AB, Crespo-Gimenez A, et al: Clinical features of patients inappropriately undiagnosed of pulmonary embolism, *Am J Emerg Med.* 31(12):1646–1650.

Urden L, Stacy K, Lough M: *Critical care nursing: Diagnosis and management,* ed 6. St. Louis, MO, 2010, Mosby.

U.S. Department of Transportation: *National emergency medical services education standards: Paramedic instructional guidelines.* Washington, DC, 2010, U.S. Department of Transportation.

U.S. Department of Transportation: *National EMS education standards: Paramedic.* Washington, DC, 2010, U.S. Department of Transportation.

Weitzenblum E: Chronic cor pulmonale. *Heart.* 89(2):225–230, 2003.

Williams B, Boyle M, Robertson N, et al.: When pressure is positive: A literature review of the prehospital use of continuous positive airway pressure. *Prehosp Disaster Med.* 28: 52–60, 2012.

Wilson SF, Thompson JM: *Mosby's clinical nursing series: Respiratory disorders.* St. Louis, MO, 1990, Mosby.

CHAPTER REVIEW QUESTIONS

© HunThomas/ShutterStock, Inc.

1. The most common sign or symptom found in patients with pulmonary embolism is:
   a. Coughing up blood
   b. Crackles in the affected lung
   c. Increased respiratory rate
   d. Pleural friction rub

2. A 52-year-old man with a history of alcoholism complains of pleuritic chest pain. He reports recent vomiting and states the pain increases when he swallows. He appears very ill and has subcutaneous emphysema around his neck. You suspect:
   a. Boerhaave's syndrome
   b. Cholecystitis
   c. Esophageal varices
   d. Pleurisy

3. A 73-year-old man awakens suddenly, complaining of dyspnea. You find him in the tripod position. Crackles are audible around his scapulae. He has a history of hypertension. You suspect his symptoms are related to:
   a. Fluid overload
   b. Increased cardiac output
   c. Left-sided heart failure
   d. Reactive airway disease

4. A 70-year-old man suspected to have a dissecting aortic aneurysm has a blood pressure of 170/102 mm Hg. This sign may indicate:
   a. Cardiac tamponade is developing
   b. Rupture of the aorta is imminent
   c. The aorta is not dissecting
   d. The renal arteries are involved

© HunThomas/ShutterStock, Inc.

5. Which of the following patients is at highest risk for pericardial tamponade?
   a. 55-year-old with end-stage lung cancer
   b. 62-year-old dialysis patient
   c. 45-year-old with influenza
   d. 72-year-old who takes warfarin

6. If you administer nitroglycerin to a patient with ST-segment elevation in leads II, III, and aVF, you should be prepared to:
   a. Administer a bolus of normal saline if the blood pressure drops
   b. Change to morphine, as nitroglycerin is rarely successful
   c. Start a dopamine drip if the patient becomes hypotensive
   d. Treat the patient for congestive heart failure

7. A 45-year-old man with a history of hypertension complains of chest "pressure" that he rates about a 5 on a pain scale of 1 to 10, for 20 minutes. He just "wants to be checked out." Vital signs and 12-lead ECG are normal. You have already administered oxygen and aspirin. You should next:
   a. Administer nitroglycerin, 0.4 mg sublingually
   b. Advise him that his ECG is normal and no further care is needed
   c. Monitor and transport to the hospital for further evaluation
   d. Perform a right-sided electrocardiogram

8. An 82-year-old woman complains of chest heaviness. She has sinus tachycardia. Her vital signs include a blood pressure of 108/72 mm Hg (equal in both arms); pulse rate, 98 beats/min; and respirations, 20 breaths/min. Her breath sounds are clear in all fields. Aside from myocardial infarction, which diagnosis should you suspect?
   a. Aortic dissection
   b. Congestive heart failure
   c. Esophageal rupture
   d. Pulmonary embolism

9. A 40-year-old has chest pain described as an "elephant sitting on my chest." He confides that he snorted cocaine 5 minutes before his pain began. You should first administer:
   a. A fibrinolytic drug
   b. Lorazepam, 2 mg IV
   c. Metoprolol, 5 mg IV
   d. Naloxone, 2 mg IV

10. A 65-year-old woman complains of chest pain that feels like "aching" in her chest. It has become progressively worse over several days. Her temperature is 101°F (38.3°C). Which finding will help narrow your differential diagnosis to pericarditis?
    a. Pleural friction rub is audible.
    b. Pulsus alternans is present.
    c. S_3 gallop is auscultated.
    d. ST-segment elevation is apparent in every lead.

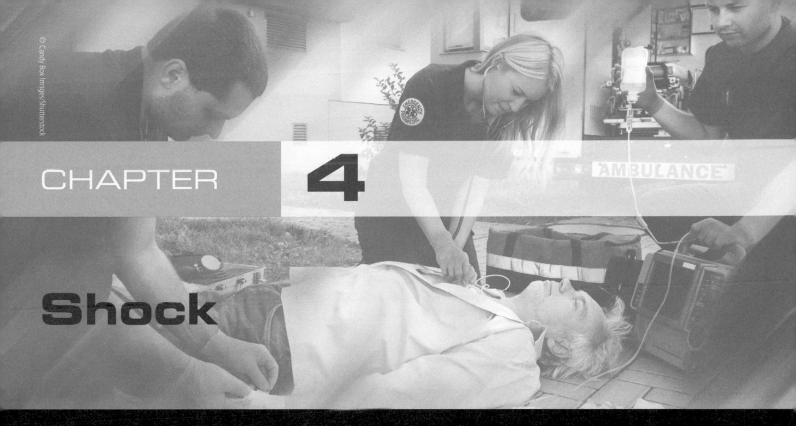

CHAPTER 4

Shock

This chapter takes a close look at perfusion, the function that fails in patients who are in shock. The chapter reviews the anatomy and physiology of tissue perfusion and describes the pathophysiology of hypoperfusion, or shock. The types of shock are discussed and compared so you will be able to recognize shock at any stage. The Advanced Medical Life Support (AMLS) assessment pathway offers tools for the assessment and emergency treatment of shock in general and of each particular type of shock.

LEARNING OBJECTIVES

At the conclusion of this chapter, you will be able to:

- Describe the anatomy and physiology of body systems as they relate to shock.

- Describe the pathophysiology of shock.

- Identify the key features of each type of shock.

- Assess the patient for life-threatening findings during the primary and secondary surveys and ongoing management.

- List effective ways of obtaining information on a patient's allergies, current medications, incident and past medical history, and last oral intake, then correlate them to each of the categories of shock.

- Describe laboratory and diagnostic tests used to verify diagnoses associated with shock.

- Apply appropriate treatment modalities for the management, monitoring, and continuing care of the patient in shock.

- Compare and describe the following types of shock: hypovolemic, distributive, cardiogenic, and obstructive.

- Formulate a differential diagnosis, demonstrate sound clinical reasoning skills, and apply advanced clinical decision making in caring for the patient in shock who has an emergent cardiovascular, respiratory, or hematologic condition.

- Describe how the AMLS pathway can be used to address problems found during the assessment of the shock patient.

SCENARIO

© HunThomas/ShutterStock, Inc.

Your patient is a 54-year-old man whose chief complaint is chest discomfort. When you examine him, you note an increased respiratory rate with increased work of breathing. He is pale. His skin is cool and moist. He tells you he had a heart catheterization 2 weeks ago. His medical history includes emphysema and a myocardial infarction 2 years ago, and he is currently taking antibiotics for an upper respiratory infection. Breath sounds are decreased in the bases with a few crackles. His blood pressure is 86/68 mm Hg; pulse rate, 126 beats/min; respirations, 22 breaths/min and slightly labored; and oxygen saturation, 94%.

- What is your initial impression?
- Which differential diagnoses are you considering based on the information you have now?
- Which additional information will you need to narrow your differential diagnosis?
- What are your initial treatment priorities as you continue your patient care?
- On the basis of your findings, what is your refined differential and why?

Shock is a progressive state of cellular hypoperfusion in which insufficient oxygen is available to meet tissue demands, which results in inadequate energy production to perform cellular activities. Either oxygen intake, absorption, or delivery fails, or the cells are unable to take up and use the oxygen to carry out cellular functions. Shock is a mechanism used by the body when the body is stressed and no longer able to compensate or meet the metabolic demands. It is key to understand that when the shock response occurs, the body is in distress. The shock response is used to maintain systolic blood pressure and brain perfusion during times of physiological distress. The response can accompany a broad spectrum of events, ranging from heart attacks, to major infections, to allergic reactions, to motor vehicle crashes. As a healthcare provider, you must understand the pathophysiology, assessment, and management of this condition, because each year in the United States more than 1 million people arrive at emergency departments (EDs) in varying states of shock. Expertise in critical thinking and decision making are essential tools to use when you encounter a critical patient in shock. This process involves a rapid assessment, providing life-saving treatment, and developing a differential field diagnosis.

The initial signs of shock can be subtle and the progression of shock insidious. If not treated promptly, shock will injure the body's vital organs and ultimately lead to death. The rapid recognition of the physiologic state of shock is an essential skill for every healthcare provider. It begins with an understanding of the anatomy and physiology of tissue perfusion.

Anatomy and Physiology of Perfusion

The word **perfusion** derives from the Latin verb *perfundere*, meaning "to pour over." In the body, the blood supplies oxygen to cells as it spills over them by way of the circulatory system.

To keep the blood moving continuously through the body, the cardiovascular system requires three main components: a functioning pump (the heart), adequate fluid volume (the blood and body fluids), and an intact system of tubing (the blood vessels) capable of reflex adjustments such as constriction and dilation, in response to changes in pump output and fluid volume (**Figure 4-1**). Intravascular volume is the amount of circulating blood in the vessels.

The Heart

The heart is a cone-shaped muscular organ situated in the mediastinum, posterior to the inferior aspect of the sternum. It lies at an oblique angle, with two-thirds of its mass to the left of the body's midline and one-third to the right of the body's midline. The heart comprises four chambers: the left and right atria, which are located at the base of the heart, and the left and right ventricles, which make up the apex.

The left and right atria are smaller than the more muscular ventricles. Deoxygenated blood enters the heart through the right atrium and then flows through the tricuspid valve into the right ventricle. From the right ventricle, the blood travels through the pulmonary valve into the pulmonary artery. Once the blood has been oxygenated in the lungs, it proceeds through the pulmonary vein to the left atrium. (The four pulmonary veins, two for each lung, are the only veins in the body that carry oxygenated blood.) The mitral (bicuspid) valve allows blood to pass from the left atrium to the left ventricle, where the blood is then pumped to the aorta through the aortic valve to the remainder of the body.

A complete heartbeat is called a **cardiac cycle**. Systole (contraction) and diastole (relaxation) in all four chambers, atria and ventricles, are the components of the cardiac cycle. The contraction of the heart occurs in stages. The ventricles relax (ventricular diastole) and the blood flows from the atria into the ventricles. Then the atria contract (atrial systole) to squeeze blood into the ventricles. The contraction of the atria is call the "atrial kick." As atrial contraction completes and the

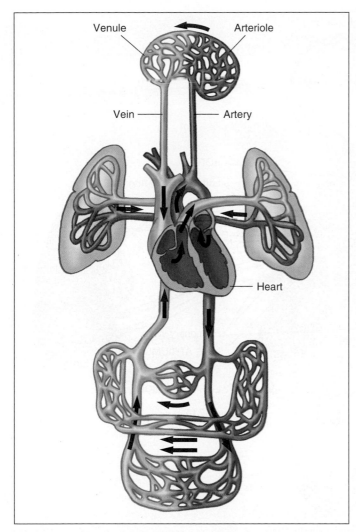

Figure 4-1 The cardiovascular system requires continuous operation of its three components: the heart (or pump), the blood vessels (or container), and the blood and body fluids (or contents).

atrioventricular valves close and atria relax (atrial diastole), the much stronger ventricles contract (ventricular systole) to pump blood to the lungs and body. The heart's contractility allows it to increase or decrease the volume of blood it pumps with each contraction, also known as the **stroke volume**. The heart can also vary the speed at which it contracts by raising or lowering the pulse rate.

Cardiac Output

For blood to "pour" through the body, it must be pumped. In a healthy person, the heart is remarkably efficient at moving oxygenated blood through the body, ensuring adequate perfusion. **Cardiac output** is the volume of blood that the heart can pump per minute and is dependent on several factors. First, the heart must have adequate strength, which is largely determined by the ability of the heart muscle to contract (**Figure 4-2**). Second, the heart must receive adequate blood to pump. As the volume of blood flowing to the heart increases, the precontraction pressure

in the heart builds up. The precontraction pressure is known as **preload**. The preload is the initial stretching of the cardiac muscles prior to contraction. It is related to the chamber volume of blood just prior to contraction. As preload increases, the volume of blood within the ventricles increases, which causes the heart muscle to stretch. When the muscle is stretched, myocardial contractility increases, leading to greater force of contraction and increased cardiac output. Lastly, the resistance to flow in the peripheral circulation must be appropriate. The force or resistance against which the heart pumps is known as **afterload**.

Cardiac output is usually expressed as liters per minute (L/min). The cardiac output of a healthy adult varies from 3 to 8 L/min, with 5 L/min being about average. Cardiac output is determined by stroke volume—the volume of blood ejected with each contraction of the heart—and pulse rate. The equation is as follows:

CO = Stroke volume × Heart rate

The stroke volume of a healthy adult is typically about 70 mL, but the amount is variable because of individual physiologic differences. The primary mechanical variable that affects stroke volume is explained by Starling's law, also known as the Frank-Starling mechanism. Starling's law describes the ability of cardiac muscle fibers to stretch and contract to regulate the strength of the heart's contraction. According to this law, the more the heart is stretched, the more strongly it contracts, but only up to a point. Think of the heart as a rubber band; the farther you stretch it, the farther it will shoot when released. Once the heart muscle has stretched beyond its optimal elasticity (like an old rubber band), the contraction will become weaker and less effective.

Neural and endocrine mechanisms also influence stroke volume through neurotransmitters. Sympathetic nerve fibers in the cardiac nerves release norepinephrine, and the adrenal medulla releases epinephrine. These two adrenergic agents boost the strength of the contraction.

Inadequate cardiac output is one cause of hypoperfusion. To generate adequate cardiac output, the heart must be able to contract with sufficient vigor, and the heart rate must be within an effective range. Details of the primary factors that determine stroke volume and cardiac output are as follows:

- *Preload.* The stretch of the myocardial tissue by the blood in the ventricles just before the start of a contraction. You can grasp the concept of preload by comparing it with the tension created when a bowstring is drawn back. If there is not enough tension on the string, the arrow will drop to the ground near the archer's feet. A strong pull, in contrast, will propel the arrow toward its target. In the heart, the pull or stretch on the muscle is from the volume of blood returning to the heart and accumulating in the ventricle prior to a contraction. Starling's law holds that the greater the stretch—up to a point—the stronger the cardiac contraction and the greater the output.

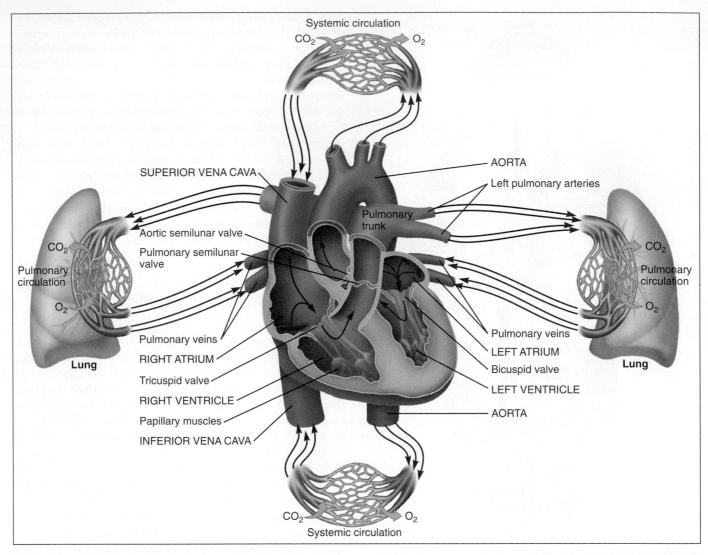

Figure 4-2 Circulation begins in the heart muscle.

- *Afterload.* The force the ejected blood meets as it exits the ventricle. You may think about afterload as the pressure it takes to push through a swinging door. If someone or something is pushing against the other side of the door, it takes more pressure to open it. In the systemic circulation, afterload is represented by aortic systolic pressure and systemic vascular resistance. Increasing or decreasing the afterload alters the cardiac output. The other factor that affects afterload is the thickness or viscosity of the blood. When the blood is thicker, it can impair the afterload as well because it takes more force to move the thick blood through the vascular system.

- *Contractility.* The force of cardiac contraction for a given level of preload. Positive inotropic stimulation, such as that provided by administration of epinephrine or dopamine, heightens the force and velocity of contraction. This stronger contraction will in turn increase

the stroke volume for a given level of preload. A drawback of increasing contractility is that it will increase the oxygen demand of the heart.

- *Synchrony.* To pump effectively, cardiac contractions must be synchronized to make the cycle function efficiently, the atria contract to fill the ventricles, and the ventricles contract to pump blood to the lungs and heart. Loss of atrioventricular synchrony, such as occurs during atrial fibrillation or conduction disorders such as a bundle branch block, alters the effectiveness of the heart as a pump. Atrial fibrillation does not allow the atria to fully contract and pump blood to the ventricles, causing a decrease in ventricular preload and potentially decreasing cardiac output. Conduction disorders such as atrioventricular blocks disturb coordination among the atria and ventricular muscle fibers, reducing the efficiency of contraction, which may result in a decrease in cardiac output.

The Vascular System

The vascular system is similar to the plumbing in a house. It is a conduit for moving blood throughout the body. The arteries and arterioles, which make up the arterial vascular system, carry oxygenated, nutrient-rich blood. The veins and venules, which make up the venous system, return deoxygenated blood to the heart and transport waste products to be eliminated from the body. The capillaries communicate between the blood and tissues by acting as the site of transfer of oxygen and other nutrients to the tissues and removal of wastes from the tissues. The precapillary sphincters dilate to allow blood to flow into the capillaries when a fresh supply is needed.

In fact, all parts of the vascular system can contract (vasoconstrict) and dilate (vasodilate) in response to various stimuli. The arteries and arterioles constrict and dilate more vigorously than the veins and venules do because their vessel walls are stronger. The increased pressure of the blood in the arteries relative to the veins keeps the blood flowing quickly. Because the residual pressure is lower in the venous system, valves are necessary to prevent the backflow of blood.

Blood

Blood has two main functions: transportation of oxygen and nutrients to the body's cells and removal of waste from the body. Hemoglobin, an iron-containing protein in red blood cells (RBCs), carries oxygen to the tissues. Carbon dioxide (CO_2), one of the primary waste products of metabolism, is dissolved in the plasma and must be eliminated quickly, since a buildup of CO_2 contributes to a state of **acidosis**.

Other components of the blood include the following:

- *White blood cells (WBCs)* Help defend the body against infection by bacteria, fungi, and other pathogens
- *Platelets* Initiate the process of clotting
- *Proteins* Perform various functions involving blood clotting, immunity, wound healing, and transport
- *Hormones* Control organ system function, regulate growth and development, and perform other vital functions
- *Nutrients* Fuel cells so that they can function properly (Glucose, for example, is a nutrient carried by the blood to cells throughout the body.)
- *Plasma* Carries the solid components in blood; this fluid is composed of about 92% water and 7% protein

An equilibrium must be maintained between the interstitial (extracellular) fluid, which occupies the spaces between the cells, and the intracellular fluid, which remains inside the cells. Plasma proteins are critical in the regulation of fluid equilibrium. The plasma proteins albumin and globulin are large and cannot easily pass out of the vessels. Their presence within the vessels creates an osmotic pressure that draws fluid back into the vasculature.

Blood Pressure

Blood pressure is the pressure the blood exerts against the walls of the arteries. Blood pressure is usually carefully controlled by the body so sufficient circulation in the various tissues and organs occurs; it is also considered a rough measure of perfusion. For perfusion to be effective, the heart must continue to force fluid into the system, and the arterial vessels must maintain their tone. This resistance of blood flow through the circulatory system is called *peripheral vascular resistance*, and it is determined by the degree of vasoconstriction of distal arteries and arterioles. Vasoconstriction exerts compressive force on the blood, which increases pressure within the vascular space. When peripheral resistance increases, arterial blood pressure rises, promoting blood flow through capillary beds and effectively perfusing the tissues.

As vessels shrink in diameter, friction—and thus resistance—increases. Friction is created as blood, a viscous fluid, courses along the vessel walls and through the vessels. RBCs are responsible for much of the blood's viscosity, but protein molecules contribute as well. When the composition of blood changes, it becomes more or less viscous. For example, the percentage of the fluid component of blood, called *plasma*, may increase or decrease. If the plasma level drops, evidenced by an increased hematocrit level, the blood becomes more viscous.

As the volume of blood ejected from the heart increases, so does the arterial blood pressure. Thus arterial blood pressure is an indirect indicator of tissue perfusion. The amount of pressure exerted against the arterial wall, stated in millimeters of mercury (mm Hg), determines the measured pressure. Blood pressure is expressed as the systolic pressure over the diastolic pressure. The systolic blood pressure represents the volume and pressure of blood ejected from the ventricle and the response of the arterial system to that ejection. The diastolic pressure represents the residual pressure in the arterial system after the ventricles relax.

Mean arterial pressure (MAP) is generally considered to be the patient's blood pressure and takes into consideration the systolic blood pressure as well as the diastolic blood pressure. However, MAP is ultimately the blood pressure required to sustain organ perfusion and is roughly 70 mm Hg. If the MAP falls significantly below 70 mm Hg for an appreciable amount of time, the result will be ischemia of the organs from lack of perfusion. Thus, the MAP needs to be greater than 60 mm Hg to ensure that the brain, coronary arteries, and kidneys remain perfused. Patients may have higher or lower MAPs in response to their medical conditions. Patients with chronic hypertension may require a pressure higher than the average to maintain adequate perfusion. The formula used to calculate the MAP is as follows:

$$\text{MAP} = \text{Diastolic pressure} + (1/3 \times \text{Pulse pressure})$$

Pulse pressure is the difference between the systolic and diastolic pressures. The pulse pressure is normally about

40 mm Hg. Changes in cardiac output or vascular resistance are responsible for changes in pulse pressure. The body's response to hypovolemic shock is an example of the effect of each on pulse pressure. A decrease in cardiac output and an increase in peripheral vascular resistance present as a narrowing pulse pressure. As volume is lost, a decrease in blood returning to the heart causes a decrease in cardiac output. The body responds by activating the sympathetic nervous system, which secretes epinephrine. This causes an increase in heart rate, an increase in contractility, and vasoconstriction. The result is an increase in diastolic blood pressure in the presence of a lower systolic blood pressure, causing a narrowing pulse pressure. The changes may be subtle and easily missed. For example, the blood pressure may change from 118/68 mm Hg to 108/82 mm Hg. This represents a decrease in pulse pressure of nearly 50% (50 to 26). When looking at the blood pressure alone, the decline in pulse pressure may not be noticed, but when the pulse pressure is calculated, a significant decrease is noted. A decline of greater than 50% indicates a 50% downturn in stroke volume. Pulse pressure is a helpful indicator of shock, especially when the measurement is taken repeatedly so that an emerging pattern can be identified. Like any other sign or symptom, it should be a part of the whole assessment and be used to direct you to collect other findings to confirm the patient's status.

The Autonomic Nervous System

The body is perfused via the cardiovascular system. Control of the cardiovascular system is a function of the autonomic nervous system, which is composed of competing subsystems. One of the subsystems, the sympathetic nervous system, helps maintain normal body functions and allows the body to respond to threats that demand an instant reaction—the so-called fight-or-flight response. During such events, the sympathetic nervous system plays a direct role in tissue perfusion by temporarily redirecting blood away from nonessential functions, such as digestion, and toward the heart and brain. The other subsystem of the autonomic nervous system is the parasympathetic nervous system, which is responsible for rest and regeneration. Table 4-1 summarizes the functions of the sympathetic and parasympathetic nervous systems.

Pathophysiology of Shock

Shock begins at the cellular level. The cellular changes that occur during shock have an impact on every system of the body, including the gastrointestinal (GI), endocrine, and neurologic systems. The symptoms of shock are consistent with the degree of metabolic impairment, but they are generally similar regardless of etiology. In other words, the compensatory mechanisms of the body tend to respond in the same way to enhance organ and tissue perfusion no matter which type of shock is presenting. Shock can result from inadequate cardiac output, decreased peripheral vascular resistance, or the inability of red blood cells to deliver oxygen to tissues. If there is a disturbance in the transportation of oxygen and removal of carbon dioxide, dangerous waste products will build up, leading to cellular death and eventually death of the entire organ.

The mitochondria are the first cellular component affected by shock. Most of the oxygen in the body is consumed by mitochondria, which produce 95% of the aerobic energy used by every body system. When oxygen has been depleted in the mitochondria, the cells undergo anaerobic metabolism, resulting in an increased production of lactate, thereby creating an acidic

Table 4-1 Functions of the Sympathetic and Parasympathetic Nervous Systems		
	Sympathetic System	**Parasympathetic System**
Cardiac muscle	Increased rate and strength	Decreased rate and strength
Coronary blood vessels	Constriction (alpha receptors) Dilation (beta receptors)	Dilation
Bronchioles	Relaxation (beta)	Constriction
Digestive tract	Decreased peristalsis	Increased peristalsis
Urinary bladder	Relaxation	Contraction
Skin	Sweat	No effect
Adrenal medulla	Increased epinephrine secretion	No effect

environment. An elevated lactate level in the blood, then, is a red flag for shock.

Metabolic Acidosis

During normal cell metabolism of glucose, oxygen is consumed. This process is called *aerobic metabolism*. When insufficient oxygen is present, glucose is metabolized through an alternative pathway that does not require oxygen. This process is termed *anaerobic metabolism*. The anaerobic pathway is much less efficient, yielding less energy (in the form of adenosine triphosphate [ATP]) per molecule of glucose and generating many more waste products, primarily lactic acid.

When the body tissues no longer have ample oxygen and cells begin producing lactic acid as a by-product of anaerobic metabolism, metabolic acidosis sets in. If shock persists, this alternative pathway will not be able to generate enough ATP, the primary means of energy storage. A deficiency of ATP impairs the function of the sodium potassium pump. The result is a buildup of sodium in the cell and a buildup of potassium in the serum. As a result, lactic acidosis and hyperkalemia (high blood potassium levels) develop. The edema forming within the cells and mitochondria eventually damages each of the components. Ischemic cells create lactate, free radicals, and inflammatory factors that increase damage to the cells. These toxins are flushed back into the circulatory system when perfusion is restored, contributing to damage to other organs as well. If the damage is severe, no amount of reoxygenation and perfusion can repair the damage, and cellular death occurs.

Three events may compromise cellular oxygen use: activation of the clot formation, lysosomal enzyme release, and a drop in circulatory volume. Each of these events triggers a cycle that progressively impairs the body's ability to maintain adequate oxygenation. As each state advances, a greater response is activated. As the body's circulatory volume becomes compromised and these states continue to advance, the body responds by activating additional compensatory mechanisms.

Compensatory Mechanisms

When any event results in decreased perfusion, such as in blood loss, myocardial infarction, or tension pneumothorax, the body must respond immediately to preserve the vital organs. A number of compensatory mechanisms can be activated to help maintain adequate oxygenation: increased minute ventilation, increased cardiac output (increased pulse rate and/or contractility), and vasoconstriction. Increased minute ventilation raises arterial oxygen content. The body boosts cardiac output by elevating the pulse rate, increasing cardiac contractility, or both. Constriction of vessels improves perfusion pressure in the tissues. In the aortic arch and carotid arteries, sympathetic nerve fibers called *baroreceptors* constantly monitor arterial blood pressure. Baroreceptors sense the decreased blood flow and activate the vasomotor center in the medulla oblongata, which oversees changes in the diameter of blood vessels, to begin constriction of the vessels and, therefore, increase blood pressure. The physiologic result of these mechanisms is vasoconstriction. The additional sympathetic response stimulates the heart resulting in an increase in pulse rate and cardiac contractility.

Compensatory mechanisms are effective only up to a point. Once that critical threshold has been reached, hypoxia develops, and shock overtakes the body. Ultimately, the oxygen levels available are insufficient to meet the oxygen demands throughout the body. If left untreated, multiple organ dysfunction and death are inevitable.

Adrenal Response

The adrenal glands, located on top of the kidneys, release epinephrine and norepinephrine in response to declining cardiac output. These hormones stimulate alpha and beta receptors in the heart and blood vessels. Alpha 1 triggers vasoconstriction, and beta 1 stimulates heart rate and cardiac contractility (Table 4-2). Receptor distribution usually leads to greater constriction in noncritical tissues such as fat, skin, and tissues of the digestive tract. Vasoconstriction also occurs within the kidneys.

Table 4-2 **Alpha-Beta Response to Shock**		
	Location	**Action**
Alpha 1	Arterioles in skin, viscera, mucous membranes Veins Bladder sphincters	Constriction, increased peripheral vascular resistance
Alpha 2	Digestive system	Decreased secretions, peristalsis
Beta 1	Heart, kidneys	Increased heart rate, force of contraction, oxygen consumption Release of renin
Beta 2	Arterioles of the heart, lungs, and skeletal muscles Bronchioles	Dilation with increased organ perfusion Dilation

Pituitary Response

The anterior pituitary gland releases antidiuretic hormone (ADH) in response to shock. ADH, which is synthesized in the hypothalamus, is released during early shock when symptoms are difficult to detect. As it circulates to the distal renal tubules and the collecting ducts in the kidneys, ADH causes fluid to be reabsorbed. Intravascular volume is maintained, and urine output decreases. ADH is also called *vasopressin* (from *vaso-*, meaning "vessel," and the Latin verb *pressor*, meaning "to press"). ADH stimulates smooth-muscle contraction in the digestive tract and blood vessels.

Renin-Angiotensin System Activation

The kidneys are vital to maintaining blood pressure. When blood flow to the kidneys is restricted, the renin-angiotensin system is activated. Renin is an enzyme released from the juxtaglomerular cells in the kidneys. It converts angiotensinogen to angiotensin I, which is in turn converted to angiotensin II in the lungs by angiotensin-converting enzymes (ACEs). Angiotensin I and II are proteins that stimulate the production and secretion of aldosterone from the adrenal cortex, which causes the kidneys to reabsorb sodium from the renal tubules. The sodium carries water back into the vasculature instead of excreting it in the urine, thereby increasing vascular volume and driving up blood pressure. The release of aldosterone signals the kidneys to halt the release of renin and restore perfusion to the kidneys. Aldosterone secretion also creates the sensation of thirst, one of the early signs of shock.

Angiotensin II is a potent but short-lived vasoconstrictor. During shock, it triggers constriction of the vessels farthest from the heart, creating resistance that increases the heart's afterload. The shunting of blood from the less essential organs allows for a greater return of blood to the heart, which increases preload. This selective perfusion occurs during the ischemic phase of shock. While perfusion of essential organs—the brain, heart, lungs, and liver—is enhanced, organs that are less essential become ischemic.

The Progression of Shock

Shock occurs in three successive phases—compensated, decompensated, and irreversible (Table 4-3). Your goal is to recognize the clinical signs and symptoms of shock in its earliest phase and begin immediate treatment before permanent damage occurs.

Table 4-3 Stages of Shock

Stage	Vital Signs	Signs and Symptoms	Pathophysiology
Compensated	Normal blood pressure Normal to slightly increased heart rate Tachypnea Delayed capillary refill	Cool hands and feet Pale mucous membranes Restlessness, anxiety Oliguria	Vasoconstriction maintains blood flow to essential organs, but tissue ischemia occurs in less essential areas.
Decompensated	Blood pressure decreasing Tachycardic > 120 beats/min Tachypneic > 30–40 beats/min	Waxen, cool, clammy skin Pale or cyanotic mucous membranes Profound weakness Metabolic (lactic) acidosis Anxiety Absent or decreased peripheral pulses	Blood pressure decreases as vascular tone decreases. Dysfunction to all organs is imminent. Anaerobic metabolism ensues, causing lactic acidosis.
Irreversible	Profound hypotension	Lactate > 8 mEq/L	Metabolic acidosis causes postcapillary sphincters to open and release stagnant and coagulated blood. Excessive potassium and acid causes dysrhythmias. Cellular damage is irreversible.

To do so, you must be aware of the subtle signs exhibited while the body is compensating and treat the patient aggressively (Table 4-4). Begin by anticipating the potential for shock based on the scene size-up and evaluation of the mechanism of injury. As your assessment progresses, you need to recognize the signs of poor perfusion that precede hypotension, and do not rely on any one sign or symptom to determine the phase of shock the patient is going through. Always err on the side of caution when you are treating a potential shock patient by initiating rapid assessment, immediate intervention, and transportation to preserve any chance of survival.

Altered mental status changes such as confusion and lethargy are late indicators because a key purpose of the shock syndrome is to keep the brain well perfused. Sometimes "alert" patients may be agitated or anxious during the compensated phase, but this is not considered an altered mental status.

Compensated Shock

The earliest stage of shock, in which the body can still compensate for decreased perfusion, is called compensated shock. In compensated shock, the body responds to an event that is causing anaerobic metabolism and a buildup of lactic acid by releasing chemical mediators. The chemical mediators, which are released by the autonomic nervous system, act to compensate for the potential catastrophic event. They stimulate the vascular system to contract, causing the arterial pressure to remain normal or slightly elevated. To address the need for oxygen and the developing acidosis, the system increases the rate and depth of respirations to assist the body to bring in more oxygen and remove more carbon dioxide. At this stage of shock, the body attempts to maintain the acid–base balance by creating respiratory alkalosis to offset the metabolic acidosis. You may see this as a decrease in capnography readings and an elevated lactate level if these measurements are assessed.

During the compensated phase of shock, blood pressure is maintained. Blood loss in hemorrhagic shock can be estimated to be at 15% to 30% at this point. A narrowing of the pulse pressure (the difference between the diastolic and systolic pressures) also occurs. The pulse pressure reflects the tone of the arterial system and is more indicative of changes in perfusion than the systolic or diastolic blood pressure alone. Patients in the compensated phase will also have a positive orthostatic test result. It is key to remember that patients in compensated shock are in shock and should be treated accordingly.

Decompensated Shock

The next stage of shock, when blood pressure is falling, is decompensated shock. In hemorrhagic shock, decompensated shock occurs when blood volume drops by more than 30%. The compensatory mechanisms are no longer able to support the progressing catastrophic event, and signs and symptoms become much more obvious. The cardiac output falls dramatically, leading to further reductions in blood pressure and cardiac function. The signs and symptoms become more obvious as blood is shunted to the brain and heart. The kidneys respond by autoregulating their own blood flow. When the cardiac output drops, the arterioles perfusing (afferent) the capillaries of the kidneys dilate and the arterioles leaving (efferent) the glomerular capillaries constrict. This allows for perfusion of the kidneys. Once the blood pressure drops, this process cannot be maintained and the perfusion of the kidneys is severely compromised. At this point, vasoconstriction can have a disastrous effect if allowed to continue. Cells in the nonperfused tissues become hypoxic, leading to anaerobic metabolism and cell death. Aggressive intervention at this stage may result in recovery.

Blood pressure may be the last measurable factor to change in shock. The body has several automatic mechanisms to compensate for initial loss of perfusion and to help maintain blood pressure. Thus, by the time you detect a drop in blood

Table 4-4 **Signs of Compensated versus Decompensated Shock**	
Compensated Shock	**Decompensated Shock**
Agitation, anxiety, restlessness	Altered mental status (verbal to unresponsive)*
Sense of impending doom	Hypotension
Weak, rapid (thready) pulse	Labored or irregular breathing
Clammy (cool, moist) skin	Thready or absent peripheral pulses
Pallor with cyanotic lips	Ashen, mottled, or cyanotic skin
Shortness of breath	Dilated pupils
Nausea, vomiting	Diminished urine output
Delayed capillary refill in infants and children	Impending cardiac arrest
Thirst	
Normal blood pressure	

*Mental status changes are late indicators.

pressure, shock is well developed. This is particularly true in infants, children, and pregnant women whose blood pressure may be maintained until they have lost more than 35% to 40% of their blood volume. For all hypotensive patients in whom you suspect shock, consider their situation an emergency, initiate lifesaving interventions, and start transport in less than 10 minutes, providing fluid resuscitation en route to the most appropriate ED.

Irreversible (Terminal) Shock

The last phase of shock is irreversible shock, when the condition has progressed to a terminal stage. Arterial blood pressure is abnormally low (typically in hemorrhagic shock there is a 40% or greater blood volume loss). A progressive deterioration of the cardiovascular system that cannot be reversed by compensatory mechanisms or medical interventions results in multisystem organ failure. Life-threatening reductions in cardiac output, blood pressure, and tissue perfusion are observed. Blood is shunted away from the liver, kidneys, and lungs to keep the heart and brain perfused. Cells begin to die. Even if the cause of shock is treated and reversed, vital organ damage cannot be repaired, and the patient may eventually die. Providing aggressive treatment at this stage does not usually result in recovery; however, because it is difficult to determine who will or will not survive, you should provide aggressive treatment en route to the appropriate facility.

AMLS Assessment Pathway

▼ Initial Observations

The AMLS assessment pathway for shock helps you efficiently recognize, evaluate, and manage a patient in shock. Early recognition and intervention of shock correlate directly with the likelihood your patient will survive the life-threatening incident. Your initial observations should center on recognizing the presence or potential for hypoperfusion. Because shock may be pronounced or insidious, you may recognize shock at multiple points during the pathway. The key is maintaining a high level of suspicion for shock because it is a life threat that may progress rapidly.

Scene Safety Considerations

Scene safety is critical in approaching any patient. When dealing with a patient who appears critical, it is easy to miss a safety issue, so take the time to ensure the scene remains safe for you and all involved.

Patient Cardinal Presentation/Chief Complaint

Initial presentations may vary in patients in shock. A patient with gastrointestinal bleeding, for example, may complain of abdominal pain, a patient with a thoracic aortic dissection may complain of back pain, and a patient with a tension pneumothorax may complain of respiratory distress. All of these patients may be in shock, but each patient's cardinal presentation is different. Each patient's treatment evolves as new diagnostic information is discovered. In the patient whose condition is critical, your immediate focus should be on airway, breathing, and circulation until definitive care is reached. If you see or suspect trauma, protect the cervical spine while initiating assessment or treatment.

For the patient suspected of shock, you must determine the following:

- Do I see any signs of a life threat as I approach my patient? Altered level of consciousness or respiratory distress?
- Does the patient's skin show signs of shock? Pale, gray-appearing, diaphoretic, blotchy, or hives?
- Do the surroundings suggest the possibility of shock? Vomitus, blood?

Primary Survey

You should focus your assessment and history collection on the components that will help you identify and treat the life threats and complete these interventions once the patient's condition stabilizes. Unexplained signs and symptoms of shock warrant immediate transport. Support oxygenation, ventilation, and circulation, maintain a normal body temperature, monitor cardiac status, and conduct pulse oximetry and capnography.

Level of Consciousness

Any patient who has an altered level of consciousness or seems anxious, combative, or confused should be evaluated for hypoxia and signs of shock. Assessing the patient using the AVPU mnemonic and the Glasgow Coma Scale can help you determine whether the patient has altered mentation. Consider oxygen administration and addressing life-threatening causes if an alteration in consciousness is identified.

Airway and Breathing

If the patient is unable to maintain a patent airway, you should provide basic airway management until definitive care is achieved, whether it is on scene or en route to the receiving facility. The key is to focus on the patient's needs and meet them in a timely manner. If you suspect cardiac arrest, use the CAB (circulation/compressions, airway, breathing) approach. Otherwise, assess the ABCs.

Once you have secured the patient's airway, you should direct your attention to improving oxygenation. Remember, the patient's oxygen level may drop significantly before symptoms of hypoxia become apparent. An escalation in the rate and depth of respiration, often the earliest sign of shock, can be confused with anxiety. Increased work of breathing should lead you to rule out a life threat as well. The patient's breathing may provide you with clues of acidosis. Prevention and prompt treatment of early acidosis can greatly improve patient outcome. If the ventilatory rate is slow in the presence of shock, shock has reached an advanced stage.

Circulation/Perfusion

Circulatory status can be rapidly assessed. Begin by looking for obvious bleeding as you approach the patient. Bloody vomitus or stool should raise suspicion of internal bleeding. Bright red blood in the stool indicates active bleeding from the lower GI tract. Dark red or maroon stool, called *melena*, is due to upper GI bleeding. Dark or black blood in the stool may indicate either old bleeding or the presence of digested blood. You may also smell the presence of GI bleeding before you see evidence. If the patient is unable to speak, ask bystanders what they have witnessed.

As you assess the patient's pulse ask yourself the following questions:

- Are the radial, carotid, and femoral pulses strong, or are they weak and thready?
- Is the rate too fast or too slow?
- Is the rate regular or irregular?

Since blood pressure is maintained in the early stages of shock, the quality of the pulse is a more useful tool to use when evaluating perfusion. Evaluating pulse quality will give you more information in less time. A weak, thready pulse is an indicator of hypoperfusion. A bounding, strong pulse suggests adequate perfusion. As you assess the patient's pulse, note the color and temperature of the skin—cool pale skin due to peripheral vasoconstriction is common in shock. For the most part, the presence of tachycardia indicates the patient may be in shock. Patients with bradycardia may have a cardiac arrhythmia contributing to shock. Bradycardia may also be present in neurogenic shock. Action should be taken to address the problem found, administering fluid and treating the cause of the pulse rate. Do not delay transport of a patient in shock.

If you must expose an area of the patient's body to assess properly for further illness or injury, take care to keep the patient warm. Shock causes diminished peripheral perfusion. Shunting of blood to the essential organs, together with the switch to anaerobic metabolism, make it difficult for the patient to retain body heat. Consider placing blankets under and over the patient and administering warmed IV fluids to help maintain the patient's temperature. Any IV fluid that is cooler than normal body temperature will have to be warmed by the patient's body, putting additional demands on an already strained metabolism.

▼ First Impression

Your first impression is key to identifying a patient in shock. For example, the initial appearance of a prostrate patient who is pale and lethargic should warrant a quick movement to the patient's side to rule out threats to the patient's life, including shock. Interventions focusing on life threats are a priority at this time.

▼ Detailed Assessment

History Taking

In a high-priority patient, history taking can be done en route to the ED along with the secondary survey and any ongoing management. Time is of the essence in shock patients. Focus on transporting the patient to the ED and keep the on-scene care to the essential items that must be done before moving the patient, such as evaluating airway, breathing, and circulation.

Obtaining a thorough history, including an account of the present illness and a comprehensive past medical history, is essential to determining the type of shock, but keep in mind that the interventions that add time to the scene must be justified by the benefits they will produce for the patient. The SAMPLER and OPQRST mnemonics can be used to obtain historical information. You may be selective initially as you are obtaining a history. For example, in a patient with signs and symptoms of shock who is complaining of "trouble breathing," you may rapidly focus on allergies, recent medication, foods ingested (allergies, medications, and last meal from SAMPLER) and ask how severe (severity from OPQRST) the patient's allergic reactions have been in the past as you initiate care and move to a physical exam. Historical data, in combination with physical exam findings, will help you modify the diagnosis and select appropriate interventions. Table 4-5 lists hypoperfusion considerations in the patient history, and Table 4-6 details medications affecting shock. Once the life threats are managed, a complete history can be obtained.

Secondary Survey

Vital Signs

Vital signs (blood pressure, pulse rate, respiratory rate, and temperature) are essential to determining the patient's stability and pinpointing the type of shock. Most types of shock are characterized by hypotension, tachycardia, tachypnea, and cool skin, but there are several exceptions. Because the blood vessels are dilated in distributive shock, the patient will have hypotension and tachycardia, but his skin may be warm. In cardiogenic shock, the patient's pulse rate may be bradycardic or tachycardic, depending on the underlying cause. In neurogenic shock, the patient is often both bradycardic and vasodilated. Vital signs will also help you determine the stages of shock and the patient's response to interventions, so trends are important.

Table 4-5 **History Taking for Hypoperfusion**
History of Volume Loss?
<ul><li>Vomiting</li><li>Diarrhea</li><li>Excessive sweating</li><li>Excessive urination</li><li>Blood loss—internal or external (hemorrhagic)</li></ul>
Obstructive Shock
Tension Pneumothorax<ul><li>Breath sounds—decreased on one side</li><li>Jugular venous distention (JVD)</li><li>Increasing respiratory distress</li></ul>**Pulmonary Emboli**<ul><li>Risk factors</li><li>Sudden onset</li><li>Hypoxia</li><li>Chest pain</li></ul>**Cardiac Tamponade**<ul><li>Risk factors</li><li>Muffled heart tones</li><li>JVD</li></ul>
Distributive Shock
Neurogenic<ul><li>Cord injury (traumatic and nontraumatic)</li><li>Recent trauma</li><li>Flushed skin</li></ul>**Anaphylaxis**<ul><li>History of exposure to allergen</li><li>Angioedema</li><li>Breath sounds—wheezing</li><li>Hives</li></ul>**Sepsis**<ul><li>History of infection (pneumonia)</li><li>Receiving antibiotics</li><li>Fever (possible)</li><li>Wounds, Foley catheter, drains, IV</li><li>Depressed immune system</li></ul>
Cardiogenic Shock
<ul><li>Cardiac history</li><li>Acute myocardial infarction (AMI)</li><li>12-lead ECG changes</li><li>Breath sounds—crackles in lungs</li><li>JVD</li><li>Peripheral edema</li></ul>
Other
<ul><li>Toxic exposure</li><li>Drug overdose</li></ul>

Physical Exam

Performing a physical exam in a patient with signs and symptoms of shock focuses on determining the cause and selecting the proper intervention. For example, as you approach a patient with an initial presentation of chest pain and signs of shock, you see distended neck veins. You know that distended neck veins may be possible with cardiac tamponade, tension pneumothorax, and cardiogenic shock due to right-sided heart failure. Your next step may be to listen to the lungs. You note decreased breath sounds on one side. This points you to the possibility of a developing tension pneumothorax and obstructive shock.

Diagnostics

Diagnostic tools used to evaluate patients with signs of shock include monitoring (pulse oximetry, cardiac rhythm, glucose monitoring, possibly hemodynamics), electrocardiography, and laboratory testing. When end-tidal carbon dioxide ($ETCO_2$) testing is available, it is a valuable adjunct to monitor acidosis and respiratory status. In the hospital, laboratory studies, computed tomography (CT), ultrasonography, and radiographic studies are essential. Table 4-7 outlines laboratory studies typically used to evaluate patients in shock.

Pulse Oximetry

A pulse oximeter is one of the simplest assessment tools to use. It requires placing a sensor on the patient's finger or skin, but despite its apparent straightforwardness, pulse oximetry presents many possibilities for error. If the pulse oximetry monitor does not display a waveform, you should question the accuracy of the reading. As blood pressure drops, peripheral vascular constriction increases and may make obtaining a pulse oximetry reading difficult to obtain. Due to the time it takes for blood to circulate, a delay in a change of the reading may occur, so a patient may be more hypoxic or less hypoxic than the actual reading. Patient care should never be delayed or withheld based on a pulse oximetry reading when other signs and symptoms indicate poor tissue perfusion is present.

Capnography

Capnography is useful in identifying shock. When the cardiac output drops suddenly, less blood is delivered to the lungs resulting in less carbon dioxide being delivered, which results in a sudden drop in $ETCO_2$ readings. The drop is seen even though the respiratory rate is maintained. A drop in $ETCO_2$ reading occurs when a ventilation-perfusion ($\dot{V}/\dot{Q}$) mismatch is present. As discussed later in the septic shock section, capnography is a valuable tool in the identification of sepsis. It is also a predictor of mortality associated with shock. Further research of capnography and its association with shock and metabolic acidosis may make this a valuable tool for identification of shock in the future.

Table 4-6 Medications Affecting Shock

Medication	Effect	Shock
Steroids	May mask signs of infection; decrease potential for early recognition	Sepsis
Beta-blockers	Block an increase in heart rate, decreasing ability to compensate	All types
Anticoagulants/antiplatelets	Increase potential for bleeding	Hemorrhagic
Calcium channel blockers	Inhibit vasoconstriction, decreasing ability to compensate	All types
Hypoglycemic agents	May impair blood glucose regulation	All types
Herbal preparations	May contribute to bleeding May increase workload on the heart	Hemorrhagic Cardiogenic specifically, but all types may be affected
Diuretics	Long-term diuretic therapy may cause hypokalemia and contribute to a dehydration state.	All types

Table 4-7 Laboratory Tests for Patients in Shock

Test	Normal Values	Abnormal Values	Indications for Test
Glucose	70–110 mg/dL (3.8–6.1 mmol/L)	Increase indicates hyperglycemia, diabetic ketoacidosis, steroid use, stress. Decrease indicates hypoglycemia, decreased reserves.	All types of shock
Hemoglobin (Hb)/hematocrit (Hct)	Hb, male: 14–18 g/dL (8.7–11.2 mmol/L) Hb, female: 12–16 g/dL (7.4–9.9 mmol/L) Hct, male: 42%–52% (0.42–0.52) Hct, female: 37%–47% (0.37–0.47)	Decrease indicates severe blood loss. Increase indicates plasma loss, dehydration.	All types of shock
Gastric/stool hemoglobin	Negative	Positive result indicates GI bleeding.	Suspected GI bleeding

(continues)

Table 4-7 Laboratory Tests for Patients in Shock (*continued*)

Test	Normal Values	Abnormal Values	Indications for Test
Lactic acid	Venous: 5–20 mg/dL (0.6–2.2 mmol/L)	Increase indicates tissue hypoperfusion and acidosis, prolonged use of tourniquet.	All types of shock
Complete blood cell count	Total WBC count 5,000–10,000/mm³ (5–10 × 10⁹/L)	Increased (excessive) WBC count indicates sepsis.	More important in septic shock
Acid–base balance	pH 7.35–7.45	Increased pH indicates alkalosis. Decreased pH indicates acidosis and impaired perfusion.	All types of shock
	Hco₃ 21–28 mEq/L	Decreased bicarbonate levels indicate it is being lost or used up rapidly in conditions such as diarrhea, intestinal fistula, or in response to increased acid such as renal failure, DKA, salicylate overdose. Increased bicarbonate levels indicate excessive intake of bicarbonate or antacids, lactate administration, or loss of acid from conditions such as vomiting, gastric suctioning, potassium deficiency, diuretic use.	
Arterial blood gases	Pco₂ 35–45 mm Hg Po₂ 80–100 mm Hg	Increased Pco₂ levels indicate CO₂ retention, hypoventilation, pneumonia, pulmonary infections, pulmonary emboli, CHF, conditions that impair respiratory effort. Decreased Pco₂ levels indicate decrease in CO₂ levels, hyperventilation, anxiety, fear, pain, CNS lesions, pregnancy, conditions that increase respiratory ventilation. Also occurs in response to metabolic acidosis (i.e., DKA) Decrease in O₂ levels indicates hypoxia.	All types of shock

(continues)

Table 4-7 Laboratory Tests for Patients in Shock (*continued*)

Test	Normal Values	Abnormal Values	Indications for Test
Serum electrolytes	Na (Sodium) 136–145 mEq/L (136–145 mmol/L) K (Potassium) 3.5–5 mEq/L (3.5–5 mmol/L)	Increased Na levels may be present with osmotic diuresis. Increased K levels are common in acidosis, vomiting, diarrhea, and DKA. Increased K levels may cause an abnormal ECG; peaked T waves may be present.	All types of shock
Renal function	Serum urea nitrogen 10–20 mg/dL (3.6–7.1 mmol/L) Creatinine 0.5–1.2 mg/dL (44–97 mmol/L)	Increased levels of serum urea nitrogen indicate severe dehydration, shock, sepsis. Increased serum creatinine levels (> 4 mg/dL [0.2 mmol/L]) indicate impaired renal function.	All types of shock
Blood/urine cultures	Negative	Positive result indicates infection.	Septic shock

CHF, congestive heart failure; *CNS*, central nervous system; *CO_2*, carbon dioxide; *DKA*, diabetic ketoacidosis; *ECG*, electrocardiogram; *GI*, gastrointestinal; *Hco_3*, bicarbonate; *K*, potassium; *Na*, sodium; *O_2*, oxygen; *Pco_2*, partial pressure of carbon dioxide; *Po_2*, partial pressure of oxygen (oxygen saturation); *WBC*, white blood cell.

This article was published in Mosby's Diagnostivc and Laboratory Test Reference, 9 ed., Pagana KD, Pagana TJ. Copyright Mosby 2009.

Electrocardiogram

An ECG is helpful in assessing heart rhythm, ischemia, injury, and certain electrolyte abnormalities. Leads must be properly placed, the findings interpreted or transmitted, and the results used to guide transport of the patient to an appropriate health-care institution. Because shock may be the result of a myocardial infarction or shock may contribute to a myocardial infarction, a multilead, diagnostic ECG should be completed in the secondary survey but early enough to help determine the patient's destination for definitive care (e.g., cardiac catheterization and intervention lab).

Laboratory Studies

Establish appropriate vascular access, and draw blood for laboratory analysis according to local protocols if you can do so without delaying appropriate care. Many facilities will not accept prehospital blood draws, so know the policies of your facility. Point-of-care testing is becoming more common in the prehospital setting, but, once again, transporting a patient in shock to an appropriate facility is your priority. Because of an increase in a person's metabolism during shock, glucose can become periously low without warning. A bedside glucose test should be done if the patient's mental status is altered. Glucose may also be elevated, as may lactate in a shock patient. Suspect septic shock in nondiabetic patients with elevated lactate and glucose levels. Elevated lactate levels due to acidosis are indicative of shock.

In the hospital, interfacility, or critical care transport setting, urine output should be maintained at a minimum of 0.5 to 1 mL/kg/h in adults (1 to 2 mL/kg/h in children) who do not have kidney disease. Urine output is an important metric because it indicates renal perfusion.

▼ Refine the Differential Diagnosis

You may have determined in your primary survey that the patient was in shock but may not have determined the cause or the disease process causing the shock. The components of the secondary survey will bring you to the stage of refining your differential diagnosis and determining the severity of the patient's condition. It is important to move quickly through this assessment with calculated purpose to help you identify the cause of shock and to initiate the necessary interventions. You may initiate care all along the way to manage the life threats, which may be identified immediately or may appear later in the assessment as your patient moves through the stages of shock. Regardless of when a life threat appears in a patient in shock, it is essential to return to the ABCs of the primary survey and then progress through your secondary survey during transport to refine the differential diagnosis as time and patient condition allows.

▼ Ongoing Management

The rule of thumb is to assess, intervene, and reassess. During your ongoing management, revisit the primary assessment, the vital signs, the chief complaint, and any treatment you have administered, including oxygen administration. Always consider the possibility of trauma, and protect the cervical spine if you suspect the patient may have been injured. Proper positioning depends on initial complaints and symptoms. If a patient is unable to tolerate the supine position because of respiratory distress or intolerable pain—or for any other reason—place the head as low as can be tolerated to ease the heart's workload and enhance perfusion.

To ensure adequate perfusion, optimal oxygenation must be maintained. Many patients become hypoxic before the symptoms of shock are overt. Critically ill or injured patients should receive oxygen. If the respiratory rate is inadequate, you may need to deliver 100% oxygen through a nonrebreathing mask or a bag-mask device. If these measures are ineffective, consider using advanced airway techniques such as intubation. Generally the goal is to administer oxygen to maintain a pulse oximetry of 94% to 98%.

Begin maintaining the patient's circulatory status by stopping any obvious bleeding. Although hemorrhagic hypovolemic shock is one of the most common types of shock, it is not the only cause of hypoperfusion. Most perfusion problems have complex causes that are difficult to reverse, so your treatment may be limited to symptomatic care until the underlying etiology can be addressed at the receiving facility. En route to the ED, initiate vascular access.

Fluid Resuscitation

Initiate administration of isotonic crystalloid fluid in patients with hypovolemic shock, but be mindful that it may be insufficient because it does not carry oxygen, hemoglobin, clotting factors, or any other essential blood components. Also remember that isotonic crystalloid fluid works as a temporary volume expander, but if too much is administered, the existing blood volume will become more dilute, compounding the edema that is already present. Frequent evaluation during administration therefore is essential. Obtaining initial lab work early will assist in fluid resuscitation needs.

An initial bolus of 20 to 30 mL/kg (1,000 to 2,000 L) of isotonic fluid should be given if the patient shows no signs of fluid overload (e.g., crackles on lung auscultation). If the patient is at risk for fluid overload, a more modest bolus of 250 to 500 mL, followed by a reassessment, is appropriate. The purpose of fluid resuscitation should be to enhance perfusion to maintain an MAP at 60 to 70 or a systolic pressure at 80 to 90 mm Hg.

Colloids, whole blood, packed RBCs, fresh-frozen plasma, platelets, dextran, and albumin are other volume expanders. If bleeding is suspected, administration of blood products is indicated. Blood products replace blood volume while offering the additional advantage of oxygen-carrying capacity, but the presence of antibodies in human blood presents some risk. It is preferred that blood be typed and crossmatched, but if time does not allow, uncrossmatched type O-negative blood can be given. If massive transfusions are required, early administration of fresh-frozen plasma and platelets has been shown to improve survival.

Dextran is a synthetic volume expander. It stays in the vessels longer than isotonic fluid, but it has no oxygen-carrying capability. Albumin is a human blood product that does not require typing or crossmatching, but it has no oxygen-carrying capacity, either. These fluids are controversial but may be indicated at some point during shock management. Isotonic fluid should be considered in the initial management.

Temperature Regulation

The body expends a great deal of energy on maintaining a normal temperature. Vasoconstriction shunts blood away from peripheral tissues, and the body will expend valuable energy trying to stay warm. To help conserve metabolic reserves, keep the patient warm. The ambulance or resuscitation room should be kept very warm, and the patient should be covered with a blanket when practical. This can be difficult during the physical exam, but it should be a high priority. Administration of warmed fluids will assist in maintaining body temperature and should be initiated when feasible.

Vasopressor Administration

Vasopressors, which are medications that raise reduced blood pressure, are an efficient adjunct treatment in patients with certain types of hypoperfusion. In cardiogenic shock, the heart isn't functioning effectively, and inotropic agents can improve cardiac output by bolstering cardiac contractility and raising blood pressure. Distributive shock, especially neurogenic shock, is characterized by hypotension and bradycardia. Although volume replacement can be helpful, vasopressors may be required to arouse the responsiveness of the veins for the patient in neurogenic shock. It is essential to ensure volume replacement has occurred prior to vasopressor initiation. The following vasoconstrictors and inotropes may be administered:

Vasoconstrictors
- Epinephrine
- Norepinephrine
- Dopamine

Inotropes
- Dopamine
- Dobutamine
- Epinephrine
- Isoproterenol
- Norepinephrine

Administration of Blood Products

Blood administration may be a viable option in the prehospital setting. When the patient is considered anemic, is in shock, or has a serious bleeding disorder, administration of blood products is indicated. As already noted, the overriding goal of a blood product transfusion is to increase the blood's oxygen-carrying capacity. Selection of the appropriate blood products will depend on the patient's underlying condition.

If blood products are stored as whole blood, the shelf life would be very brief, and the platelets within would deactivate quickly. The preferred process is to separate the blood components out and provide specific products with longer shelf life. For blood transfusions, packed red blood cells are generally used. These packed cells have 80% of the plasma removed and a preservative added. Table 4-8 describes available blood products and their clinical applications.

Transfusion Reactions

There are generally two complications of blood product administration: infection and immune reactions. Improved methods of screening donors and blood products have decreased problems with the spread of infections. There remains a small risk, especially for cytomegalovirus, which is a common virus that is rarely serious in the general population. Some pathogens can infect blood even during cold storage.

Hemolytic Reactions

When the recipient's antibodies recognize and react to transfused blood as an antigen, the donor RBCs are destroyed or hemolyzed. This hemolytic reaction can be quick and aggressive or slower, depending on the immune response.

Errors in the blood administration process can create fatal hemolytic reactions. When this occurs, most transfused cells are destroyed in an overwhelming immune response. When an immune response occurs, the coagulation cascade is also engaged, potentially creating bleeding disorders such as disseminated intravascular coagulation (DIC). With DIC and anaphylactic response, symptoms may include back pain, IV site pain, headache, chills and fever, hypotension, dyspnea, tachycardia, bronchospasm, pulmonary edema, coagulopathic bleeding, and renal failure.

At the first sign of transfusion reaction, the blood products must be stopped and appropriate lab analysis completed. Immediate supportive treatment is instituted and the blood bank notified. Every institution that credentials personnel to administer blood products has strict policies and procedures that guide the provider in these cases.

Febrile Transfusion Reactions

During the transfusion or shortly thereafter, fever that is usually responsive to antipyretics may develop. Monitoring the patient's temperature is a standard of care during blood administration. Those patients prone to febrile reactions may be given diphenhydramine and acetaminophen as the transfusion is begun.

Allergic Transfusion Reaction

An onset of hives and/or rash is usually self-limiting during transfusion of blood products, but some cases will progress to bronchospasm and anaphylaxis. Treatment may include

Table 4-8 **Blood Products**	
Product	**Clinical Application**
Packed red blood cells	Low hemoglobin (usually < 7.0)
Platelets	Prevent bleeding
	Thrombocytopenia
Fresh-frozen plasma (FFP)	Coagulation deficiencies in liver failure, warfarin overdose, disseminated intravascular coagulation, or massive transfusion
Cryoprecipitate (cold FFP with fibrinogen, factor VIII, and von Willebrand factor)	For bleeding disorder, massive transfusion
Massive transfusion	Aggressively bleeding patients where > 10 units of blood given over 24 hours; coagulation factors and platelets added. Patient at risk for hypothermia, hypocalcemia.

antihistamines. In case of a more severe reaction, treatment for anaphylaxis should be initiated.

Transfusion-Related Acute Lung Injury

Transfusion-related acute lung injury (ALI) is a rare but complex immune response during or after transfusion, with subsequent development of noncardiogenic pulmonary edema, or ARDS/ALI, which is described in the *Acute Respiratory Distress Syndrome or Acute Lung Injury* section of this chapter.

Hypervolemia

For those patients with limited cardiovascular reserve (elderly, infants), transfusion of blood products can increase circulating volume and create problems for the patient's cardiovascular system with symptoms of dyspnea, hypoxia, and pulmonary edema.

Pathophysiology, Assessment, and Management of Specific Types of Shock

Shock can be categorized into four types: hypovolemic, distributive, cardiogenic, and obstructive, depending on which portion of the cardiovascular system fails (Table 4-9). Failure can occur in any of the three major components of the cardiovascular system: the pump (the heart), the pipes (the blood vessels), or the fluid within them (the blood).

Hypovolemic Shock

It is easy to remember the cause of inadequate tissue perfusion in hypovolemic shock by taking a closer look at the term **hypovolemia** itself. The prefix *hypo-* means "below" or "low," *vol-* refers to volume, and the combining form *-emia* means "in or pertaining to the blood."

Inadequate circulating fluid leads to a diminished cardiac output, which results in an inadequate delivery of oxygen to the tissues and cells. The classic signs and symptoms of hypovolemic shock are tachycardia, hypotension, and increased respiratory rate, but signs will vary depending on how much fluid has been lost. Bleeding, vomiting, diarrhea, and many other conditions can lower the volume of circulating fluid (**Figure 4-3**). There are hemorrhagic and nonhemorrhagic causes of hypovolemic shock.

Hemorrhagic Shock

Hemorrhagic shock is a common cause of hypovolemic shock. Significant blood loss can occur without obvious bleeding. Internal or external hemorrhage can accompany traumatic injuries or medical problems such as ruptured or dissected aortic aneurysm, ruptured spleen, ectopic pregnancy, GI bleeding, or other causes of significant blood loss. The bleeding may be obvious, as in a patient vomiting blood, or insidious, as in a patient with internal GI bleeding that has been occurring over time. In hemorrhagic shock, oxygen-carrying capacity diminishes as red blood cells are depleted.

Table 4-9 Types of Shock			
Category	**Initial Signs**	**Causes**	**Management**
Hypovolemic Shock			
Hemorrrhagic/ nonhemorrhagic	Cool, clammy skin Pale, cyanotic skin Decreased BP Altered LOC Decreased capillary refill	Hemorrhage: trauma, GI bleeding, ruptured aortic aneurysm, pregnancy-related bleeding Severe dehydration: gastroenteritis, diabetic ketoacidosis, adrenal crisis	Administer oxygen. Stop the bleeding. Give IV fluid bolus. Splint fractures. Transport to appropriate facility for surgical intervention.
Distributive Shock			
Septic	Hyperthermia or hypothermia Decreased BP Altered LOC	Infection	Administer oxygen. Give IV fluid bolus. Administer antibiotics. Consider vasopressors.

(continues)

Table 4-9 Types of Shock (*continued*)

Category	Initial Signs	Causes	Management
Anaphylactic	Pruritus, erythema, urticaria, angioedema Increased pulse rate Decreased BP Anxiousness Respiratory distress, wheezing	Antibody-antigen hypersensitivity response	Give epinephrine 1:1,000, 0.3–0.5 mg IM. May repeat as needed. Epinephrine 1:10,000, 0.3–0.5 mg IV if no response to IM administration over 3–10 min, and repeat every 15 min as needed. Epinephrine should not be withheld in order to start an IV. Intravenous fluid bolus Diphenhydramine, 1–2 mg/kg IV (max, 50 mg) Consider corticosteroid treatment. Consider vasopressor treatment. Consider H_2 administration.
Neurogenic	Warm, dry, pink skin Decreased BP Alert Normal capillary refill time		Administer oxygen. Give IV fluid bolus. Consider norepinephrine or dopamine.
Toxins	Based on specific agent (See Chapter 10 for a discussion of toxic agents.)	(See Chapter 10.)	Based on specific agent (See Chapter 10.)
Cardiogenic Shock			
	Cool, clammy skin Pale, cyanotic skin Tachypnea Tachycardia or other abnormal rhythm Decreased BP Altered LOC Decreased capillary refill time	Pump failure: AMI, cardiomyopathy, myocarditis, ruptured chordae tendineae, papillary muscle dysfunction, toxins, myocardial contusion, acute aortic insufficiency, ruptured ventricular septum Dysrhythmia	Administer oxygen. Give IV fluid bolus. Rate correction (medication or pacing/cardioversion) Inotropes Vasopressors Intra-aortic balloon pump
Obstructive Shock			
	Decreased blood pressure Difficulty breathing, tachycardia, tachypnea JVD, unilateral decreased breath sounds, muffled heart tones	Massive pulmonary embolus, tension pneumothorax, acute pericardial tamponade	Administer oxygen. Perform needle decompression for tension pneumothorax. Perform a pericardiocentesis for a pericardial tamponade. Transport to appropriate facility for surgical intervention.

AMI, Acute myocardial infarction; *BP,* blood pressure; *GI,* gastrointestinal; *IM,* intramuscular; *IV,* intravenous; *JVD,* jugular venous distention; *LOC,* level of consciousness.

Hemorrhagic hypovolemic shock is best treated by stopping the bleeding. External bleeding can be more readily controlled in the prehospital setting than internal bleeding. In the presence of external bleeding, direct pressure should be applied. If direct pressure or a pressure dressing to an extremity is ineffective, a tourniquet should be used. In the past, concern about tissue and nerve destruction discouraged tourniquet application. Although such damage is a possibility, survival of the whole person outweighs survival of an extremity. When possible, it is key to apply the tourniquet before signs and symptoms of shock present to increase the rate of patient survival. Use of hemostatic dressings and wound packing may be considered to control external bleeding as well.

Nonhemorrhagic Shock

Loss of fluids other than blood can also cause hypovolemic shock. For example, extreme interstitial fluid loss may follow vomiting, diarrhea, and massive diuresis in patients with diabetes mellitus or diabetes insipidus. Excessive plasma loss in patients with significant burn injuries and inadequate fluid replacement may result in shock. Shock in these patients is often delayed due to the time it takes for the fluids to shift.

The severity of shock depends on the percentage and rate of fluid loss. Insidious fluid loss gives the body time to compensate. In a healthy adult, a 10% to 15% blood loss is well tolerated. Children and older adults are more sensitive to even a small amount of volume loss, and compensatory mechanisms or medications may delay outward signs. **Table 4-10** summarizes the stages of hypovolemic shock.

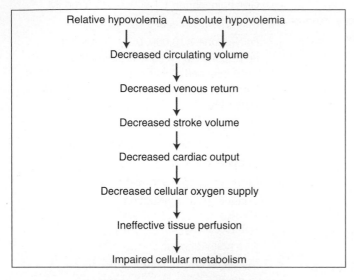

Figure 4-3 Pathophysiology of hypovolemic shock.

This article was published in Thelan's critical care nursing: Diagnosis and management, ed 5, Urden LD. Copyright Mosby 2006.

Table 4-10 **Classes of Hypovolemic Shock**							
	% Blood Loss	**Stage of Shock**	**Mental Status**	**Blood Pressure**	**Pulse Rate**	**Respiratory Rate**	**Skin**
Class I	<15%	Compensated	Slightly anxious	Normal	Normal	Normal	Pink, normal
Class II	15%–30%	Compensated (early)	Mildly anxious	Low normal	Mild tachycardia	Mild tachypnea	Pale, cool skin, >2 sec capillary refill
Class III	30%–45%	Decompensated (late)	Altered, lethargic	Hypotension	Severe tachycardia	Moderate tachypnea	Pale, mild cyanosis, cool, >3 sec capillary refill
Class IV	>45%	Irreversible	Extremely lethargic, unresponsive	Severe hypotension	Severe tachycardia to bradycardia	Severe tachypnea to agonal	Pale, central and peripheral cyanosis, cold, >5 sec capillary refill

The treatment of hypovolemic shock includes administering isotonic fluids (lactated Ringer's or normal saline solution) via intravascular or intraosseous routes. Fluid should be administered in 500- to 1,000-mL increments in adults (20 mL/kg in children). It is important to reassess the patient after each bolus to determine how the patient is tolerating the fluids and whether the patient's condition is stabilizing. Stabilization is indicated by a decrease in pulse rate and improvement of blood pressure and respiratory status. In general for adults, the fluid should be administered to titrate to a blood pressure of 80–90 mm Hg systolic. If bleeding is present, administration of blood may be indicated as well.

As new tools such as the compensatory reserve index are developed and researched, earlier detection of shock may be a possibility.

Distributive Shock

Distributive shock is also due to an inadequate volume of blood to fill the vascular space, but the problem does not stem from blood or fluid *loss*, but from a precipitous *increase* in vascular capacity as blood vessels dilate and the capillaries leak fluid. This fluid leaks into extravascular and interstitial spaces, which is called the "third space." Such vasodilation and capillary leakage can occur in sepsis, anaphylaxis, neurogenic shock, toxic shock syndrome, and toxin exposure. Too much vascular space translates into too little peripheral vascular resistance and a decrease in preload, which in turn reduces cardiac output and sets the stage for shock.

Septic Shock

Septic shock is the result of a massive systemic inflammatory response to infection by gram-negative or gram-positive aerobes, anaerobes, fungi, or viruses. Gram-negative organisms appear to be the primary cause of sepsis, especially in hospitalized patients.

Several changes in health care have contributed to a recent rise in the incidence of sepsis. More patients are remaining at home and have medical devices inserted, making the patients prone to infection. Many of these patients also have compromised immune systems, putting them at even greater risk for sepsis. In addition, infection by antibiotic-resistant gram-positive organisms such as *Staphylococcus aureus* and *Streptococcus*

pneumoniae is increasing in incidence. The following factors predispose a patient to septicemia:

Inadequate Immune Response
- Patients with diabetes mellitus, liver disease, or HIV/AIDS
- Neonates
- Older adults
- Pregnant women
- Persons with alcoholism

Primary Infections
- Pneumonia
- Urinary tract infection
- Cholecystitis
- Peritonitis
- Abscess

Iatrogenic Sources
- Indwelling vascular catheter
- Foley catheter
- Major abdominal or pelvic surgery

The basis of septic shock and systemic inflammatory response syndrome (SIRS) is a complex process of inflammatory response and multisystem organ failure. Two or more of the following criteria must be met for a diagnosis of SIRS:

- Temperature > 100°F (38°C) or < 97°F (36°C)
- Pulse rate > 90 beats/min
- Respiratory rate > 20 breaths/min or $Paco_2$ < 32 mm Hg
- White blood cell count > 12,000/mm^3, < 4,000/mm^3, or > 10% band neutrophilia

Sepsis syndrome is a precursor to septic shock. In a patient who has SIRS compounded by organ dysfunction or hypotension, sepsis can be said to have progressed to septic shock when the hypotension continues despite adequate fluid resuscitation. Sepsis may present in the hyperdynamic phase or the hypodynamic phases, described later. The Robson Prehospital Severe Sepsis Screening tool (Table 4-11) has a 75% success rate in identifying sepsis. It can be adapted to the prehospital or hospital setting. It is key that prehospital providers relay the potential for sepsis to hospital personnel. Early recognition and intervention for sepsis has been shown to improve survival rates.

Table 4-11 Robson Prehospital Severe Sepsis Screening Tool*
- Temperature > 100.9°F (38.3°C) or < 96.8°F (36.0°C) - Heart rate > 90 beats/min - Respiratory rate > 20 breaths/min - Acutely altered mental status - Plasma glucose > 6.6 mmol/L (119 mg/dL) unless diabetic

*If these findings are present in a patient with a history that is suggestive of infection, sepsis should be considered.

Ulrika Wallgren, Maaret Castrén, Alexandra Svensson, et al, Identification of adult septic patients in the prehospital setting: a comparison of two screening tools and clinical. European Journal of Emergency Medicine 2014 Aug;21(4):260–5.

Care of the patient in septic shock can be complicated. Relative hypovolemia develops in sepsis because the vasculature dilates. Actual hypovolemia may develop secondary to massive GI fluid loss or if third-spacing of fluid from capillary leakage occurs.

Heart function is depressed in sepsis even in the early hyperdynamic phase. This phase, formerly known as "warm shock," is characterized by decreased systemic vascular resistance and occasionally by elevated cardiac output. As inflammatory mediators circulate, the heart bears the brunt of the impact. Inflammation and altered metabolism can cause heart muscle injury. The pulse rate may increase, and a fever may be present. The patient's skin will still be warm.

In the hypodynamic phase, (formerly "cold shock,") hypotension becomes evident, and an altered level of consciousness develops. In this phase, the patient's skin will feel cool and clammy.

Prehospital treatment of septic shock must be aggressive. You should ensure adequate oxygenation and rapid fluid infusion. Pay close attention to airway management. Simple oxygen therapy may be adequate, but some patients require advanced airway support measures such as intubation. Establish vascular access (intravenous [IV] or intraosseous [IO]), and administer isotonic fluid in 500- to 1,000-mL increments in adults (20 mL/kg in children), and reassess the patient after each bolus. The goal of fluid resuscitation is to restore perfusion, as indicated by a decreased heart rate, revived blood pressure, and diminished respiratory distress. If the patient's blood pressure doesn't improve, repeat the fluid challenge up to 2,000 mL. Up to 30 mL/kg may be indicated in the first 3 hours of treatment. Perform fluid resuscitation cautiously, as fluid overload is possible, particularly in older adults and children. If resuscitation is ineffective, a vasopressor and/or inotrope infusion titrated to effect may be beneficial. These medications may include norepinephrine, epinephrine, phenylephrine, or dopamine.

Other tools that can be used to identify sepsis include capnography, serum glucose testing, serum lactate testing, ultrasonography, and central venous pressure.

- *Capnography.* The end-tidal carbon dioxide (ETCO$_2$) reading may be used by healthcare providers to identify severe sepsis. In sepsis, the ETCO$_2$ level decreases. The decrease is due to two components. The first is a response to lactic acid production. As the body undergoes anaerobic metabolism, lactate builds up and a metabolic acidosis develops. The body increases the respiratory rate to compensate for the metabolic acidosis, which causes the ETCO$_2$ to decrease. The second factor that contributes to the decrease in expired carbon dioxide is hypoperfusion. As the body enters the shock state, cardiac output drops and less blood is delivered to the lungs. The decrease in delivery of blood to the lungs results in less carbon dioxide to exhale, contributing to a low ETCO$_2$ level. Studies have found that low ETCO$_2$ levels correlate with elevated lactate levels in septic patients. The low ETCO$_2$ rates predict metabolic acidosis and are also predictive of mortality rates.

- *Serum glucose.* Elevation of serum glucose above 120 mg/dL or 6.6 mmol/L in nondiabetic patients has been found to be predictive of possible sepsis when present with other findings.

- *Serum lactate.* Elevated lactate (lactic acid) levels are also predictors of sepsis. The Robson tool suggests a level greater than 2 mmol/L as significant in identifying sepsis. The "Surviving Sepsis" campaign uses a lactate level greater than 4 mmol/L due to the higher mortality rate associated with this level. Serial lactate levels are useful in determining the success of fluid resuscitation and reversal of anaerobic metabolism. A lactate level that is greater than 4 mmol/L and drops to less than 4 mmol/L after fluid administration would indicate an improvement in the patient's status. Lactate has a half-life of approximately 20 minutes, so if a repeat lactate is drawn and is still elevated, it is because the patient is still producing lactate through anaerobic metabolism, not because the body cannot rid itself of the lactate. Lactate levels are more commonly determined in the facility, but some EMS systems are evaluating point-of-care finger-stick lactate levels. Regardless of where the lactate level is determined, the key point is to monitor the trend to determine the success of interventions. There are other causes of elevated lactate levels, such as muscle injury and leaving a tourniquet on too long, so repeat levels and evaluation for other causes should be considered.

- *Ultrasonography.* Ultrasonography is used to measure the size of the vena cava and compare the change that occurs on inspiration. If the inferior vena cava is less than 2.1 cm and collapses more than 50% during inspiration, the patient has a central venous pressure of 3 mm Hg. This suggests hypovolemia or distributive shock, and fluid resuscitation is recommended until collapse of the inferior vena cava is less than 50%.

- *Central venous pressure (CVP).* Central venous access can be useful in managing patients in septic shock. The goal of management is maintaining the CVP greater than 8 mm Hg through fluid administration. CVP measurements are primarily in-hospital tools, but may be used during interfacility transports by appropriately trained transport teams.

During transport, communicate the possibility of sepsis or SIRS to the receiving facility so the protocol to address these patients can be initiated as soon as possible. Once the patient arrives at the hospital, appropriate cultures should be collected *before* antibiotics are infused, so long as there is no significant delay. The cultures typically include two sets of blood cultures and a urine culture. In certain instances, ED personnel will collect a wound culture or a culture of a medical device (e.g., Foley catheter or central line). Typically, two broad-spectrum antibiotics will be initiated, and a more targeted antibiotic will be used when the results of the cultures become available. Research has found that when the ED performs these four bundled activities, the survival rates from sepsis improve. The recommendation is that once the patient is in the ED, the following should occur: (1) Obtain blood cultures before antibiotics, and (2) draw a lactate level before 90 minutes; assure intravenous (IV) antibiotics before 180 minutes, and administer 30 mL/kg of IV fluids before 180 minutes for hypotension or lactate ≥ 4 mmol/L. EMS can assist with this by identifying potential sepsis patients and relaying the information to the ED.

Ongoing care to be completed within 6 hours should include the following to improve survival:

- Apply vasopressors (for hypotension that does not respond to initial fluid resuscitation—the goal is to maintain a mean arterial pressure [MAP] ≥ 65 mm Hg).
- If arterial hypotension persists despite volume resuscitation or an initial lactate level ≥ 4 mmol/L (36 mg/dL), document reassessment of volume status and tissue perfusion with: EITHER
  - A repeat focused exam after initial fluid resuscitation (vital signs, cardiopulmonary, capillary refill, pulse, and skin findings). OR two of the following:
  - *Measure central venous pressure (CVP)*. The goal is to maintain a CVP of 8–12 mm Hg.
  - *Measure the central venous oxygen saturation (ScVO$_2$)*. Attempt to maintain an ScVO$_2$ ≥ 70%—consider blood administration if you are unable to keep the ScVO$_2$ at the desired level.
  - *Perform bedside cardiovascular ultrasound.*
  - *Perform dynamic assessment of fluid responsiveness with passive leg raise or fluid challenge.*
- Reassess the lactate level if the initial level was elevated.

Recombinant human activated protein C (rhAPC) has been approved for use in sepsis along with antibiotics. Activated C protein inhibits thrombin production, which is important because stimulation of the coagulation cascade is believed to promote the inflammatory process in patients with sepsis.

Anaphylactic Shock

For patients with known hypersensitivities, anaphylaxis is a frightening possibility. Signs and symptoms such as hypotension, tachycardia, difficulty breathing, wheezing, crackles, rhonchi, anxiety, urticaria, and pruritus can begin within minutes or up to 1 hour after exposure to the antigen. Gastrointestinal symptoms such as nausea and vomiting are also prominent. Once the symptoms have resolved, they can return 1 to 12 hours later, at which time they may be either milder or more severe. Yet despite the sudden onset and dramatic nature of an anaphylactic reaction, the condition precipitates only 400 to 800 deaths per year in the United States.

An antibody-antigen hypersensitivity response is the primary cause of anaphylactic shock. Not all hypersensitivity reactions evolve into shock. Most allergic reactions produce only mild symptoms such as pruritus and urticaria. Patients with allergic reactions may be managed with diphenhydramine and monitoring for additional symptoms. Not all people have repeated anaphylactic reactions to additional exposures, but of the 40% to 60% who do, the most common trigger is the sting

of an insect belonging to the *Hymenoptera* order—wasps, bees, and ants. Almost any substance can provoke a reaction in a sensitive individual, but some other common triggers of anaphylaxis are eggs, milk, shellfish, and peanuts (Table 4-12).

Latex allergy is a trigger that has become increasingly common among patients and healthcare workers since 1987, when the Centers for Disease Control and Prevention issued

Table 4-12 Some Triggers of Anaphylactic Shock

Foods

- Eggs
- Milk
- Fish and shellfish
- Nuts and seeds
- Legumes and cereals
- Citrus fruits
- Chocolate
- Strawberries
- Tomatoes
- Avocados
- Bananas

Food Additives

- Food coloring
- Preservatives

Diagnostic Agents

- Iodine contrast material

Biological Agents

- Blood and blood components
- Gamma globulin
- Vaccines and antitoxins

Environmental

- Pollen, mold, spores
- Animal hair
- Latex

Drugs

- Antibiotics
- Aspirin
- Narcotics

Animal/Insect Venom

- Bees, wasps
- Snakes
- Jellyfish

recommendations for universal precautions to prevent the transmission of blood-borne pathogens. Several patient populations are at risk for latex allergy:

- Patients with neural tube defects, such as spina bifida
- Patients with congenital urologic disorders
- Persons who have had cumulative exposure to latex, including patients who have undergone multiple surgeries, healthcare professionals, and workers in rubber manufacturing (including glove manufacturing)

Remember, simply inhaling invisible latex proteins can cause a life-threatening anaphylactic reaction in sensitive persons. Asking about a latex allergy when taking the patient's history is important so that latex substitutes can be used if necessary.

During anaphylaxis, biochemical mediators such as histamine, eosinophils, chemotactic factor of anaphylaxis, heparin, and leukotrienes are released. Vasodilation, increased capillary permeability (including pulmonary capillary permeability), bronchoconstriction, excessive mucus secretion, coronary vasoconstriction, inflammation, and cutaneous reactions ensue. The cutaneous reaction may be observed as flushed, warm skin resulting from vasodilation and urticaria.

As with other causes of distributive shock, peripheral vasodilation in anaphylaxis causes a relative hypovolemia. This is due to vasodilation and leaking at the capillary level. The sudden loss of volume and resistance causes cardiac output to drop. Cardiovascular collapse and or airway obstruction are typically the direct cause of death.

Because shock can quickly overwhelm such patients, prompt intervention is critical. As the ABCs—airway, breathing, circulation—are initiated, it is important to ascertain the following:

- Does the patient have a history of previous allergic reactions? Does the patient use an EpiPen?
- Has the patient been exposed to an offending agent? If so, when?
- Is there a complaint of urticaria, rash, throat swelling, or shortness of breath? Laryngeal edema can have a rapid onset, so intervention must be swift.
- When did the symptoms begin? The more rapid the onset, the more likely it is the reaction will be severe.
- How long have the symptoms lasted? Symptoms typically resolve within 6 hours.

The treatment of anaphylactic shock requires removing the allergen and reversing the effects of the biochemicals that have been released (**Figure 4-4**). Epinephrine should be administered without delay. It may be necessary to support vital functions by

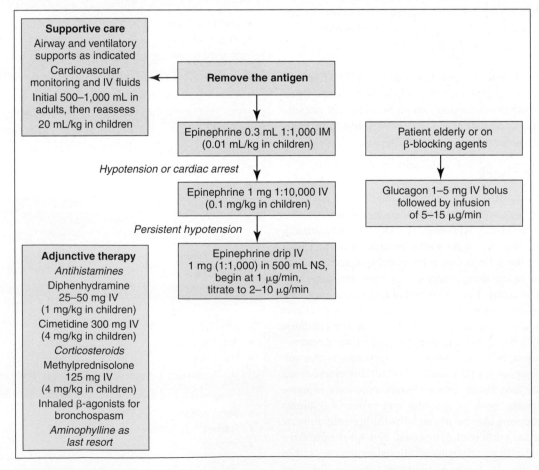

Figure 4-4 Management of anaphylaxis.

This article was published in Haddad and Winchester's clinical management of poisoning and drug overdose, ed 4, Shannon M, Borron S, Burns M, Copyright Saunders 2007.

providing oxygen, initiating intubation or mechanical ventilation, and administering IV fluids. Corticosteroids can stabilize the capillary membranes and reduce angioedema and bronchospasm, but because they do not take effect quickly, their use is limited to preventing or ameliorating the late-phase component of anaphylaxis, not to treating an initial attack. The two most common drugs used to treat anaphylaxis, epinephrine and diphenhydramine, are summarized in Table 4-13. In patients receiving beta-blockers, glucagon administration should be considered. Glucagon has ionotropic and chronotropic properties and has the ability to reverse bronchospasm. H_2 blockers may be used with diphenhydramine to address GI and dermal anaphylactic symptoms. Patients with severe symptoms and/or sudden onset of anaphylaxis should be monitored for an extended period as a repeat onset of symptoms may occur and will require immediate intervention.

Neurogenic Shock

Neurogenic shock is a rare form of distributive shock. When signal transmission in the sympathetic nervous system is interrupted, the body cannot mount an appropriate fight-or-flight response. Spinal cord injury, usually at the sixth thoracic vertebra (T6) or higher, often leads to neurogenic shock. Vessels do not receive the sympathetic nervous system message to constrict and instead dilate due to the unopposed vagal stimulus. For this reason, neurogenic shock is sometimes called *vasogenic shock*. The dilated vessels make the patient's skin warm and pink. Blood pressure slackens, peripheral vascular resistance falls, and the circulatory system below the level of injury fails to return enough venous blood to the heart. The heart rate slows—bradycardia is highly characteristic

of neurogenic shock, but not an absolute finding—because of the lack of sympathetic stimulation. Arterial pressure diminishes, and tissue ischemia sets in at values below 50 to 60 mm Hg.

If the patient with neurogenic shock is also a trauma patient, the cervical spine must be protected. Ensure that the airway is patent and offer support as necessary. Maintain oxygenation by providing supplemental oxygen or assisting respiration as indicated. Establish vascular access and initiate fluid resuscitation. If the patient does not respond to fluid resuscitation, consider vasopressor agents such as norepinephrine or dopamine. Be sure to keep the patient warm and monitor the patient for increased intracranial pressure and other neurologic dysfunction; associated head injury may be present. Transport the patient as quickly as possible to definitive care.

Vasodilation may also occur as a result of exposure to a toxin, poison, or medication overdose. In these cases, provide supportive care as you address the exposure. See Chapter 10 for details of AMLS management of exposure to toxins.

Cardiogenic Shock

Cardiogenic shock occurs when the heart is unable to circulate sufficient blood to maintain adequate peripheral oxygen delivery. Either the right or left ventricle may be the site of the cause, which may include a rhythm disturbance, a cardiac structural disorder such as ruptured chordae tendineae, or the action of certain toxins. The most common cause is myocardial infarction with greater than a 40% loss of heart muscle. This is usually due to a massive infarction of the anterior wall of the heart, but it can be caused by many smaller infarctions throughout the heart. Risk factors for cardiogenic shock include advancing age, female sex, congestive heart failure, previous myocardial infarction, and diabetes.

Table 4-13 Common Agents Used to Treat Anaphylaxis

Epinephrine

- **Class**: catecholamine, sympathomimetic, adrenergic, inotrope
- **Action**: binds with alpha and beta receptors, thereby increasing blood pressure, pulse rate, and bronchodilation
- **Dosage**:
  - 1:1,000: 0.3–0.5 mg for rapidly progressing or severe reactions. Repeat every 5–15 minutes as needed. Do not delay administration to provide other treatments.
  - 1:10,000: 0.3–0.5 mg over 3–10 minutes for severe reactions. Repeat every 15 minutes as needed. IM administration should be completed while awaiting IV access.
- **Route**:
  - 1:1,000: intramuscular
  - 1:10,000: intravenous (IV)
- **Adverse effects**: palpitations, tachycardia, hypertension, anxiety, nausea, vomiting

Diphenhydramine

- **Class:** antihistamine, anticholinergic, histamine-1 (H_1) receptor antagonist
- **Action:** binds and blocks H_1 receptors. Provides symptomatic relief but does not reverse anaphylaxis.
- **Dosage:** 1–2 mg/kg (maximum 50 mg) IV every 4 to 8 hours
- **Route:** oral, IV, intramuscular
- **Adverse effects:** hypotension, palpitations, drowsiness, anxiety, chest tightness

In patients with cardiogenic shock, blood is no longer effectively pumped because of a diminished stroke volume or a heart rate that is too slow or too fast. When the left side of the heart fails, the blood overloads the pulmonary vasculature, causing pulmonary edema and impaired gas exchange.

The signs and symptoms of cardiogenic shock are diverse and difficult to diagnose in the field. The patient's respiratory rate is increased, and crackles caused by pulmonary edema can be heard on auscultation. Because of the ineffective myocardium, diminished stroke volume, and dwindling cardiac output, the pulse rate may be greater than 100 bpm, heart sounds are diminished, and the pulse is weak and thready. Dysrhythmias may be present. The patient's skin will be cool, moist, and pale. The patient may have an altered level of consciousness. Systolic blood pressure will be low, and the patient may complain of chest pain and shortness of breath.

Cardiogenic shock requires early identification of the cause and initiation of decisive supportive care. An electrocardiogram (ECG) assists in diagnosing ischemia or infarction and arrhythmia. At the receiving facility, a chest radiograph can be performed to detect pulmonary edema and pleural effusion. Cardiac markers such as creatine kinase-MB (CK-MB) and troponin should be sent for laboratory analysis. In addition, a test for the presence of elevated levels of a hormone called *brain-natriuretic peptide* (BNP) in the patient's serum should be done, which may indicate heart failure. In certain patients, BNP is released in response to the stretch of the atria and ventricles. The vasodilation that occurs causes natriuresis (release of excessive sodium into the urine) and a reduction in blood volume. When BNP is elevated beyond the normal level of 100 pg/mL (< 100 ng/L [SI units]), it is typically a sign that the patient's difficulty breathing is related to congestive heart failure. If the BNP level is normal, the difficulty in breathing is more likely pulmonary in origin, not cardiac.

Your initial treatment of a patient in cardiogenic shock must focus on stabilization. Prolonged efforts to stabilize the condition of the patient in the field, however, are not recommended. Managing the airway is always of paramount importance. Correct hypoxia as rapidly as possible and obtain vascular access. If an acute myocardial infarction has occurred, administer aspirin and heparin unless a contraindication exists. Use nitroglycerin and morphine only if the patient has an adequate blood pressure. Although beta-blockers may be used in myocardial infarction, they are inappropriate in cardiogenic shock until the patient's condition has been stabilized.

If hypotension is present, consider initiating small isotonic fluid challenges, about 250 mL each, before progressing to a vasopressor infusion. Fluid must be administered cautiously, especially if high central venous pressure or pulmonary edema is present. Initiate a vasopressor and titrate to effect. If using dopamine, administer the lowest effective dose to limit the spike in pulse rate dopamine often causes. If tachycardia is present with hypotension, use a norepinephrine or phenylephrine infusion. Use dobutamine and/or milrinone if the patient's systolic blood pressure is 80 to 100 mm Hg. Emergency treatment of cardiogenic shock centers on maintaining the heart's pumping ability without significantly affecting the pulse rate. Manage cardiogenic shock with signs of pulmonary congestion by placing the patient in semi-Fowler's position with the feet

dependent unless this causes more severe hypotension. Oxygen should be administered to patients with breathlessness, signs of heart failure, shock or an oxygen saturation less than 94%. Use of continuous positive airway pressure (CPAP) or bilevel positive airway pressure (BiPAP) may assist in relieving pulmonary congestion at the alveolar level but is relatively contraindicated in hypotension. Follow local protocols to guide this decision.

An intra-aortic balloon pump may be required to support the heart and promote revascularization of the coronary arteries. In a patient with cardiogenic shock as a result of an ST elevation myocardial infarction (STEMI), timely transport to a cardiac center with percutaneous coronary intervention (PCI) capabilities is essential and increases survival.

Obstructive Shock

Obstructive shock occurs when blood flow in the great vessels or heart is occluded. Common causes are acute pericardial tamponade, massive pulmonary embolus, and tension pneumothorax. Common signs and symptoms of patients in obstructive shock are shortness of breath, anxiety, tachypnea, and tachycardia. Breath sounds may be diminished if a pulmonary cause is involved. In later stages, the patient becomes hypotensive, and a declining level of consciousness and cyanosis become apparent. Pulsus paradoxus may occur with cardiac tamponade or tension pneumothorax.

Reversal of obstructive shock requires support of vital functions and removal of the obstruction, so the treatment of the patient will depend on the specific cause of the obstruction. Initial management should focus on increasing vascular volume with fluid resuscitation and vasopressors as needed to maintain perfusion until a definitive diagnosis and treatment plan can be established.

Cardiac Tamponade

Cardiac tamponade is seen when fluid or blood accumulates in the pericardial sac surrounding the heart, diminishing the heart's ability to function. Trauma, ventricular rupture, and infection are possible causes of cardiac tamponade. The speed of fluid accumulation (blood or effusion) in the pericardium creates either a rapid deterioration with smaller amounts or a slow, chronic presentation with much larger amounts of fluid in the sac. It may help to remember Beck's triad, the classic indicator of cardiac tamponade: jugular venous distention, hypotension, and muffled heart sounds. But this is a late sign, present in only 10% to 40% of patients, and it is difficult to differentiate clinically.

Cardiac tamponade may be treated by inotropic medications and by pericardiocentesis, which involves inserting a needle attached to a syringe into the chest far enough to penetrate the pericardium and then withdrawing fluid, but treatment depends on the cause and rate of fluid accumulation.

Pulmonary Embolus

A pulmonary embolus is a life-threatening condition that occurs when a thrombus (a blood clot, cholesterol plaque, or air bubble) travels through the vasculature and lodges in the pulmonary artery. If a large component of the pulmonary vasculature is occluded, reduced blood flow back to the heart decreases cardiac output, resulting in hypoperfusion.

Pulmonary embolus interventions focus on oxygenation and ventilation. Be prepared to support the vasculature with fluids. The primary therapy is systemic anticoagulation with heparin or fractionated heparin medications such as enoxaparin (Lovenox). Thrombolytics may be considered for severe cases with shock.

Tension Pneumothorax

The most treatable cause of obstructive shock is tension pneumothorax. A tension pneumothorax develops when air becomes trapped outside the lung between the visceral and parietal pleura and applies pressure to the contents of the chest cavity. This pressure causes the mediastinum to shift to the unaffected side and interferes with respiration. The increased intrathoracic pressure causes compression of the vena cava, diminishing venous return to the heart and leading to inadequate cardiac output. Although trauma is a common cause of a pneumothorax, the condition can develop spontaneously or as a result of positive-pressure ventilation. Patients with chronic obstructive pulmonary disease have weakened areas of the lungs and are thus vulnerable to the effects of excessive pressure. Pneumothorax can also be caused by overzealous ventilation in an otherwise healthy patient; patients being ventilated with positive pressure are at increased risk for a tension pneumothorax.

Avoid treatment using positive-pressure ventilation if possible. Usually the only action that can prevent eventual death from a tension pneumothorax is decompression of the injured side of the chest. Needle or tube thoracostomy must be performed on patients with this life-threatening emergency.

Complications of Shock

Acute Renal Failure

During shock, blood is initially shunted from the least vital organs to the brain and heart. Because blood flow to the kidneys is reduced, acute renal failure is common. If circulation is impaired for too long, cellular dysfunction can be permanent. More specifically, if the renal tubules receive insufficient quantities of oxygen for more than perhaps 45 to 60 minutes—depending on the individual—irreversible damage is done. This phenomenon is known as "acute tubular necrosis." Once kidney failure occurs, the body can no longer remove electrolytes, acids, or excess fluid from the bloodstream, so dialysis will be required either temporarily or indefinitely.

Acute Respiratory Distress Syndrome or Acute Lung Injury

During shock, capillary permeability allows proteins, fluid, and blood cells to seep from the capillaries and collect in the alveoli, thereby impairing ventilation and adequate oxygenation.

Inflammation and diffuse alveolar injury cause widespread edema in the lungs. Other mediators released by neutrophils cause pulmonary vasoconstriction. This constellation of events is known as acute respiratory distress syndrome (ARDS) or acute lung injury (ALI). ARDS/ALI can have many causes other than shock, including pneumonia, aspiration, pancreatitis, and drug overdose. Despite advances in treatment, the syndrome continues to carry a high mortality rate. If the patient does survive, he or she may require mechanical ventilation for an extended period.

Coagulopathies

Late shock can trigger an overstimulation of the clotting cascade in which clotting and bleeding begin to occur simultaneously. This condition is known as **disseminated intravascular coagulation (DIC)**. Some of the clots can clog the vessels and cut off the blood supply to major organs such as the liver or brain. Platelets bind where the blood is pooling, further promoting viscosity. Over time, the clotting factors that are normally present are rapidly exhausted and the person has a high risk of bleeding. Bleeding begins as the coagulation components are broken down and the fibrinolytic system is activated. This condition can be acute or chronic. The following conditions may cause DIC:

Acute
- Abruptio placentae, HELLP syndrome, or eclampsia in pregnant women
- Massive transfusions
- Obstructive jaundice
- Acute liver failure
- Aortic balloon pump
- Burns
- Trauma/hemorrhage

Chronic
- Cardiovascular disease
- Autoimmune disease
- Hematologic disorder
- Inflammatory disorder
- HIV/AIDS

Manifestations include rapid development of hemorrhage (e.g., oozing from venipuncture sites and bruising), shock that is more severe than is consistent with the apparent amount of blood loss, and a positive D-dimer lab test. Microvascular clotting may present with signs of ischemia in distal tissues. In isolation, standard laboratory coagulation tests, such as prothrombin time and partial thromboplastin time (PT/PTT), are unreliable. A low platelet count, prolonged thrombin time, and a low fibrinogen level in addition to a prolonged PT/PTT provide a more convincing diagnostic picture.

Treatment depends on the cause of DIC and will vary among patients. Management goals, though, are generally to reduce bleeding, discourage excess coagulation, and improve perfusion by eliminating the underlying etiology and restoring homeostasis.

Hepatic Dysfunction

Liver failure, as evidenced by persistently elevated liver enzyme levels, glucose abnormalities (hyperglycemia or hypoglycemia), unremitting lactic acidosis, and jaundice may occur if shock is left untreated. The liver is essential in any shock state because of its ability to regulate glucose (which the body converts to energy) and manufacture clotting factors (which are important in healing from injury). The liver can become ischemic, however, as blood is shunted to more essential organs. Elevated hepatic transaminase levels and a serum bilirubin of greater than 2 mg/dL (18 μmol/L [SI units]) indicate dysfunction. Liver failure is typically a late development that may be prevented with efficient early care.

Multiple Organ Dysfunction Syndrome

An uncontrolled inflammatory response can set in motion a progressive sequential dysfunction of interdependent organ systems. This calamitous condition, known as multiple organ dysfunction syndrome (MODS), is a progressive condition characterized by combined failure of two or more organs or organ systems that were initially unharmed by the acute disorder or injury that caused the patient's initial illness. It typically occurs in response to injury or severe illness and carries a grim prognosis. In fact, it is the leading cause of death in intensive care units, with a mortality rate as high as 54% if only two organ systems have failed. Mortality is greater than 80% if five organ systems have failed.

Sepsis and septic shock are the most common causes of MODS, but it can be brought on by any pathologic process that initiates a massive systemic inflammatory response. MODS is often precipitated by severe trauma, major surgery, acute pancreatitis, acute renal failure, ARDS, and the presence of necrotic tissue (e.g., eschar in a patient with burns). Older adults, those with preexisting medical disease, and those with extensive tissue damage are at the greatest risk for MODS.

MODS can be divided into primary and secondary stages. Primary MODS is evident immediately after a discrete insult such as chest trauma or overwhelming infection. Diminished perfusion is local and generalized, making it difficult to detect. A low-grade fever, tachypnea, dyspnea, acute respiratory distress syndrome, altered mental status, and hypermetabolism may be present. Cardiovascular signs include tachycardia, increased systemic vascular resistance, and increased cardiac output. Gastrointestinal indicators include abdominal distention, ascites, paralytic ileus, upper and lower gastrointestinal bleeding, diarrhea, ischemic colitis, and decreased bowel sounds. Jaundice, right upper quadrant pain, and elevated serum ammonia and liver enzyme levels indicate hepatic involvement.

A latent period occurs after the initial insult. Then, as macrophages and neutrophils are activated in response to the initial organ dysfunction, organs unaffected by the original insult begin to collapse. This systemic response constitutes secondary MODS. As the vascular endothelium becomes dysfunctional, coagulation and fibrin cascades are touched off, causing disseminated intravascular coagulation and thrombocytopenia. This systemic response leads to uncontrolled hypermetabolism, increased capillary permeability, and vasodilation. Cardiac output drops, and tissue perfusion becomes progressively more impaired as the imbalance between oxygen supply and demand widens. Ultimately, tissue hypoxia, myocardial dysfunction, and metabolic failure result in widespread total organ dysfunction.

Special Populations
Older Adult Patients

Older adults are living longer and staying more active into their later years. Paradoxically, living longer makes a person more likely to become severely ill or injured.

The use of medications to control chronic disease states can complicate both the body's ability to save itself and your ability to recognize disorders such as shock. Platelet-inhibiting drugs can cause bleeding even when therapeutic levels are present; for example, gastrointestinal bleeding may develop in a patient. Excessive bleeding may result if too much medication is taken or if trauma occurs. Because platelet-inhibiting drugs affect the body's ability to stop bleeding, it is important to identify these or any other drugs that may prolong bleeding and understand their potential to contribute to shock. Recognizing the need to control bleeding and possibly reverse the effects of certain drugs with antagonists or blood products is part of early intervention. Ask older patients whether they take any drugs that inhibit platelet activity, including acetylsalicylic acid (aspirin) and clopidogrel (Plavix). Many older adults are also on anticoagulation therapy with warfarin (Coumadin). Recently, the blood thinners dabigatran (Pradaxa) and rivaroxaban (Xarelto) have been introduced and must be considered as part of your assessment. Early notification to the receiving facility of the use of these medications is important if bleeding is suspected to allow the facility time to prepare interventions. Patients may also be taking supplements that increase bleeding, including vitamin E, ginkgo biloba, ginseng, dong quai, feverfew, garlic, ginger, and omega-3 fatty acids.

Some antihypertensive and vasoactive drugs limit the ability of the heart to increase its rate in response to a shock state. Beta-blockers and calcium channel blockers are two examples of medications that may keep the patient's pulse rate low despite normal compensation mechanisms that would create tachycardia.

Other factors can complicate the early diagnosis of shock in an older adult patient. As a person ages, pulmonary and cardiac reserves diminish. The alveoli stiffen, and tidal volume becomes shallower. Resting cardiac output declines, as does the basal metabolic rate. Shock-related compensatory mechanisms are more sluggish and less effective. The amount of adipose tissue decreases, muscle mass begins to atrophy, and it becomes more difficult to maintain body heat.

Obstetric Patients

When caring for a pregnant patient, it is important to realize that the survival of two patients depends on maintaining adequate perfusion. Pregnancy normally lasts about 40 weeks, and a woman's body undergoes tremendous change during that time. The maternal heart rate accelerates by 10 to 15 beats/min to compensate for the additional perfusion demands of the fetus. Blood volume expands by almost 1.5 times, and cardiac output surges by 30%.

As the fetus grows, it places additional pressure on the internal organs, diaphragm, and vena cava. Because of the increased cardiac output and intravascular volume, signs of hypoperfusion in pregnant patients may be delayed. Vascular changes attributable to pregnancy can mask early signs of shock.

During the second half of pregnancy, place the patient in the left-lateral recumbent position to avoid hypotension caused by pressure on the vena cava. Maintain adequate oxygenation, and initiate IV fluid therapy.

Pediatric Patients

Children have a great capacity for compensation when in shock due to their ability to increase cardiac output by greatly increasing their heart rate; hypotension is a late finding. Fluid replacement with boluses of isotonic fluids such as saline or lactated Ringer's solution is necessary until the patient is at the hospital for definitive care and blood transfusions. Other diseases also predispose children to shock.

Sickle Cell Disease

Sickle cell disease is a genetically inherited autosomal-recessive disorder of red blood cells. It usually presents in childhood in people of African-American descent. Up to 1 out of every 500 African-Americans will have this disorder which results in abnormal sickling of the red blood cells in the microvasculature, resulting in occlusion and leading to ischemia and painful crises. Other groups with a high incidence of sickle cell disease include individuals whose families have come from Mediterranean countries, Central America, the Caribbean Islands, India, and Saudi Arabia.

Bleeding Disorders

Thrombocytopenia Thrombocytopenia occurs when the body has an abnormally low number of platelets in the blood. The risk of bleeding is proportional to the degree of thrombocytopenia. Platelet counts below 100,000 per microliter of blood are associated with impaired ability for the blood to form clots, and platelet counts below 20,000 can lead to spontaneous bleeding.

Thrombocytopenia can have many causes, including infections, cancers such as leukemia, rheumatologic diseases such as lupus, and splenic sequestration (pooling of blood in the spleen). Some inherited conditions may also cause low platelet counts. Besides spontaneous bleeding or prolonged bleeding with injury, patients with low levels of platelets may exhibit petechiae or purpura. Large bruises may develop from minimal injuries or with no history of injury. Physical abuse should always be considered in children with unexplained bruising until proven otherwise.

Treatment of patients with bleeding secondary to thrombocytopenia includes treating the underlying cause if present, and transfusing platelets if bleeding cannot be controlled with local measures.

Hemophilia Hemophilia is a bleeding disorder that occurs when there is a deficiency in clotting factors, or proteins in the blood that work with platelets to help blood to clot. There are two main types of hemophilia, hemophilia A and hemophilia B. Hemophilia is a genetic disorder usually inherited from the mother. Hemophilia A and B have the same signs and symptoms. Affected patients usually have a bleeding disorder history in the family or, if new in onset, early and severe bleeding is experienced with minor trauma, especially in the joints and muscles. There is a common pattern to the bleeding in the patient's history as well. Bleeding into the joints is very common and leads to subsequent joint damage. Bleeding into the muscle body can cause compartment syndrome, and bleeding into the mouth can progress rapidly to airway compromise. Central nervous system bleeding may present as a new-onset headache with localized neurologic signs.

Treatment of hemophilia A and B entails factor replacement in those patients with known disease. Patients should carry at least one dose with them at all times. It is important to ask about this medication if the patient's history uncovers a diagnosed bleeding disorder. Pain control is also a treatment goal, while avoiding intramuscular injection of analgesics.

Von Willebrand's Disease Von Willebrand's disease is the most common heritable disorder of coagulation, and its presentation can mimic hemophilia A. Von Willebrand's disease is characterized by missing or deficient von Willebrand's factor, which, like other clotting factors, helps platelets stick or clump together. These patients may have abnormal menstrual bleeding, bleeding of the gums, epistaxis, bruising, and petechiae.

Treatment includes use of the synthetic hormone desmopressin (1-deamino-8-D-arginine-vasopressin [DDAVP]).

Obese Patients

The obese patient in shock presents many challenges to the healthcare provider. Among these challenges will be managing the airway, gaining venous access, and obtaining diagnostics and vital signs, such as BP, pulse oximetry, and an accurate ECG. Due to these many challenges of assessment and management, a high index of suspicion for shock must be maintained when managing an obese patient.

Putting It All Together

Early, accurate identification of the patient's stage and type of shock is essential in managing this condition. Seasoned clinical reasoning skills, a thorough assessment, and judicious interpretation of diagnostic findings are necessary to provide effective treatment for the patient in shock.

SCENARIO SOLUTION

© HunThomas/ShutterStock, Inc.

- This patient is sick.
- Differential diagnoses may include sepsis-related upper respiratory infection, cardiogenic shock due to previous cardiac issues, pericardial tamponade due to recent heart catheterization, pulmonary emboli, or a tension pneumothorax.
- To narrow your differential diagnosis, you will need to complete the history of past and present illness. Perform a physical exam that includes assessment for jugular venous distention, tracheal deviation, muffled heart sounds, and pulsus paradoxus. Perform capnography, a 12-lead ECG, and blood glucose evaluation, and obtain the patient's body temperature. Your findings are distended neck veins; trachea, midline; heart tones, strong; ETCO₂, 35 mm Hg; 12-lead ECG, ST elevation in Rv4, II, III, and aVf; blood glucose, < 112 mg/dL (6.6 mmol/L); and temperature, 98.8°F (37°C).

- The patient has signs of shock and hypoxia. Take immediate measures to secure his airway and administer oxygen. If tension pneumothorax is suspected, decompress the chest. Establish vascular access, and administer IV fluids. Monitor the ECG and obtain a 12-lead ECG. Transport to the closest appropriate healthcare facility. During transport, it is important to relay to the facility if sepsis or SIRS is suspected, because some facilities are beginning sepsis intervention based on EMS findings.
- Your patient is most likely suffering from cardiogenic shock because of the ECG findings. Sepsis is not as likely due to the patient's normal temperature, glucose level < 112 mg/dL, and ETCO₂ level of 35 mm Hg, but his history of infection makes it a consideration. Pericardial tamponade is not as likely because the ECG showed a myocardial infarction and normal heart sounds. Pulmonary emboli is possible due to hypoxia. Tension pneumothorax is not likely due to the presence of bilateral breath sounds.

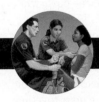

Summary

- Understanding inadequate tissue perfusion requires a thorough knowledge of the anatomy, physiology, and pathophysiology of shock.
- Shock is a progressive state of cellular hypoperfusion in which too little oxygen and too little energy is available to meet tissue demands in multiple organ systems.
- The three primary stages of shock are compensatory, decompensated, and irreversible.
- The three main determinants of cellular perfusion are cardiac output, intravascular volume, and vascular capacitance.
- Cardiac output is determined by stroke volume and heart rate.
- The four primary determinants of stroke volume are preload, afterload, contractility, and synchrony.
- Mean arterial blood pressure is an indirect indicator of tissue perfusion. Higher mean arterial pressures may be required for adequate perfusion in patients with a history of hypertension.
- Narrowing pulse pressures are indicators of decreased cardiac output and a helpful indicator of shock.
- Blood transports oxygen to and wastes from the body's cells. Hemoglobin, an iron-containing protein in RBCs, carries oxygen to the tissues.
- Underlying chronic medical illnesses, age, obesity, and immunosuppression adversely affect compensatory mechanisms of shock.
- Compensatory mechanisms include increasing minute ventilation, increasing cardiac output, and vasoconstriction.
- The types of shock are hypovolemic, obstructive, distributive, and cardiogenic.
- When the body no longer has ample oxygen and cells begin producing lactic acid as a by-product of anaerobic metabolism, metabolic acidosis sets in.
- During the ischemic phase of shock, perfusion of the brain, heart, lungs, and liver is enhanced, while less essential organs become ischemic.
- Anxiousness, combativeness, and confusion may be early signs of shock.

Summary (CONTINUED)

- Most types of shock are characterized by tachycardia, tachypnea, cool skin, and hypotension. In distributive shock, however, the skin may be warm. Bradycardia can accompany cardiogenic or neurogenic shock.
- Assessment tools used to evaluate patients suspected of being in shock include pulse oximetry, electrocardiography, serum glucose testing, end-tidal carbon dioxide testing, and lactate levels. In the hospital, laboratory studies, CT, ultrasonography, and radiographic studies are used.
- Complications of shock include acute renal failure, ARDS, coagulopathies, hepatic dysfunction, and MODS.
- Initial treatment of shock consists of supportive measures, supplemental oxygen, fluid resuscitation, temperature regulation, and administration of vasopressors. Specific interventions are based on the underlying cause.

KEY TERMS

© HunThomas/ShutterStock, Inc.

acidosis An abnormal increase in the hydrogen ion concentration in the blood, resulting from an accumulation of an acid or the loss of a base, indicated by a blood pH below the normal range.

afterload In the intact heart, the pressure against which the ventricle ejects blood. It is impacted by peripheral vascular resistance and the physical characteristics and volume of blood in the arterial system.

cardiac cycle A complete cardiac movement or heartbeat. The period from the beginning of one heartbeat to the beginning of the next; from diastole through systole.

cardiac output The effective volume of blood expelled by either ventricle of the heart per unit of time (usually volume per minute); it is equal to the stroke volume multiplied by the heart rate.

disseminated intravascular coagulation (DIC) A disturbance of blood coagulation as a result of activation of the coagulation mechanism and simultaneous clot lysis.

hypovolemia Abnormally decreased volume of circulating blood in the body; the most common cause is hemorrhage.

mean arterial pressure (MAP) The average pressure within an artery over a complete cycle of one heartbeat.

perfusion The act of pouring over or through, especially the passage of a fluid through the vessels of a specific organ.

preload The mechanical state of the heart at the end of diastole, it reflects venous return and the stress or stretch on the ventricular wall.

pulse pressure The difference between the systolic and diastolic blood pressures.

shock A condition of profound hemodynamic and metabolic disturbance characterized by failure of the circulatory system to maintain adequate perfusion of oxygen and nutrients to vital organs. It may result from inadequate blood volume, cardiac function, or vasomotor tone.

stroke volume The amount of blood ejected by the ventricle at each heartbeat. It varies with age, sex, and exercise.

BIBLIOGRAPHY

© Hun Thomas/ShutterStock, Inc.

Aehlert B: *Paramedic practice today: above and beyond.* St. Louis, MO, 2009, Mosby/JEMS.

American Academy of Orthopaedic Surgeons: *Nancy Caroline's emergency care in the streets*, ed 7. Burlington, MA, 2013, Jones & Bartlett Learning.

American College of Surgeons: *ATLS student course manual*, ed 8. Chicago, IL, 2008, American College of Surgeons.

Boschert S: Is it septic shock? Check the lactate level. *ACEP News/ Elsevier Global Medical News.* November 2007. http://www. acep.org/Clinical---Practice-Management/Is-It-Septic-Shock--Check-Lactate-Level/

Cairns CB: Rude unhinging of the machinery of life: Metabolic approaches to hemorrhagic shock. *Curr Opin Crit Care.* 7(6):437–443, 2001.

Centers for Disease Control and Prevention: *Guide to infection prevention for outpatient settings: Minimum expectations for safe care.* http://www.cdc.gov/HAI/settings/outpatient/out-patient-care-gl-standared-precautions.html

Copstead-Kirkhorn LE, Banasik JL: *Pathophysiology.* Philadelphia, PA, 2010, Saunders.

Darovic GO: *Handbook of hemodynamic monitoring*, ed 2. Philadelphia, PA, 2004, Saunders.

Gaugler MH: A unifying system: Does the vascular endothelium have a role to play in multi-organ failure following radiation exposure? *Br J Radiol.* 78:100–105, 2005.

Hamilton GC: *Emergency medicine: An approach to clinical problem-solving*, ed 2. Philadelphia, PA, 2003, Saunders.

Hirschl M, Wollmann C, Mayr H: 30 day survival of patients with STEMI and cardiogenic shock. *Crit Care Med.* 41(12), 2013. doi: 10.1097/01.ccm.0000439211.53447.b9

Hudak CM, Gallo BM, Morton PG: *Critical care nursing: A holistic approach*, ed 7. Philadelphia, PA, 1998, Lippincott.

Hunter CH: End-tidal carbon dioxide may be used in place of lactate to screen for severe sepsis. *JEMS.* (March):134, 2014.

Hunter CL, Silvestri S, Dean M, et al.: *End-tidal carbon dioxide levels are associated with mortality in emergency department patients with suspected sepsis.* October 1, 2011. http://med. ucf.edu/media/2011/10/i2-poster-dean-matthew.pdf

Hunter CL, Silvestri S, Ralls G, et al.: The sixth vital sign: Prehospital end-tidal carbon dioxide predicts in-hospital mortality and metabolic disturbances. *Am J Emerg Med.* 32(2):160-165, 2014.

Kolecki P, Menckhoff C: *Hypovolemic shock treatment and management.* http://emedicine.medscape.com/article/760145 treaent#a1126, updated February 27, 2014.

Kragh JF Jr, Walters TJ, Baer DG, et al.: Survival with emergency tourniquet use to stop bleeding in major limb trauma. *Ann Surg.* 249:1–7, 2009.

Link MS, Berkow LC, Kudenchuk PJ, et al. Part 7: Adult Advanced Cardiovascular Life Support: 2015 American Heart Association Guidelines Update for Cardiopulmonary Resuscitation and Emergency Cardiovascular Care. Circulation, 132(18 Suppl 2), S444–64, 2015. http://doi.org/10.1161/CIR.0000000000000261

Marshall JC: The multiple organ dysfunction syndrome. In Holzheimer RG, Mannick JA, Eds. *Surgical treatment: Evidence-based and problem-oriented.* Munich, Germany, Zuckschwerdt, 2001. http://www.ncbi.nlm.nih.gov/books/NBK6868/

Marx JA, Hockberger RS, Walls RM: *Rosen's emergency medicine: Concepts and clinical practice*, ed 6. St. Louis, MO, 2006, Mosby.

McCance KL, Huether SE: *Pathophysiology: The biologic basis for disease in adults and children*, ed 5. St. Louis, MO, 2006, Mosby.

Miller RD, Eriksson L, Fleisher L, et al.: *Miller's anesthesia*, ed 7. Philadelphia, PA, 2009, Churchill Livingstone.

Moultan SL, Mulligan J, Grudic GZ, et al.; Running on empty? The compensatory reserve index. *J Trauma Acute Care* Surg. 75(6): 1053–1059, 2013.

Mustafa S, Kaliner A: *Anaphylaxis medication.* http://emedicine. medscape.com/article/135065-medication, updated December 15, 2014.

National Association of Emergency Medical Technicians (U.S.), Pre-Hospital Trauma Life Support Committee & Trauma, American College of Surgeons: *PHTLS prehospital trauma life support.* St. Louis, MO, 2007, Mosby/JEMS.

Pagana KP: *Mosby's diagnostic and laboratory test reference*, ed 9. St. Louis, MO, 2008, Mosby.

Patton KT, Thibodeau GA: *Anatomy and physiology*, ed 7, St. Louis, MO, 2010, Mosby.

Seif D, Perera P, Mailhot T, et al.: Review article: Bedside ultrasound in resuscitation and the rapid ultrasound in shock protocol. *Crit Care Res Pract.* (Article ID 503254), 2012. doi:10. 1155/2012/503254. http://emcrit.org/wp-content/uploads/2011/ 03/New-RUSH-Review-Article1.pdf

Society of Critical Care Medicine: *Surviving sepsis: Bundles.* http:// www.survivingsepsis.org/Bundles/Pages/default.aspx

Solomon EP: *Introduction to human anatomy and physiology*, ed 3. Philadelphia, PA, 2009, Saunders.

Stanton BA, Koeppen BM.: *Berne and Levy physiology*, ed 6. St. Louis, MO. 2008, Mosby.

Surviving Sepsis Campaign: *6-hour bundle.* http://www.survivingsepsis.org/SiteCollectionDocuments/Bundle-6Hour-Step2a-CVP.pdf

Swan KG Jr, Wright DS, Barbagiovanni SS, et al.: Tourniquets revisited, *J Trauma.* 66:672–679, 2009.

Tintinalli JE, Kellen GD, Stapczynski S, et al.: *Tintinalli's emergency medicine: A comprehensive study guide*, ed 6. New York, NY, 2003, McGraw-Hill.

Urden LD, Stacy KM, Lough ME: *Thelan's critical care nursing: diagnosis and management*, ed 5. St. Louis, MO, 2006, Mosby.

Wallgren UM, Castrén M, Svensson AEV, et al.: Identification of adult septic patients in the prehospital setting: A comparison of two screening tools and clinical judgment. *Eur J Emerg Med Off J Eur Soc Emerg Med.* 28(6):573-579, 2013.

CHAPTER REVIEW QUESTIONS

1. A 44-year-old man presents with a history of vomiting bright red and coffee ground-colored emesis. His initial vital signs included a blood pressure of 118/78 mm Hg; pulse rate, 126 beats/min; and respirations, 22 breaths/min. Which of the following findings on repeat assessment would indicate that shock is developing?
   a. End-tidal CO_2, 35 mm Hg
   b. Pulse rate, 118 beats/min
   c. Mean arterial pressure, 86 mm Hg
   d. Pulse pressure, 32 mm Hg

2. Which response is directly responsible for vasoconstriction in shock?
   a. Beta 1
   b. Beta 2
   c. Angiotensin II
   d. Renin

3. Which of the following is predictive of septic shock?
   a. Pulse rate < 90 beats/min
   b. Lactate level < 2 mmol/L
   c. $Paco_2$ level < 32 mm Hg
   d. Glucose level < 120 mg/dL (6.6 mmol/L)

4. Your patient is presents with a pulse rate of 58 beats/min and a blood pressure of 84/60 mm Hg. The skin on her abdomen and legs is warm and dry. Which type of shock do you suspect?
   a. Hypovolemic
   b. Obstructive
   c. Cardiogenic
   d. Neurogenic

5. You are caring for a patient who is lethargic, tachycardic, hypotensive, and has a capillary refill of >3 seconds. This patient is in which stage of shock?
   a. Class I, compensated shock
   b. Class II, compensated shock
   c. Class III, decompensated shock
   d. Class IV, irreversible shock

6. Which diagnostic tests most accurately assess the presence and magnitude of anaerobic metabolism?
   a. Capnography and lactic acid
   b. Hemoglobin and oxygen saturation
   c. Glucose and capnography
   d. Serum potassium and creatinine

7. All of the following patients are hypotensive and tachycardic. Which patient is most likely presenting with signs of obstructive shock?
   a. A 26-year-old man with a sudden onset of respiratory distress and absent breath sounds on one side
   b. A 52-year-old with a history of vomiting and diarrhea for several days
   c. A 65-year-old woman with chest pain for several days and currently presenting with bilateral crackles
   d. A 67-year-old who has black tarry stools

8. A 20-year-old woman is flushed and itches after eating a salad with crab legs. Her vital signs include a blood pressure of 110/64 mm Hg; pulse rate, 108 beats/min; and respirations, 20 breaths/min, with a few wheezes noted in the bases of the lungs. She tells you her throat feels tight. She is allergic to shellfish but has not had an anaphylactic reaction before. Which intervention is indicated first?
   a. Albuterol updraft
   b. Intravenous diphenhydramine
   c. Intramuscular epinephrine
   d. Normal saline bolus

9. Your patient is a 72-year-old woman in a long-term care facility. Her skin is warm and pale. She has a blood pressure of 76/60 mm Hg and a pulse rate of 122 beats/min. Which of the following should be initiated first?
   a. Acetaminophen administration
   b. A 250- to 500-mL isotonic fluid bolus
   c. Norepinephrine infusion
   d. Dextran administration

10. Shock related to cardiac tamponade is most directly related to:
    a. Decreased afterload
    b. Hypovolemia
    c. Hypoxemia
    d. Pressure on the heart

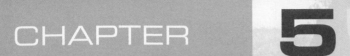

CHAPTER 5

Neurologic Disorders

Assessing and treating patients with neurologic problems can be some of the most challenging cases you will encounter. This is particularly true of the patient with an altered mental status. The many causes of altered mental status and the frequent inability of patients to communicate effectively can present unique difficulties. This chapter will assist you by providing tools to complete a basic neurologic exam and formulate a differential diagnosis using the AMLS assessment pathway.

LEARNING OBJECTIVES

At the conclusion of this chapter, you will be able to:

- Recognize the signs and symptoms of altered mental status and abnormal neurologic function.

- Gather pertinent historical data related to neurologic complaints.

- Perform a basic neurologic exam.

- Treat immediate life threats.

- Recognize the signs that indicate the patient's condition is stable, unstable, or may soon become unstable.

- Provide physical and emotional supportive care on the scene and en route.

- Apply the neurologic exam findings to help formulate a diagnosis using the AMLS assessment pathway.

- Consider the appropriate differential diagnosis.

- Explain the importance of performing a blood glucose test on every patient that has altered mental status to rule out the possibility of hypoglycemia being a contributing factor.

- Consider special transport alternatives on the basis of the likely diagnosis.

SCENARIO

As you pull up to a well-kept bungalow, you see a man and woman seated in folding chairs on the front porch. Your patient is a 68-year-old woman. Her husband explains that she normally has some memory problems but today she seems even more confused. She's also been complaining of a severe headache and says that things look "fuzzy." You notice a walker next to her, and her husband hands you a bag full of her medications. He says he is not really sure what she takes them for. "Oh my," you think, "this is going to be a big puzzle to solve."

- What specific assessments should you perform on this patient?
- What conditions are in your differential diagnosis?

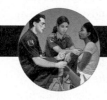

This chapter builds on your current knowledge foundation for patients with altered mental status to develop the clinical judgment necessary to form a differential diagnosis, treat immediate life threats, monitor a patient's status, and intervene with appropriate treatment. Any decrease in a person's alertness, difficulty with cognition, or behavior that departs from what is normal for that person constitutes **altered mental status**. Behavior that is normal for one person might not be typical of another, so altered mental status manifests differently from one individual to the next. The signs of altered mental status range from mild confusion to significant cognitive deficit.

Altered mental status is a common sign of morbidity in the prehospital setting, and early recognition and treatment of its underlying cause can be life saving. The condition is often associated with comorbid conditions such as trauma and infection. Identification of these conditions is helpful in determining the patient's course of treatment.

Patients with neurologic problems are vulnerable and can be in danger. Many of the reflexes that protect an awake person can be temporarily inactive when the nervous system is depressed by any cause. The eyelids do not blink away dust and irritants. The larynx does not cause gagging and coughing in reaction to secretions oozing down the airway. The airway is at risk.

Providing appropriate emergency care and formulating a differential diagnosis for any patient depends on having a solid understanding of the human body and obtaining a methodical, detail-oriented assessment. To carry out an adequate neurologic assessment of the patient with altered mental status, you cannot rely on vital signs alone. Close observation of the patient's symptoms and behavior, a skillful physical examination, and additional diagnostic tests, such as blood glucose and end-tidal carbon dioxide ($ETCO_2$) measurements, can help give you a clearer picture of the cause of a patient's distress.

Anatomy and Physiology
The Brain and Spinal Cord

The brain represents only 2% of body weight, yet it defines who we are. Billions of neurons allow us to interact with the world around us, regulate our thoughts and behavior, determine our intelligence and temperament, make it possible for us to perceive pleasure and pain, mold our personalities, and store a lifetime of memories. The brain is not fully developed until after 20 years of life, and new evidence suggests that even an adult brain can create new neurons in a process called *neurogenesis*. Thanks to advances made in neurologic research—including revolutionary functional and structural imaging modalities—we now know more about the brain than at any other time in human history.

Protective Anatomic Structures

The central nervous system (CNS), which consists of the brain and spinal cord, accounts for 98% of all neural tissues of the body. The brain itself is composed of nervous tissue (called white matter or gray matter, depending on its location and function) and occupies about 80% of the cranial vault, or skull. The average adult brain weighs about 1.5 kg (approximately 3 lb) and is cushioned inside the skull by **cerebrospinal fluid (CSF)**. CSF is a transparent, slightly yellowish fluid that acts as a shock absorber for the brain. It is made up primarily of water but also contains proteins, salts, and glucose. The flow of CSF within the skull is shown in **Figure 5-1**.

Additional protection for the brain and spinal cord is provided by the three membrane layers called *meninges* (**Figure 5-2**). Each layer of the meninges is called a *meninx*, from a Greek word meaning "membrane." The innermost meninx, which attaches directly to the brain's surface, is a delicate membrane called the *pia mater* (meaning "tender mother" or "soft mother"). The pia mater is highly vascular, containing the blood vessels that supply the surfaces of the brain and spinal cord. The middle

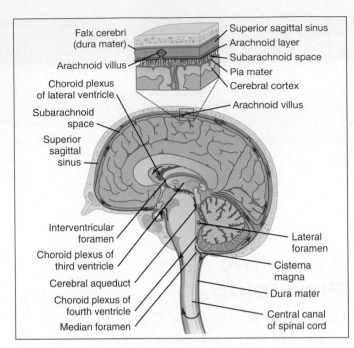

Figure 5-1 Flow of cerebral spinal fluid.

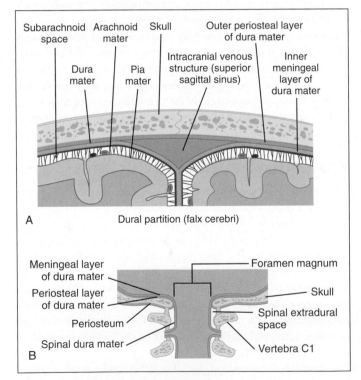

Figure 5-2 The dura mater, arachnoid mater, and pia mater are the three layers of the meninges. **A.** Superior coronal view. **B.** Continuity with the spinal meninges.

layer of the meninges is a tangle of collagen and elastin fibers that takes its name from its appearance. The meshlike vascular network of this meninx resembles a cobweb, so it is known as the *arachnoid* (meaning "spiderlike") *membrane*. CSF circulates in

the space between the arachnoid and the pia mater (the subarachnoid space), protecting the brain against mechanical injury and providing an immunologic shield. The outermost meninx, which lines the cranial vault, contains arteries that supply the bones of the skull. It is called, appropriately, the *dura mater*—"tough mother." Composed of two fibrous layers, the dura mater is the most impregnable layer of the meninges. The epidural space is between the dura mater and the skull, and the subdural space is between the dura and the subarachnoid membranes.

Blood Supply

Maintaining the critical functions of the brain requires that adequate perfusion is maintained. The brain requires a constant supply of oxygen and glucose to function properly and does not have any storage capability.

Four major arteries supply blood to the brain: two internal carotid arteries anteriorly and two vertebral arteries posteriorly. The vertebral arteries merge to become the basilar artery just inside the base of the skull, which provides branches to the brainstem and cerebellum. The basilar artery divides and joins branches of the internal carotid arteries to form the circle of Willis on the undersurface of the brain, as shown in **Figure 5-3**.

Cerebral blood flow is maintained and regulated independently of systemic blood pressure both globally and regionally based on metabolic demands by constriction or dilation of cerebral vessels. This capability is effective as long as the **cerebral perfusion pressure** (roughly equivalent to systolic blood pressure) is between 60 and 160 mm Hg. It is therefore critical to maintain a systolic pressure of at least 60 to 70 mm

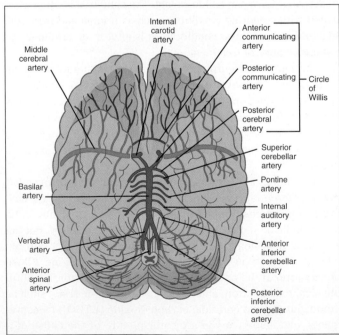

Figure 5-3 Cerebral circulation and the circle of Willis at the base of the brain.

Hg and less than 160 mm Hg to ensure preservation of cerebral perfusion. Many types of brain injury lead to impairment of this mechanism, in which case maintaining normal levels of systemic blood pressure is even more crucial.

Cerebral blood flow is also affected by the serum level of carbon dioxide (CO_2). Hypocarbia (such as with hyperventilation) causes cerebral vasoconstriction, thus leading to decreasing perfusion but also decreased intracranial pressure due to decrease in total intracranial blood. Alternatively, hypercarbia causes vasodilation. Thus, close monitoring of $ETCO_2$ is important to avoid an unwanted impact on cerebral perfusion. Understanding cerebral vasoactivity, which is the constriction or dilation of blood vessels, is important in managing patients with altered mental status or suspected traumatic brain injury or stroke.

The capillaries that nourish the brain have a special lining with tight junctions between cells forming a protective barrier between blood and the brain's extracellular fluid, known as the **blood–brain barrier (BBB)**. This barrier prevents certain particles (including bacteria, some proteins and toxins, but also antibodies and many antibiotics) from flowing into the brain while still allowing and actively facilitating the passage of oxygen, water, and glucose. Head trauma and certain infections and illnesses disrupt the BBB, often causing secondary brain injury.

Functional Regions of the Brain

The brain is a complex organ with many components and functional areas. The brain can be divided into four main regions: the cerebrum, the cerebellum, the diencephalon, and the brainstem. The limbic system, which contains a group of structures—the amygdala and the hippocampus—plays an important part in human emotions.

Cerebrum

The cerebrum comprises the cortex (divided into lobes) and subcortex. The cortex, also called the *neural cortex* or *gray matter*, is the outermost layer of the cerebrum and is the highest functioning part of the brain, comprising more than two-thirds of its mass. Because of its many convolutions, grooves, and ridges, the surface area of the cerebral cortex is actually 30 times larger than the space it occupies. Each ridge, or gyrus, and groove, or fissure, is associated with a specific cognitive function. **Figure 5-4** depicts the cerebrum and the other major structures of the brain.

The structure and function of the brain hemispheres and lobes are as follows:

- *Right and left hemispheres.* The cerebrum is divided into left and right hemispheres. Structurally and functionally, they control opposite sides of the body. The hemispheres are interconnected by constantly communicating nerve fibers (in the corpus callosum) that transmit as many as 4 billion impulses per second.

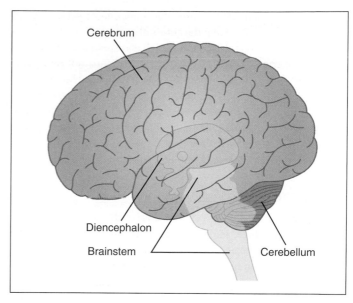

Figure 5-4 The four primary areas of the brain are the brainstem, diencephalon, cerebrum, and cerebellum.

The brain's structure is not identical from one individual to the next. In more than 90% of right-handed people and more than 70% of left-handed people, the interpretive speech center is located in the left hemisphere. The left hemisphere, often called the *logical brain*, is also responsible for reading, writing, mathematical calculation, and sequential and analytic tasks. The right hemisphere, known as the "creative brain," interprets sensory information and processes spatial awareness. Interestingly, many musicians, dancers, and artists are left-handed, and the right hemisphere of the cerebral cortex in such people appears to be more active than the left.

- *Lobes.* The cerebrum is further subdivided into lobes, each of which is named for the cranial bone that lies above it. For example, the frontal lobe lies beneath the frontal bone. The other lobes are the parietal, temporal, and occipital. Each lobe and its corresponding region of the cerebral cortex has a specific function. The frontal lobe controls motor function, determines personality, and elaborates thought and speech; the parietal lobe interprets bodily sensations; the temporal lobe stores long-term memory and interprets sound; and the occipital lobe is responsible for sight.

Cerebellum

The second largest part of the brain, the cerebellum, lies above the brainstem and posterior to the cerebrum (see **Figure 5-4**). The cerebellum coordinates movements, balance, and posture.

Diencephalon

Near the center of the brain is the diencephalon (see **Figure 5-4**). The diencephalon includes the thalamus and the hypothalamus.

The thalamus, composed of gray matter, connects sensory input between the spinal cord and the cerebral cortex and houses much of the reticular activating system, which is responsible for arousal (sleep/wake transitions). The tiny hypothalamus, not much bigger than a cherry pit, is responsible for maintaining homeostasis in the body. It links the sympathetic and parasympathetic nervous systems by way of the pituitary gland. The hormones of the hypothalamus stimulate or inhibit the release of hormones from the pituitary gland to regulate circadian rhythm (the body's innate sleep cycle), thirst and hunger, and other functions.

Brainstem

Connecting the spinal cord to the brain is the brainstem, which includes the medulla, midbrain, and pons (see **Figure 5-4**). The medulla controls basic physiologic functions such as breathing and heart rate. The midbrain is involved in regulation of vision, hearing, and body movement. The pons (meaning "bridge") connects the cerebellum to the medulla and is involved in posture and movement, as well as sleep.

Limbic System

Surrounding the thalamus are the structures of the primitive brain, known collectively as the *limbic system* (**Figure 5-5**). The limbic system comprises two structures: the amygdala and the hippocampus. The system is connected to the prefrontal cortex of the frontal lobe.

The limbic system is referred to as the primitive brain because it controls basic survival instincts and many of the behavioral responses that constitute key features of our personalities, such as whether we have a positive or negative outlook.

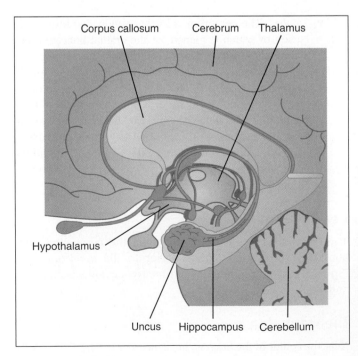

Figure 5-5 The limbic system.

Labels: Corpus callosum, Cerebrum, Thalamus, Hypothalamus, Uncus, Hippocampus, Cerebellum

The system is responsible for intense feelings—fear, frustration, anxiety, tension, anger, rage, sexual desire, appetite, the desire or ability to bond, and the storage of our emotional memories. The limbic system allows us to interpret events as they are happening and helps us predict the consequences of actions or events.

Ventricles

The ventricles (meaning "little bellies") are cavity-like spaces filled with circulating CSF, which is constantly produced by the capillary network within the ventricles.

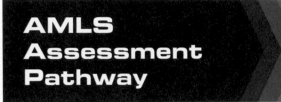

AMLS Assessment Pathway

▼ Initial Observations

Scene Safety Considerations

For your own safety as well as that of the patient, make sure the scene is safe before you approach. If you are called to a scene at which the patient shows signs of altered mental status and a gun or knife is reported or seen, the patient may be violent, delirious, or confused, make sure the scene has been secured by law enforcement personnel before you approach. If the scene is initially safe, observe the patient from a distance and note any physical movements and verbal comments. If the patient is becoming agitated or aggressive, take this behavior into account as part of your scene safety evaluation and immediately call for appropriate backup or assistance.

Gloves are a necessary standard approach for all patients. Remember that patients who have seizures may be incontinent. The standard precautions you use should be based on the procedures you use and the likelihood of being contaminated. A patient with a neurologic disease may not be able to communicate with you.

Patient Cardinal Presentation/Chief Complaint

A brief overview of some of the most common cardinal presentations or chief complaints in patients with neurologic dysfunction follows. Many disease processes have similar presentations, or one finding may mask another. For example, delirium may lead to hypoglycemia, hypoglycemia may cause a seizure, and a seizure may mask a stroke. In addition, although a patient's neurologic symptoms may seem pressing, sometimes they indicate more serious medical conditions that should be considered in the differential diagnosis. Syncope (fainting), for example, may indicate a pulmonary embolism.

Altered Mental Status

Patients with altered mental status may show signs of confusion or exhibit changes in their typical behavior. In a patient with altered mental status, it is often difficult to sort out cause and effect. Hypoglycemia and electrolyte abnormalities (such as hyponatremia) can be responsible for disorientation, and depression, intoxication, and overdose can trigger unusual or disturbing behavior. Such behavioral alterations should be confirmed by a family member or someone else who knows the patient well.

A patient who has a significantly depressed mental status or is comatose and cannot give a history requires immediate resuscitation. A mental decline of this sort can be ominous and attributable to hemorrhagic stroke, overdose, and other grave conditions.

Delirium

Delirium is an acute alteration in cognition characterized by waxing and waning impairment of awareness, orientation and cognition, and sometimes associated with hallucinations or delusions. It is seen more often in women than men and is often associated with illness in the very young and those older than 60 years. These alterations can cause decrements in alertness, orientation, emotional or behavioral response, perception, language expression, judgment, and activity. Causes of delirium include intoxication, infection, trauma, seizure, endocrine disorders, organ failure, stroke, shock, infection, conversion disorder, intracranial bleeding, and tumors.

Dementia is sometimes confused with delirium but represents a chronic loss of brain function, particularly short-term memory function. It also affects thinking, language, judgment, and behavior. Unlike delirium, dementia is degenerative, occurring over time, and is usually irreversible.

In a patient with delirium, short-term memory becomes clouded, and the person becomes disoriented to time or place. Level of awareness may fluctuate over brief periods, and speech may be incoherent, tense, or rambling. The patient usually has no discernible focal neurologic deficit. Nevertheless, infection, intoxication, dehydration, cardiac dysrhythmia, thyroid problems, and medication issues (such as overdosing and underdosing) may cause alterations in vital signs and physical exam findings.

The patient who demonstrates any level of delirium must be fully evaluated. Appearance, vital signs, hydration, and evidence of trauma should all be taken into account. A mini-mental state exam can be given to document the severity, nature, and progress of mental status changes. When you encounter an individual in an acute delirious state, remember that the patient is confused and is likely to have poor judgment. Your safety and that of the patient are the highest priorities. The patient may require physical or chemical restraints, using a benzodiazepine or antipsychotic agent.

Perform appropriate airway management measures to maintain an open airway and reduce the risk of aspiration if the patient is unconscious, has poor gag reflex, or you note snoring or noisy breathing. Provide supplemental oxygen if oxygen saturation is < 94% or the patient appears to be in respiratory distress. If you suspect a traumatic injury, take precautions to protect the cervical spine. Also be sure to test the patient's serum glucose level. The patient will be evaluated in the emergency department (ED) with the aid of laboratory and radiologic studies. The patient may need a surgical, neurologic, or psychiatric evaluation.

In a syndrome called *agitated delirium*, the patient initially appears to be grossly psychotic and may exhibit strength out of proportion to your expectations. The patient may be extremely distraught, hyperstimulated, and uncontrollable. Attempts to physically restrain the agitated delirium patient may only worsen these findings. When restrained physically or with electrical devices (Taser devices), the patient's violent struggling may suddenly cease. The patient with agitated delirium may then have an irregular respiratory pattern followed shortly (typically within a few minutes) by death. Cardiac dysrhythmias have been noted in these patients, but asystole is the primary presenting rhythm. They may be hyperthermic and often have elevated circulating levels of epinephrine and metabolic acidosis. All patients who exhibit signs of agitated delirium must be medically evaluated and should not be restrained in a prone position, which is thought to exaggerate the acidosis by impeding ventilation. Chemical restraint with appropriate sedative such as a benzodiazepine, neuroleptic or ketamine is often appropriate. Monitor the patient's cardiac rhythm and use continuous pulse oximetry. If active struggling stops abruptly, be immediately on the lookout for respiratory arrest, usually followed by cardiac arrest. Aggressive airway management and cardiac support may be lifesaving.

Syncope/Light-Headedness

Syncope, a transient loss of consciousness associated with decreased brain perfusion, has many possible causes. Light-headedness, near-syncope, and syncope have the same differential diagnosis. It includes conditions such as aortic valve stenosis, hypertrophic cardiomyopathy, cardiac dysrhythmia, hypovolemia (dehydration, ectopic pregnancy rupture, aortic aneurysm rupture), CNS event (e.g., subarachnoid hemorrhage), pulmonary embolism, and vasovagal reflex (often due to situational or emotional triggers).

Dizziness/Vertigo

When patients complain of dizziness, it is essential to differentiate whether the patient is referring to a feeling of light-headedness (or near-syncope) versus vertigo, a feeling of spinning or abnormal sensation of movement.

Patients who report alterations in **proprioception** (spatial orientation of one's own body) and balance are usually able to give a history of such experiences. You may not be able to assess intermittent alterations such as those secondary to transient ischemic attack (TIA). Many patients, however, including those with stroke, positional vertigo, overdose, vertebral artery dissection, and electrolyte abnormalities, may still be symptomatic as you complete your assessment.

Vertigo is a symptom. It originates in the CNS or vestibular organs. Central vertigo may be caused by hemorrhagic or ischemic insult (stroke), concussion, tumors, infection, migraine headache, multiple sclerosis, toxic ingestion or inhalation, Wernicke-Korsakoff syndrome, or lesion of the eighth cranial nerve nucleus in the brainstem. Peripheral vertigo is due to a disruption in the vestibular system or eighth cranial nerve.

A patient with vertigo has a feeling of imbalance or difficulty maintaining an upright posture and may complain of feeling drunk or that the room is spinning around. The patient may have nausea or vomiting. The vertigo may have an abrupt onset, and the patient may also complain of tinnitus, a buzzing or ringing in the ears. It is important to question the patient about a history of stroke, atrial fibrillation, and hypertension, because this history can suggest stroke-related vertigo. A patient may have a decreased LOC, or the eyes may be moving quickly back and forth, a condition known as "nystagmus." Nystagmus may be horizontal, vertical, or rotatory and may or may not diminish spontaneously. Nystagmus can result from a lesion in the cerebellum, brainstem, or vestibular organs.

Patients who have vertigo lasting longer than 24 hours, accompanied by a loss of balance and difficulty maintaining their posture, standing, and walking are often found to have a cerebellar infarction. Transient symptoms not triggered by motion may indicate a TIA. The patient who has other cranial nerve deficits needs to be evaluated for brainstem or cerebellar issues.

Vertigo may also be due to dysfunction of the vestibular system, usually the inner ear. This is commonly referred to as *peripheral vertigo*. Symptoms may be more acute, abrupt, severe, and of shorter duration than central vertigo and are often worsened or triggered by movement or change in position of the head. Brief, recurrent episodes of vertigo associated with a change in position that resolve with cessation of movement suggests benign positional vertigo. Patients may prefer to face one side or the other during transport and may not want to turn toward you to answer questions, because it exacerbates symptoms.

Seizure

You may be able to obtain a history from patients who have had a seizure if their mental status has improved sufficiently. Usually in the immediate postictal period, however, you will have to rely on bystanders for information. The seizure may be generalized (involving loss of consciousness), associated with tonic-clonic movements, incontinence, and tongue biting, or it may be a focal seizure that affects only one part of the body without loss of consciousness but with possible decreased awareness.

During your scene survey, you may notice antiseizure medications or a medical alert bracelet. In addition to epilepsy, it is important to consider that this seizure may have been precipitated by other conditions such as head injury, stroke, meningitis, or toxins.

Headache

Headache can be an ambiguous, puzzling symptom. Provided there has been no loss of consciousness, as may happen with ischemic stroke or intracranial hemorrhage, the patient will probably be able to describe the symptoms to you. Pay special attention to the patient's description of the onset, nature, and location of the pain. This information can be useful in pinpointing specific etiologies such as temporal arteritis and migraine.

Note any associated symptoms such as vision changes—for example, ipsilateral vision changes (on the same side of the body as the headache) occur with temporal arteritis. Patients with a migraine may have photophobia (light sensitivity) and phonophobia (sound sensitivity), and they may perceive flashing lights. Patients who have experienced trauma and complain of headaches may have a subdural or epidural hematoma or a vertebral artery dissection. A severe headache that has a sudden onset, with or without vomiting, may indicate subarachnoid bleeding. A history of comorbidities (coexisting medical problems), such as hypertension and vascular abnormalities, points to bleeding or aneurysm. A history of intravenous (IV) drug use or improper cleaning of implanted port sites before accessing may suggest epidural abscess. Finally, be alert for abnormal vital signs, including fever, which could indicate meningitis.

Ataxia/Gait Disturbance

Ataxia refers to a loss of muscular control and coordination causing truncal instability, gait unsteadiness, abnormal eye movements, or difficulty with precision of movements of the extremities, such as distance-finding or rapid alternating movements. This may be due to brain dysfunction, often of the cerebellum, or pathology of the spinal cord, peripheral nerves, or inner ear, or muscle weakness. The patient or a family member may report that the patient is unable to walk normally, and any of the following may be noted:

- Has trouble coordinating movements
- Double vision or irregular eye movements
- Feels weak or unstable (off balance or about to fall) when walking or standing

Associated symptoms such as incontinence or altered mentation (as occurs with normal-pressure hydrocephalus) or nausea, vomiting, and visual changes (as may occur with a posterior-circulation stroke) may also be present. Causes of ataxia are summarized in **Table 5-1**.

Focal Neurologic Deficit

Focal neurologic deficit refers to any localized loss of neurologic function, such as weakness or numbness in part or all of an extremity or one side of the face. Unless the patient has an associated neurologic insult that hinders speech, a condition known as **expressive aphasia**, he or she will probably be able to describe the onset of the deficit. Stroke is a particularly

Table 5-1 Causes of Ataxia

Gait Disturbance	Description	Differential Diagnosis
Broad-based gait	Person walks with an abnormally wide distance between the feet, which increases stability Patient may hesitate, freeze, lurch, or be unable to walk in a straight line	Acute alcohol intoxication Cerebellar atrophy caused by chronic alcohol abuse Diabetic peripheral neuropathy Stroke Ingestion of antiseizure medications such as phenytoin (Dilantin) Normal-pressure hydrocephalus Increased intracranial pressure
Propulsive (festinating) gait	Stooped, rigid posture, with the head and neck bent forward Shuffling gait Often accompanied by urinary incontinence	Advanced Parkinson's disease Carbon monoxide poisoning Chronic exposure to manganese (in those who handle pesticides and in welders and miners) Ingestion of certain medications such as antipsychotics
Spastic gait	Characterized by stiffness and foot dragging Caused by long-term unilateral muscle contraction	Stroke Liver failure Spinal cord trauma or tumor Brain abscess or tumor Head trauma
Scissors gait	Crouching posture, with legs flexed at the hips and knees Knees and thighs brush together in a scissors-like movement when patient walks Patient takes short, slow, deliberate steps Patient may walk on toes or on balls of feet	Stroke Liver failure Spinal cord compression Thoracic or lumbar tumor Multiple sclerosis Cerebral palsy
Steppage gait	Characterized by foot drop; foot hangs down, causing toes to scuff the ground while walking	Guillain-Barré syndrome Lumbar disk herniation Peroneal nerve trauma

time-sensitive etiology of focal neurologic deficits. The history may reveal a preceding illness (e.g., Guillain-Barré syndrome) or chronic neurologic disorder (e.g., neuromuscular degenerative disease [Lou Gehrig disease], multiple sclerosis, or myasthenia gravis). Be sure to ask about bowel and bladder function, because incontinence typically accompanies the lower extremity weakness of cauda equina syndrome. Note any change in the patient's ability to understand or follow instructions. Such deficit may indicate stroke, intoxication, electrolyte abnormality, or hepatic encephalopathy.

Primary Survey

The primary survey includes an evaluation of the patient's airway, breathing, and circulation, as well as interventions for immediate life threats. Blood glucose levels should be checked in *every patient* with any change in mental status or behavior, even if another cause seems obvious.

Level of Consciousness

If the patient has a decreased level of consciousness (LOC), the airway may also be compromised. In most cases, a patient who is able to speak has a patent airway, but any neurologic condition that impairs mental status may quickly progress to the patient being unable to maintain a functional airway. Once an individual becomes unconscious, the tongue or secretions can obstruct the airway. Listen for snoring, gurgling, or stridor and ensure there is good airflow. Keeping the airway open is of the utmost importance. It might become necessary to provide interventions such as suctioning, patient positioning, placement of an oral or nasopharyngeal airway, and intubation or placement of an advanced airway adjunct.

Airway and Breathing

Evaluation of the patient's respiratory rate, depth, and pattern may also indicate the underlying cause of altered mental status. Acidosis, stroke, metabolic disease, and other pathologic conditions cause changes in breathing patterns. Hypoventilation may indicate CNS depression, which might be attributable to drug overdose, stroke, or intracranial swelling. If possible, obtain a baseline oxygen saturation measurement (with the patient breathing ambient air) before you provide assistance, but in cases of respiratory distress, do not delay treatment just to obtain a baseline reading. Provide oxygen and ventilatory support to maintain an oxygen saturation of at least 94%. Monitor the patient's response to oxygenation and ventilation. Adequacy of ventilation (minute ventilation) is best assessed by measuring the partial pressure of carbon dioxide ($Paco_2$) in blood. In the field and in other emergency settings, you can approximate $Paco_2$ by measuring the $ETCO_2$. The goal should be to maintain an $ETCO_2$ of 30 to 40 mm Hg ($ETCO_2$ is about 5 mm Hg lower than serum Pco_2) unless there is a clear reason to do otherwise, such as setting a lower $ETCO_2$ goal in patients with metabolic acidosis or definite signs of cerebral herniation. In intubated patients in particular there is a strong tendency for providers to hyperventilate the patient, which directly correlates with increased brain injury from decreased cerebral perfusion.

Circulation/Perfusion

In this component of the primary survey, you first want to ensure that the patient has a palpable pulse. As blood pressure drops, pulses are usually lost first in the distal extremities (radial and pedal), then more proximally (femoral and antecubital), and, last, the carotid. One can assess the strength of the pulse and also check for other signs of adequate perfusion, including capillary refill and skin color and temperature. Mental status is perhaps usually the best indicator of adequate perfusion, but for this chapter it is assumed to be abnormal and thus not helpful.

Assessment of pulse rate and rhythm can also help you pinpoint the cause of an altered mental status. Primary dysrhythmias such as atrial fibrillation with rapid ventricular response, tachyarrhythmias, and bradyarrhythmias can directly cause hypoperfusion. Tachycardia (rapid pulse rate) could be a sign of infection, temperature elevation, postictal (postseizure) state, drug withdrawal or toxicity, or hypovolemia (low blood volume). Bradycardia may suggest cerebral herniation, hypothermia, or drug toxicity. An irregular pulse should lead you to consider cardiac dysrhythmia, which may be triggered by an acute coronary syndrome, electrolyte disturbance, acidosis, hypoxia, or ingestion of a toxic substance.

While blood pressure is relied on heavily in determining the cause of an altered mental status, and this should be obtained as part of your examination, it is important to not use this parameter alone to confirm adequate perfusion. You must rely on all the manifestations of perfusion as previously described and recognize that automated devices may yield false readings as well.

▼ First Impression

When you are trying to determine whether your patient has a neurologic problem, look for both obvious and subtle changes that can indicate disease. Take in the surroundings. Being alert will help keep you safe and could suggest a diagnosis. Is the area clean and neat, or is it dirty and untidy? Is there any evidence that the patient is a victim of neglect or abuse? Send your partner to investigate (ask permission of a family member if necessary) the cabinets and refrigerator to see whether there seems to be enough food. If not, or if the food on hand appears to be spoiled, the patient's condition could be attributable to malnutrition or electrolyte abnormalities. Look for insulin or oral hypoglycemic medications. Are there empty or nearly empty pill bottles lying scattered about? Are the prescription labels out of date? If so, an accidental or intentional overdose might be responsible for the patient's altered mental status. Who is the patient's caregiver if he or she does not live independently or is a minor? Be alert to objects in the patient's environment (e.g., oxygen canisters or drug paraphernalia) that can help you formulate a differential diagnosis. Check for anything out of place in the room. Is the phone on the floor, as if the patient had attempted to call 9-1-1 but dropped the receiver before doing so? This may tip you off to consider stroke as a potential diagnosis.

Life-Threatening Presentations

Hypoglycemia

A patient with hypoglycemia often presents with confusion and abnormal behavior but may also seem depressed, sluggish, or dull witted. He may have focal weakness or seizure or be completely unresponsive. If the patient is awake enough to swallow without risk of aspiration, oral glucose in some form may be given. When the patient has decreased level of consciousness, dextrose should be administered IV according to local protocol. If the patient is unconscious, or if there is any delay or difficulty in checking the blood glucose level, it is preferable to give the IV dextrose rather than withhold it until the level can be obtained. When IV access is not available, glucagon should be administered by IM injection.

Hypoventilation (CO₂ Narcosis)

A patient requires ventilatory assistance if unconscious or if respiratory effort is compromised, which may be due to a stroke, accidental or intentional medication overdose, or trauma or a medical event. When ventilation is impaired, $Paco_2$ climbs to dangerous levels, causing confusion, drowsiness, tremors, and **convulsions**. This condition is known as "CO_2 narcosis," and it will lead to death if ventilatory assistance is not provided. Such assistance may be given with a bag-mask or advanced-airway device or by intubating the patient. Initially the ventilation rate can be slightly higher than normal to bring down the $Paco_2$ level quickly, but the patient's condition must be monitored carefully to prevent alkalosis. Capnography is essential to both making the diagnosis and assessing treatment.

Hypoxia

Severe hypoxia may lead to confusion and decrease in mental status, so measurement of oxygen saturation is an essential component of the assessment of every patient with AMS. Depression of consciousness may also be associated with hypoventilation leading to hypoxia. Supplemental oxygen will be required if the Spo_2 is < 94%, and assisted ventilation must be provided if the patient is hypoventilating (best determined by the $ETCO_2$ measurement). Providers should be aware of several situations in which Spo_2 is not accurate. Perhaps the most common of these is related to carbon monoxide poisoning, in which case pulse oximetry readings show hemoglobin bound to CO is oxygenated. Methemoglobinemia, which is caused by certain drugs such as benzocaine, also leads to a slightly higher than actual reading, and with a characteristic reading of 85% in severe cases. Finally, cyanide may block oxygen utilization at the cellular level despite fully saturated blood level.

Hypoperfusion with Cerebral Ischemia

Many acute medical conditions, major trauma, and certain kinds of medications can cause hypoperfusion that leads to cerebral ischemia (lack of blood flow to the brain). The cause of the shock should be quickly discerned and targeted treatment implemented when possible. Chapter 4 offers an in-depth discussion of what to do in cases of shock.

Intracranial Hypertension

Elevated intracranial pressure (ICP) can significantly compromise perfusion to the brain, especially with significant acute elevations. ICP elevation may be due to mass effect, such as from acute hemorrhage or edema, or malfunction of a ventriculoperitoneal shunt. If pressure becomes too high, herniation of the brain into the lower skull or through the foramen magnum may occur. This condition is often characterized by a unilateral blown pupil and unconsciousness, and has a high mortality.

Treating intracranial hypertension with hyperventilation must be done very cautiously. Hyperventilation decreases the amount of CO_2 dissolved in the blood, which induces cerebral vasoconstriction. Vasoconstriction decreases blood volume in the brain, thereby reducing ICP. However, vasoconstriction also decreases blood flow. The net effect on perfusion is difficult if not impossible to predict, so the patient's neurologic status must be monitored closely. In deciding whether to perform hyperventilation, follow local protocol and the preference of the receiving hospital. In life-threatening situations with herniation, mild to moderate hyperventilation may be indicated as a short-term measure. Adequate oxygenation and systemic perfusion ($ETCO_2$, about 30 mm Hg [no lower than 25 mm Hg]) must be maintained.

▼ Detailed Assessment
History Taking

Patients with altered mental status may not be able to give a clear history or understand the caregiver. It is helpful to have other family members around if possible to collect additional information at the scene that could prove useful. If the patient is able to give some history, it should be obtained as soon as possible because a person's mental status can deteriorate within only a few minutes. If you are working with a partner, the history and physical exam can often be conducted simultaneously.

When you treat a patient with altered mental status, gather information from witnesses or bystanders that might help describe the patient's baseline mental status and how it has changed recently. Ask about the degree of change, and inquire when the patient was last seen or known to be acting normal. Collect any other potential clues to the cause of the mental status change, such as information about the patient's medication regimen, blood pressure, and any recent trauma that might have been sustained. Ask about and observe for signs of abnormal body movements, smells, speech, or automatisms.

OPQRST and SAMPLER

The OPQRST and SAMPLER mnemonics should be used to obtain the patient's complete history using a systematic approach. Talk to the patient directly when the neurologic status allows. Ask the patient what's wrong and allow the patient to describe his or her concerns in an open-ended fashion. Patients may give you valuable historical clues that will help generate your differential diagnosis. A teenage girl may tell you she has a fever and a stiff neck. An older man may admit he took the wrong medication by mistake. Conversely, if the patient has difficulty speaking, a stroke or other severe medical problem becomes a stronger possibility.

Secondary Survey

After you have stabilized the patient and treated any life threats, form a general impression of the patient's status and develop a list of possible differential diagnoses. Before you perform the secondary survey and the detailed physical exam, you should try to get an idea of how distressed the patient is, taking into account your general assessment findings as well as vital signs, the results of the serum glucose test, and pulse oximetry readings. Decide whether the patient must be immediately transported to the hospital or if you can take more time for evaluation on scene. Because the conditions of patients with altered mental status tend to be unstable and may decompensate quickly, much of the rest of your evaluation and examination may be performed en route to the hospital. Remain alert for traumatic injuries and for any information that could prove diagnostically useful, such as unusual sights, sounds, and odors. Note the patient's positioning and any clues in visual appearance that may suggest causes of distress.

The secondary survey is meant to help generate a more complete set of differential diagnoses that can then be ruled in or out with the aid of sound clinical reasoning. Document a history of the complaint and related issues, a time line indicating when each of the patient's symptoms began, and a list of exacerbating factors.

During the physical examination, identify any injuries or other abnormalities in the patient's physical condition, and complete as much of a neurologic exam as possible. During your initial contact with the patient, you will have completed your evaluation of the patient's LOC, ability to speak, and general orientation, but other neurologic functions should be tested, including the presence or absence of cranial nerves functions, motor function in the upper and lower extremities, and sensation and strength in those extremities. Document incontinence if present, and, if the patient is able to walk, document whether the gait is normal.

Diagnostics

The types of diagnostic tools in an ambulance or helicopter are limited, but the tools you do have, along with careful observation, often allow you to detect critical and treatable conditions. The easiest and most widely used means of evaluation is the AVPU mnemonic, which classifies the patient's LOC as alert, responsive to verbal stimuli, responsive to painful stimuli, or unresponsive. The Glasgow Coma Scale is another tool used to evaluate LOC and mental status (Table 5-2). Scores are obtained on the basis of three responses: eye opening, motor response, and verbal response (Table 5-3). This tool is often used to assess for brain injury in patients with head trauma.

As noted earlier, vital signs, including temperature when possible, blood glucose, oxygen saturation, and end-tidal carbon dioxide measurements, should be taken and recorded, and appropriate treatment should be administered. Cardiac monitoring and, if indicated, a 12-lead electrocardiogram (ECG) should be performed. Some blood analyses may be carried out using a portable device. In addition, some services may be equipped with portable ultrasound.

The mnemonics in the Rapid Recall boxes may assist you in formulating a differential diagnosis on the basis of history, physical exam, and laboratory findings.

RAPID RECALL

Causes of Decreased Level of Consciousness: AEIOU-TIPS

A Alcohol, anaphylaxis, acute myocardial infarction

E Epilepsy
Endocrine abnormality
Electrolyte imbalance

I Insulin (glucose)

O Opiates

U Uremia

T Trauma

I Intracranial (tumor, hemorrhage, or hypertension)
Infection

P Poisoning

S Seizure
Stroke
Syncope

Table 5-2 **Glasgow Coma Scale**		
Responses	**Adult**	**Pediatric (< 5 years)**
Eye opening	4. Spontaneous 3. Voice 2. Pain stimulation 1. None	4. Spontaneous 3. To shout/voice 2. Pain stimulation 1. None
Verbal	5. Oriented 4. Disoriented 3. Inappropriate words 2. Incomprehensible 1. None	5. Smiles, speech/interaction appropriate for age 4. Cries but consolable, inappropriate words/interactions 3. Difficult to console 2. Restless and inconsolable 1. None
Motor	6. Obeys 5. Localizes pain 4. Withdraws from pain 3. Decorticate 2. Decerebrate 1. None	6. Spontaneous 5. Localizes pain 4. Withdraws from pain 3. Decorticate 2. Decerebrate 1. None

Table 5-3 Interpretations of Glasgow Coma Scale Scores			
Score	**Severity**	**Treatment**	**Facility**
13–15	Mild	Ensure adequate oxygen, glucose, and temperature to promote proper nervous system functioning	Patient's or family's choice
9–12	Moderate	Close airway assessment Watch for decreasing consciousness	Closest appropriate facility
8 or less	Critical	May need airway/ventilation control Decrease scene time	Closest appropriate facility

RAPID RECALL

Assessment of Acute Mental Status Changes: SMASHED

S Substrates—Substrates may include hyperglycemia, hypoglycemia, and thiamine

Sepsis

M Meningitis and other CNS infections

Mental illness

A Alcohol—Intoxicated or in withdrawal

S Seizure—Ictal (active) or postictal phase

Stimulants—Anticholinergic agents, hallucinogens, or cocaine

H Hyper—Hyperthyroidism, hyperthermia, hypercarbia

Hypo—Hypotension, hypothyroidism, hypoxia

E Electrolytes—Hypernatremia, hyponatremia, or hypercalcemia

Encephalopathy—Hepatic, uremic, hypertensive, or others

D Drugs—Any type

RAPID RECALL

Initial Assessment of Altered Mental Status: SNOT

Remember this mnemonic when performing initial assessment in the prehospital setting:

S Sugar

Stroke

Seizure

N Narcosis (CO_2, opiates)

O Oxygen

T Trauma

Toxins

Temperature

Be aware that this list is not a comprehensive survey of all possible causes of altered mental status.

Courtesy Vince Mosesso, MD

▼ Refine the Differential Diagnosis

The components of the primary and secondary survey will help you refine your differential diagnoses and determine the severity of the patient's condition. Manage any life threats as they appear during the assessment process. Remember that most diseases or conditions, including neurologic disorders, are caused by more than one factor. The specific conditions described later will provide an approach for helping you determine the differential diagnosis and recognize key findings.

▼ Ongoing Management

Managing patients with suspected neurologic dysfunction should be approached in a systematic manner. During your ongoing management, revisit the primary assessment, the vital signs, the cardinal presentation/chief complaint, and any treatment you have administered, including oxygen administration. As always, you should monitor airway, breathing, and circulation. Maintain the patient's oxygenation (94% oxygen saturation is the minimal level acceptable in stroke patients without supplemental oxygen, but oxygen at 2 to 6 liters per minute [LPM] by nasal cannula is almost always appropriate). Check for hypoglycemia, which can mimic many neurologic disorders, and even if IV fluids are not needed, place an IV with a saline lock in case the patient decompensates. If you have any suspicion that the patient may have suffered traumatic injury, protect the cervical spine.

A calm, supportive professional demeanor is of the utmost importance because the patient is usually frightened. A physiologic function he or she may have taken for granted is not working properly or no longer working. In addition, the patient may be confused and lash out physically or verbally. Use a composed, reassuring manner at all times.

Your team must decide which hospital can best treat the patient. You may select a stroke center, a trauma center, or another center that offers advanced specialized care. If the patient's condition is life threatening, transport the patient to the closest facility, where the medical staff can stabilize and transfer the patient for more definitive care if needed. If the decision is made not to transport the patient to the nearest hospital, the destination should be chosen on the basis of local point-of-entry protocols, each hospital's respective capabilities, and the patient's medical needs. Online medical control can be a resource for additional guidance if needed.

Specific Diagnoses
Stroke

A **stroke**, sometimes called a *brain attack*, is a brain injury that occurs when blood flow to the brain is obstructed or interrupted, causing brain cells to die. According to the National Stroke Association, the term **cerebrovascular accident (CVA)** is no longer is being used by the medical community because stroke is considered to be a preventable event, not an accident.

Strokes are classified as either ischemic or hemorrhagic, as shown in **Figure 5-6**. An **ischemic stroke** occurs when a thrombus or embolus obstructs a vessel, diminishing blood flow to the brain. A **thrombus** is a blood clot or a cholesterol plaque that forms in an artery, occluding blood flow. An **embolus** is a clot or plaque that forms elsewhere in the circulatory system, breaks off, and obstructs blood flow when it becomes lodged in a smaller artery. Rarely, an embolus may be composed of fat from a broken bone or an air bubble introduced during IV therapy, surgery, trauma, or severe decompression sickness. Ischemic stroke is much more common than **hemorrhagic stroke**, which occurs when a diseased or damaged vessel ruptures.

Pathophysiology

During an ischemic stroke, blood flow to a portion of the brain is disrupted, and ischemia of the brain occurs (see Figure 5-6, B). Ischemia is insufficient blood flow to an organ or tissue—in this case the brain—causing inadequate perfusion. Death of neurons and cerebral infarction (tissue death) follow. Blood flow may be restricted by an embolism or thrombus, or cerebral blood flow can be decreased by blood pressure relative to ICP or shock.

A blood clot, or embolus, may arise from the heart or its vessels and travel to the smaller vessels of the brain. The most common sites of thrombotic stroke are in the branches of the cerebral arteries, the circle of Willis, and the posterior circulation. When lack of perfusion to a portion of the brain causes infarction, an area of potentially reversible ischemia surrounds the region. The goal of treatment is to reverse or stop the ischemia in order to prevent further destruction and permit oxygenation of affected brain tissue.

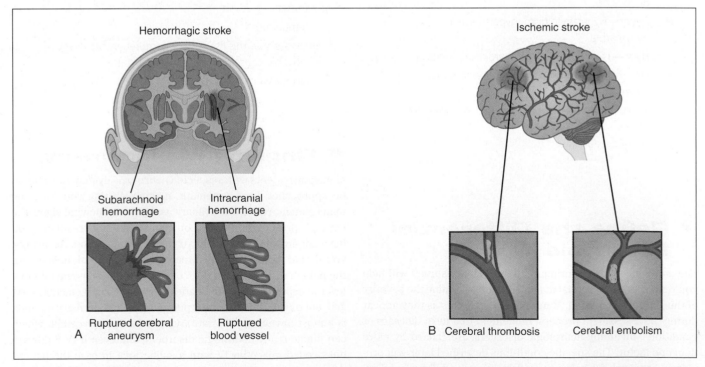

Figure 5-6 Causes of stroke. **A.** Hemorrhagic stroke is the result of bleeding caused by an intracerebral hemorrhage or a subarachnoid hemorrhage, usually a result of a ruptured cerebral aneurysm. **B.** Ischemic stroke is the result of a blocked blood vessel caused by a cerebral thrombosis or cerebral embolism.

Strokes in the middle cerebral artery typically produce **hemiparesis**, or unilateral weakness, on the opposite side of the body from the stroke (**Figure 5-7**). Patients often show a gaze preference toward the side of the lesion. If the ischemic lesion is in the dominant hemisphere, the patient may have receptive or expressive aphasia. A stroke in the nondominant hemisphere may cause neglect of or inattention to one side of the body. Usually, weakness is more pronounced in the arm and face than in the lower extremity. A stroke in the distribution of the anterior cerebral artery can cause altered mental status and impaired judgment, opposite-side weakness (greater in the leg than in the arm), and urinary incontinence.

Posterior cerebral artery occlusion impairs thought processes, clouds memory, and causes visual field deficits. Finally, vertebrobasilar artery occlusions may cause vertigo, syncope, ataxia, and cranial nerve dysfunction, including nystagmus, double vision, and difficulty swallowing.

Patients with atherosclerosis may have turbulent blood flow, which increases the risk of blood clot formation and platelet adherence within the arteries. In addition, patients who have blood disorders such as sickle cell anemia, protein C deficiency, and polycythemia (a hereditary disorder characterized by an abundance of circulating red blood cells) also have properties of the blood that increase the risk of stroke.

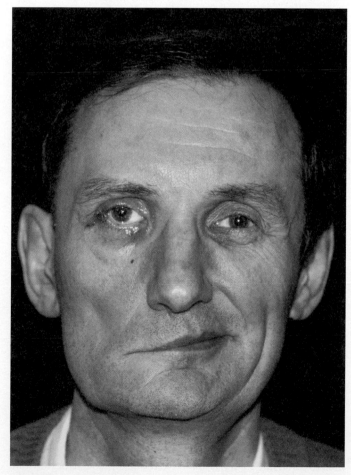

Figure 5-7 Facial droop.
Dr. P. Marazzi / Science Source

Signs and Symptoms

Any patient who presents with an acute neurologic deficit should be evaluated for a stroke, whether the deficit is focal, such as a loss of strength or sensation in a particular body region, or diffuse, such as altered mental status.

A patient having a stroke usually experiences an abrupt onset of significant weakness on one side of the face, in one arm or leg, or on the entire one side of the body. A sudden decrease in or loss of consciousness altogether may also occur. A patient may lose vision in one or both eyes and have nausea or vomiting, a headache, or trouble speaking. This difficulty speaking may take the form of **dysarthria** or expressive or receptive aphasia.

Symptoms of stroke can occur alone, but patients usually have an array of symptoms. The presentation of a stroke can be either subtle or dramatic. A stroke can even occur while sleeping, and the patient does not feel any symptoms until he or she awakens. Sometimes the symptoms are incapacitating, and the patient cannot use a telephone or summon other help because of an altered mental status, aphasia, or **hemiplegia** (paralysis on one side of the body).

A very important point to differentiate here is the time the patient was last seen acting normally and the time the symptoms are discovered. If a patient is sitting with a family member and suddenly cannot speak or has acute weakness on one side of the body (or other stroke symptoms), the time of discovery of symptoms and the time last seen normal are the same. If the patient went to bed the night before and was acting normally but woke up in the morning with stroke symptoms, the time the patient was last seen acting normally was the night before. The same applies if a patient seemed normal when a family member left the house to go out but was showing symptoms of a stroke when the family member returned a few hours later. The time the patient was last seen normal is prior to the family member's leaving the house, not the time of arrival home. This is a critical distinction as the time limit for administration of tissue plasminogen activator (TPA) is based on *when the patient was last known to be normal.* Further, if a patient has suffered a stroke in the past, it is important to know the patient's baseline functioning and mental status. At the hospital, the patient will probably undergo a computed tomography (CT) scan and magnetic resonance imaging (MRI), and the physician will decide whether to administer a thrombolytic agent. Key findings include the following:

- Unilateral weakness
- Speech disturbance
- Vertigo or loss of balance
- Altered mental status

Differential Diagnosis

It is difficult to distinguish one kind of stroke from another in the field, but certain other causes of altered mental status can be quickly ruled out. A hypoglycemic episode, for example, can mimic a stroke. For this reason, blood glucose levels should be checked in any patient who exhibits altered mental status or weakness. The symptoms of traumatic brain injury may also be similar to those of a stroke. Migraine headaches or migraine equivalents, electrolyte abnormalities, CSF infections such as encephalitis and meningitis, demyelinating diseases of the nervous system such as multiple sclerosis or Guillain-Barré syndrome, and psychiatric disorders also have strokelike symptoms, but making these diagnoses will require further testing at the hospital.

Other differential diagnoses to consider include acute intoxication with alcohol or other drugs, Bell's palsy, abscess or other infection, delirium, amnesia, carotid or vertebral artery dissection, intracranial bleeding attribuff to trauma, and postictal state following a seizure.

A transient ischemic attack (TIA) mimics a stroke, but the symptoms resolve within 24 hours, with a majority resolving in 1 hour. According to the National Stroke Association, about 10% of these patients will suffer a stroke in 90 days and about half of those do so within 2 days. A TIA is a red flag that should not be ignored. However, a TIA precedes only one of every eight strokes. For most people then, a stroke occurs without warning.

Treatment

The immediate priority in the prehospital setting is to consider stroke and transport the patient to a stroke center as quickly as possible if you believe the patient is having or has had a stroke. A stroke scale will help you determine the presence of a stroke and indicate whether it warrants transport to a **stroke center designation**:

- The Cincinnati Stroke Scale compares facial droop and arm drift on each side of the body and takes into account slurred speech.
- The Los Angeles Prehospital Stroke Screen measures smile or grimace, hand grip, and arm weakness on each side of the body and also factors in historical information about age, presence of a seizure disorder, duration of symptoms, glucose measurement, and ambulation at baseline.
- The National Institutes of Health Stroke Scale is a tool for more detailed evaluation of the neurologic and neuromotor deficits in stroke patients (Table 5-4). It also allows hospital providers to follow the patient's course.
- The FAST mnemonic is a quick identification tool to recognize stroke victims. F stands for facial drooping; A, arm weakness; S, speech difficulties; and T, time. EMS training has included FAST since 1998.
- The MEND stroke assessment is being used by many states. MEND is an acronym for the Miami Emergency Neurologic Deficit exam, and is a more detailed assessment than the Cincinnati Stroke Scale.

Evaluate airway, breathing, and circulation and intervene as necessary. Check the patient's blood glucose level and correct if necessary, according to protocol. Provide supplemental oxygen if the patient's oxygen saturation dips below 94%. At the hospital, patients treated with fibrinolytic agents within 3 hours of the last time they are definitely known to be acting normally (not time found with deficit) tend to have improved neurologic

functioning and a lower mortality rate. Recent evidence suggests extending the time window for fibrinolytic treatment to 4½ hours for certain patients. Other interventions available at some centers to remove or dissolve clots include mechanical devices and directed intra-arterial fibrinolytics, which can often be done beyond the 3- to 4½-hour window for intravenous therapy. New research has shown improved outcomes with intra-arterial interventions, particularly in patients with large vessel occlusion (LVO).

Patients should be kept in a comfortable position, either a low-Fowler's or supine position with slight head elevation if an ischemic stroke is suspected. Regulate the patient's blood pressure to maintain a **mean arterial pressure (MAP)** of at least 60 mm Hg, which will allow for cerebral blood flow. Do not lower the patient's blood pressure unless after multiple readings it exceeds 220/120 mm Hg or the decision has been made (usually on hospital arrival) to treat the patient with thrombolytics. The patient's temperature should be lowered if it is higher than normal because hyperthermia accelerates ischemic brain injury. Seizure-control medications may be administered as directed by medical control or per local protocol.

Patients who are believed to be having a stroke should be transported to a stroke center. For patients with symptoms of less than 3 hours, it is usually best to go to the closest primary stroke center. Patients who have acute symptoms of longer duration or who are not eligible for peripheral fibrinolytic therapy, however, may be best served by transport to a comprehensive stroke center or hospital where additional intravascular interventions can be performed. Patients who have a severe headache or known intracerebral lesion (e.g., tumor, arteriovenous malformation, or aneurysm) should be transported to a hospital with neurosurgical capabilities in the event the stroke is found to be hemorrhagic and the patient requires emergency surgery.

Carotid Artery Dissection

The internal carotid arteries supply the brain with oxygenated blood. Carotid artery dissection begins with a tear in the innermost layer of the artery. Circulating blood enters the tear, quickly dissecting (separating) the innermost and middle layers. This mechanical process compresses the lumen (the hollow interior space) of the artery so that blood can no longer circulate through it, triggering an ischemic stroke.

Carotid artery dissection is an unusual cause of ischemic stroke (see **Figure 5-6**, B). This kind of stroke can occur in any age group but tends to appear most often in people younger than age 50. Carotid artery dissection represents about a quarter of all strokes that occur in teens and young adults, often striking while they are engaged in physical activity. Men and women are roughly equally affected.

Pathophysiology

The initial tear in the inner layer of the artery wall may be attributable to traumatic injury, connective tissue disease, hypertension, atherosclerosis, or some other pathologic process. In addition, the weakened outer layer of the diseased or damaged artery can

Table 5-4 National Institutes of Health Stroke Scale

Instructions	Scale Definition
1a. Level of Consciousness: The investigator must choose a response if a full evaluation is prevented by such obstacles as an endotracheal tube, language barrier, orotracheal trauma/bandages.	**0 = Alert;** keenly responsive **1 = Not alert but arousable** by minor stimulation **2 = Not alert;** requires repeated stimulation to attend **3 = Responds** only with reflex motor or autonomic effects or totally unresponsive, flaccid, and areflexic
1b. LOC Questions: The patient is asked the month and his/her age. The answer must be correct—there is no partial credit for being close.	**0 = Answers** both questions correctly **1 = Answers** one question correctly **2 = Answers** neither question correctly
1c. LOC Commands: The patient is asked to open and close the eyes and then to grip and release the nonparetic hand. Substitute another one-step command if the hands cannot be used.	**0 = Performs** both tasks correctly **1 = Performs** one task correctly **2 = Performs** neither task correctly
2. Best Gaze: Only horizontal eye movements will be tested. Voluntary or reflexive (oculocephalic) eye movements will be scored, but caloric testing is not done.	**0 = Normal** **1 = Partial gaze palsy;** gaze abnormal in one or both eyes **2 = Forced deviation,** or total gaze paresis not overcome by the oculocephalic maneuver
3. Visual: Visual fields (upper and lower quadrants) are tested by confrontation, using finger counting or visual threat, as appropriate.	**0 = No visual loss** **1 = Partial hemianopia** **2 = Complete hemianopia** **3 = Bilateral hemianopia (blind)**
4. Facial Palsy: Ask—or use pantomime to encourage—the patient to show teeth or raise eyebrows and close eyes.	**0 = Normal** symmetrical movements **1 = Minor paralysis** (asymmetry on smiling) **2 = Partial paralysis** (total or near-total paralysis of lower face) **3 = Complete paralysis** of one or both sides
5. Motor Arm: The limb is placed in the appropriate position: extend the arms (palms down) 90 degrees (if sitting) or 45 degrees (if supine). Drift is scored if the arm falls before 10 seconds. **5a.** Left arm **5b.** Right arm	**0 = No drift;** limb holds position for 10 seconds **1 = Drift;** limb holds position but drifts down before full 10 seconds **2 = Some effort against gravity;** limb cannot get to or maintain position, drifts down to bed, some effort against gravity **3 = No effort against gravity;** limb falls **4 = No movement** **UN = Amputation** or joint fusion
6. Motor Leg: The limb is placed in the appropriate position: hold the leg at 30 degrees (always tested supine). Drift is scored if the leg falls before 5 seconds. **6a.** Left leg **6b.** Right leg	**0 = No drift;** leg holds position for full 5 seconds **1 = Drift;** leg falls by the end of the 5-second period but does not hit bed **2 = Some effort against gravity;** leg falls to bed; by 5 seconds, has some effort against gravity **3 = No effort against gravity;** leg falls to bed immediately **4 = No movement** **UN = Amputation** or joint fusion

(continues)

Table 5-4 National Institutes of Health Stroke Scale (*continued*)

Instructions	Scale Definition
7. Limb Ataxia: The finger-nose-finger and heel-shin tests are performed on both sides with eyes open.	**0 = Absent** **1 = Present in one limb** **2 = Present in two limbs** **UN = Amputation** or joint fusion
8. Sensory: Sensation or grimace to pinprick when tested, or withdrawal from noxious stimulus in the obtunded or aphasic patient.	**0 = Normal;** no sensory loss **1 = Mild to moderate sensory loss;** feels pinprick is less sharp or is dull on the affected side; or there is a loss of superficial pain with pinprick, but aware of being touched. **2 = Severe to total sensory loss;** patient is not aware of being touched in the face, arm, and leg.
9. Best Language: Patient is asked to describe what is happening in an attached picture, to name the items on an attached naming sheet, and to read from an attached list of sentences. Comprehension is judged from responses here, as well as to all of the commands in the preceding general neurologic exam.	**0 = No aphasia;** normal **1 = Mild to moderate aphasia;** some obvious loss of fluency or facility of comprehension, without significant limitation on ideas **2 = Severe aphasia;** all communication is through fragmentary expression; great need for inference, questioning, and guessing by the listener. **3 = Mute, global aphasia;** no usable speech or auditory comprehension
10. Dysarthria: An adequate sample of speech must be obtained by asking patient to read or repeat words from a list.	**0 = Normal** **1 = Mild to moderate dysarthria;** patient slurs some words; can be understood with some difficulty. **2 = Severe dysarthria;** patient's speech is so slurred as to be unintelligible; or is mute/anarthric. **UN = Intubated** or other physical barrier
11. Extinction and Inattention (Formerly Neglect): Sufficient information to identify neglect may be obtained during prior testing. If the patient has a severe visual loss preventing visual double simultaneous stimulation, and the cutaneous stimuli are normal, the score is normal.	**0 = No abnormality** **1 = Visual, tactile, auditory, spatial, or personal inattention** or extinction to bilateral simultaneous stimulation in one of the sensory modalities **2 = Profound hemi-inattention or extinction to more than one modality;** does not recognize own hand or orients to only one side of space

Administer stroke scale items in the order listed. Record performance in each category after each subscale exam. Do not go back and change scores. Follow directions provided for each exam technique. Scores should reflect what the patient does, not what the clinician thinks the patient can do. The clinician should record answers while administering the exam and work quickly. Except where indicated, the patient should not be coached (i.e., repeated requests to patient to make a special effort).

Modified from National Institute of Neurological Disorders and Stroke at the National Institutes of Health: *NIH stroke scale.* 2003. www.ninds.nih.gov

begin to bulge, forming an aneurysm that may cause stenosis (narrowing) of the artery. In rare cases, the artery ruptures. A carotid aneurysm and a carotid dissection, however, are considered to be distinct pathologic processes.

The dissection of the internal carotid artery can occur inside or outside the skull. Extracranial dissection occurs most frequently because the skull tends to absorb the force of any traumatic impact. Sophisticated imaging studies are often required to make this diagnosis, since the signs and symptoms of the condition are ambiguous.

Signs and Symptoms

Patients with carotid artery dissection may complain of unilateral headache, neck, or facial pain, and they may report a recent traumatic injury. You may note a Horner syndrome on the affected side, characterized by ptosis (drooping) of the eyelid, miosis (a constricted pupil), and facial anhidrosis (a lack of perspiration). The syndrome is usually the result of unilateral sympathetic nerve compression due to tumor, trauma, or vascular disorders.

The patient may present after physical activity or after an event that is normally innocuous, such as coughing or sneezing. Pain, usually in the head, back, or face, is often the initial symptom of a spontaneous, nontraumatic dissection. The headache is described as constant, severe, and unilateral. Transient vision loss may occur, and the patient may report a decreased sensation of taste. Physical findings may include hemiparesis, massive nosebleed, neck hematoma, cervical spine trauma, cervical bruit, or cranial nerve palsy. Key findings include the following:

- Unilateral pain in head or neck
- Vision changes
- Pupil constriction, especially unilaterally

Differential Diagnosis

The differential diagnosis for a carotid artery dissection includes neck trauma, other causes of stroke (either hemorrhagic or ischemic), subarachnoid hemorrhage, intoxication or toxicity, TIA, electrolyte abnormality, headache, cervical spine fracture, near-hanging injury, vertebral artery dissection, and retinal artery or vein occlusion.

Treatment

If trauma preceded the dissection, immobilize the patient's spine. Provide supportive care and monitor airway, breathing, and circulation. At the emergency department, blood pressure should be regulated, and the physician may choose anticoagulation or surgical/neuroradiologic intervention on the basis of an MRI or angiographic findings.

The patient should be transported to a hospital that has neurologic and vascular capabilities and is able to perform interventional radiologic procedures.

Intracerebral Hemorrhage

The term *intracerebral hemorrhage* is used interchangeably with *hemorrhagic stroke* (see Figure 5-6, A). In a hemorrhagic stroke, small arteries rupture and bleed directly into the tissues of the brain. Intracerebral hemorrhage accounts for 10% to 15% of all strokes and carries a higher likelihood of mortality than

ischemic stroke. Mortality during the first month after this kind of stroke ranges from 40% to 80%. About half of all deaths, however, occur within 48 hours of presentation. Only 20% of patients with intracranial hemorrhage regain full functional independence.

Certain conditions place people at higher risk of intracerebral hemorrhage: anticoagulation, hypertension, atherosclerosis, and use of cocaine or amphetamines.

Pathophysiology

The stage is set for intracranial hemorrhage when small intracerebral arteries—that is, arteries within the brain rather than on its surface—are damaged by disease processes such as hypertension and atherosclerosis. In patients who have had a previous stroke, the vascular tissue may be weaker and more friable and bleed more readily. Smoking may also weaken blood vessels. In fact, smokers with a systolic blood pressure greater than 150 mm Hg are nine times more likely to suffer a hemorrhagic stroke than nonsmokers.

Bleeding most often occurs in the thalamus, putamen, cerebellum, or brainstem. Brain tissue beyond the immediate area of the bleeding may be damaged by pressure produced by the mass effect of the hemorrhage itself. This mass effect increases intracranial pressure, which may cause symptoms such as nausea, vomiting, altered mental status, coma, respiratory depression, and/or death.

Signs and Symptoms

A patient with intracerebral hemorrhage is likely to have an altered mental status. Frequent complaints include headache, nausea, and vomiting. The patient may have a seizure, with or without marked hypertension. However, in the prehospital setting, it is very difficult to distinguish between intracranial bleeding and an ischemic stroke. That determination will have to be made on arrival at the emergency department by obtaining a CT scan of the brain. Key findings include the following:

- Alteration in vital signs (hypertension, pulse, and respiration changes)
- Altered LOC
- Stiff neck or headache
- Focal neurologic deficit (weakness, gaze preference)
- Difficulty with gait, fine motor control
- Nausea, vomiting
- Dizziness or vertigo
- Abnormal eye movements

Differential Diagnosis

The differential diagnosis of a hemorrhagic stroke includes ischemic stroke, migraine headache, tumor, and metabolic abnormalities. Vomiting may be gastrointestinal in origin, but it may also suggest increased intracranial pressure, as occurs with an intracerebral hemorrhage. A TIA may also mimic the presentation of intracranial bleeding.

Treatment

The most important thing to do when hemorrhagic stroke is suspected is transport the patient as quickly as possible. Recognize the signs and symptoms of stroke, and be able to take control of any difficulties that arise with airway, breathing, or circulation. Patients who do not have a patent airway or who have signs of respiratory dysfunction, including apnea, require intervention. Protocol may mandate that you use a stroke scale or ask specific questions about anticoagulation and bleeding problems. Treating life-threatening problems should take precedence over gathering information.

Many patients who have intracerebral bleeding also have hypertension. In general, blood pressure will not be treated in the field unless otherwise ordered by protocol or by medical control. However, you should minimize stimuli that could further increase the patient's intracranial pressure. Monitor the patient, establish IV access, and check the blood glucose level because hypoglycemia may mimic stroke symptoms and has been associated with poor outcomes in stroke patients.

Patients with intracranial bleeding may have ECG changes or seizures. The receiving hospital will perform an immediate CT scan on the patient. Other possible imaging includes CT angiography, CT perfusion, and MRI (including MR angiography and venography). Patients who are on anticoagulants or are hypocoagulable from other causes may be treated by a number of different modalities. Vitamin K, fresh-frozen plasma, or recombinant factor VIIa may be administered in an attempt to limit bleeding. Blood pressure may be tightly controlled for the same reason. Emergent neurosurgical consultation may be necessary.

Patients believed to have had a hemorrhagic stroke should be brought to a stroke center that has neurosurgical capabilities.

Subarachnoid Hemorrhage

Subarachnoid hemorrhage occurs when arteries on the brain's surface bleed into the subarachnoid space, the area between the pia mater and the arachnoid. The blood often seeps into the ventricles, causing irritation. The volume of blood may also cause a mass shift. This kind of bleeding can be triggered by trauma such as a car accident, but more often occurs when a cerebral aneurysm or arteriovenous malformation ruptures (see Figure 5-6, A).

Pathophysiology

A cerebral aneurysm is a pouch that develops in the weakened wall of a diseased or damaged vessel. An arteriovenous malformation is a genetic developmental defect of the vascular system in which certain arteries connect directly to veins rather than to a capillary bed, creating a tangle of vessels that can rupture. However, any part of the brain that has a tumor, thrombosis, or an abnormal blood vessel malformation may bleed. Uncontrolled hypertension and congenital aneurysms can be predisposing factors. Patients who have certain systemic diseases, such as Ehlers-Danlos syndrome, Marfan syndrome, aortic anomalies, or polycystic kidney disease, may also be at increased risk of subarachnoid hemorrhage. Patients with vessel-wall deficits due to age, hypertension, smoking, or atherosclerosis are also at risk.

Signs and Symptoms

Subarachnoid hemorrhage should be suspected in any patient who describes a sudden, severe headache that came on like a thunderclap. Loss of consciousness may have occurred. About half of patients who present with subarachnoid bleeding have elevated blood pressure. Middle cerebral artery bleeding may cause seizures, motor deficits, nausea and vomiting, neck stiffness, back pain, photophobia, and visual changes.

About 30% to 50% of patients have a sentinel hemorrhage, a small amount of bleeding into the subarachnoid space. The headache often has the same characteristics as that of a larger subarachnoid hemorrhage, particularly a sudden onset and pain perceived as worse than usual, but may improve fairly quickly and there may be no evident neurological deficits or symptoms. It is critical to recognize these initial small amounts of bleeding as an anticipatory sign of a subsequent, often catastrophic larger hemorrhage. There are five grades of hemorrhage.

- *Grade 1*. Mild headache, with or without meningeal irritation
- *Grade 2*. Severe headache and nonfocal examination, with or without pupillary change
- *Grade 3*. Mild alteration in neurologic examination
- *Grade 4*. Depressed level of consciousness or focal deficit
- *Grade 5*. Comatose, with or without posturing

Key findings include the following:

- Sudden onset of severe headache
- Weakness (focal) or neglect
- Altered mental status
- Nausea/vomiting
- Vision changes/nystagmus
- Neck stiffness with associated headache

Differential Diagnosis

The differential diagnosis of subarachnoid hemorrhage includes any pathologic occurrence that could lead to headache, nausea and vomiting, loss of consciousness, and altered mental status, including stroke, migraine headache, tumor, infection, medication use, overdose, and trauma.

Treatment

During prehospital treatment, support of the patient's airway, breathing, and circulation is of utmost importance. If at all possible, do not sedate the patient en route. Obtain IV access and prepare to secure the airway if the patient exhibits an acute change in mental status or consciousness. Blood pressure control is usually not recommended in the field, but any stimuli that might increase the patient's intracranial pressure should be minimized.

At the hospital, a CT scan will be performed, and perhaps an MRI or cerebral angiogram will be done to locate the source of the bleeding. A patient with no obvious bleeding on initial imaging studies may receive a lumbar puncture to look for blood in the CSF or for changes consistent with blood being degraded in the CSF (xanthochromia), which is usually seen 12 hours after the onset of bleeding.

Appropriate triage and transport of the patient to a hospital that has CT scanning and neurosurgical support capabilities are critical.

Subdural Hematoma

A subdural hematoma is a collection of blood between the dura mater and arachnoid membrane. The hematoma may be acute, subacute, or chronic. The acute period is measured from the time of the injury to the third day. The subacute period lasts from day 3 to about 2 weeks after the injury, and the chronic phase begins 2 to 3 weeks after the injury. Subdural hemorrhage has a mortality rate of about 20% and usually occurs in patients older than age 60.

Pathophysiology

Subdural hemorrhage is usually caused by a tearing of the bridging veins that communicate between the cerebral cortex and the venous sinuses. This is usually precipitated by direct trauma or acute deceleration. The blood then clots in the subdural space. In the subacute phase of a subdural bleed, the clotted blood may liquefy and thin out. In the chronic phase, the blood has disintegrated, and serous fluid remains in the subdural space.

The phenomenon of coup–contrecoup injury can lead to subdural hematoma. The coup, or blow, causes trauma to the brain directly under the area of the skull that absorbs the direct force of impact. After the impact, the brain recoils within the closed container of the skull and is injured on its opposite side (contrecoup) when it rebounds against the cranium. This may cause bleeding or neurologic damage on both sides of the brain and generate separate but distinct findings on physical exam and imaging studies of the brain.

The elderly may have a smaller brain volume as a result of the aging process and be at greater risk for tearing of the bridging veins between the skull and brain during any type of traumatic or deceleration injury leading to subdural bleeding, and because there is increased empty intracranial space the hemorrhage may also be less symptomatic.

Signs and Symptoms

After blunt head trauma, the patient may present with a subdural hematoma, often accompanied by loss of consciousness or amnesia for the event. The patient may either be asymptomatic or have personality changes, signs of increased intracranial pressure (headache, visual changes, nausea, or vomiting), hemiparesis, or hemiplegia. Patients with bleeding abnormalities, such as hemophilia, and patients taking anticoagulant medications may develop a subdural hematoma after only minor trauma, as can alcoholics and older adults. Key findings include the following:

- Headache
- Loss of or alteration in LOC
- Focal or general weakness
- History or signs of trauma

Differential Diagnosis

The differential for subdural hematoma is the same as that for any other intracranial hemorrhage, infections such as meningitis, or ischemic stroke. Intracranial neoplasm may also have a similar presentation.

Treatment

Evaluate the patient in the prehospital setting to assess for a change in mental status. Focal neurologic deficits can be a sign of subdural hematoma. Check the patient's blood glucose level, and correct it if necessary. If the patient has an altered LOC or airway compromise, take corrective action. If external trauma is evident, alert the physician to the possibility of associated injury and use proper procedures to protect the cervical spine. Because of the potential for a worsening mental status, watch carefully for any signs of increasing confusion or airway compromise.

The patient should be transported to a trauma center or, if that's not possible, taken to a hospital where neurosurgical backup is available.

Epidural Hematoma

An epidural hematoma is an accumulation of blood between the inner table of the skull and the dura mater, the outermost of the meninges. This condition is usually caused by trauma to the arteries in the epidural space, and thus leads to high pressure mass effect. Frequently there is an associated skull fracture, usually in the area of the middle meningeal artery on the temporal aspect of the skull. Prompt surgical decompression is necessary for patients with significant neurologic dysfunction. The likelihood of recovery is directly related to the patient's preoperative neurologic condition.

Pathophysiology

About 80% of epidural hematomas are located in the temporoparietal region over the middle meningeal artery or its branches. The condition is usually precipitated by direct trauma to the head. Epidural hematomas in the frontal and occipital regions account for about 10% of epidural hematomas. Most of the time, the bleeding is arterial, but in a third of patients, it's the result of venous injury. Venous bleeding occurs almost exclusively with depressed skull fractures, and the resulting hematoma tends to be smaller and more benign.

The pressure associated with arterial epidural bleeding can result in a midline shift and herniation of the brain. Compression of the third cranial nerve can cause contralateral hemiparesis and ipsilateral pupil dilation. Although epidural hematomas usually attain their maximum size rapidly, in about 10% of patients, the size of the hematoma increases during the first 24 hours after injury.

Signs and Symptoms

The patient may or may not lose consciousness after the trauma, or may lose consciousness and then awaken (the so-called lucid interval) for a period of time until again becoming obtunded or unresponsive. During the lucid interval, the patient may feel fine and be acting appropriately and wish to refuse treatment. Special care must be taken to explain that this period may precede the onset of symptoms. The patient may decompensate after refusal.

The patient may complain of severe headache and have vomiting or seizures. Increased ICP may cause **Cushing's triad**: systolic hypertension, bradycardia, and irregular respiratory pattern; this patient will be unresponsive, and this reaction indicates death is imminent.

A pupil that is dilated, fixed, or slow to respond on the same side of the injury may indicate herniation due to increased ICP. The classic symptoms of an increasing herniation are coma, fixed and dilated pupil, and decerebrate posturing. Key findings include the following:

- Trauma
- Altered mental status
- Nausea/vomiting
- Dizziness/generalized weakness
- Altered LOC
- Unilateral dilated pupil
- Cushing's triad

Differential Diagnosis

The differential diagnosis of an epidural hematoma includes other types of intracranial hemorrhage, diffuse axonal injury, and concussion.

Treatment

In all patients with suspected epidural hematoma, start an IV line, administer oxygen, and place the patient on a cardiac monitor. Do not administer fluids unless the patient's blood pressure is low, and then only in small boluses. Maintain the oxygen saturation above 94%, and recheck the vital signs frequently. Take precautions to protect the cervical spine as indicated. If the patient has a decrease in LOC, secure the airway and take steps to ensure hemodynamic stability.

Some studies of head-injured patients have associated increased mortality with prehospital intubation, and this has become a topic of intense debate within the EMS community. The best current recommendation is for advanced providers to maintain a high level of proficiency at advanced airway intervention through continued training and quality assurance procedures. Effective bag-mask ventilation is a skill that all providers must maintain, and it may be an option for difficult airways in lieu of endotracheal intubation.

In the ED, the patient will be evaluated according to trauma protocol, and a CT scan is usually performed. Further management includes neurosurgical consultation and control of ICP. Dilantin or another anticonvulsant may be given to reduce the incidence of early seizures but will not prevent development of a seizure disorder in the future.

Patients with suspected epidural hematoma should be brought to a trauma center with neurosurgical capability.

Tumors

A brain tumor, or intracranial neoplasm, is the inappropriate proliferation of cells forming a mass that invades and compresses the surrounding healthy parenchymal tissue. Tumors are classified as either primary or metastatic and benign or malignant. *Primary* means the tumor originates in the brain. A metastatic tumor arises when cells migrate from a tumor elsewhere in the body, such as cutaneous melanoma or lung cancer, travel through the bloodstream, and begin to grow in the brain. Primary malignant lesions account for about half of all intracranial tumors and tend to be aggressive, invasive, and life threatening. Primary benign tumors tend to grow more slowly and are less aggressive, but they can still be life threatening if they arise in vital areas such as the brainstem.

Tumors are often classified by cell type, such as meningioma or glioma, but prehospital treatment is the same regardless of cell type.

Pathophysiology

Brain tumors may damage neural pathways by mass effect or infiltration of normal brain tissue. Tumors that arise near the third and fourth ventricles may obstruct the flow of CSF, causing hydrocephalus. Blood vessels that form to support the tumors may disrupt the blood–brain barrier and cause edema or may rupture, leading to hemorrhage.

Signs and Symptoms

The signs and symptoms of a brain tumor are nonspecific. The patient may have headache, altered mental status, nausea, vomiting, weakness, alterations in gait, or even subtle behavioral changes. Focal seizure, visual changes, speech deficit, and sensory abnormalities are also possible. The patient may not notice symptoms, even as the tumor grows rather large, but often seeks treatment when an acute change in symptoms occurs. Such a change is often precipitated by an obstruction of CSF flow or hemorrhage.

Tumors in the frontal lobe may cause behavioral disinhibition, memory loss, decreased alertness, or a diminished sense of smell. Tumors in the temporal lobe may lead to emotional changes and behavioral disturbances. Pituitary tumors may cause visual changes, impotence, or changes in the menstrual cycle. Tumors in the occipital lobe may produce visual field deficits. Brainstem or cerebellar tumors can cause cranial nerve palsies, reduced coordination, nystagmus, and sensory deficits on either side of the body. Key findings include the following:

- Focal weakness
- Visual changes
- Dizziness/vertigo
- Nausea/vomiting

Differential Diagnosis

The differential diagnosis for brain tumor includes infection, stroke, and intracranial bleeding.

Treatment

Provide supportive care on the basis of the patient's symptoms. Edema, hydrocephalus, intracranial hemorrhage, pituitary infarction, infarction of the parenchyma (usually caused by compression of blood vessels), and seizures can cause the patient to deteriorate abruptly. Be prepared to intervene in the event the patient's LOC suddenly diminishes or a seizure occurs.

Patients with suspected brain tumor should be brought to a hospital that has oncology and neurosurgical backup.

Idiopathic Intracranial Hypertension

Idiopathic intracranial hypertension used to be known as "pseudotumor cerebri," or "false tumor," because its symptoms mimic those of a brain tumor. The condition is characterized by the poor resorption of cerebrospinal fluid (CSF) from the subarachnoid space. Idiopathic intracranial hypertension predominantly affects obese women in their childbearing years. Papilledema, or the swelling of the optic nerve, is the most worrisome problem and is due to chronically elevated intracranial pressure. Papilledema leads to progressive optic nerve atrophy and blindness.

Pathophysiology

The cause of idiopathic intracranial hypertension, as its name suggests, remains elusive. Some studies have found a decreased outflow of CSF into the dural venous sinus. Others suggest that increased blood flow impedes the brain's ability to drain CSF.

Signs and Symptoms

Elevated intracranial pressure may lead the patient to seek medical attention for headaches that are nonspecific and tend to vary in type, location, and frequency. Pulsatile ringing in the ears and horizontal diplopia (double vision) are other symptoms. Uncommonly, the patient may have pain that radiates into the arms. Affected individuals may have orthostatic hypotension after bending over and standing up again, causing episodes of syncope. Papilledema may lead to intermittent dimming or blacking out of

the vision in one or both eyes. The patient may have progressive loss of peripheral vision, usually starting in the nasal lower quadrant and then moving to the central visual field, followed by loss of color vision. Key findings include the following:

- Headache
- Vision disturbance and papilledema
- Younger, obese female patients

Differential Diagnosis

The differential diagnosis for idiopathic intracranial hypertension includes aseptic meningitis, Lyme disease, vascular tumors such as meningioma, arteriovenous malformation, stroke, hydrocephalus, intracranial abscess, intracranial bleeding, migraine headache, and lupus.

Treatment

Little can be done for the patient in the prehospital arena. Prehospital care is typically supportive only. The patient should be transported to an institution that offers ophthalmologic, neurologic, and neurosurgical specialty care.

At the hospital, visual acuity testing, direct ophthalmologic examination, lumbar puncture, and imaging studies may be required. Blood and CSF must be examined to rule out differential diagnoses. The patient may be placed on medication and may require drainage of CSF by lumbar puncture or surgical care, including placement or adjustment of an intracranial shunt.

Brain Abscess

A brain abscess is an infection that begins when an organism from a site beyond the CNS penetrates the blood–brain barrier to enter the brain. Initially, inflammation occurs, turning into a collection of pus around which a well-vascularized capsule usually forms.

Pathophysiology

Certain bacteria (*Streptococcus*, *Pseudomonas*, *Bacteroides*) typically enter from the sinuses, mouth, middle ear, or mastoid (area located behind the ear) through veins that drain directly into the brain from these sites. Other bacteria (*Staphylococcus*, *Streptococcus*, *Klebsiella*, *Escherichia*, *Pseudomonas*) usually spread via the blood vessels from distant sites. Direct spread from penetrating trauma or surgical procedures may also be a source of bacterial infection (*Staphylococcus*, *Clostridium*, *Pseudomonas*) in the brain. About a fourth of abscesses have no clear source. Patients who have compromised immune systems, use IV drugs, have prosthetic valves, or are chronic steroid users, as well as near-drowning patients and patients who have extensive dental procedures, are at risk for brain abscesses caused by the spread of bacteria.

Signs and Symptoms

A patient who has a brain abscess most often complains of a headache. A focal neurologic deficit consistent with the site of infection may be present. The triad of headache, fever, and focal neurologic deficit is seldom seen. Seizures, altered mental status, nausea or vomiting, and stiff neck may also indicate a brain abscess. A sudden worsening of the headache may indicate rupture of the abscess into the CSF. Patients who are immunocompromised, either due to medication or underlying illness such as AIDS, are at particular risk of having a brain abscess. Key findings include the following:

- Fever
- Altered mental status, such as confusion or diminished LOC
- Neck stiffness/meningismus
- Headache
- Nausea/vomiting
- Focal deficit consistent with the location of the abscess

Differential Diagnosis

Beyond the wide range of bacterial infections that must be considered, the differential diagnosis for a brain abscess includes headache, hypertension, intracranial bleeding, fungal infection, and tumor.

Treatment

Brain abscesses are life threatening. With early recognition and intervention, however, morbidity and mortality have declined. Provide supportive care for the patient. Monitor the patient's airway, breathing, and circulation, administer oxygen, and give IV fluids. If the patient has a seizure or decompensates, be prepared to provide the appropriate interventions. Although these patients are at risk of dying as a result of the mass effect of the abscess, its interference with brain function, and sepsis, this rarely happens acutely. Nevertheless, the abscess may rupture or cause bleeding in the brain, and the patient's condition may quickly deteriorate.

A patient suspected of having a brain abscess should be transported to an institution where neurosurgical services and a neurologic intensive care unit are available. At the hospital, laboratory and radiologic studies and possibly a lumbar puncture or brain biopsy will be performed, and antibiotics will be administered.

Encephalitis

Encephalitis is a general inflammation of the brain that causes focal or diffuse brain dysfunction. This disorder has signs and symptoms similar to those of meningitis, including lethargy and headache. The key distinguishing feature is that encephalitis usually causes some alteration of brain function—disorientation, behavior change, motor or sensory deficits—whereas meningitis does not. However, keep in mind patients may have both conditions at once.

Pathophysiology

Encephalitis is most often a viral infection that damages brain parenchyma. A virus can enter the body by many different vectors. Some viruses are transmitted by humans, some are mosquito or tick borne, and some are transmitted by animal bites. A common culprit is herpes simplex virus type 1, known more commonly for causing cold sores. Patients with compromised immune systems are more likely to contract certain viruses, such as cytomegalovirus and varicella zoster. This latter virus, also known as "herpes zoster," lies dormant in sensory nerve ganglia after initial infection (chickenpox) and is reactivated under circumstances that are still obscure, causing shingles. Rabies must be considered if there was potential exposure such as an animal bite or contact with a bat. Geography plays a role as well, with persons in North America at risk for St. Louis encephalitis and those in Asia for Japanese encephalitis.

Usually the virus replicates outside the CNS and enters through the bloodstream or a neural pathway. Once the virus has crossed over into the brain and entered the neural cells, the cells begin to malfunction. Hemorrhage, inflammation, and perivascular congestion all occur more frequently in the gray matter.

Postinfectious encephalitis is an immune-related disorder in which the body's immune response attacks brain tissue after a viral infection. This is difficult to distinguish clinically from acute viral infection at the time of initial presentation.

Signs and Symptoms

The course of encephalitis varies widely among patients. The acuity and severity of presentation usually correlate with the prognosis. Generally the patient reports a history of having a virus consistent with the common cold or flu as an early symptom. It might include fever, headache, nausea and vomiting, myalgia, or lethargy. The patient may also have behavioral or personality changes, decreased alertness or altered mental status, a stiff neck, photophobia, lethargy, generalized or focal seizures, confusion or amnesia, or flaccid paralysis. In the case of encephalitis associated with one of the viruses that causes chickenpox, measles, mumps, cold sores or Epstein-Barr, the patient may have a rash, lymphadenopathy, or glandular enlargement. Because of the effect of the infection on the CNS, the patient may be agitated or violent. Remember that any patient with psychiatric symptoms may have an underlying medical problem. Infant patients may have skin, eye, or mouth lesions, a rash, decreased alertness, increased irritability, seizures, poor feeding, and shocklike symptoms. Human immunodeficiency virus (HIV) infection may predispose patients to encephalopathy secondary to toxoplasmosis infection. Key findings include the following:

- Fever
- Altered mental status, such as confusion or diminished LOC
- Headache

Differential Diagnosis

The differential diagnosis for encephalitis includes bacterial, viral, fungal, and protozoal infections, reactive autoimmune disease, and noninfectious illnesses and conditions that can cause encephalopathy such as renal failure, liver failure, chronic autoimmune diseases, seizures, cerebral hemorrhage/edema, electrolyte abnormalities, intoxication, stroke, syphilis, trauma, and brain abscess.

Treatment

The mortality rate for encephalitis is up to 75%, and those fortunate enough to survive often have long-term motor or mental disabilities. In the case of rabies encephalitis, the mortality is thought to be 100%.

Patients with encephalitis may decompensate quickly, so be ready to take control of the airway and provide resuscitative support of blood pressure. Patients who have a seizure or are in status epilepticus should be treated according to protocol. Antiviral medications will usually be given in the ED early in the course of treatment. Signs of hydrocephalus and increased intracranial pressure will usually be treated conservatively at first and then with more aggressive methods including diuresis, mannitol, and corticosteroids and placement of an external ventricular drain.

If you suspect a patient has encephalitis, protect yourself by wearing a mask, gown, and gloves to prevent airborne transmission of particles. As with any patient who may have an infectious disease, the prehospital provider should practice strict blood and body fluid isolation precautions and should wear a mask at all times. For additional safety, a mask should also be placed on the patient.

The patient should be transported to a facility that has intensive care, a neurologist, and neurosurgery backup (in case a brain biopsy has to be performed). An infectious disease specialist, if available, may be of assistance. Pediatric patients should be transported to a pediatric facility with intensive care capabilities. In the hospital, the patient will undergo a series of blood tests, radiologic and other imaging studies, and CSF studies, including viral serologies. A brain biopsy may be performed.

Meningitis

Meningitis is an inflammation of the meninges, the membranes that surround the brain and spinal cord. By extension, the CSF will also show signs of infection and inflammation. Meningitis has many different infectious and noninfectious causes, but life-threatening acute meningitis is frequently a bacterial infection.

Pathophysiology

Bacterial meningitis usually occurs when bacteria migrate from the bloodstream to the CSF. If there is not an obvious source of infection, invasion of the CSF is usually presumed to have been caused by the bacteria that colonize the nasopharynx. In some cases, bacteria may spread from contiguous structures (e.g., sinuses, nasopharynx) that are infected or have been disrupted by trauma or surgical instrumentation.

Once in the CSF, the lack of antibodies and white blood cells allows bacteria to proliferate. The presence of bacterial components in the CSF makes the blood–brain barrier more permeable and allows toxins to enter. As the bacteria multiply, inflammatory cells respond, changing the cell count, pH, lactate, protein, and glucose composition of the CSF. Intracranial pressure may rise as inflammation develops, causing occlusion of CSF outflow.

At a certain point, pressure in and around the brain reverses the flow of CSF. This development is associated with further deterioration of mental status. Ongoing damage to the brain triggers vasospasm, thrombosis, and septic shock, and the patient usually dies from diffuse ischemic injury.

Meningitis in neonates and infants is usually caused by group B streptococcus or *Escherichia coli*. In children beyond the first year, *Streptococcus pneumoniae* and *Neisseria meningitidis* become increasingly common; these bacteria are the most common in adult meningitis as well. *Haemophilus influenzae* type B, once the most prevalent cause in children, is rarely seen since the advent of immunization for this organism, but there are some cases caused by different *Haemophilus* subtypes in children and adults. Other causative bacteria in adults include *Listeria monocytogenes* (particularly in the elderly), *Staphylococcus aureus*, various other streptococci, and gram-negative species. A different spectrum of bacteria are seen in meningitis after neurosurgical procedures; these include various staphylococci, streptococci, and gram-negative rods, including *Pseudomonas* and *Aeromonas*.

Signs and Symptoms

Patients with acute bacterial meningitis may decompensate quickly and require emergency care and antibiotics. The classic symptoms of meningitis include headache, nuchal rigidity (resistance to flexing/extending the neck), fever and chills, and photophobia. The infection can also cause seizures, altered mental status, confusion, coma, and death. The condition is usually precipitated by an upper respiratory illness.

Nearly a fourth of patients with bacterial meningitis present acutely within 24 hours of the onset of symptoms. Most patients with viral meningitis have symptoms that develop slowly over the course of a week. Patients who have a fever and headache should be examined for nuchal rigidity or discomfort with flexion of the neck, Kernig's sign (positive when the leg is flexed at the hip and knee, and subsequent extension of the knee is painful, leading to resistance and flexion of the torso), and Brudzinski's sign (involuntary flexing of the legs in response to flexing of the neck; **Figure 5-8**).

Altered mental status is often seen and can range from irritability or confusion to coma. Because of the effect of the infection on the CNS, the patient may be agitated or violent. Remember that any patient with psychiatric symptoms may have an underlying medical problem. In infants, the patient may present with

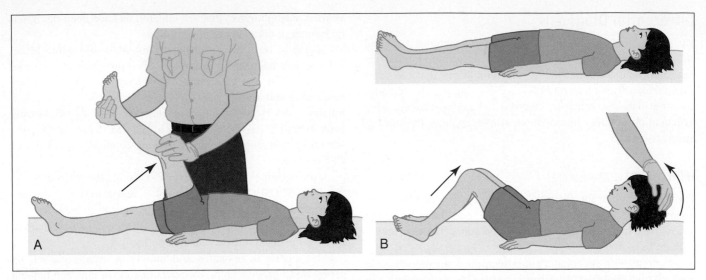

Figure 5-8 A. Kernig's sign. Meningeal irritation results in the inability to straighten the leg with the hips flexed. **B.** Brudzinski's sign. Meningeal irritation results in an involuntary flexion of the knees when the head is flexed toward the chest.

a bulging fontanelle, decreased tone, and paradoxical irritability (calm when left alone, crying when held). Meningitis should be considered in older adults and in young children, especially those with diabetes, renal insufficiency, or cystic fibrosis. Patients with immune system suppression, those who live in crowded conditions (e.g., military recruits, inmates at correctional facilities, and college dorm residents), splenectomy patients, patients with alcoholism or other cirrhotic liver disease, patients receiving chemotherapy, patients who use IV drugs, and patients who have been exposed to others with meningitis are all at high risk of contracting this illness.

If you suspect the patient has meningitis, you should protect yourself, using droplet precautions including a mask, gown, and gloves to prevent airborne transmission of particles. Potential exposures of crew to patients should be reported immediately to a supervisor or the occupational health department. Prophylactic antibiotics are needed if there is a high likelihood a provider has been exposed to bacterial meningitis due to meningococcus (*N. meningitidis*); prophylaxis for meningitis due to other organisms is not indicated. Key findings include the following:

- Fever
- Altered mental status, especially confusion or diminished LOC
- Meningismus (a triad of nuchal rigidity, photophobia, and headache)

Differential Diagnosis

The differential diagnosis for meningitis includes brain abscess or tumor, encephalitis, delirium tremens, bleeding, and stroke.

Treatment

Be sure that the patient's airway, breathing, and circulation have been stabilized, and begin IV fluids to treat the patient for shock or hypotension. Because patients with meningitis are at high risk

for seizures, take seizure precautions, and administer treatment according to protocol. If the patient does have altered mental status, consider airway protection. If the patient is alert and may have an early stage of meningitis, monitor closely, administer oxygen, establish IV access, and transport rapidly to the ED. A patient with meningitis may decompensate en route, so be prepared to control airway and breathing and treat seizures if they occur.

Patients with suspected meningitis can be treated in most EDs. If the patient is younger than 14 years of age, consider transport to a pediatric hospital if within reasonable distance. While at the ED, the patient will be stabilized, and a head CT scan may be performed to rule out stroke and bleeding. Testing will usually include a lumbar puncture for evaluation of CSF. If bacterial meningitis is suspected, the patient will receive IV antibiotics. The patient may also receive corticosteroids.

Normal-Pressure Hydrocephalus

Normal-pressure hydrocephalus is characterized by an excessive volume of CSF in the ventricles but normal CSF pressure when determined by lumbar puncture. The classic triad of symptoms includes urinary incontinence, abnormal gait, and cognitive disturbance, which are often reversible.

Pathophysiology

A patient with normal-pressure hydrocephalus has an increased volume of CSF in the ventricles. The excess CSF is believed to put pressure on the nerve fibers exiting the cerebral cortex, leading to the clinical findings. CSF accumulation is generally believed to be due to inadequate absorption across the arachnoid membrane into the dural sinuses.

Signs and Symptoms

The patient with normal-pressure hydrocephalus typically presents with the triad of gait disturbance, urinary incontinence, and cognitive impairment. The patient tends to have a shuffling, widened gait and usually has difficulty taking the first step, much like a patient with Parkinson's disease. Urinary incontinence rather than bowel incontinence is experienced, and in the early stages, the patient may have urinary urgency and frequency. Cognitive impairment typically consists of apathy, psychomotor slowing, decreased attention span, and inability to concentrate. Key findings include the following:

- Altered gait
- Urinary incontinence
- Altered mental status

Differential Diagnosis

The differential diagnosis for normal-pressure hydrocephalus includes Alzheimer's disease and other causes of dementia, stroke, Parkinson's disease, electrolyte abnormalities, toxicity, and idiopathic increased intracranial pressure.

Treatment

On the scene and during transport, provide physical and emotional support to the patient. Once the diagnosis has been made by means of radiologic and laboratory studies in the inpatient setting, the patient may have CSF fluid removed and a shunt placed to allow continuous CSF shunting to decrease volume and pressure.

Careful monitoring and documentation of vital signs, historical data, and physical exam findings will be useful to the ED team at the receiving facility. Emergency interventions are usually not necessary, but remain alert in case the patient has a seizure.

Transport the patient to a hospital that offers neurosurgical support.

Cerebral Venous Thrombosis

Cerebral venous thrombosis (CVT) is a blood clot that forms in the veins and dural sinuses of the brain. The condition, once thought to be rare because it could be diagnosed only at autopsy, has been shown with advanced imaging techniques to be more common than previously believed. It affects women more often than men, and it tends to occur in early adulthood or middle age.

Pathophysiology

CVT typically occurs in persons with an underlying risk factor, such as a hypercoagulable state (an abnormally increased tendency to form blood clots, which can occur during pregnancy and with the use of oral contraceptives), facial or sinus infection, or head trauma. The clotted blood can be in a localized area or involve large areas of the venous system. CVT can lead to cerebral edema and/or increased intracranial pressure and thereby result in global or focal neurological dysfunction.

Signs and Symptoms

The most common chief complaint, occurring in 90% of patients with CVT, is headache, which may be localized initially and then more diffuse as the condition progresses. Thunderclap headache has been reported. Local effects on the brain can lead to strokelike symptoms, while increased intracranial pressure will lead to more generalized effects and visual disturbances. Cranial nerve palsies can be seen with cavernous sinus thrombosis. Nausea and vomiting are frequently present, and seizure may occur. Other symptoms may include hemiparesis, aphasia, ataxia (altered gait), dizziness, tinnitus (ringing in the ears), diplopia (double vision), and facial weakness. Key findings include the following:

- Headache
- Nausea/vomiting
- Visual changes
- Tinnitus

Differential Diagnosis

The differential diagnosis for venous thrombosis includes acute stroke, head injury, idiopathic intracranial hypertension, nerve palsy, seizure, infection, and lupus.

Treatment

Provide supportive care en route to the hospital. As with a stroke, airway patency and adequate ventilation should be ensured. To prevent aspiration if the patient has an altered mental status or hemiplegia, do not provide the patient anything to eat or drink. Fluids may be given intravenously, and supplemental oxygen may be placed. Treat seizures according to protocol. At the hospital, the patient will usually undergo computed tomography or magnetic resonance imaging, and infectious processes will be ruled out. Laboratory studies, including a lumbar puncture, may be done, and the patient may be placed on blood thinners to prevent further clotting.

The patient should be transported to a hospital that has neurologic consultative services. Because patients with blood clots in the venous sinuses are often given thrombolytic agents using a surgically placed microcatheter, interventional radiology or neurosurgery backup at the hospital is recommended.

Hypertensive Encephalopathy and Malignant Hypertension

Hypertensive emergencies involve damage to the brain, kidney, or heart in the setting of severe hypertension. *Hypertensive encephalopathy* describes the neurologic symptoms associated with an extremely elevated blood pressure; malignant hypertension comprises retinal hemorrhage and papilledema. These symptoms are usually reversible when blood pressure is lowered.

Most patients with hypertensive encephalopathy already have a history of hypertension. For those who don't, history taking may require specifically focused questions to identify the cause of the high blood pressure, including the use of drugs.

Pathophysiology

In healthy patients, cerebral autoregulation preserves steady-state cerebral blood flow through a range of mean arterial pressure, roughly from 50 to 150 mm Hg. In chronically hypertensive patients, the range of effective autoregulation is shifted to a higher range to allow protection at higher blood pressures. When blood pressure elevates dramatically, cerebral autoregulation is overcome, leading to increased pressure in the intracranial vessels, vascular damage, and compromise of the BBB. These events lead to capillary fluid leak and resultant cerebral edema. In the eye, increased ICP can cause retinal hemorrhages and lead to edema of the optic nerve, called *papilledema*.

Signs and Symptoms

The patient may have a headache, confusion, visual disturbances, seizure, nausea, or vomiting. Be alert for other end-organ damage, such as aortic dissection, congestive heart failure, angina, palpitations, papilledema, or hematuria (blood in the urine).

Key findings include the following:

- Hypertension
- Headache
- Nausea/vomiting
- Visual changes
- Altered mental status or focal neurologic deficits

Differential Diagnosis

A patient who has symptoms consistent with hypertensive encephalopathy may also have renal disease, pheochromocytoma, or preeclampsia or eclampsia (in pregnant patients). The patient may have ingested a specific food or medication that caused a blood pressure spike or may be in withdrawal from antihypertensive agents or alcohol. Bleeding in the brain, trauma, and stroke should also be considered as part of the differential diagnosis.

Treatment

Give supplemental oxygen and start an IV. Specific intervention to lower blood pressure is generally warranted only if the systolic blood pressure is above 220 mm Hg or the diastolic blood pressure is above 120 mm Hg. Medications commonly used for this purpose include IV boluses of labetalol and hydralazine, IV drips of nitroprusside, nicardipine, and nitroglycerin, and orally administered clonidine. For most ground EMS, the only medication available is nitroglycerin SL, although some are now carrying ACE inhibitors such as captopril for sublingual administration

and enalapril, which is given by the IV route. Remember to be cautious if antihypertensive medications are initiated, because lowering blood pressure rapidly can cause serious complications such as ischemic stroke or myocardial infarction. Blood pressure should not be lowered by more than 25% acutely, with a diastolic blood pressure of 100 mm Hg a reasonable goal within 6 hours.

Because patients who are acutely hypertensive may have a sudden intracranial hemorrhage and lose consciousness or become unable to protect their own airway, be prepared to take appropriate steps if the airway is lost.

The patient should be transported to a facility that has cardiology consultation and an intensive care unit.

Wernicke's Encephalopathy and Korsakoff's Syndrome

Wernicke's encephalopathy and Korsakoff's syndrome are thought to be different stages of the same pathologic process, with the former progressing to the latter. Acute deficiency of thiamine, or vitamin B_1, can cause the disorder known as **Wernicke's encephalopathy**, which is characterized by a triad of symptoms: acute confusion, ataxia, and **ophthalmoplegia** (abnormal function of the eye muscles). However, only a third of affected patients demonstrate all three features of the triad.

Korsakoff's syndrome is the term given to the symptoms in the late stages of the disease, especially memory loss. The syndrome is often seen in alcoholics, but it can occur in any patient who has malnutrition, such as those on long-term hemodialysis and patients with acquired immunodeficiency syndrome (AIDS). The average age at diagnosis of the syndrome is about 50, but the syndrome can occur in younger patients who have metabolic disorders, receive parenteral nutrition, or have a diet deficient in thiamine or other vitamins.

Pathophysiology

Thiamine plays a key role in the metabolism of carbohydrates. If too little thiamine is available, these cellular systems fail, leading to inadequate usable energy and subsequent cell death. The systems most critically affected are those that have rapid turnover because of high metabolic needs, such as the brain. Energy production decreases, and neuronal damage occurs, causing cellular edema and further nervous system injury.

Signs and Symptoms

A diagnosis of Wernicke's encephalopathy should be considered for any patient who has evidence of alcohol abuse or malnutrition and acute symptoms of confusion, ocular dysfunction, and memory disturbance. The ocular problems most commonly seen are nystagmus, bilateral lateral rectus palsies, and dysconjugate gaze. Blindness is not usually seen.

The encephalopathy may manifest as global confusion, apathy, agitation, or inattentiveness. Significant mental status changes, such as coma or low LOC, are rarely seen. About 80% of patients have some peripheral neuropathy. Hypotension, nausea, and temperature instability may also be caused by thiamine deficiency. Infants may have constipation, agitation, vomiting, diarrhea, anorexia, eye disorders, or altered mental status, including seizures and loss of consciousness. Key findings include the following:

- Ascending and peripheral weakness moving upward and inward
- Mixed upper and lower motor neuron findings

Differential Diagnosis

The differential diagnosis includes alcohol or illicit drug intoxication, delirium, dementia, stroke, psychosis, closed head injury, encephalopathy secondary to liver failure, and postictal state.

Treatment

At the hospital, the patient will undergo an array of possible laboratory and radiologic tests, such as blood tests, electrolyte measurement, lumbar puncture, arterial blood gas readings, and a CT scan and MRI to evaluate differential diagnoses.

Focus on stabilizing the airway, ensuring oxygenation, and maintaining blood pressure and volume control. If the condition is suspected, empirical thiamine replacement should be initiated. Thiamine can be given orally, but to ensure absorption, it is often administered IV or intramuscularly (IM). The initial dose of thiamine is typically 100 mg, but over time as much as 500 mg may be needed to reverse the encephalopathy.

Some clinicians have expressed concern about giving patients dextrose before administering thiamine if they are in a thiamine-deficient state. The concern is that dextrose will exacerbate the encephalopathy. However, this effect is seen only in patients receiving long-term dextrose administration without concurrent thiamine administration. It is safe to give dextrose alone in the prehospital setting for hypoglycemic events, even if thiamine is not immediately available.

Thiamine and glucose should be given to patients who have an altered mental status if there is a chance that Wernicke's encephalopathy is being considered as a diagnosis.

No special transport decisions must be made. The patient may be brought to any hospital, but children should be brought to a pediatric specialty center if one is available.

Migraine Headaches

Migraine headaches are severe, recurrent headaches accompanied by incapacitating neurologic symptoms such as cognitive or visual disturbances, dizziness, nausea, and vomiting. The headache may be either unilateral or bilateral. Migraines often begin in childhood and become more frequent during adolescence.

About 80% of patients experience their first migraine before age 30 years, and the headaches tend to become less frequent after age 50. Common migraine triggers are as follows:

- Stress
- Illness
- Physical activity
- Changes in sleep pattern
- High altitude and other barometric pressure changes
- Skipping meals
- Use of certain medications (such as oral contraceptives)
- Ingestion of caffeine, alcohol, and certain foods
- Exposure to bright lights, loud noises, or unpleasant odors

Pathophysiology

The pathophysiology of migraine headaches is not completely understood. Recent research shows that **neurotransmitters** in the brain, such as serotonin and dopamine, stimulate an inflammatory cascade that causes vasodilation, which is responsible for the pain. Some of the symptoms associated with migraine headaches, such as nausea and vomiting, are also associated with dopamine receptor activation. Many dopamine antagonists have been clinically shown to be effective in treating migraines.

Signs and Symptoms

An aura consisting of dizziness, tinnitus, a perception of flashing lights or zigzagging lines in the visual field may signal or accompany the migraine. The headache is often described as throbbing and unilateral and accompanied by photophobia and/or phonophobia, although a wide variety of neurologic symptoms have been associated with or attributed to migraine syndrome. Subtypes of migraine include ocular (scotomata or transient blindness), hemiplegic (some of which lead to permanent weakness with brain infarction) and brainstem (associated with vertigo, dysarthria, tinnitus, diplopia, or ataxia). Migraines usually last 4 to 72 hours, and the patient often prefers to be in a quiet, dark room and may initially attempt to treat the headache with over-the-counter medication. Key findings include the following:

- Headache
- Photophobia
- Nausea/vomiting
- Increased sensitivity to sound or smell
- History of migraines

Differential Diagnosis

The differential diagnosis for migraine headaches includes headaches of a different cause, infections (such as meningitis and sinusitis), temporal arteritis, and ischemic or hemorrhagic stroke or bleeding. In addition, increased intracranial pressure from a brain tumor, idiopathic intracranial hypertension, a leaking aneurysm, or opiate withdrawal may also cause headaches that resemble migraines.

Treatment

Although patients may appear to be uncomfortable, their conditions are usually stable. Opioid analgesia should be withheld until the patient can be fully evaluated by a physician. Treatment with antiemetics may help break the cycle and intensity of the migraine as well as treat the accompanying nausea. IV fluids may be helpful if the patient has been vomiting.

Patients with a history of migraine headaches may mistake a stroke or other emergent condition for an especially bad migraine. Be alert for sudden changes in neurologic status should one of these other conditions be present.

Because the differential diagnosis includes stroke and intracranial hemorrhage, transport the patient to a facility that can care for these medical conditions. Patients may prefer to be transported without lights or sirens or with their eyes closed or covered because they may be highly sensitive to light and sound. Supportive care is usually all that is necessary during transport.

Temporal Arteritis

Temporal arteritis, also known as "giant cell arteritis," is an inflammation of the temporal arteries that causes throbbing or burning pain in the area of the temples, often accompanied by difficulty swallowing or chewing, visual disturbances, and other symptoms. Other arteries may be inflamed as well. The condition tends to affect adults age 50 years and older, especially women in their 70s.

Pathophysiology

The exact pathophysiology of temporal arteritis is unknown. Some researchers speculate that it has an infectious cause, but this has never been proven. Another hypothesis implicates an autoimmune response that stimulates T-cell proliferation in the arterial walls.

Signs and Symptoms

The patient usually reports a headache and scalp tenderness in the area of the temporal artery. The headache has an acute onset but affects only one side of the head. In addition, the patient typically has jaw claudication and a swollen area in the temporal region, difficulty swallowing, hoarseness, and cough. Fever is also common. A frequent and very concerning complication is visual disturbance in the ipsilateral eye. Sometimes the patient reports hearing loss or vertigo. Other signs and symptoms include diaphoresis, anorexia (loss of appetite) with accompanying weight loss, muscle aches, fatigue, weakness, mouth sores, and bleeding gums. Key findings include the following:

- Headache (usually unilateral and temporal)
- Visual changes (usually in one eye)
- Older adult

Differential Diagnosis

The differential diagnosis for temporal arteritis includes other inflammatory rheumatic diseases, malignancies, migraine headache, tumor, and infection.

Treatment

Provide supportive care and monitor the patient's airway, breathing, and circulation. At the receiving facility, the patient may undergo a battery of tests, including blood tests, radiologic studies, and temporal artery biopsy. Patients who are believed to have temporal arteritis are usually prescribed corticosteroids to reduce vascular inflammation.

The patient should be transported to a hospital at which ophthalmologic care is available.

Seizures

A **seizure** is a transient occurrence of abnormal excessive or synchronous neuronal activity in the cerebral cortex of the brain that can cause loss of or alteration in consciousness, convulsions or tremors, incontinence, behavior changes, subjective changes in perception (taste, smell, fears), and other symptoms.

Seizures are a common nonspecific manifestation of neurologic injury and disease, and may occur as a primary condition or secondary to an underlying abnormality. Seizures can be caused by fever, infection, drug ingestion/withdrawal, acute neurologic insult (e.g., stroke, trauma), structural changes (e.g., brain tumor, degenerative diseases), pregnancy complications, metabolic disturbances, electrolyte imbalances, and congenital conditions. Seizures (reflex seizures) can also be caused by light flickers, certain visual patterns, or even brushing the teeth. Nearly 70% of all seizures have no known cause (idiopathic).

Those with a history of seizures can have seizure frequency and severity exacerbated simply due to menstrual hormonal changes (catamenial epilepsy). Other triggers for those with a history of seizures are failure to take medication correctly, changing from a brand name to generic medication, sleep deprivation/fatigue, stress/illness, and even dehydration.

Epilepsy is a condition in which a persistent abnormality in the brain leads to recurrent seizures; this may a congenital or acquired structural, metabolic or genetic abnormality. Seizure due to transient abnormalities such as hyponatremia are not considered epilepsy.

Seizures can be classified as generalized or focal. A generalized seizure quickly involves both cerebral hemispheres and is associated with loss of consciousness. A focal seizure involves only or primarily one cerebral hemisphere so wakefulness is usually maintained but there may be changes in mentation, responsiveness or behavior. Within generalized seizures are absence, atonic, tonic, clonic, and tonic/clonic types. The classification of focal seizures is discussed later.

Pathophysiology

Seizures are thought to occur when there is an imbalance between the excitatory and inhibitory forces within the brain, and the scales tip in favor of the excitatory forces. Researchers believe seizures are caused by either a decrease of gamma-aminobutyric acid (GABA), an inhibitory neurotransmitter in the cerebral cortex of the brain, or by an increase of glutamate, an excitatory neurotransmitter. Benzodiazepines, commonly used to stop active seizure activity, increase GABA release and thus inhibit neuronal activity.

Seizures have three distinct phases, the preictal, ictal, and the postictal phase. Depending on the type of seizure, not all phases are observed. Some patients may even experience a symptom several hours or days before a seizure warning them that a seizure will occur. The preictal phase is the period immediately prior to observable seizure activity and may include an aura or warning of the impending seizure. The aura is a very small focal seizure lasting only a few seconds or minutes. Although anti-seizure medications may obscure or alter the aura, patients may say they felt weak, hot or cold, or had abnormal epigastic sensations just prior to the seizure. Others describe their auras to be a sudden sense of fear, with difficulty speaking or understanding speech, a headache, hearing sounds and smelling unpleasant odors that are not there, a tongue-tingling sensation, or visual hallucinations. The ictal phase is the actual seizure activity, when the transient occurrence of abnormal excessive or synchronous neuronal activity in the cerebral cortex takes place and can be recorded on an electroencephalogram (EEG). The various observable clinical manifestations are related to the location of the abnormal electrical activity. The postictal phase immediately follows the ictal phase as seizure activity subsides and is considered the recovery period after the seizure. Some patients recover immediately whereas others may take minutes to hours to feel like their usual selves, depending on the type of seizure, how long it lasted, and the location of the activity within the brain. Patients can be aware of the seizure or wake up afterwards not knowing what happened. Generalized seizures involve complete loss of consciousness, whereas focal seizures typically do not. During a generalized seizure, the patient cannot talk, reach out, or perform purposeful activity. Following a generalized tonic-clonic seizure, the postictal phase is more severe and may manifest as amnesia, confusion, fatigue, or coma.

Most seizures, including generalized tonic-clonic seizures terminate prior to 2 minutes with a small percentage prolonged up to 5 minutes or more. A single, short-duration seizure is usually not a life-threatening event. However, a prolonged seizure, called status epilepticus (discussed later in this chapter), is a life-threatening medical and neurologic emergency that requires prompt diagnosis and immediate treatment.

Signs and Symptoms

Most often, a family member or bystander will call EMS to report a person exhibiting convulsive activity or acting confused or disoriented or wandering aimlessly. People may activate EMS if they believe they are about to have a seizure. For many years seizures were classified as generalized or partial, but in 2010 the International League Against Epilepsy (ILAE) commission published a revised classification (Table 5-5) that retains the term *generalized seizure* but changed *partial* to *focal* and replaced subtypes of focal with descriptive phrases.

Generalized seizures, according to the 2010 ILAE classifications, originate at some point within, and rapidly engage, bilaterally distributed networks. Generalized seizures initially start with a loss of consciousness, which may be brief or extended, but continues through to the postictal phase.

There are multiple subtypes of generalized seizures. The tonic-clonic form tends to start out tonic (flexion or extension of the head, trunk, or extremities), then become clonic (rhythmic motor jerking of the extremities or neck), and then resolve with the patient becoming postictal. Other forms of generalized seizure include tonic only, clonic only, myoclonic jerking, atonic, and absence.

During a generalized seizure the patient may experience airway obstruction or may not breathe adequately. Providers should be prepared to maintain the airway and assist ventilation.

Table 5-5 **Classification of Seizures***
Generalized seizures
Tonic-clonic (in any combination)
Absence
Typical
Atypical
Absence with special features
Myoclonic absence
Eyelid myoclonia
Myoclonic
Myoclonic
Myoclonic atonic
Myoclonic tonic
Clonic
Tonic
Atonic
Focal seizures
Unknown
Epileptic spasms

*Seizures that cannot be clearly diagnosed into one of the preceding categories should be considered unclassified until further information allows their accurate diagnosis. This is not considered a classification category, however.

From Berg AT, Berkovic SF, Brodie MJ, et al.: Revised terminology and concepts for organization of seizures and epilepsies: Report of the ILAE Commission on Classification and Terminology, 2005–2009, *Epilepsia.* 51(4):676, 2010.

Focal seizures, according to the ILAE, originate within networks limited to one hemisphere, which may be discretely localized or more widely distributed. Focal seizures are the most common type of seizure experienced by people with epilepsy and usually last only 1 to 3 minutes. The two subsets of focal seizures are as follows:

- *Focal seizure with retained consciousness and awareness.* This seizure usually starts and stays within a very small, defined area of one hemisphere leading to abnormalities that can be identified as coming from that area of the brain. For example, a seizure starting and staying within the right motor area of the cerebral cortex may cause rhythmic movement in the left arm, leg, or face. The patient will usually always be awake and aware of the seizure activity. If the patient is unconscious or has altered mental status, consider and investigate other causes for the decreased consciousness state.

- *Focal seizure with impaired consciousness or awareness or responsiveness.* This seizure also takes place in only one hemisphere but usually involves a larger area or the entire hemisphere. Patients remain conscious but are not aware of their surroundings, dangerous situations, or able to identify friends. They may sit quietly and exhibit automatisms or they might start to scream, take off their clothes, or even walk into traffic. EMS responders should be extremely careful when approaching and caring for patients exhibiting focal seizures. Patients with this type of seizure are known to be aggressive and may violently resist any physical touch or restraint. Many individuals with this disorder (old terminology was complex partial seizure) have been injured while EMS and law enforcement personnel have tried to subdue them believing the patient was intoxicated, willfully belligerent, and unresponsive to their commands. This has led to lawsuits for violating the individual's legal rights listed under the American's with Disability Act. Many patients with this disorder wear medical jewelry identifying them with this seizure disorder. Usually no medical treatment is required as the seizure will correct itself within a few minutes.

"Observe, contain, and don't restrain" is the easiest way to treat a person with a focal seizure. Approach the patient cautiously, and speak calmly. Again, avoid triggering violent behavior by minimizing physical contact. Talk with bystanders to hear their observations. Was the change from normal to the current situation slow or rapid? Focal seizures come on quickly, and, if observed, there will usually be a rapid change from normal behavior. The type of behavior change is different from the slow change caused by drugs or alcohol. However, a person can still be intoxicated and have focal seizure activity at the same time. Document any reported altered awareness, blank staring, confusion, inability to respond, mumbling, emotional outbursts, automatisms, and/or wandering. With termination of the seizure, patients usually relax and their level of consciousness and awareness returns. Patients may be tired and stay confused for another 15 minutes, and may not return to full functioning for hours.

Although consciousness is maintained during a focal seizure, a focal seizure may evolve into unconsciousness and generalized seizure. Key findings of a focal seizure include the following:

- Altered mental status
- Focal or generalized rhythmic, uncontrolled movements
- Staring spell or drop attack, eyelid flutter
- Grunting sounds, repeating of words or phrases, laughter, screams, crying
- Taking clothes off, walking into traffic, wandering about without purpose
- Automatisms
- Postictal state described by family, friends, or caregivers

Status epilepticus (SE) is defined as convulsions lasting for 5 or more minutes or recurrent episodes of convulsions in a 5-minute interval without return to preconvulsive neurologic baseline. SE is further classified into convulsive and nonconvulsive types, based on the presence of tonic and/or clonic movement of the patient's extremities. SE is a life-threatening medical and neurologic emergency that requires prompt diagnosis and immediate treatment. During SE, cerebral glucose and oxygen supplies can be depleted. Systemic hypoxia, hypercarbia, acidosis, blood pressure changes, hyperthermia, neurogenic pulmonary edema, and rhabdomyolysis can occur. After 30 minutes of SE, pathologic changes in the brain take place, and after 60 minutes neurons start to die.

A nonconvulsive SE (NCSE) is defined as a mental status change from baseline of at least 30 to 60 minutes' duration associated with continuous or near-continuous ictal discharges on an EEG. This type of seizure occurs frequently after acute traumatic brain injury and has been reported in 8% to 20% of critically ill patients. Delayed diagnosis and treatment of NCSE may lead to increased mortality.

NCSE may present as absence, focal, or only observed on an EEG. For this reason, if there is no improvement in level of consciousness or awareness after 5 to 10 minutes postictal, the EMS provider should consider the possibility of the patient to be in NCSE and treat per protocol and/or contact medical control.

A psychogenic nonepileptic seizure (PNES) may look like generalized seizure activity with abnormal motor movements and altered mentation, but it is not caused by abnormal neuronal activity. A PNES is considered primarily due to stress-related or emotional causes. Without EEG monitoring, a PNES is nearly impossible to diagnose and as such, it is the most common condition misdiagnosed as epilepsy. It is also possible to have an EEG diagnosed seizure disorder and still exhibit a PNES at other times. Withholding treatment and anti-seizure medication believing your patient to be "faking a seizure," however, could be dangerous and is not recommended. Contact medical control.

A PNES should not affect the medulla or a patient's respirations because it is not caused by a generalized seizure or abnormal electrical discharges. The patient will usually continue to breathe. The use of capnography to monitor the patient's respirations and CO_2 status is an excellent assessment tool to help potentially help differentiate seizure-like activity.

Differential Diagnosis

The differential diagnosis for seizure includes stroke, hypoglycemia, hyperthermia, migraine, amnesia, hemorrhage, tumor, metabolic abnormality, sleep disorders, movement disorders, pseudoseizure and psychiatric conditions.

Treatment

Oxygenation, ventilation, and protection from harm are the most important interventions in the prehospital scenario. Protect the patient from injury by placing padding or removing hazards. Administer oxygen via blow-by for infants and/or cannula for all others. Oxygen masks strapped down to the patient should be used cautiously due to the possibility of vomiting and aspiration. Consider the placement of a nasal airway. Provide ventilatory assistance if the patient's respiratory rate or ventilatory effort is inadequate or if the patient becomes hypoxic. Obtain IV access if seizure is prolonged or after the seizure if transporting so another seizure can be treated. Blood glucose levels should be checked in all patients, and dextrose administered as needed. If the patient is hyperthermic, begin temperature management measures, but do not allow the patient to shiver. Placing patients on their side or in the recovery position helps to protect the airway from aspiration. As with any patient with an uncontrolled airway, never give oral antiseizure medication to an actively seizing patient.

Patients actively seizing for more than 5 minutes should be considered to be in SE and treated aggressively with a benzodiazepine to stop the seizure. If an attempt to start an IV has not been successful or is delayed, consider other routes for initial medication administration, including IM, IN, IO, and rectal. This should be based on the specific benzodiazepine used. The provider should know the characteristics of the specific drugs he or she has available, such as that diazepam should not be given by the IM route. A recent trial found that intramuscular midazolam and intravenous lorazepam were equally safe and effective in adults. Intranasal administration (IN) of specific benzodiazepines, such as midazolam, has also been shown to be a safe and effective means of managing acute repetitive seizures in children and adults. Another route often used by parents and child care providers for infants and young children is rectal administration of diazepam gel. As all benzodiazepines can cause respiratory depression, EMS responders should ask about any medications or treatments given to the patient prior to their arrival.

If adequate and repeated doses of benzodiazepine are not effective at stopping the seizure activity, then second-line agents such as phenytoin (Dilantin) and phenobarbital should be administered. These medications are typically not carried by ground EMS but may be available in air medical and critical care transport units. There is evidence that ketamine, for those EMS agencies that carry this medication, can effectively control status epilepticus, especially if it is resistant to phenobarbital. The last resort are general anesthetic agents, including propofol. During the postictal state, supportive care is the best treatment. Postictal patients will probably be confused, upset, and perhaps aggressive or violent. Be reassuring, and try to explain what happened. If the patient is in public, consider the patient's need for privacy and the possibility of incontinence and opened or torn clothes. Not all adult patients that have an out-of-hospital seizure need to be transported to the hospital for evaluation. If the postictal patient is regaining his or her level of consciousness, some EMS systems allow crews to stay on-scene for up to 15 minutes to monitor the patient's return to baseline behavior. If the patient is of legal age, returns to an awake stage, is fully oriented and mentating normally, and is judged to understand and accepts the risks of not going to the hospital for evaluation, the patient has the right to refuse transport. Ideally, the patient is under current medical care for their seizure disorder and is taking their medications and has a plan of action for when 'break through' seizures occur. EMS crews should encourage the patient to contact their personal physician to inform them of this seizure episode. It is possible, due to a number of factors (e.g., illness, exercise, diet, etc.), that the AED the patient has been prescribed is no longer at a therapeutic level and needs to be adjusted.

Patients who suffered a seizure for the first time should be always be transported to a hospital for evaluation. Similarly if the seizure is due to trauma, if possible aspiration occurred or the seizure took place in water, if the patient is elderly, diabetic, or pregnant, if the seizure lasted longer than 5 minutes or occurs in series, or if during the postictal phase there is no obvious improvement in level of consciousness within 5 to 10 minutes. If the seizure is thought to have been precipitated by trauma, due to the decreased level of conscious, a trauma center or hospital with surgical/trauma treatment abilities is recommended.

Febrile seizures are convulsions brought on by a fever in children between the ages of 6 months and 3 years and are particularly common in toddlers. Approximately one in every 25 children will have at least one febrile seizure. The vast majority of febrile seizures are harmless. Most last for only a few seconds to 15 minutes, with the majority less than two minutes. There is no evidence that short febrile seizures cause brain damage although certain children who have febrile seizures face an increased risk of developing epilepsy. As the child does not breathe during the seizure, the child's color can turn dark or cyanotic. This observation, along with the seizure activity, can be very scary for parents and observers who have never witnessed a seizure before.

EMS responders should be aware that a seizure thought to be due primarily to hyperthermia (e.g., illness, infection) might be caused by another disorder (e.g., hypoglycemia, trauma), so considering and assessing for other pathologies causing seizure are important. Blood glucose levels should always be checked and treated appropriately. During your workup, ask about medical history, ask about other family members and look for signs at the scene. During your physical examination, look closely at the skin for signs related to a contagious disease (e.g., petechial rash) and evidence of trauma. Assess for focal neurologic abnormalities and consider the possibility of poisoning or electrolyte imbalance from vomiting/diarrhea.

If the child is wrapped in or wearing clothing holding in body heat, open up or remove the clothing, but do not allow the child to shiver and generate more heat. Cooling measures and antipyretic administration might make the febrile child more comfortable but have not been shown in studies to decrease the initial occurrence or recurrence of febrile seizures. Maintain airway, give oxygen and monitor that the child is continuing to improve.

If the seizure has continued longer than 5 minutes, consider the patient to be in febrile status epilepticus (FSE) and aggressively treat per protocol. FSE rarely stops spontaneously, is fairly resistant to medications, and even with treatment persists for a significant period of time. Give benzodiazepines by IM, IN, IO, or rectally if unable to start or a delay in starting an IV is likely. Maintain airway control and reparatory status. Monitor saturation and capnography. Early aggressive treatment results in shorter total seizure duration. Contact medical control if FSE continues after initial treatment.

In general, all pediatric patients who have had a seizure should be transported by ALS personnel to a hospital emergency room for evaluation. Most children who have a febrile seizure do not need to be hospitalized. However, if the seizure is prolonged or is accompanied by a serious infection, or if the source of the infection cannot be determined, a doctor may recommend that the child be hospitalized for observation.

Bell's Palsy

Bell's palsy is a unilateral facial paralysis that has an abrupt onset and uncertain cause. It is one of the most common cranial neuropathies, but it may frighten the patient by mimicking a stroke. Bell's palsy accounts for about half of cases of peripheral facial nerve palsy, with the other half associated with specific causes.

Pathophysiology

Bell's palsy refers to unilateral facial weakness due to dysfunction of the seventh cranial nerve itself, as opposed to the nucleus of the nerve which lies in the brain stem. Inflammation and swelling of the sheath of the nerve is typically present where it passes through the temporal bone. By definition, when the etiology is unknown, the condition is termed *Bell's palsy*, and there is increasing evidence of specific causes, most notably infection, particularly due to herpes simplex and a variety of other viruses.

Signs and Symptoms

A patient with Bell's palsy typically calls EMS or comes to the ED after having facial weakness that leads the person to believe he or she has had a stroke. Some patients have pain in the mastoid region or external ear, decreased tearing of the eye on the affected side, and an altered sense of taste.

On exam, weakness or paralysis of the entire face on the affected side may be present, and the eye may not close completely on that side. If you watch carefully, you may see that the eye on the affected side rolls upward and inward. Facial signs of a stroke differ in that only the lower half of the face will be weak, but the forehead and upper eyelid retain normal motor function. In some patients, this can be difficult to differentiate, and in these cases the patient should be treated as having had a stroke until proven otherwise. Key findings include the following:

- Unilateral weakness of entire side of face
- No arm or leg weakness
- Difficulty closing eyes

Differential Diagnosis

Facial nerve palsy has a variety of potential causes other than Bell's palsy. These include Lyme disease, shingles, acute HIV infection, tumor, and otitis media. It is important to rule out a CNS cause (also called *upper motor neuron*) such as stroke. A person who has had a stroke will usually have some wrinkling of the forehead.

Treatment

The management of Bell's palsy in the prehospital setting is primarily providing patient transport, supporting vital signs, and offering emotional support to the patient. Because of the impaired eyelid closure on the affected side, you should protect the affected eye with an eye shield or gauze taped lightly over the eye to keep it closed. Periodically placing a small amount of normal saline in the eye or on the gauze to keep it moist is also an acceptable option. In the ED, after ruling out other causes previously mentioned, corticosteroids and antiviral agents may be prescribed, with neurologic follow-up for further testing and observation.

Bell's palsy is not life threatening and is usually self-limiting. For this reason, emergency transport is not necessarily indicated, but if there is any question whether the patient may be having an acute stroke, he or she should be transported urgently to the nearest stroke center.

Cauda Equina Syndrome

Cauda equina syndrome is a disorder in which the nerve roots exiting from the end of the spinal cord in the lower lumbar and sacral region of the spine become compressed, causing lower extremity pain, weakness or paralysis, bladder and bowel incontinence, and loss of sexual function. This syndrome is an emergent condition, and surgical intervention is necessary to prevent permanent loss of function.

Pathophysiology

Anatomically, the cauda equina resembles a horse's tail. It is formed by the nerve roots distal to the end of the spinal cord between T12 and L2. Cauda equina syndrome may be due to any compression of the nerve roots, including compression caused by trauma, disk herniation, tumors and other spinal cord lesions, and spinal stenosis (narrowing of the spinal canal). The nerve roots in the lumbar part of the spinal cord are susceptible to injury because they lack a well-developed covering, or epineurium, which may protect against stretch and compression injury.

Signs and Symptoms

The patient affected by cauda equina syndrome may have low back pain, sciatica on either side or sometimes bilaterally, saddle sensory disturbances in the area of the perineum, and bowel or bladder dysfunction. Variable lower extremity motor and sensory changes caused by compression of the nerve roots may also be present, and lower extremity reflexes may be diminished or absent. Back pain is the most common complaint. If the patient doesn't voluntarily relate a history of urinary or bowel incontinence or retention, or of weakness, numbness and tingling in lower extremities, be sure to ask. Key findings include the following:

- Low back pain, often with radiation down legs
- Bowel or bladder incontinence or retention
- Recent manipulation of the spine (such as during a lumbar puncture or surgery)
- Trauma

Differential Diagnosis

The differential diagnosis includes back pain attributable to trauma and other causes, tumor, Guillain-Barré syndrome, spinal cord compression, metabolic abnormality, and other nerve disorders.

Treatment

Prehospital care is mainly supportive, including pain control if needed. Although prehospital intervention is not usually necessary, and cauda equina syndrome is not fatal, neurologic impairment may be permanent if not treated with emergency surgery. On arriving at the ED, various imaging studies (x-ray, CT, or MRI) can be done and are most diagnostic.

A patient suspected of having cauda equina syndrome may require spinal immobilization for transport in case there is an underlying traumatic cause that could be worsened with movement. The patient should be transported to a hospital where orthopedic or neurosurgical spinal surgery can be performed.

Neuromuscular Degenerative Disease

Neuromuscular degenerative disease is known in the United States as **Lou Gehrig disease** or **amyotrophic lateral sclerosis (ALS)**. The disease is characterized by degeneration of the upper and lower motor neurons, which causes voluntary muscles to weaken or atrophy. Patients usually die 3 to 5 years after diagnosis, which is commonly made between ages 40 and 60. More men than women are affected.

Pathophysiology

Neuromuscular degenerative disease has no single known cause. Scientists have recently identified a mutation in a gene that controls protein synthesis and synaptic function of motor neurons in some patients. However, this explanation accounts for only a small percentage of cases of neuromuscular degenerative disease. Glutamate toxicity, mitochondrial dysfunction, and autoimmunity may all play a role in ALS, but researchers are still trying to find out precisely how.

Signs and Symptoms

Upper motor neuron findings in patients with neuromuscular degenerative disease include spasticity and hyperreflexia. Lower motor findings include weakness, ataxia, and fasciculations. Death is attributable to respiratory muscle weakness and aspiration pneumonia. Medical complications of immobility add to the morbidity and mortality of patients with this disorder.

The patient may seek acute medical care for limb weakness, difficulty speaking and swallowing, visual disturbances, and limb spasticity. Motor problems typically present from the periphery inward, starting with wrist drop, loss of finger dexterity, foot drop, and tongue fasciculations. The patient's lack of control over emotions may be present and may cause the patient to overreact to sad or humorous events or comments. Ocular, sensory, and autonomic dysfunction occur late in the disease, usually in patients who require ventilatory support. Weakness is often asymmetric and begins in the arms or legs. Difficulty chewing and swallowing occurs late in the illness. Key findings include the following:

- Ascending and peripheral weakness moving upward and inward
- Mixed upper and lower motor neuron findings

Differential Diagnosis

The differential includes Guillain-Barré syndrome, multiple sclerosis, myasthenia gravis, spinal cord tumor, and stroke.

Treatment

Prehospital care requires transport of the patient and support of the patient's airway, breathing, circulation, and vital signs.

Administer oxygen and fluids for general weakness according to protocol.

At the hospital, the patient will undergo a battery of tests, including neurology consults and nerve conduction studies. Care is mainly symptomatic, and emotional support should be available to the patient and family. The patient's living will or DNR orders should be followed. Complications such as pneumonia or other infections, deep vein thrombosis, or respiratory problems are common. These problems should be managed according to protocol.

Patients with neuromuscular degenerative disease may decompensate from extreme weakness in the respiratory muscles, and corrective action must be taken. If the decision is made to intubate, the patient and family need to be informed that it is unlikely the patient will be able to be weaned from the ventilator.

The patient should be brought to the hospital and cared for by a neurologist, especially if the condition is chronic. As with most patients who have an altered mental status, the patient should be brought to a stroke center or a center that has neurologic and neurosurgical backup, because the diagnosis of neuromuscular degenerative disease is usually made during the course of a hospital stay.

Guillain-Barré Syndrome

Guillain-Barré syndrome refers to a group of acute immune-mediated polyneuropathies, demyelinating disorders that cause weakness, numbness, or paralysis throughout the body. The incidence of Guillain-Barré is 1 to 3 per 100,000 people in the United States. Although the syndrome can occur at any age, it is usually found in young adults and older adults. The condition affects men and women equally.

Pathophysiology

Guillain-Barré syndrome is believed to represent an autoimmune response to a recent infection or to many different types of medical problems. Researchers believe the body forms antibodies against the peripheral nerves, in particular the axons, which become demyelinated, leading to motor weakness and in some cases sensory loss. Recovery is typically associated with a brief remyelination period. It has been shown that many patients with Guillain-Barré syndrome are seropositive for *Campylobacter jejuni*.

Signs and Symptoms

The patient with Guillain-Barré often is seen initially with lower extremity muscle weakness, mainly in the thighs. The weakness usually appears a few weeks after a respiratory or gastrointestinal illness. Over the course of hours to days, the weakness may progress to involve the arms and chest muscles, facial muscles, and respiratory muscles. Approximately 12 days from onset, most patients will be at their worst and then will gradually begin to improve during the next few months.

Many patients with Guillain-Barré syndrome require mechanical ventilation during their illness to compensate for respiratory muscle weakness. In many cases, patients cannot stand or walk even though they feel strong. Lack of deep tendon reflexes is a relatively strong indicator of Guillain-Barré. In addition, the patient may have paresthesias in the feet, initially, then the hands. Pain may be present with the most minimal movements and is most impressive in the shoulder, back, buttocks, and thighs. The patient may experience a loss of ability to sense vibration, loss of proprioception and touch, and impressive autonomic dysfunction, including wide variation in vital signs, heart rate, and blood pressure. The patient may also have urinary retention, constipation, facial flushing, hypersalivation, anhidrosis, and tonic pupils. Key findings include the following:

- Progressive, symmetric weakness of legs, arms, face, and trunk
- Areflexia (absence of reflexes)
- Preceding illness

Differential Diagnosis

The differential diagnosis of Guillain-Barré is the same as that of a spinal cord infection or injury. Electrolyte abnormalities such as hyperkalemia and hypokalemia can cause weakness. Infections such as meningitis, encephalitis, and botulism, as well as tick-borne infections, also mimic this disease. In the early stages of the disease, Guillain-Barré may also be mistaken for multiple sclerosis; myasthenia gravis; toxic ingestion of alcohol, heavy metals, or organophosphates; diabetes; and HIV neuropathy.

Treatment

In the prehospital setting, management of airway, breathing, and circulation, administration of oxygen, and assisted ventilation (if needed) are of primary importance. Other prehospital treatments include IV placement and cardiac monitoring devices. If the patient does have autonomic dysfunction, hypertension is best treated with short-acting agents; symptomatic bradycardia is best treated with atropine, and hypotension usually responds to IV fluids. Temporary cardiac pacing may be required if the patient has a second- or third-degree heart block.

Because this is a rapidly progressing disease, it is important to recognize the likelihood that a patient will decompensate. Provide airway control and maintenance as necessary.

Transport should be to a tertiary care center when possible; rapid imaging and neurologic consultation are often required.

Acute Psychosis

The patient with acute psychosis has disturbances in thinking, behavior, and perception but not in orientation. He or she may have delusions, hallucinations, speech problems, flattened affect, withdrawal, and apathy.

Pathophysiology

Psychosis is primarily associated with abnormalities of brain chemistry and development. Genetics may play a role in the development of psychosis, but psychosocial stressors are thought to serve as triggering factors. It is believed that overactivity of the dopamine receptors in the brain, ones that are blocked by antipsychotic drugs, may cause the active hallucinations and delusions that characterize acute psychosis. Decreased activity in the prefrontal cortex of the brain related to serotonin transmission may be associated with symptoms such as flattened affect and social withdrawal.

Signs and Symptoms

About 50% of patients have an acute onset of psychosis. The patient may have a period of worsening mental health before the acute break occurs. That period is usually characterized by declining functioning at home, at work, and in public. Some patients with acute psychotic issues will seek medical care for medication reactions, such as hypotension, dry mouth, sedation, and difficulty with urination or sexual activity. Other patients may not have taken medications prescribed for psychosis for some period of time. Key findings include the following:

- Agitation and behavioral changes
- Abnormal thought content, often with delusions and/or hallucinations
- Labile mood

Differential Diagnosis

The differential diagnosis for acute psychosis includes delirium, depression, panic disorder, intoxication, brain tumor, and infection.

Treatment

Your safety and that of the patient are of utmost concern when treating a person with psychotic issues. The patient may require chemical sedation or physical restraint or police escort, depending on local protocol. Monitor the patient's vital signs if possible, and provide emotional support. If the patient becomes medically unstable, initiate appropriate treatment per protocol.

Because a medical issue may be responsible for the patient's alteration of mental status, the blood glucose level should be checked, a traumatic injury assessment should be performed, and vital signs, including pulse oximetry, should be carefully evaluated and treated if necessary. In addition, a history of the precipitating events should be carefully taken to evaluate for poisoning, intoxication, and inappropriate or accidental medication ingestion.

Transport the patient to a facility that has both medical and psychiatric consultation services.

Acute Depression/Suicide Attempt

Suicide occurs when a person deliberately ends his or her own life. A suicide attempt occurs when a person tries to commit suicide but is unsuccessful. According to the National Institute of Mental Health, for every person who commits suicide, 12 to 25 attempts are made. Among teens, possibly as many as 200 attempts are made for every suicide. A suicide attempt can take many forms, and emergency care must be administered on the basis of the self-inflicted harm the person has committed.

Although teen suicide pacts and other sensational suicides dominate the news on this topic, the rate of suicide among older adults is much higher than that among teens, primarily because older adults select more lethal means of ending their lives. According to the Institute on Aging, firearms, hanging, and poisoning (including toxic overdose), in that order, are the first, second, and third most common methods of suicide chosen among adults aged 65 and older. About 1 in 4 suicide attempts among this age group is successful. White men aged 80 and older have a higher risk of suicide than people in any other age, gender, or ethnic group.

The rate of suicide has increased steadily among adults aged 35 to 64, however, and is now about equal to the rate among older adults. Suicide remains the third leading cause of death among teens aged 15 to 19. Men are at much higher risk than women, and their attempts succeed much more often because they tend to choose more lethal means. The ethnic groups at highest risk are American Indians, Alaska Natives, and non-Hispanic whites.

According to the Centers for Disease Control and Prevention, in 2010, there were 38,364 suicides in the United States. The goals of treatment are to stabilize the patient, identify any underlying medical conditions, evaluate mental health status, and provide appropriate referrals.

Pathophysiology

The pathophysiology of depression is multifactorial, but it is believed to involve changes in the neurotransmitters of the limbic system. Serotonin, norepinephrine, and dopamine have all been investigated as possible causes of depression. A family history of depression is frequently encountered, including among those who attempt suicide, but no definitive genetic link to depression has been found. Alcohol and other substance abuse is also a risk factor for depression. Emotional stressors such as physical or sexual abuse, suicide in the immediate family, family violence or divorce, incarceration, and prior suicide attempts may also accompany or precipitate depression or thoughts of suicide.

Signs and Symptoms

Depression can manifest in many different ways. Some patients become withdrawn, others appear agitated. Eating behavior and sleeping patterns are affected. The patient may feel fatigued, hopeless, helpless, or worthless, and no longer take pleasure in activities that were once enjoyed. He may become forgetful, have changes in appetite or weight, and experience physical symptoms that have no obvious cause. The patient may have a slowing of normal functions, such as thinking and speech, and often has poor concentration. In severe cases of depression, the patient may come to the attention of medical providers when he or she attempts suicide.

Key findings included the following:

- Flat or depressed affect
- History of depression/suicidal ideation
- Trauma (such as cutting or strangling oneself)
- Ingestion of a toxic substance

Differential Diagnosis

The differential diagnosis for depression includes intoxication, anxiety, abuse or violence, electrolyte abnormality, headache, psychosis, infection, tumor, and other stressors.

Treatment

Initiate supportive interventions, staying alert for a decreasing LOC, especially if the patient is suspected of having taken a drug overdose or has otherwise attempted to commit suicide. In these cases, management of airway, breathing, and circulation are the highest priorities. Provide treatment consistent with the manner in which the patient has attempted suicide. For example, take spinal precautions if the person has attempted hanging or jumping from a height, provide oxygenation for carbon monoxide poisoning, and use trauma packaging in patients with penetrating or blunt trauma. Look for stridor in hanging, deceleration injuries from jumps, and electrolyte and rhythm abnormalities from ingestions. For potential poisonings, monitor the patient's cardiac rhythm and watch for QRS widening on the ECG.

Any suicide attempt should be taken seriously. The patient should not be left alone at any time. It is important to secure the back doors of the ambulance and to make sure the patient does not have easy access to potentially lethal objects in the back of the ambulance.

The patient should be transported to a hospital with psychiatric facilities unless trauma or medical issues are present, or as based on local guidelines. These patients should not be allowed to refuse transport, as they typically do not have the mental capacity to make such decisions. In some cases, police or a third party may elect to initiate the involuntary commitment process in order to ensure full legal authority to transport the patient against his or her will.

Panic Attack/Hyperventilation Syndrome

Panic disorder is a distressing phenomenon for patients. The diagnosis is challenging because it must be made by ruling out other more serious disorders. Asthma, arrhythmia, pneumonia, chronic obstructive pulmonary disease, pneumothorax, pulmonary embolism, and pericarditis are all conditions that may mimic panic disorder. Be sure to consider hormonal disorders such as thyroid storm, pheochromocytoma, and hypoglycemia as well.

Panic disorder is estimated to have a 1% to 5% prevalence in the U.S. population, and it is about twice as prevalent in women as in men. It may be present with other psychiatric illness, such as personality disorder, schizophrenia, or agoraphobia.

Pathophysiology

The underlying cause of panic disorder is psychiatric, that is, a functional disorder in the brain related to an imbalance of neuronal stimulation and neurotransmitter release and uptake. This is a variant of anxiety marked by sudden onset of severe (unfounded) fearfulness.

Signs and Symptoms

A personal or family history of similar episodes may be elicited. Abuse of drugs, especially methamphetamine, cocaine, PCP, ecstasy, and LSD can exacerbate symptoms and the frequency of their occurrence. Over-the-counter (OTC) medications such as caffeine, stimulants, and weight-loss products can also exacerbate the disorder. Key findings include the following:

- Sudden onset of fear or anxiety
- Palpitations
- Shaking
- Dyspnea
- A smothering sensation
- Chest pain or discomfort
- Dizziness
- Light-headedness
- Chills or hot flashes
- A dread of dying

Differential Diagnosis

Many symptoms are similar to those of cardiovascular disease, such as a myocardial infarction and pulmonary embolus. Exclude acute coronary syndromes before narrowing down the diagnoses to a panic attack.

Treatment

A physical exam may show only tachycardia and anxiety. The patient may hyperventilate, but not dramatically. Evaluation is directed at excluding life-threatening illness. Treatment is symptomatic only. Treatment used to include having the patient breathe into a paper bag to limit the amount of carbon dioxide removed from the body, but this remedy is no longer recommended because of the potential to retain excessive CO_2 in patients trying to blow it off, as seen with DKA or metabolic acidosis. Supplemental oxygen should not be necessary, but a dip in oxygen saturation suggests you should investigate other diagnoses.

Putting It All Together

The patient with alterations in mental status or acute neurologic changes is often challenging for healthcare providers. When a person's mental function is altered, it is difficult to obtain an accurate history and perform a reliable examination, so you must be especially observant and astute in looking for diagnostic clues and interpreting the information obtained. After assessing the patient's airway, breathing, and circulation for life threats, it is critically important to check every patient for those fundamental conditions that can be rapidly identified and managed. The SNOT mnemonic may help you do so. Once screening for these threats has been completed, guided by the patient's chief complaint, more detailed evaluation using the SAMPLE/OPQRST mnemonic for history should be carried out, the secondary survey should be conducted, and a differential diagnosis developed. This stepwise process allows prioritization of diagnostic testing and treatment interventions and, in the prehospital setting, determination of the most appropriate transport destination. Repeated reassessment until care is transferred at the receiving facility is particularly important in patients with acute neurologic conditions and accompanying altered mental status.

SCENARIO SOLUTION

© HunThomas/ShutterStock, Inc.

- After you ensure that the patient has a patent airway, is breathing adequately, and has adequate perfusion, you should obtain her vital signs. Your full-body assessment should include examination of her pupils, her vision (including peripheral vision), and her extraocular movements. Ask if she has photophobia. Note any redness, swelling, or tenderness in her temporal area. Evaluate the symmetry of her face. Auscultate her carotid arteries for bruits. Determine if she has any nuchal rigidity. Assess her extremities for pulse, sensory function, and motor strength. Obtain additional history to determine whether she has sustained trauma. Evaluate her medications to obtain clues regarding her past medical history. Perform a stroke scale. Consider other diagnostic tests based on your findings. Blood glucose levels should be checked in *every patient* with any change in mental status or behavior, even if another cause seems obvious.

- Differential diagnosis for this patient could include stroke, intracranial hemorrhage, temporal arteritis, meningitis, and migraine headache.

Summary

- Neurologic disorders can be serious because depressed reflexes leave the airway and other body systems vulnerable.
- The central nervous system has two central structures: the brain and the spinal cord, which account for 98% of all neural tissues of the body.
- Each portion of the brain is responsible for specific functions. The occipital lobe receives and stores images. The temporal lobe makes language and speech possible. The frontal lobe controls voluntary motion. The parietal lobe allows perception of the sensation of touch and pain. The diencephalon filters out unneeded information from the cerebral cortex. The midbrain helps to regulate the level of consciousness. The brainstem regulates the blood pressure, pulse rate, and respiratory rate and pattern. The hypothalamus and pituitary control the release of epinephrine and norepinephrine from the endocrine system. The cerebellum allows unconscious management of complex motor activity.
- The AMLS assessment pathway can be used to rule in or out differential diagnoses based on a patient's cardinal presentation/chief complaint.
- It is critical to determine when the patient was last seen acting normally because the amount of time elapsed since the onset of symptoms will dictate the treatments available.
- The neurologic exam findings will help refine the differential diagnoses.
- A variety of disease processes can cause neurologic dysfunction, including cancer, degenerative conditions, developmental anomalies, infectious diseases, and vascular conditions.
- Most neurologic diseases are thought to be multifactorial—that is, a number of factors combine to induce vulnerability to a particular disease process.
- Physical and emotional supportive care are vital on the scene and en route to the treatment facility.

KEY TERMS

© HunThomas/ShutterStock, Inc.

altered mental status Any decrease in normal level of wakefulness, change in mentation or behavior that is not normal for a particular patient.

amyotrophic lateral sclerosis (ALS) The disease characterized by degeneration of the upper and lower motor neurons, which causes voluntary muscles to weaken or atrophy. Also known as Lou Gehrig disease.

ataxia Loss of coordination of muscle control, which can lead to gait disturbance or extremity clumsiness. May be due to many causes, including peripheral nerve, spinal cord, or brain dysfunction, often of the cerebellum, which controls coordination.

blood brain barrier (BBB) A filtering mechanism of the capillaries that carry blood to the brain and spinal cord tissue, blocking the passage of certain substances.

cerebral perfusion pressure (CPP) Represents the pressure gradient driving cerebral blood flow (CBF) and therefore oxygen and metabolite delivery; it is the difference between the mean arterial pressure (MAP) and the intracranial pressure (ICP). CPP=MAP-ICP.

cerebrospinal fluid (CSF) A transparent, slightly yellowish fluid in the subarachnoid space around the brain and spinal cord.

cerebrovascular accident (CVA) Another term for *stroke*.

convulsion The visual clinical manifestation of a seizure.

Cushing's triad Hypertension, bradycardia, and rapid, deep, or irregular respirations.

dysarthria Garbled speech (but of one's intended words) due to cranial nerve dysfunction (distinguish from expressive and receptive aphasia).

embolus A particle that travels in the circulatory system and obstructs blood flow when it becomes lodged in a smaller artery. A blood clot is the most common type of embolus, but fat (after long bone fracture), atherosclerotic, and air (diving) emboli can also occur.

expressive aphasia Inability to speak intended words due to dysfunction of the cerebral speech center (Broca's area) in the left frontal lobe (distinguish from dysarthria).

hemiparesis Unilateral weakness, usually occurring on the opposite side of the body from the stroke.

hemiplegia Paralysis or severe weakness on one side of the body.

hemorrhagic stroke Damage to the brain from bleeding in the brain tissue (intracerebral) or into the subarachnoid space, usually due to rupture of an aneurysm or arteriovenous malformation.

ischemic stroke A stroke that occurs when a thrombus or embolus obstructs a vessel, diminishing blood flow to part of the brain.

Korsakoff's syndrome Chronic and irreversible condition involving cognitive dysfunction, especially memory loss, due to prolonged thiamine deficiency.

Lou Gehrig disease *See* amyotrophic lateral sclerosis (ALS).

mean arterial pressure (MAP) The average pressure in a patient's arteries during one cardiac cycle, an indicator of perfusion to vital organs; to calculate MAP, double the diastolic blood pressure and add the sum to the systolic blood pressure, then divide by 3.

neurotransmitter A chemical substance that is released at the end of a nerve fiber by the arrival of a nerve impulse (action potential) and, by diffusing across the synapse or junction, causes the transfer of the impulse to another nerve fiber, a muscle fiber, or some other structure.

ophthalmoplegia Abnormal function of the eye muscles.

proprioception Sensory function that provides the awareness of the location of body parts relative to the rest of the body.

seizure A transient occurrence of abnormal excessive or synchronous neuronal activity in the cerebral cortex of the brain that can cause loss of or alteration in consciousness, convulsions or tremors, incontinence, behavior changes, subjective changes in perception (taste, smell, fears), and other symptoms.

stroke Sometimes called a *brain attack* or *cerebrovascular accident* (CVA), a stroke is a brain injury that occurs when blood flow to a part of the brain is obstructed or interrupted, or when bleeding in the brain damages brain cells from increased pressure.

stroke center designation There are currently 4 levels of stroke center designation: Basic Stroke Capable Hospital, Advanced Stroke Capable Hospital, Primary Stroke Center, and Comprehensive Stroke Center. Both Primary and Comprehensive stroke centers are certified by The Joint Commission to be fully capable of delivering acute stroke treatment and rehabilitation services, and are held to higher standards of care and reporting. A Comprehensive Stroke Center is the highest level of stroke center designation and provides, including those services of a Primary Stroke Center, the following:

KEY TERMS (CONTINUED)

© HunThomas/ShutterStock, Inc.

(1) availability of advanced imaging techniques, including MRI/MRA, CTA, DSA, and TCD, (2) availability of personnel trained in vascular neurology, neurosurgery, and endovascular procedures, (3) 24/7 availability of personnel, imaging, operating room, and endovascular facilities, (4) ICU/neuroscience ICU facilities and capabilities, (5) experience and expertise treating

patients with large ischemic strokes, intracerebral hemorrhage, and subarachnoid hemorrhage.

thrombus   A blood clot that forms in a blood vessel.

Wernicke's encephalopathy   A disorder often caused by deficiency of thiamine, or vitamin B_1, and characterized by a triad of symptoms: acute confusion, ataxia, and ophthalmoplegia.

BIBLIOGRAPHY

© HunThomas/ShutterStock, Inc.

American Academy of Orthopaedic Surgeons: *Nancy Caroline's emergency care in the streets*, ed 7. Burlington, MA, 2013, Jones & Bartlett Learning.

American Brain Tumor Association: *About brain tumors. A primer for patients and caregivers*. Des Plaines, IL, 2009, The Association. www.abta.org/index.cfm?contentid=170, modified January 2009.

Arzimanoglu A, Blast T, Jaume C, et al., eds.: Prolonged epileptic seizures: Identification and rescue treatment strategies, *Educational Journal of the International League Against Epilepsy*. Suppl 1(Oct), 2014.

Baslet G: Treatment of psychogenic nonepileptic seizures: Updated review and findings from a mindfulness-based intervention case, *Neuroscience*. December 2, 2014.

Berg AT, Berkovic SF, Brodie MJ, et al.: Revised terminology and concepts for organization of seizures and epilepsies: Report of the ILAE Commission on Classification and Terminology, 2005–2009, *Epilepsia*. 51(4):676, 2010.

Borris DJ, Bertram EH, J: Ketamine controls prolonged status epilepticus, *Epilepsy Res*. 42(2-3):117–122, 2000.

Brandt J, Puente A: Update on psychogenic nonepileptic seizures: Special Reports, Cognitive Behavioral Therapy, Neuropsychiatry, Psychopharmacology, Psychotherapy, Somatoform Disorder. *Psychiatric Times*. February 27, 2015.

Buck ML: Intranasal administration of benzodiazepines for the treatment of acute repetitive seizures in children, *Pediatr Pharm*. 19(10), 2013.

Centers for Disease Control and Prevention: *Suicide: Facts at a glance*. 2012. www.cdc.gov/violenceprevention/pdf/suicide-datasheet-a.pdf

Devinsky O, Cilio MR, Cross H, et al.: Cannabidiol: Pharmacology and potential therapeutic role in epilepsy and other neuropsychiatric disorders, *Epilepsia*. 55(6):791–802, 2014.

England MJ, Liverman CT, Schultz AM, et al., eds.: *Epilepsy across the spectrum: Promoting health and understanding*. Washington, DC, 2012, Institute of Medicine (US) Committee on the Public Health Dimensions of the Epilepsies, National Academies Press (US).

Hackam DG, Kapral MK, Wang JT, et al.: Most stroke patients do not get a warning: A population-based cohort study, *Neurology*. 73:1074, 2009.

Hills D: The psychological and social impact of epilepsy, *Neurology Asia*. 12(Suppl 1):10-12, 2007.

Institute on Aging: *Suicide and the elderly*. San Francisco, CA. https://encore.berkeley-public.org/iii/encore/record/C__Rb1504342__Ssuicide%20and%20the%20elderly__Orightresult__X1?lang=eng&suite=pearl

Kapur J: Prehospital treatment of status epilepticus with benzodiazepines is effective and safe. *Epilepsy Curr*. 2(4):121–124, 2002.

Klein P, Tyrlikova I, Mathews GC: Dietary treatment in adults with refractory epilepsy: A review, *Neurology*. Nov 18;83(21):1978-1985, 2014.

Laccheo I, Sonmezturk H, Bhatt AB, et al.: Non-convulsive status epilepticus and non-convulsive seizures in neurological ICU patients. *Neurocrit Care*. 22(2):202-211, 2015.

Lee J, Huh L, Korn P, et al.: Guidelines for the management of convulsive status epilepticus in infants and children, BCMJ. 53(6):279-285, 2011.

National Institute of Mental Health: *Suicide in the U.S.: Statistics and prevention*. NIH Publication No. 06-4594. www.nimh.nih.gov/health/publications/suicide-in-the-us-statistics-and-prevention/index.shtml, modified July 27, 2009.

National Stroke Association: *National Stroke Association's complete guide to stroke*, Centennial, CO, 2003, The Association.

National Stroke Association: *What is TIA?* www.stroke.org/site/PageServer?pagename=TIA

Pearce JMS: Meningitis, meninges, meninx, *Eur Neurol*. 60:165, 2008. http://content.karger.com/ProdukteDB/produkte.asp?-Doi=145337. doi: 10.1159/000145337.

BIBLIOGRAPHY
(CONTINUED)

© HunThomas/ShutterStock, Inc.

Ruoff G, Urban G: *Standards of care for headache diagnosis and treatment*, Chicago, IL: 2004, National Headache Foundation. www.guideline.gov/summary/summary.aspx?doc_id=6578&nbr=004138&string=migraine

Ryvlin P, Nashef L, Lhatoo SD, et al.: Incidence and mechanisms of cardiorespiratory arrests in epilepsy monitoring units (MORTEMUS): A retrospective study, *Lancet Neurol.* 12(10):966–977, 2013.

Seinfeld S, Shinnar S, Sun S, et al.: Emergency management of febrile status epilepticus: Results of the FEBSTAT study. *Epilepsia.* 55(3):388–395, 2014.

Silbergleit R, Durkalski V, Lowenstein D, et al.: Intramuscular versus intravenous therapy for prehospital status epilepticus, *NEJM.* 366(7):591–600, 2012.

Silbergleit R, Lowenstein D, Durkalski V, et al.: Neurological Emergency Treatment Trials (NETT) Investigators. RAMPART (Rapid Anticonvulsant Medication Prior to Arrival Trial): a double-blind randomized clinical trial of the efficacy of intramuscular midazolam versus intravenous lorazepam in the prehospital treatment of status epilepticus by paramedics, *Epilepsia.* 52 (11;Suppl 8):45-47, 2011.

Substance Abuse and Mental Health Services Administration: *2008 National survey on drug use and health: Suicidal thoughts and behaviors among adults.* September 17, 2009. http://oas.samhsa.gov/2k9/165/Suicide.htm

Theodore W, Spencer S, Wiebe S, et al.: Epilepsy in North America: A report prepared under the auspices of the Global Campaign against Epilepsy, the International Bureau for Epilepsy, the International League Against Epilepsy, and the World Health Organization. ILEA Report, *Epilepsia.* 1–23, 2006.

Thurman DJ, Hesdorffer DC, French JA: Sudden unexpected death in epilepsy: Assessing the public health burden, *Epilepsia.* 55:1–7, 2014.

Vespa PM, McArthur DL, Xu Y, et al.: Nonconvulsive seizures after traumatic brain injury are associated with hippocampal atrophy, *Neurology.* 75(9):792, 2010.

Warden CR, Zibulewsky J, Mace S, et al.: Evaluation and management of febrile seizures in the out-of-hospital and emergency department settings, *Ann Emerg Med.* (Feb)41:2, 2003.

CHAPTER REVIEW QUESTIONS

© HunThomas/ShutterStock, Inc.

1. Which of the following describes a behavior that represents normal mental status? A person who:
   a. Asks you repeatedly what day of the week it is
   b. Does not respond when you call her name, but pushes your hand away when you perform a sternal rub
   c. Is drowsy and slow to respond to questions after awakening from a nap
   d. Is oriented to person, place, and time and has voices telling her she is evil

2. Which assessment evaluates at least one aspect of cranial nerve function?
   a. Blood glucose analysis
   b. Cincinnati Prehospital Stroke Scale
   c. Glasgow Coma Scale
   d. Mini-mental state examination

3. A 72-year-old man had a syncopal episode in church. He is now awake but confused. His wife said he has been complaining of a headache for about a week. He has early Alzheimer's disease. His medications include Lipitor and Exelon (rivastigmine). Which of the following questions may help narrow your differential diagnosis?
   a. Did he fall or hit his head recently?
   b. Does he have any allergies?
   c. Did he take his prescribed medication this morning?
   d. When was he diagnosed with Alzheimer's disease?

4. A 56-year-old woman experiences a sudden onset of headache and blurred vision during yoga class. Her right eyelid is drooping, and the pupil on that side is small compared to the left pupil. You should take her to a hospital with:
   a. A STEMI center
   b. Ophthalmology surgical capability
   c. Psychiatric specialists
   d. Specialized neurologic and vascular capability

5. A 32-year-old man complains of headache and dizziness. He vomited once and is walking with a staggering gait. His blood pressure is 148/72 mm Hg; pulse, 92 beats/min; and respirations, 20 breaths/min.

He has a steady stare up toward his right ear. Which sign or symptom makes you consider an intracerebral hemorrhage more strongly than a migraine headache as a cause of his emergency?

a. Abnormal gaze
b. Blood pressure
c. His age
d. Dizziness and vomiting

6. Which is the most reliable indicator that ventilation should be assisted in a patient with altered mental status?

a. Blood glucose level of 600 mg/dL
b. End-tidal CO_2 of 60 mm Hg
c. Glasgow Coma Scale score of 10
d. Oxygen saturation of 80%

7. A 24-year-old man complains of a sudden explosive headache. He asks you to lower the lights. He has vomited once. Which of these findings would increase your index of suspicion for subarachnoid hemorrhage?

a. Bradycardia
b. Hypotension
c. Pupil dilation
d. Stiff neck

8. Which of the following findings indicates the need to increase the rate of ventilation in an intubated patient you suspect to have an epidural hematoma?

a. Flexion to painful stimulus
b. Hypotension
c. Positive Babinski sign
d. Unilateral blown pupil

9. A 25-year-old woman who was wearing a helmet was thrown from a horse. She is complaining of weakness in her upper extremities. You ask her to close her eyes and identify whether you are moving her thumb up or down. She is unable to do so. This indicates she does not have normal:

a. Fine motor movement
b. Proprioception
c. Sensation of touch
d. Spinal accessory nerve function

10. A 44-year-old man is postictal after a witnessed grand mal seizure. He reacts to light pain and is presently snoring. His vital signs include a blood pressure of 142/86 mm Hg; pulse, 120 beats/min; respirations, 20 breaths/min; and Spo_2, 98%. You should:

a. Assist ventilation with a bag mask
b. Insert a nasopharyngeal airway
c. Prepare to intubate the trachea
d. Place the patient in a supine position

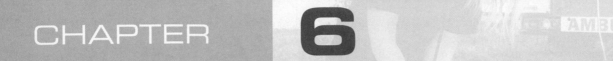

CHAPTER 6

Abdominal Disorders

The causes of abdominal discomfort can have origins in any system of the human body. The severity of a given illness can range from innocuous to dire, yet limited treatment is available in the field. Diagnosing and treating abdominal discomfort requires you to draw on all your skills as a provider. It is essential to identify patients who are critically ill as soon as possible. Patients with abdominal complaints exhibit a wide range of signs and symptoms. Formulating a broad differential diagnosis and then arriving at a working diagnosis is challenging for the most expert of clinicians. This chapter will increase your expertise by examining the clues that add up to an accurate diagnosis, beginning with a review of the gastrointestinal system and the functions of the digestive organs. The signs, symptoms, and treatment of various abdominal disorders you are likely to encounter most often in the field are discussed. Common causes of abdominal discomfort that originate in body systems other than the gastrointestinal system are covered.

LEARNING OBJECTIVES

At the conclusion of this chapter, you will be able to:

- Describe the anatomy and physiology of the following systems as they relate to abdominal disorders: cardiovascular, respiratory, gastrointestinal, genitourinary, reproductive, neurologic, and endocrine.

- List effective ways of obtaining the SAMPLER history and determine how this information will affect patient care.

- Correlate the finding of pain as it relates to abdominal discomfort based on location, referral, and type—visceral or somatic—using the OPQRST mnemonic.

- Apply the AMLS assessment pathway to assist in formulating a differential diagnosis using sound clinical reasoning skills and advanced clinical decision making in caring for patients presenting with abdominal discomfort.

- Evaluate patients for life-threatening conditions during the primary, secondary, and ongoing assessments.

- Apply appropriate treatment modalities for the management, monitoring, and continuing care of patients with abdominal discomfort/disorders.

SCENARIO

You are dispatched to a local tavern for a sick call. When you arrive, a 40-year-old woman is curled up in the fetal position on the floor. Chunky yellow vomitus is pooled beside her and has sprayed onto the nearby wall. Her medical history includes sickle cell disease, hypertension, and high cholesterol. The bartender and other patrons call her by name and say she wasn't herself this evening, but she hates to miss coming in each day. The patient tells you "this is the worst pain I've ever had." As you roll her to her back, she moans loudly and holds her abdomen. Her vital signs include a blood pressure of 98/50 mm Hg; pulse rate, 124 beats/min; and respirations, 24 breaths/min. You note that she is pale, and small beads of sweat have welled up on her forehead.

- What differential diagnoses are you considering based on the information you have now?
- What additional information will you need to narrow your differential diagnosis?
- What are your initial treatment priorities as you continue your patient care?

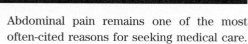

Abdominal pain remains one of the most often-cited reasons for seeking medical care. In 2012, a report from the U.S. Centers for Disease Control and Prevention found that abdominal complaints were second only to chest pain in patients aged 15 years and older. In children younger than 15 years, abdominal complaints are less frequent. Given the varied anatomy and physiology of the **gastrointestinal (GI)** system, the causes of abdominal signs and symptoms are extremely diverse.

Anatomy and Physiology

The GI tract links the organs involved in the consumption, processing, and elimination of nutrients. It begins at the mouth, moves to the esophagus, travels through the chest cavity into the abdomen, and terminates in the pelvic girdle at the rectum. Along this lengthy path, many problems can arise. Patients' complaints are often nonspecific, so arriving at a diagnosis can be challenging even with advanced diagnostic tools at your disposal.

Upper Gastrointestinal Tract

The GI system begins in the mouth with the tongue and salivary glands (**Figure 6-1**). The process of digestion starts with mastication, or chewing. Mastication is the process by which the teeth and saliva break down solid food to facilitate its passage into the esophagus. The next step in digestion takes place in the esophagus, a hollow, muscular organ posterior to the trachea that passes distally through the chest, progresses through the diaphragm, and terminates at the stomach. The muscular wall of the esophagus propels food toward the stomach from the mouth. Because the esophagus lacks a rigid framework, it is easily compressible. At the termination of the esophagus is the lower esophageal sphincter, a muscular band that prevents the reflux of gastric contents from the stomach into the esophagus.

The stomach lies inferior to the diaphragm, just below the left lobe of the liver, and is protected by the rib cage. When empty, the stomach has numerous folds, or rugae, that allow it to expand to accommodate 1 to 1.5 liters of food and fluid. Three layers of smooth muscle enhance its expansion and the processing of food. Glands within the stomach produce digestive enzymes to aid digestion and protect the body from potentially harmful microorganisms that enter with the food. The speed at which the stomach empties its contents into the lower digestive tract, known as the "rate of gastric emptying," depends on the type and amount of food ingested and on other factors such as the person's age and medical condition.

Lower Gastrointestinal Tract

Digestion continues from the stomach into the small intestine, the first structure in the lower GI tract. When stretched out, the small intestine is about 22 feet long, but in the body it is looped tightly within the relatively small abdominal cavity. The duodenum, the jejunum, and the ileum are the three sections of the small intestine. The duodenum extends from the stomach. At just a foot in length, it is the shortest portion of the small intestine. The duodenum receives the semifluid, partially digested stomach contents, or chyme, as well as exocrine secretions from the liver and pancreas. The jejunum is about 8 feet long and is responsible for most of the chemical digestion and absorption of nutrients. The ileum is the final section of the small bowel and is the longest section at 13 feet. It is responsible for nutrient absorption as well. The large intestine includes the cecum, colon, and rectum. The cecum is a pouch that receives the products of digestion from the small intestine. The vermiform appendix attaches to the cecum. The large intestine is primarily responsible for the reabsorption of water and absorption of vitamins. The rectum is responsible for expelling stool.

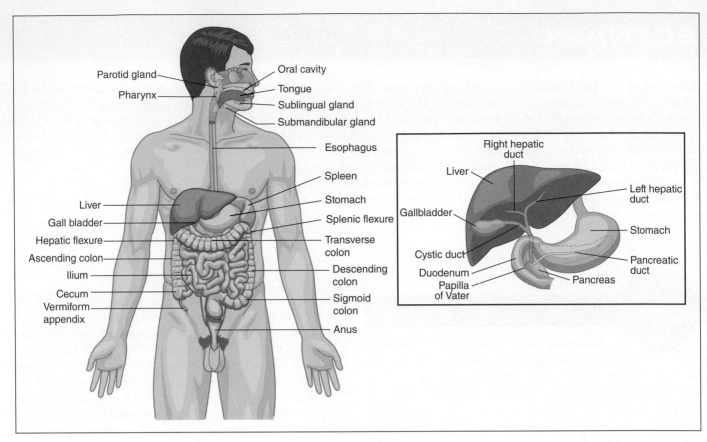

Figure 6-1 Digestive organs.

Accessory Organs

Liver The liver lies in the right upper quadrant of the abdominal cavity distal to the diaphragm. The specific functions of the liver are broad and include bile production and metabolic and hematologic regulation. The liver performs more than 200 functions in the body, several of which are listed in **Table 6-1**.

The liver is a dense, heavy organ, weighing about 1.5 kg (3.3 lb). It is divided into left and right lobes made up of lobules, masses of cells that comprise the basic structural units of the liver. The liver contains about 100,000 lobules. It is an

extremely vascular organ. In fact, as the largest reservoir of blood in the body, even a small laceration can cause extensive blood loss.

Gallbladder The gallbladder is a pear-shaped organ housed below the liver. Its function is to modify and store bile. Excessive precipitation of bile salts can cause painful gallstones to form.

Pancreas The pancreas lies posterior to the stomach between the first part of the duodenum and the spleen in the midepigastric area, joining the common bile duct and emptying into the duodenum. It functions in digestion as an exocrine organ, secreting digestive enzymes, bicarbonate, electrolytes, and water. The

Table 6-1 **Functions of the Liver**		
Metabolic	**Hematologic**	**Other Major Functions**
Extraction of nutrients from blood	Removal of aged or damaged red blood cells	Secretion of bile
Extraction of toxins from blood	Synthesis of plasma proteins	Absorption and breakdown of hormones
Removal and storage of excess nutrients such as glucose	Synthesis of clotting factors	
Maintenance of normal glucose levels		
Storage of vitamins		

pancreas performs an endocrine function that is not directly involved in digestion by secreting the following:

- Glucagon, to raise glucose levels
- Insulin, to promote movement of glucose into the tissues
- Somatostatin, to regulate other endocrine cells in the pancreatic islets

Functions of the Gastrointestinal System

To process or digest nutrients effectively, the four chief functions of the GI system—motility, secretion, digestion, and absorption—must be intact. These functions require a complex interaction among the nervous system, the endocrine system, the musculoskeletal system, and the cardiovascular system.

Motility

Food progresses through the GI tract by a process called *motility*. This process also mixes food components and reduces particle size so food can be digested and nutrients absorbed. A structured, coordinated muscular response known as "peristalsis" is required for the process to be successful. The neurologic system—specifically, the sympathetic and parasympathetic nervous systems—orchestrates this effort.

The vagus nerve, part of the parasympathetic nervous system, innervates the GI tract to the level of the transverse colon. This nerve plays a pivotal role in gastric emptying by affecting the motility of the GI tract by controlling the contraction and dilation of sphincters and smooth muscle. In addition, the nerve has a secretory function and helps stimulate vomiting. Bradycardia is often present when a person vomits because the vagus nerve also helps regulate the heart rate. The pelvic nerve stimulates the descending colon, sigmoid colon, rectum, and anal canal. The vagus and pelvic nerves innervate the striated muscle in the upper third of the esophagus and the external anal sphincter.

The sympathetic nervous system focuses on the major ganglia (celiac, superior mesenteric, inferior mesenteric, and hypogastric), the secretory and endocrine cells.

Secretion

The digestive tract is lined with cells that secrete fluids to aid in motility and digestion. These cells secrete up to 9 liters of water, acids, buffers, electrolytes, and enzymes in a 24-hour period. A majority of this fluid is reabsorbed, but when diarrhea occurs and is severe or extended, significant fluid loss can occur, and dehydration and shock may ensue.

Digestion

Digestion is the process of breaking down food into components to be used for nutrition for the body at the cellular level. Digestion involves the mechanical and chemical breakdown of the food we ingest.

Absorption

The small intestine is the primary site for absorption of fluid and nutrients, and the large intestine is the primary site of absorption of water and salts.

Pain

The most common GI complaint is abdominal pain. Despite or perhaps because of the frequency of the complaint, determining its cause can challenge even a seasoned healthcare provider. Often the complaint of abdominal pain is vague and ill defined. To obtain the necessary information from the patient and arrive at a diagnosis, you must know GI system pathophysiology and understand how to take a history and perform an assessment in a reassuring and supportive way. Because an accurate diagnosis is not always immediately apparent, patients can become frustrated and feel as if you don't believe them. Establishing an environment of trust can allow you to acquire much needed information, including precipitating factors and a description of additional symptoms that may point to a probable diagnosis.

The very young and the elderly may have difficulty relaying pain to clinicians. Both have a different perception of pain, and both localize pain differently. Older adult patients may get confused about where pain actually originates and often live with chronic pain that may affect their perception. Pediatric patients poorly localize the exact pain location and may have difficulty verbalizing their pain.

One complicating factor in the diagnosis of abdominal pain is that the perception of discomfort varies widely, depending on its cause and the patient's individual level of tolerance. In addition, abdominal pain often evolves over time, becoming better defined as the disease process progresses. Abdominal pain can be divided into three categories: visceral pain, parietal pain, and referred pain.

Visceral Pain

Visceral pain occurs when the walls of the hollow organs are stretched, thereby activating the stretch receptors. This kind of pain is characterized by a deep, persistent ache ranging from mild to intolerable. Common descriptors include cramping, burning, and gnawing.

Visceral pain is difficult to localize, since the abdominal organs transmit pain signals to both sides of the spinal cord, but it's typically felt in the epigastric, periumbilical, or suprapubic region. Epigastric visceral pain typically comes from the stomach, gallbladder, liver, duodenum, or pancreas. Periumbilical pain tends to be related to the appendix, small bowel, or cecum, while suprapubic pain arises from the kidneys, ureters, bladder, colon, uterus, or ovaries (**Figure 6-2**).

The patient may have trouble finding a comfortable position, so he or she will shift frequently or need to be adjusted during transport. Depending on the cause, diaphoresis, nausea, vomiting, restlessness, or pallor may be present. Table 6-2 outlines a small number of the possible differential diagnosis of abdominal discomfort in patients with nausea and vomiting.

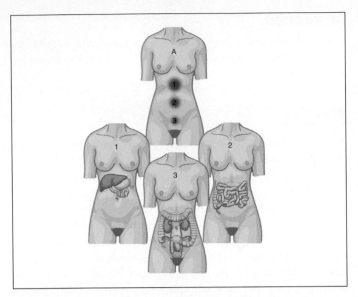

Figure 6-2 Localization of visceral pain. Pain arising from organ areas depicted in 1, 2, and 3 is felt in the epigastrium, midabdomen, and hypogastrium, respectively, as shown in A.

Somatic (Parietal) Pain

Somatic (parietal) pain is caused by an irritation of the nerve fibers in the parietal peritoneum or other deep tissues, such as those of the musculoskeletal system. The origin of somatic pain is easier to pinpoint than visceral pain. Physical findings include sharp, discrete, localized pain accompanied by tenderness to palpation, guarding of the affected area, and rebound tenderness.

Somatic pain usually emerges later in the disease process. Since the parietal peritoneum surrounds the organs involved, it takes longer for the affected structures to become irritated and painful. The dorsal root ganglia in the spine activate peritoneal pain, so the pain is typically on the same side and in the same dermatome as the affected organ. Dermatomes represent the relationship between the spinal nerve and portion of the body they innervate (**Figure 6-3**).

Referred Pain

When pain emanates from a site other than that of its origin, it is said to be **referred pain**. In other words, the pain is "referred" from its origin to another location. Overlapping neural pathways

Table 6-2 Differential Diagnosis of Abdominal Discomfort with Nausea and Vomiting

			Neurologic		
Intracerebral bleeding	Bleeding within the brain tissue	Trauma, stroke, hypertension, smoking, alcohol abuse	Hemiparesis, hemiplegia, nausea, headache, altered level of consciousness, Cushing's triad	CTA, CBC, coagulation studies, electrolytes, glucose	Maintain airway. Administer oxygen. Establish IV access. Place a 12-lead ECG.
Meningitis	Bacterial, viral, or fungal infection of the meninges	—	High fever, headache, stiff neck, seizures Resembles flu Can progress over several days	CBC, electrolytes, blood cultures, lumbar puncture	Maintain airway. Administer oxygen. Place a 12-Lead ECG. Establish IV access. Administer isotonic fluid. Give antibiotics if the infection is bacterial.
			Cardiac		
Acute MI	Necrosis of the heart muscle	Coronary artery disease, smoking, high cholesterol, history of MI	Chest, midepigastric, back, and neck pain Nausea Difficulty breathing	Serial 12-lead ECG, x-ray, CBC, coagulation studies, electrolytes	Administer oxygen. Establish IV access. Administer nitroglycerin, ASA, and anticoagulants. Angiography will be performed at the receiving facility. For hypotension, use caution with the administration of nitroglycerin and consider RV, MI, and 15 lead for normal or nondiagnostic findings.

(continues)

(continued)

Table 6-2 Differential Diagnosis of Abdominal Discomfort with Nausea and Vomiting (*continued*)

Gastrointestinal

Boerhaave's syndrome	Spontaneous rupture of the esophagus	Explosive vomiting, coughing, seizures, childbirth, status asthmaticus	Pain in the chest, neck, back, or abdomen Difficulty breathing, tachycardia, hematemesis, fever, subcutaneous emphysema	CBC, coagulation studies, type and cross-match	Treat airway compromise, hypoxia, and shock. Surgery will be performed at the receiving facility.
Mallory-Weiss tear	Longitudinal tears in the esophageal mucosa, causing severe arterial bleeding	Severe, protracted vomiting, bleeding	Severe, protracted vomiting Bleeding	Bronchoscopy, CBC, coagulation studies, type and cross-match	Treat airway compromise and shock, administer oxygen, and establish IV access. Gastric lavage and possibly surgery will be performed at the receiving facility.
Upper GI bleeding	Bleeding proximal to the junction of the duodenum and jejunum	Hematemesis (vomiting blood that is bright red or resembles coffee grounds), alcohol abuse, use of NSAIDs, liver disease, varices	Abdominal pain Red or coffee-colored vomitus or stool	Chest and abdominal x-rays, angiography CBC, Hct, Hb, PTT, platelets, coagulation studies, type and cross-match, etc.) Nasogastric tube, endoscopy	Administer oxygen. Perform an ECG. Establish IV access. Treat shock. Administer blood products.
Ischemic bowel	Necrosis of the GI tract	Severe abdominal pain, sick appearance, hypercoagulability, recent surgery, shock	Abdominal pain, tachycardia, hypotension, fever, restlessness	CBC, coagulation studies, electrolytes, type and cross-match	Administer oxygen. Perform an ECG. Establish IV access. Treat shock. Radiography and CT imaging and surgery will be performed at the receiving facility.

Endocrine

Diabetic ketoacidosis	Hyperglycemia, ketosis, and acidosis	Diabetes, especially type 1, but can occur in patients with type 2 diabetes who are ill	Nausea, vomiting, polydipsia, polyuria, abdominal pain, metabolic acidosis	Blood glucose, serum electrolytes, arterial blood gas analysis, CBC	Administer oxygen. Establish IV access. Administer isotonic fluids and insulin as indicated.

ASA, acetylsalicylic acid; CBC, complete blood count; CT, computed tomography; CTA, computed tomography angiography; ECG, electrocardiogram; GI, gastrointestinal; Hb, hemoglobin; Hct, hematocrit; IV, intravenous; MI, myocardial infarction; NSAIDs, nonsteroidal antiinflammatory drugs; PTT, partial thromboplastin time.

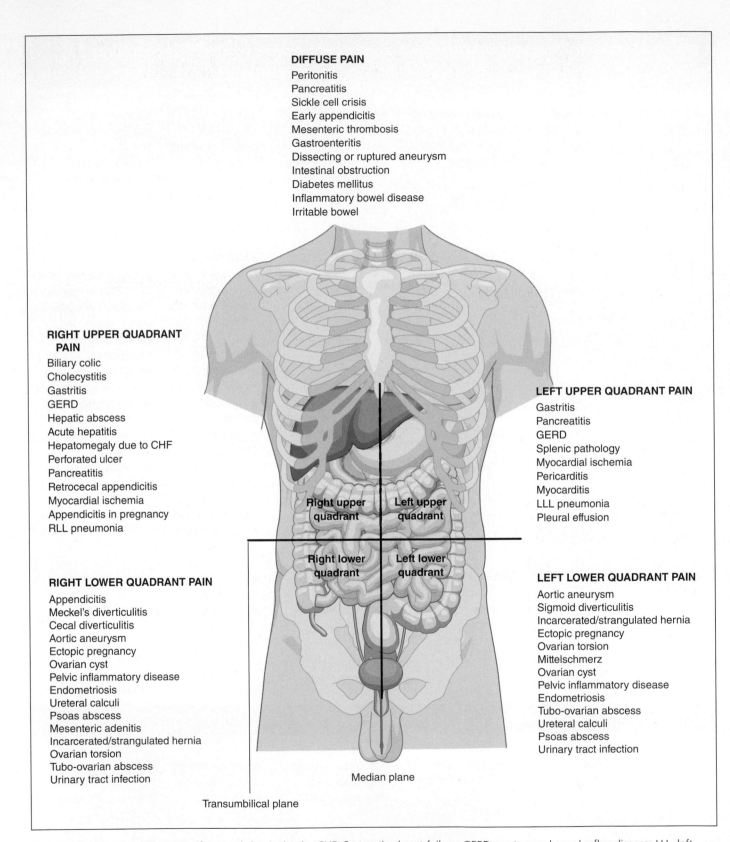

DIFFUSE PAIN
Peritonitis
Pancreatitis
Sickle cell crisis
Early appendicitis
Mesenteric thrombosis
Gastroenteritis
Dissecting or ruptured aneurysm
Intestinal obstruction
Diabetes mellitus
Inflammatory bowel disease
Irritable bowel

RIGHT UPPER QUADRANT PAIN
Biliary colic
Cholecystitis
Gastritis
GERD
Hepatic abscess
Acute hepatitis
Hepatomegaly due to CHF
Perforated ulcer
Pancreatitis
Retrocecal appendicitis
Myocardial ischemia
Appendicitis in pregnancy
RLL pneumonia

LEFT UPPER QUADRANT PAIN
Gastritis
Pancreatitis
GERD
Splenic pathology
Myocardial ischemia
Pericarditis
Myocarditis
LLL pneumonia
Pleural effusion

Right upper quadrant   Left upper quadrant

Right lower quadrant   Left lower quadrant

RIGHT LOWER QUADRANT PAIN
Appendicitis
Meckel's diverticulitis
Cecal diverticulitis
Aortic aneurysm
Ectopic pregnancy
Ovarian cyst
Pelvic inflammatory disease
Endometriosis
Ureteral calculi
Psoas abscess
Mesenteric adenitis
Incarcerated/strangulated hernia
Ovarian torsion
Tubo-ovarian abscess
Urinary tract infection

LEFT LOWER QUADRANT PAIN
Aortic aneurysm
Sigmoid diverticulitis
Incarcerated/strangulated hernia
Ectopic pregnancy
Ovarian torsion
Mittelschmerz
Ovarian cyst
Pelvic inflammatory disease
Endometriosis
Tubo-ovarian abscess
Ureteral calculi
Psoas abscess
Urinary tract infection

Median plane

Transumbilical plane

Figure 6-3 Differential diagnosis of acute abdominal pain. CHF, Congestive heart failure; GERD, gastroesophageal reflux disease; LLL, left lower lobe; RLL, right lower lobe.

From Marx JA, Hockberger RS, Walls RM, et al.: *Rosen's emergency medicine*, ed 7, St Louis, 2009, Mosby

are responsible for this phenomenon. For example, referred pain often accompanies cholecystitis, in which the patient usually feels pain in the right scapular area. It is also common in myocardial infarction, in which pain is referred to the neck, jaw, or arm.

AMLS Assessment Pathway

▼ Initial Observations

Scene Safety Considerations

Your field impression begins when you receive the dispatch information related to an abdominal complaint. Multiple patients are not a common occurrence with GI patients. When you arrive on scene, you'll be able to determine how well your field impression agrees with your initial observations. A call for assistance to an office building where several patients are reporting abdominal pain, for example, should lead you to consider a scene where a chemical or biologic agent has been released.

Follow standard precautions. Bleeding, nausea, and vomiting are hazards associated with abdominal pain and require you to use personal protective equipment to shield yourself from exposure to body fluids. In addition to gloves, gowns, and masks, the following equipment is essential to providing good patient hygiene while maintaining personal safety:

- Eye protection
- Towels and wash rags
- Extra linens
- Absorbent pads
- Emesis basin
- Disposable basin
- Biohazard bags
- Sterile water for irrigation

Proper cleaning and maintenance of equipment and uniforms soiled during a call are essential to ensuring the health of the EMS crew and the health of the patient.

Immediately address any apparent life-threatening emergencies. The primary life threat associated with abdominal discomfort is shock caused by hemorrhage, dehydration, or sepsis, as in the following circumstances:

- Internal bleeding due to a ruptured aneurysm, GI bleeding, or ectopic pregnancy
- Dehydration caused by vomiting or diarrhea from a wide range of causes
- Sepsis secondary to a ruptured appendix, an infection from an indwelling catheter, or perforated bowel

If no life threat is present, focus your assessment on identifying the cardinal presentation/chief complaint.

Patient Cardinal Presentation/Chief Complaint

Signs and symptoms associated with a range of critical, emergent, and nonemergent abdominal disorders are summarized in Table 6-3. Gather clues during your assessment and combine them to build a differential diagnosis.

Primary Survey

Your main goals are observation of standard precautions, maintenance of ABCs, and management of pain/nausea. Once you have addressed airway, breathing, and circulation, begin to narrow down your list of potential diagnoses, and continue your assessment. The patient presentation will dictate your next actions. If you have the resources to perform a more detailed assessment as you stabilize the patient's condition, then do so, but further assessment should not be done before stabilization of the patient's ABCs.

Level of Consciousness

Observing the patient's level of consciousness (LOC) can help you gauge the severity of the problem. Patients who are confused, pale, and diaphoretic may be critically ill. Pain causes some patients to pace and show other signs of agitation. Many GI complaints are associated with pain or hemorrhage, which can diminish the patient's LOC. Someone who is talking is providing you with foundational physiologic information. Talking means an open airway. To talk, the patient must also be breathing, have adequate blood pressure to maintain brain activity, and have a sufficient blood glucose level.

Airway and Breathing

Airway patency becomes more pertinent in a patient with abdominal problems. A patient who is vomiting has a greater chance of aspiration. Closely inspect the airway for foreign bodies. Remove or suction obstructions. Note any unusual odors from the mouth. Patients who have extremely advanced bowel obstructions can have breath that smells of stool.

Breathing is rarely affected by GI problems. If a breathing problem is encountered, it typically stems from a severe complication. Once you ensure the airway is clear, your ability to oxygenate and ventilate the patient will not be impaired.

Circulation/Perfusion

An assessment of the circulatory system is essential in understanding the impact of GI disease on the body. As with all patients, assess skin color, temperature, and moisture. Note any findings that indicate shock. Determine the patient's pulse rate. Evaluate the peripheral pulses and how they compare with central pulses.

Many GI disorders involve pain or hemorrhage. As the patient's blood volume begins to drop, the body compensates by releasing catecholamines (epinephrine and norepinephrine) to vasoconstrict the periphery, increase the pulse rate, and increase the force of left ventricular contraction. Pain stimulates similar body responses. Either problem can leave the patient with tachycardia, diminished peripheral pulses, diaphoresis, and pale, cool, and clammy skin.

When you are examining patients for gross bleeding, it is not unusual to find large amounts of blood. Take note of the amount of blood lost; patients often exaggerate the volume of blood lost.

Table 6-3 Critical, Emergent, and Nonemergent Disorders with Abdominal Signs and Symptoms

Disorder	Signs and Symptoms
Critical	
Gastrointestinal	
Boerhaave's syndrome	Pain, nausea/vomiting, bleeding
Ischemic bowel	Pain, nausea/vomiting, diarrhea
Mallory-Weiss tear	Pain, nausea/vomiting, bleeding
Upper gastrointestinal tract bleeding	Pain, nausea/vomiting, bleeding
Fulminant hepatic failure	Pain, nausea/vomiting, jaundice
Cholangitis	Pain, nausea/vomiting, jaundice
Neurologic	
Intracerebral bleeding	Nausea/vomiting
Meningitis	Nausea/vomiting
Cardiac	
Acute myocardial infarction	Pain, nausea/vomiting
Budd-Chiari syndrome	Pain, nausea/vomiting, jaundice
Severe congestive heart failure	Jaundice
Obstructing aortic aneurysm	Jaundice
Endocrine	
Diabetic ketoacidosis	Pain, nausea/vomiting
Reproductive	
Preeclampsia/HELLP	Jaundice
Placenta abruptio	Pain, vaginal bleeding
Placenta previa	Vaginal bleeding
Emergent	
Gastrointestinal	
Gastric outlet obstruction	Pain, nausea/vomiting
Mesenteric ischemia	Pain, nausea/vomiting, diarrhea

(continues)

Table 6-3 Critical, Emergent, and Nonemergent Disorders with Abdominal Signs and Symptoms (*continued*)

Disorder	Signs and Symptoms
Gastrointestinal	
Intestinal obstruction	Pain, nausea/vomiting, constipation, diarrhea
Bowel perforation	Pain, nausea/vomiting, constipation
Perforated viscus	Pain, nausea/vomiting, bleeding
Pancreatitis	Pain, nausea/vomiting
Ruptured appendix	Pain, nausea/vomiting
Peritonitis	Pain, nausea/vomiting
Crohn's disease	Pain, nausea/vomiting
Ulcerative colitis	Pain, nausea/vomiting, diarrhea
Cholelithiasis	Pain, nausea/vomiting
Neurologic	
Central nervous system tumor	Nausea/vomiting
Endocrine	
Adrenal insufficiency	Pain, nausea/vomiting, diarrhea
Reproductive	
Hyperemesis gravidarum	Nausea/vomiting
Genitourinary	
Testicular torsion	Pain, nausea/vomiting
Nonemergent	
Gastrointestinal	
Hepatitis	Pain, nausea/vomiting, diarrhea, jaundice
Gastroenteritis	Pain, nausea/vomiting, diarrhea
Irritable bowel syndrome	Pain, nausea/vomiting, constipation, diarrhea
Diverticulitis/diverticulosis	Pain, bleeding, constipation, diarrhea
Inflammatory bowel syndrome	Pain, nausea/vomiting, bleeding, diarrhea

▼ First Impression

The fundamental determination you must make in the field is whether the patient's condition is life threatening, as evidenced by abnormal vital signs or respiratory distress. Patients who exhibit either one must be rapidly treated and transported to an appropriate facility.

The following list gives a review of the management of life-threatening abdominal complaints after the scene has been determined to be safe and personal protective equipment is donned:

- Manage the airway as necessary using appropriate basic life support techniques. Maintain the patient's oxygen saturation at > 95% by administering additional oxygen through a nonrebreathing mask or by assisting ventilation as necessary.
- Apply a cardiac monitor (consistent with your level of training), and consider placing a serial 12-lead ECG if appropriate.
- Control obvious hemorrhage. Use gastric suctioning if indicated.
- Establish IV access and administer crystalloid fluid. Use care, however, because aggressive fluid administration can dilute the concentration of red blood cells and impede clot formation if bleeding is present. Blood pressure should be maintained at a level vigorous enough to perfuse vital organs. Use a target systolic pressure of 80–90 mm Hg. Use mental status as a gauge to assess whether perfusion is adequate.
- Administer medications per local protocol.
- Monitor the patient closely, and reassess frequently to determine the response.
- Be prepared to administer blood products if the patient shows evidence of uncontrolled bleeding or an inability to maintain adequate perfusion.
- Consider placing a Foley catheter.
- A nasogastric tube should be placed if GI bleeding is suspected. Although an aspirate that does not contain blood does not conclusively rule out upper GI bleeding, placement is still necessary. The majority of the patients require only supportive care.

If the situation is not life threatening, when you see the patient, closely examine where he or she is found. The patient's body posture or position can give you hints as to what happened. Has the patient been in bed sick for several days? Was the patient at work when a sudden bout of pain caused him or her to double over? Look to the environment for clues as to the length and degree of illness the patient is experiencing.

One aspect of your first impression of the patient with an abdominal disorder is odor. Note the smell of the room. Foul-smelling stool is often present in these disorders. Also examine the patient's living conditions. This information can help you determine whether the problem is chronic or acute and can suggest whether the patient's emergency is isolated to the GI system.

Many people with GI complaints have long-standing medical problems, so the information provided can assist you in generating an initial differential diagnosis.

▼ Detailed Assessment

History Taking

OPQRST and SAMPLER

Gathering an accurate, detailed history is essential with any patient but especially important when caring for patients with GI complaints. It can be challenging to obtain useful information, but keeping in mind the SAMPLER and OPQRST mnemonics will help you remember to ask the right questions. Demonstrating patience and taking a genuine interest in the patient will improve your rapport with him or her. Table 6-4 points out involvement of body systems for patients with abdominal discomfort. Table 6-5 lists clinical signs associated with selected abdominal disorders. Any abdominal complaint should also prompt you to ask about appetite, bowel regimen, urine, menstrual history, and discharge from reproductive organs as you gather the patient's history.

Secondary Survey

Pain Assessment

In evaluating GI complaints, your assessment must include a detailed appraisal of the patient's pain. Abdominal pain is often diffuse and difficult to categorize, and documenting it methodically can help you refine your diagnosis. The initial task is to ascertain the origin of the pain and determine its referral sites (see Figure 6-2; Figure 6-4). Knowing the time of onset will help you assess how the pain has evolved, which may indicate the severity of the illness. Be alert for any signs that typically accompany pain, such as vomiting.

Document pain in the patient's own words because they may be more revealing than the words a healthcare professional might use. Ask open-ended questions—What does your pain feel like? Can you describe your pain? Encourage candid responses, which may range from "It hurts" to "It feels like I'm being shredded apart." If the person is unable to describe the pain, offer a few helpful descriptions. Ask, is it sharp, tearing, hot, burning, dull? Ask what activities or movements worsen or improve the pain, noting any home remedies or corrective measures that were attempted even if they were ineffective.

Using a pain scale allows you to compare the patient's pain over time. People have widely different levels of pain tolerance depending on cultural norms and their own pain thresholds. The best use of a pain scale, therefore, is not in determining the severity of pain, which is largely subjective, but in tracking any improvements or worrisome trends. Ask the patient frequently to reassess the pain, taking care to document the response, and trust the patient's statements about his or her symptoms.

Table 6-4 Selected System Considerations for Assessment of Abdominal Complaints

System	History, Differential Diagnosis, and Other Assessment Considerations
Neurologic	Ask about recent accidents or trauma, particularly if the patient has an altered level of consciousness or nausea and vomiting.
Respiratory	Explore any evidence of breathing problems. Pneumonia may be associated with upper abdominal discomfort. Esophageal ruptures may present with respiratory signs and symptoms.
Cardiovascular	Indigestion and upper abdominal discomfort should prompt you to evaluate the patient for acute coronary syndrome.
Gastrointestinal, genitourinary, and reproductive	Explore any history of chronic or acute diagnoses. Question the patient about any changes in eating, bowel, or urinary habits that may suggest a diagnosis. Vaginal discharge, bleeding, and menstrual changes suggest specific disease processes.
Musculoskeletal and skin	Observe the skin for pallor, jaundice, uremia, and other changes that may suggest the cause of abdominal pain. Look for any scars, ostomies, or external devices (such as drains, tubes, and pumps) that may indicate the cause of the patient's abdominal symptoms.
Endocrine, metabolic, and environmental	Collect past medical history. Assess blood glucose level. Assess the scene or thoroughly question the patient, family, and bystanders if you are unable to observe the conditions to which the patient was subjected.
Infectious disease and hematologic	The patient's history, a foul smell, and the presence of a Foley catheter or other invasive drain may point to an infectious process. Take the patient's temperature to evaluate for fever. Assess the patient for damage to the bowel, which is associated with peritonitis and possibly sepsis. Analyze lab values that may be useful in making a hematologic diagnosis, such as white blood cell count, hemoglobin and hematocrit, prothrombin time, and partial thromboplastin time.
Toxicologic (nuclear, biological, and chemical)	Explore exposure problems. Many toxidromes have a GI component. Being familiar with a range of toxidromes and maintaining a high index of suspicion will prevent you from overlooking them in your differential diagnosis.

Physical Assessment

Analysis of the patient's vital signs is critical to making a reliable diagnosis. Fever, for example, indicates that an infection may be present; typically, a temperature of 100.3°F (38°C) or greater is considered significant. This rule does not apply, however, to older adults or to patients with compromised immune systems. In such patients, a serious infection may be present even if the patient's body temperature is normal. Low blood pressure and a rapid heart rate can point to hypovolemia. The heart rate may accelerate as body temperature rises, except in patients who take beta-blockers, because such agents reduce the heart rate. An elevated respiratory rate can be a red flag portending serious illness such as pneumonia, myocardial infarction, sepsis, or hypoperfusion.

Perform a systematic, thorough physical examination. The examination, though, can be a difficult experience for the patient.

No one likes to be poked and prodded, but discomfort or unpleasantness is magnified in the face of the anxiety often associated with illness and injury. An already uncomfortable patient may worry that the exam will be painful. Preparing the patient by explaining the procedure first may diminish uncertainty and improve cooperation.

Physical examination skills include inspection, auscultation, percussion, and palpation.

Inspection

Examination of the abdomen should always begin with inspection, because any palpation can alter the abdomen's general appearance and may provoke the patient's pain, after which further palpation may be hampered by guarding. Look for distention, pulsation, ecchymosis, asymmetry, pregnancy, scars, masses, and anything else unusual.

Table 6-5 Clinical Signs Associated with Selected Abdominal Disorders

Sign	Description	Differential Diagnosis
Hematemesis	Blood in vomitus	Upper GI bleeding
Coffee-ground emesis	Vomiting of partially digested blood	GI bleeding
Feculent vomiting	Foul-smelling vomit with a feculent odor	Bowel obstruction
Hematochezia	Red blood passed through the rectum	Lower GI bleeding
Melena	Black, tarry stool that contains digested blood	Upper GI bleeding
Hemoccult blood in stool	Laboratory identification of blood in the stool that's not obvious to the naked eye	Lower GI bleeding
White stools	White, chalky stool	Liver or gallbladder disease
Hematuria	Blood in the urine	Bladder infection Kidney disease Trauma

GI, Gastrointestinal.

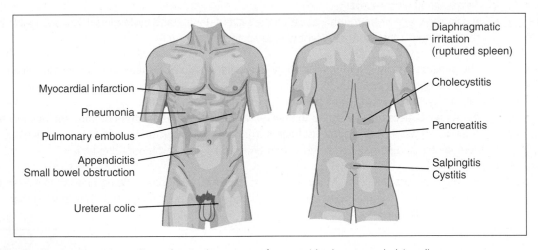

Figure 6-4 Referred pain patterns. Pain or discomfort in these areas often provide clues to underlying disease processes.

Auscultation

Auscultation is the second step in the general physical examination. Palpating the abdomen before listening to it can alter the findings by stirring bowel sounds. If time and circumstances allow, auscultate each quadrant of the abdomen for about 30 seconds. Normal bowel sounds sound like water gurgling. Without experience, it is difficult to tell whether these sounds are normal or abnormal. Hyperactive bowel sounds may signal gastroenteritis or early bowel obstruction. Hypoactive or silent bowel sounds in one quadrant can indicate an ileus. It may be impossible, however, to hear abdominal sounds in a noisy environment like the back of an ambulance. To thoroughly assess bowel sounds, an extended auscultation time period of up to 5 minutes in each quadrant is required. A shortened time is often used in the field, however, or the sounds are not auscultated because it is impractical. If a shortened auscultation time is used, it does not mean bowel sounds are absent; it means the bowel sounds may not have been heard at that time.

Percussion

Abdominal percussion indicates whether certain areas contain more gas or liquid. Borders of organs and masses may also be determined using percussion. Like auscultation, percussion requires practice. Before you perform any palpation or percussion of the abdomen, make sure the patient understands what you are doing. The procedure is easier for the patient to tolerate and produces less anxiety if you begin with the unaffected side and then progress to the areas of discomfort. Pain and tenderness may present with percussion and should be noted.

Palpation

It is important that the patient is relaxed during palpation, because abdominal rigidity and guarding caused by anxiety can make the findings less reliable. Encourage your patient to relax. During palpation of each quadrant, watch the reaction on the patient's face, and ask how the patient feels. Ideally, the patient will be distracted, and you can watch for signs of discomfort. Grimacing or tears may reveal more than verbal complaints. Attempt to elicit differences in pain before, during, and after palpation. Pain when the pressure is released, known as "rebound tenderness," is a classic sign of peritoneal irritation, but it is present in up to 25% of patients with nonspecific abdominal complaints. In some areas, clinicians may be discouraged in eliciting rebound tenderness, as the patient may be resistant to further abdominal assessment. Tapping on the heel or coughing may elicit similar pain. Each of these activities jars or stimulates the irritated peritoneum and can help to isolate the pain.

Diagnostics

With point-of-service lab testing a reality, EMS providers are now able to determine laboratory findings at the scene in as little as 3 minutes. If the function of the GI system is impaired, its ability to eliminate waste will be impaired as well. Sodium and potassium levels in particular can change rapidly and must be monitored. Handheld blood analyzers allow paramedics to test these levels in the back of the ambulance. Finding chemical imbalances early gives EMS providers needed information to institute preventive care. Laboratory parameters often measured in patients with abdominal complaints are summarized in Table 6-6. Table 6-7 summarizes radiologic studies used to diagnose abdominal disorders.

At the hospital, specific laboratory tests performed will include a complete blood count (hematocrit, coagulation studies, serum urea nitrogen, creatinine, electrolytes, glucose, liver function, and blood type and cross-match). Imaging studies will include CT and possibly endoscopy. For a critically ill patient, however, resuscitation takes precedence.

Ultrasonography and intra-abdominal pressure testing are two additional tools that may be available to the EMS provider; however, research does not support their use in the prehospital setting at this time. They are typically seen in the critical care transport setting.

▼ Refine the Differential Diagnosis

The components of the primary and secondary survey will help you refine your differential diagnoses and determine the severity of the patient's condition. Manage any life threats as they appear during the assessment process. Remember that most diseases or conditions are caused by more than one factor. The specific conditions described later and in Table 6-8 will provide an approach for helping you determine the differential diagnosis and recognize key findings.

▼ Ongoing Management

Monitor your patient for changes in condition. Routine monitoring should include pulse rate, ECG, blood pressure, respiratory rate, and pulse oximetry. If the patient has GI bleeding, continue to assess for signs of shock. Document the patient's response to treatment.

Choosing the appropriate method of transport for a patient with a GI complaint can be complicated. First you must decide whether the patient is critically ill and determine which modes of transportation the patient can tolerate. Altitude changes during flight can cause severe pain unless the pressure is relieved. The GI system contains a large amount of air. Under

---

Table 6-6 Laboratory Studies for the Diagnosis of Abdominal Complaints

Component or Parameter	Normal Values	Interpretation	Indications
Glucose	70–110 mg/dL	Above normal level indicates DKA, steroid use, stress Below normal level indicates decreased reserves, increased insulin	
Hemoglobin/hematocrit	Hb in men: 14–18 g/dL (8.7–11.2 mmol/L) Hb in women: 12–16 g/dL (7.4–9.9 mmol/L) Hct in men: 42%–52% (0.42–0.52) Hct in women: 37%–47% (0.37–0.47)	Below normal level indicates severe blood loss Above normal level indicates plasma loss, dehydration	All types of shock

(continues)

Table 6-6 Laboratory Studies for the Diagnosis of Abdominal Complaints (*continued*)

Component or Parameter	Normal Values	Interpretation	Indications
Gastric/stool hemoglobin	Negative	Positive indicates GI bleeding	Suspected GI bleeding
Lactic acid	Venous: 5–20 mg/dL (0.6–2.2 mmol/L)	Above normal level indicates tissue hypoperfusion and acidosis, as occurs with prolonged use of a tourniquet	All types of shock
Complete blood cell count	Total white blood cell count 5,000–10,000/mm^3 (5–10 × 10^9/L)	Above normal level in white blood cells indicates sepsis	More important in septic shock
Arterial blood gases	pH 7.35–7.45	Above normal pH indicates alkalosis. Below normal pH indicates acidosis, impaired perfusion.	All types of shock
	$Paco_2$ 35–45 mm Hg Pao_2 80–100 mm Hg	Below normal level of O_2 indicates hypoxia.	
	Hco_3 21–28 mEq/L	Below normal level of Hco_3 indicates metabolic acidosis.	
Serum electrolytes	Na 136–145 mEq/L (136–145 mmol/L) K 3.5–5 mEq/L (3.5–5 mmol/L)	Below normal level of Na may be present with osmotic diuresis Below normal level of K common with vomiting, diarrhea, diuretic use Above normal level of K common in acidosis, DKA Above or below normal level of K may have an abnormal ECG.	All types of shock
Renal function	Serum urea nitrogen 10–20 mg/dL (3.6–7.1 mmol/L) Creatinine W: 0.5–1.1 mg/dL M: 0.6–1.2 mg/dL (44–97 μmol/L)	Above normal serum urea nitrogen indicates severe dehydration, shock, sepsis Above normal serum creatinine indicates impaired renal function	All types of shock
Lipase	Adults younger than 60: 10–140 U/L Older than 60: 18–180 U/L	High levels may be caused by diseases of the pancreas and gallbladder, chronic kidney disease, intestinal problems, peptic ulcer disease, hepatic disease, and alcohol or drug abuse	
Blood/urine cultures	Negative	Positive result indicates infection	Septic shock
Bilirubin	Total: 0.3 mg/dL (5.1–17 μmol/L) Indirect: 0.2–0.8 mg/dL (3.4–12 μmol/L) Direct: 0.1–0.3 mg/dL (1.7–5.1 μmol/L)	Above normal level indicates liver dysfunction and jaundice, gallstones, liver metastases, large-volume transfusion, hepatitis, sepsis, cirrhosis, sickle cell anemia. Can also be caused by certain drugs, such as allopurinol, anabolic steroids, dextran, diuretics, and many others.	Septic shock
Alkaline phosphatase	50–120 units/L	Above normal level can indicate cirrhosis, biliary obstruction, liver tumor, hyperparathyroidism Below normal level can indicate hypothyroidism, malnutrition, pernicious anemia, celiac disease, hypophosphatemia	—

(continues)

Table 6-6 Laboratory Studies for the Diagnosis of Abdominal Complaints (*continued*)

Component or Parameter	Normal Values	Interpretation	Indications
Amylase	25–80 units/L	Above normal level can indicate pancreatitis, penetrating or perforated peptic ulcer, necrotic or perforated bowel, acute cholecystitis, ectopic pregnancy, DKA, duodenal obstruction	—
Ammonia	15–45 µg/dL (11–32 µmol/L)	Above normal level indicates hepatocellular disease, Reye syndrome, portal hypertension, GI bleeding or obstruction with mild liver disease, hepatic encephalopathy or coma, genetic metabolic disorder; with hepatic failure, an altered mental stautus may occur, which is often misdiagnosed as hypoglycemia or an acute cerebral event	—

DKA, diabetic ketoacidosis; GI, gastrointestinal; Hb, hemoglobin; HCO_3, bicarbonate; Hct, hematocrit; K, potassium, Na, sodium; $Paco_2$, partial pressure of carbon dioxide; Pao_2, partial pressure of oxygen.

Table 6-7 Radiologic Studies for the Diagnosis of Abdominal Disorders

Test	Description	Indications	Advantages and Disadvantages
Radiography	An upright abdominal film displays air-fluid levels. A supine abdominal film detects fluid or blood in the peritoneum or gas in bowel.	First test typically performed Can show free air, small-bowel obstruction, bowel ischemia, and foreign bodies	Inexpensive Easy to perform Causes minimal discomfort
Computed tomography (CT)	Images solid organs to detect scarring, tumors, metastasized cancers	First test performed for suspected diverticulitis, pancreatitis, appendicitis, aortic aneurysm, blunt trauma, and pancreatic cyst	Unlike radiography, a good image can be obtained no matter what the level of air or gas in the bowel Rapid test Causes minimal discomfort Not available 24 hours a day at some hospitals
Ultrasonography	Reflects and refracts sound waves as they strike fluid, air, and solid tissues in the body, allowing imaging of organs, tissues, and body cavities	First test performed for right upper quadrant pain Can detect cholelithiasis, cholecystitis, pancreatic masses, and biliary duct dilation Used in trauma when abdominal injury is suspected	Noninvasive and inexpensive Can be performed at the bedside Accurate reading depends on operator skill

normal circumstances, the pressure in the GI system is equal to the pressure in the external environment. At an elevation of 25,000 feet or higher, however, these gases expand as the barometric pressure decreases. The expanding gases in turn put pressure on the diaphragm, thereby diminishing the ability of the lungs to expand.

In a patient who has had recent abdominal surgery and is being transported by air at a high elevation, place a gastric tube or an ileus to release pressure. Empty any ostomy bags, and monitor the patient closely so the new bag does not rupture from an excessive buildup of gas. See Chapter 1 for a detailed discussion of transport and flight safety considerations.

Table 6-8 Differential Diagnosis of Abdominal Disorders with Emergent Presentations

Disorder	Causes	History	Findings	Prehospital Treatment	Hospital Testing/ Treatment
Mesenteric ischemia	Myocardial infarction, valvular heart disease, arrhythmia, peripheral vascular disease, hypercoagulability, oral contraceptive use, aortic dissection, trauma	Acute onset of severe midabdominal pain, nausea, vomiting, and diarrhea	Severe midabdominal pain, nausea, vomiting, diarrhea Pain out of proportion to tenderness	Administer oxygen. Place patient in a comfortable position. Establish IV access.	Surgical consult
Intestinal obstruction	Can be due to stool, foreign body, intussusception, adhesions, polyps, volvulus, tumors, ulcerative colitis, or diverticulitis	Abrupt onset: suspect small-bowel obstruction Onset over 1–2 days: suspect distal obstruction History of bowel obstruction, abdominal surgery, cancer, radiation therapy, chemotherapy, hernia, or abdominal illness	Crampy abdominal pain, constipation, diarrhea, inability to pass flatus, distended abdomen Absent or high-pitched bowel sounds	Administer oxygen. Place patient in a comfortable position. Establish IV access. Give nothing by mouth.	Laboratory and x-ray to determine location and extent of obstruction
Perforated viscus	Peptic ulcer disease, diverticula, trauma, use of NSAIDs, advancing age	Acute onset of epigastric pain Vomiting	Epigastric pain, vomiting, fever, shock, sepsis Elevated WBCs and amylase	Administer oxygen. Place patient in a comfortable position. Establish IV access. Give nothing by mouth.	Laboratory, x-ray, and CT to determine location and extent of perforation
Acute pancreatitis	Alcohol, cholelithiasis, trauma, infection, inflammation	Alcohol use, use of certain drugs, recent trauma, cholelithiasis	Midepigastric abdominal pain, low-grade fever, nausea, vomiting	Place patient in a comfortable position. Establish IV access. Give nothing by mouth.	Amylase/lipase levels and CT
Ruptured appendix	Obstruction, infection	Initially patient feels diffuse pain, especially in umbilical area. Later, pain settles in the right lower quadrant or lower back.	Nausea, vomiting, fever, positive Rovsing's sign	Place patient in a comfortable position. Establish IV access. Give nothing by mouth.	Laboratory, CT/ ultrasound, antibiotics, and surgical consult

CT, Computed tomography; IV, intravenous; NSAIDs, nonsteroidal antiinflammatory drugs; WBCs, white blood cells.

Gastrointestinal Causes of Abdominal Disorders

Upper Gastrointestinal or Esophageal Bleeding

Pathophysiology

Bleeding in the GI tract is a symptom of another disease, not a disease itself. Acute upper GI bleeding affects 50 to 150 people per 100,000 population, leading to 250,000 admissions per year. Men and elderly persons are at much higher risk for the disorder. Lower GI bleeding is less common overall but has a higher incidence among women. The possible causes of an upper GI bleed are extensive. Factors that heighten the risk of mortality include hemodynamic instability, repeated **hematemesis** or **hematochezia**, failure to clear blood despite gastric lavage, age older than 60, and existence of an additional organ system disease, such as cardiovascular or pulmonary disease.

Signs and Symptoms

Signs and symptoms of GI bleeding are variable. Each of the many conditions that can cause GI bleeding has its own pattern of disease progression. For example, diverticular disease has a rather gradual onset, and Mallory-Weiss syndrome has a sudden onset. Many patients do report bleeding, but others have more ambiguous initial signs and symptoms such as tachycardia, syncope, hypotension, angina, weakness, confusion, or cardiac arrest. Taking a good history may be the only way to determine the cause of such complaints.

Differential Diagnosis

To refine your diagnosis, in addition to finding out the patient's past medical history and other possible events of abdominal pain, find out the medications the patient is taking. You must ascertain whether the bleeding is an acute or chronic condition. Did the bleeding and pain begin suddenly, or did it have a delayed onset? Acute-onset GI bleeding is characterized by massive sudden hemorrhage and signs of hypovolemic shock. Chronic bleeding is more common in older adult patients and in those with chronic conditions such as renal failure. Fatigue and weakness will gradually exhaust the patient, and blood will appear in the stool. If the bleeding lasts long enough, signs of anemia may become evident. There are several questions specific to GI bleeding complaints, including: What was the onset of the bleeding? Was it gradual or sudden? Does anything make it better or worse? Has anything caused an increase—for example vomiting? What does the bleeding look like? What color is it? How much are you bleeding? From where are you bleeding? Question the patient about upper and lower GI bleeds. For example, you might ask, "On a scale of 0–10, how would you rank the bleeding? Is it increasing or decreasing in severity? How long have the

symptoms been present? Are they continuous or intermittent?" Even if the patient does not complain of pain, the OPQRST mnemonic is helpful.

Treatment

Treatment for the patient with GI bleeding consists of several general management guidelines. Fluid resuscitation is common. In most patients, even those with stable vital signs, it is prudent to establish an IV line, providing 1,000 mL of normal saline solution of lactated Ringer's using a macro drip tubing. This type of IV will allow you to quickly resuscitate the patient with fluids should conditions change.

Peptic Ulcer Disease

Pathophysiology

Peptic ulcer disease affects about 5 million people in the United States and is the most common cause of GI bleeding, representing about 60% of cases. *Helicobacter pylori* has been found to be the cause of 60% to 70% of peptic ulcers over the last decade, therefore peptic ulcer is no longer considered a chronic disease.

Duodenal, gastric, and stomal ulcers are all types of peptic ulcer disease. Because the gastric mucosa secretes hydrochloric acid and pepsinogen, the stomach is an acidic environment. This acidity is necessary for the proper digestion of protein. A delicate balance is maintained by secretion of sodium bicarbonate in the duodenum. Peptic ulcers form when this balance is upset and the acidic environment is allowed to predominate. A few of the factors that may irritate or contribute to ulcers include nonsteroidal antiinflammatory drugs (NSAIDs), smoking, excessive alcohol ingestion, and stress.

Signs and Symptoms

Bleeding in peptic ulcer disease can be severe. The patient may show signs of shock, pallor, hypotension, and tachycardia, which should be quickly documented and treated. Patients will experience a classic sequence of pain in the stomach that subsides or diminishes immediately after eating and then reemerges 2 to 3 hours later. The pain will be described as burning or gnawing. Nausea, vomiting, belching, and heartburn are common. If erosion is severe, gastric bleeding can occur with the result of hematemesis and **melena**. In rare incidents, the ulcer perforates (eats through the lining of the stomach or bowel), causing severe pain and a rigid, boardlike abdomen. Swelling of the ulcerated tissue may cause an acute obstruction.

Differential Diagnosis

The patient's past medical history is important for narrowing down the possible diagnoses. Ask about previous ulcers, whether the pain of the ulcer occurs prior to or after eating, and previous episodes of bleeding. The patient's answers will help you accurately assess the degree and blood loss and prepare to manage any hypotension that is present.

Treatment

After the patient's condition is stabilized, initiate proton pump inhibitors if the patient is not already taking them. Proton pump inhibitors (PPIs) diminish bleeding by reducing the amount of acid in the stomach. These medications can be given as an intravenous (IV) bolus followed by an IV drip. For more chronic treatment, in addition to PPIs, the patient should avoid NSAIDs because their prostaglandin inhibition can cause gastric and duodenal ulcers by hindering blood flow to the submucosa, minimizing the secretion of mucus, bicarbonate, and gastric acid. Patients should also avoid aspirin, caffeine, and alcohol. Treatment of documented *H. pylori* infection with antibiotics has been shown to promote healing and diminish the chance of recurrence, whereas smoking exacerbates the disease and slows healing time. In order to treat the *H. pylori* infection, a combination of antibiotics may be required. Antiulcer medications are used to suppress acid secretion and to form a barrier over the ulcer. These medications are summarized in Table 6-9.

Erosive Gastritis and Esophagitis

Pathophysiology

Erosive gastritis and esophagitis, as its name suggests, is due to erosion and inflammation of the gastric and esophageal mucosa. The condition can have an acute or chronic onset, and the potential causes are numerous. Nonspecific causes include alcohol, NSAIDs, corrosives, and radiation exposure. Erosive gastritis and esophagitis typically causes less bleeding than peptic ulcer disease, and the condition is self-limiting.

Signs and Symptoms

The chief signs and symptoms include indigestion, heartburn, dyspepsia, and belching. A few patients also have nausea and vomiting. The severity of symptoms does not accurately indicate the severity of the lesions.

Differential Diagnosis

A diagnosis in the field is typically difficult because of the myriad of signs and symptoms.

Treatment

Little can be done for this condition in the prehospital setting. Maintain airway, breathing, and circulation, and offer comfort measures such as proper positioning, analgesics, and **antiemetics**. Gastric lavage can be performed to assess for active bleeding. If the patient has no active bleeding, a mixture of viscous lidocaine and an antacid may provide relief. For long-term care, as with peptic ulcer disease, the patient may be placed on a PPI and should be advised to avoid aspirin, NSAIDs, caffeine, and alcohol.

Esophageal and Gastric Varices

Pathophysiology

Esophageal and gastric varices are veins that have become dilated as a result of mounting pressure that damages the veins and weakens the venous structure. Varices occur when blood flow through the liver is restricted (portal hypertension). This causes the blood to back up into the veins in the wall of the esophagus, causing the vessels to dilate. Portal hypertension,

Table 6-9 **Antiulcer Medications**		
Antisecretory Agents	**Specific Drugs**	**Mechanism of Action**
H₂ receptor antagonists	cimetidine (Tagamet) famotidine (Pepcid) nizatidine (Axid) ranitidine (Zantac)	Suppress acid secretion by blocking H₂ receptors on parietal cells
Proton-pump inhibitors	esomeprazole (Nexium) lansoprazole (Prevacid) omeprazole (Prilosec, Zegerid) pantoprazole (Protonix) rabeprazole (AcipHex)	Suppress acid secretion by inhibiting H, K-ATPase
Muscarinic antagonists	pirenzepine (Gastrozepin)	Suppress acid secretion by blocking muscarinic cholinergic receptors
Mucosal protectants	sucralfate (Carafate)	Form a barrier over ulcer

H, K-ATPase, hydrogen, potassium, adenosine triphosphatase; H₂, histamine-2.

most often associated with chronic excessive alcohol use, is the most common cause of the increasing pressure. Varices are typically asymptomatic until they rupture and bleed, causing massive blood loss. Patients who have bled from their varices have a 70% chance of bleeding again. If they do bleed a second time, 30% of the cases result in death.

Signs and Symptoms

A patient with esophageal and gastric varices exhibits signs of liver disease, including fatigue, weight loss, jaundice, anorexia, an edematous abdomen, pruritus, abdominal pain, nausea, and vomiting. The disease process is gradual, taking months to years to reach a state of extreme discomfort.

Differential Diagnosis

A differential diagnosis may include peptic ulcer disease unless the varices rupture and the patient reports an abrupt onset of discomfort in the throat, which is more definitive. Severe dysphagia, vomiting of bright red blood, hypotension, and signs of shock may also occur.

Treatment

In the prehospital setting, treat the patient according to the general guidelines as you would any GI bleeding disorder. Accurate assessment of the degree of blood loss is critical. Be prepared for a hemodynamically unstable patient needing volume resuscitation and aggressive suctioning of the airway. If the patient's level of consciousness begins to decrease, consider securing the airway to prevent aspiration.

If hemorrhage is uncontrolled, balloon tamponade may be performed in the hospital using a Sengstaken-Blakemore tube to apply pressure directly to the bleeding varices. This is a temporary solution that requires frequent monitoring. Pressure within the two balloons must be maintained at appropriate levels in order to apply the proper amount of pressure to the varices. Tension of 1 to 3 lb is applied to the tube by connecting it to a helmet the patient wears. Low intermittent suction is connected to both the gastric and esophageal ports (**Figure 6-5**). The patient must be intubated before this procedure is performed. If transportation to another facility is necessary, special precautions should be taken to protect the patient from changes in barometric pressure at higher elevations or during flight. Typically the balloons are deflated within 24 hours to diminish the risk of necrosis, but occasionally they are left in place for up to 72 hours.

Endoscopy may be performed to inject a sclerosing agent (a strong irritating solution) to promote clot formation, a procedure known as "sclerotherapy." Octreotide may be administered, but its effectiveness for variceal bleeding is limited. Vasopressin infusion is an additional pharmacologic option. Another option to promote clot formation is band therapy using rubber bands on the varices. Varices resemble polyps, and banding can prevent bleeding (**Figure 6-6**).

Mallory-Weiss Syndrome
Pathophysiology

Mallory-Weiss syndrome is a special type of esophageal condition in which severe hemorrhage can occur from longitudinal tears of the mucosa at the gastroesophageal junction, primarily at the level of the stomach. Severe, protracted vomiting can cause the tears, which then lead to arterial bleeding. Mallory-Weiss syndrome affects both men and women equally. It tends to occur in older adults and older children. The mortality rate is less than 10%.

Signs and Symptoms

This syndrome can range in severity from mild and self-limited to severe and life threatening. In serious cases, more vomiting is triggered as the person swallows blood. The initial symptom is often the severe bleeding itself; hematemesis occurs in 85% of patients with Mallory-Weiss syndrome. Aspirin use, excessive alcohol use, and bulimia (an eating disorder associated with episodes of binge eating followed by self-induced vomiting) are associated with the syndrome as well.

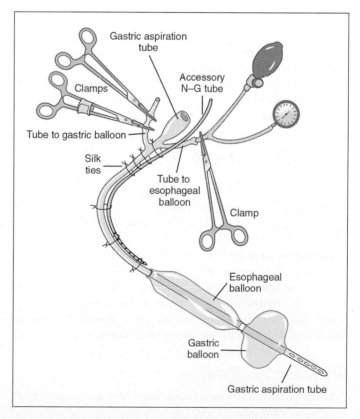

Figure 6-5 Modified Sengstaken-Blakemore tube. Note accessory nasogastric (NG) tube for suctioning of secretions above esophageal balloon, and two clamps (one secured with tape) to prevent inadvertent decompression of gastric balloon.

This article was published in Sabiston textbook of surgery: the biological basis of modern surgical practice, ed 18, Townsend CM, Beauchamp RD, Evers BM, et al, Copyright Saunders 2007.

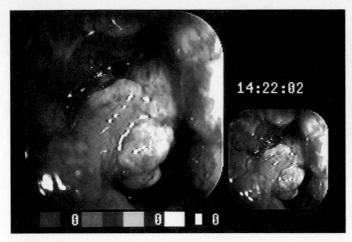
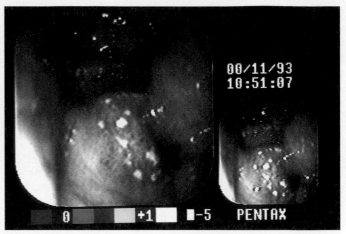

Figure 6-6 Endoscopic view of variceal ligation–related ulcers. **A.** Gastroesophageal junction is seen on a retroflexed view following ligation of multiple gastric varices, which resemble polyps. **B.** Upper endoscopy in same patient 4 weeks later demonstrates multiple ulcers at sites of prior ligation.
© CAVALLINI JAMES/BSIP SA/Alamy

Differential Diagnosis

The differential diagnosis includes esophageal and gastric varices.

Treatment

Primary management is supportive, because the bleeding usually resolves spontaneously. Gastric lavage should be performed until the bleeding has ceased. If it continues, endoscopy may be necessary. If the patient is still nauseated or vomiting, antiemetics should be considered. If the bleeding cannot be controlled, the patient must be transported to the hospital.

Perforated Viscus

Pathophysiology

A perforated or ruptured **viscus (*pl.* viscera)** is an emergent event. It often occurs when a duodenal ulcer erodes the serosa (the outermost layer of the bowel). Peritonitis ensues when the intestinal contents spill into the abdominal cavity. As the time between perforation and diagnosis lengthens, the mortality rate climbs. Rupture of the large intestine, small intestine, colonic diverticula, or gallbladder is possible but constitutes a rare event. Risk factors include advanced age, diverticular disease, use of NSAIDs, and a history of peptic ulcer disease.

Signs and Symptoms

Perforation usually causes an acute onset of epigastric pain; however, older adult patients may not have significant pain. The pain may be diffuse, with guarding and rebound tenderness. A rigid abdomen is a late sign. About half of patients experience vomiting. A low-grade fever, attributable to the peritonitis, may also be a late sign. Bowel sounds are diminished, tachycardia is common, and shock may develop with massive bleeding and sepsis.

Differential Diagnosis

Differential diagnoses include appendicitis and mesenteric ischemia, which are discussed later.

Treatment

In prehospital care, establishment of IV access and support of airway, breathing, and circulation are essential.

In the emergency department (ED), preoperative labs and diagnostic imaging should be performed. An elevated white blood cell count may be seen due to the peritonitis. In 70% to 80% of patients, an upright radiograph will show free air if an ulcer perforates. Computed tomography (CT) will reveal more information about the extent of the perforation.

Boerhaave's Syndrome

Pathophysiology

Boerhaave's syndrome is a spontaneous rupture of the esophagus as a consequence of hyperemesis gravidarum, childbirth, violent coughing, seizures, status asthmaticus, weight lifting, certain neurologic disorders, or explosive vomiting after an excessive intake of food and drink.

Signs and Symptoms

The patient typically has diffuse, severe, distracting pain in the chest, neck, back, and abdomen, as well as difficulty breathing, tachycardia, vomiting blood, and fever. If the rupture occurs in the neck, subcutaneous emphysema may be present.

Differential Diagnosis

Differential diagnoses may include a Mallory-Weiss tear, myocardial infarction, and peptic ulcer disease.

Treatment

Provide the patient oxygen, and rapidly transport the patient to the hospital. The mortality rate is as high as 50% without early surgical intervention.

Acute Pancreatitis

Pathophysiology

Diabetes is the most common disorder related to the pancreas, but pancreatitis is also common. Acute pancreatitis is an inflammatory process in which premature activation of pancreatic enzymes causes the pancreas to begin to digest itself, resulting in pain and necrosis as the inflammation spreads. The disease is thought to be caused by cholelithiasis or alcohol abuse in more than 90% of cases. Alcoholic pancreatitis is more common in men between the ages of 35 and 45. Urban EDs tend to be more familiar with the condition. In addition, certain medications, such as amiodarone (an antidysrhythmic), carbamazepine (an antiseizure medication), metronidazole (an antifungal), and quinolones (a class of antibiotics), can cause drug-induced pancreatitis.

Signs and Symptoms

The patient with acute pancreatitis experiences constant, severe midepigastric pain that radiates to the back. It is generally not exacerbated by eating. Cullen sign, a blue discoloration around the umbilicus, and Grey Turner sign, a blue discoloration around the flanks, may be present. Other symptoms may include low-grade fever, nausea, and vomiting. A systemic inflammatory response can develop, leading to shock and multiorgan failure.

Differential Diagnosis

A definitive diagnosis can be made only in pathologic analysis. CT and serum amylase and lipase values can assist in the diagnosis. No single laboratory test can diagnose pancreatitis, but lipase is thought to be more sensitive and specific than amylase. Amylase is less sensitive 36 hours after the onset of pain, because the level stays elevated for only a short time. The lipase level, on the other hand, is more specific to the pancreas and stays elevated for several days.

Treatment

Treat patients with suspected pancreatitis by establishing IV access, giving nothing by mouth, providing fluid resuscitation, and administering analgesics and antiemetics. Complications can include pancreatic hemorrhage or necrosis. The treatment of chronic pancreatitis is similar and is generally supportive.

Gastroparesis

Gastroparesis, also called delayed gastric emptying, is a medical condition consisting of a paresis (partial paralysis) of the stomach, resulting in food remaining in the stomach for an abnormally long time. Normally, the stomach contracts to move food down into the small intestine for additional digestion. The vagus nerve controls these contractions. Gastroparesis may occur when the vagus nerve is damaged and the muscles of the stomach and intestines do not properly function. Food then moves slowly or stops moving through the digestive tract. Transient gastroparesis may arise in acute illness of any kind, as a consequence of certain cancer treatments or other drugs that affect digestive action, or due to abnormal eating patterns. Gastroparesis sufferers are disproportionately female. One possible explanation for this finding is that women have an inherently slower stomach-emptying time than men. A hormonal link has been suggested, as gastroparesis symptoms tend to worsen the week before menstruation when progesterone levels are highest. Neither theory has been proven definitively.

Gastroparesis is frequently caused by autonomic neuropathy. This may occur in people with type 1 or type 2 diabetes. In fact, diabetes mellitus has been named as the most common cause of gastroparesis, as high levels of blood glucose may affect chemical changes in the nerves. The vagus nerve becomes damaged by years of high blood glucose or insufficient transport of glucose into cells resulting in gastroparesis. Other possible causes include anorexia nervosa and bulimia nervosa and damage to the vagus nerve. Gastroparesis has also been associated with connective tissue diseases such as scleroderma and Ehlers-Danlos syndrome, and neurologic conditions such as Parkinson's disease. It may also occur as part of a mitochondrial disorder.

Chronic gastroparesis can be caused by other types of damage to the vagus nerve, such as abdominal surgery. Heavy cigarette smoking is also a plausible cause because smoking causes damage to the stomach lining.

Idiopathic gastroparesis (gastroparesis with no known cause) accounts for a third of all chronic cases; it is thought that many of these cases are due to an autoimmune response triggered by an acute viral infection. "Stomach flu," mononucleosis, and other ailments have been anecdotally linked to the onset of the condition, but no systematic study has proven a link.

Gastroparesis can also be connected to hypochlorhydria and can be caused by chloride, sodium, and/or zinc deficiency, as these minerals are needed for the stomach to produce adequate levels of gastric acid in order to properly empty itself of a meal.

Signs and Symptoms

The most common symptoms of gastroparesis include chronic nausea, vomiting (especially of undigested food), and abdominal pain. Other symptoms include palpitations, heartburn, abdominal bloating, erratic blood glucose levels, loss of appetite, gastroesophageal reflux, spasms of the stomach wall, weight loss, and malnutrition. Morning nausea may also indicate gastroparesis. Vomiting may not occur in all cases, as sufferers may adjust their diets to include only small amounts of food.

Differential Diagnosis

Gastroparesis can be diagnosed with tests such as radiographs and gastric emptying scans. The clinical definition for gastroparesis is based solely on the emptying time of the stomach (and not on other symptoms), and severity of symptoms does not necessarily correlate with the severity of gastroparesis. Some patients with gastroparesis have a jejunostomy tube or implanted gastric neurostimulators ("stomach pacemakers").

Treatment

To treat a patient with gastroparesis, establish IV access, administer analgesics and antiemetics, and transport the patient to the hospital in a comfortable position.

Appendicitis

Pathophysiology

Appendicitis is typically caused by an infection or the buildup of fluid in the appendix. As the appendix becomes distended and inflamed, it may rupture, spilling toxins into the abdomen and touching off peritonitis. Bacteria can also enter the bloodstream, causing sepsis. Even if the appendix does not rupture, gangrene is a possibility and constitutes a surgical emergency. Despite a 7% incidence among the general population, there is no way of predicting when appendicitis will develop, although the condition is most common in persons aged 20 to 40.

Signs and Symptoms

Patients with appendicitis have pain localized to the right lower quadrant or right lower back. The pain classically begins in the periumbilical region, then becomes more localized in the right lower quadrant as inflammation worsens. Other signs and symptoms include fever, nausea and vomiting, and a positive psoas sign, which is quite specific to appendicitis. To assess for this sign, place the patient in the left lateral decubitus position and extend the right leg at the hip. Exacerbation of pain in the right lower quadrant is a positive psoas sign. Young children, older adult patients, pregnant women, and patients who have human immunodeficiency virus/acquired immunodeficiency syndrome (HIV/AIDS) may have an abnormal presentation of appendicitis and be at higher risk of complications. In young children, the onset of appendicitis may be delayed and nonspecific. Misdiagnosis is common because of the limitations in communicating with preverbal patients and because of the atypical presentation. As you might expect, misdiagnosis elevates the risk of perforation. In patients older than 70, the rate of misdiagnosis is as high as 50%, and early rupture is common. Appendicitis is the most common cause of extrauterine abdominal pain during pregnancy and should be suspected with GI complaints in pregnant women. Patients with HIV/AIDS have the same symptoms as other patients, but they have a much higher risk of complications. They are also more likely to delay seeking treatment for appendicitis because of the frequency of other GI problems.

Differential Diagnosis

The differential diagnosis of appendicitis is difficult because the signs and symptoms can be attributed to many conditions. Pancreatitis, Crohn's disease, and endometriosis all present with similar symptoms, to name a few. At the receiving facility, therefore, a definitive diagnosis will be made using ultrasound or CT. Laboratory studies such as a complete blood cell count and a urinalysis will be evaluated. CT is the most useful study because it can also reveal an alternative diagnosis if the patient does not have appendicitis. In fact, use of CT has been shown to reduce the number of unnecessary appendectomies in women. However, a gravid uterus makes appendicitis difficult to diagnose. To avoid radiation exposure with CT, ultrasound or MRI can aid in the diagnosis. If appendicitis is confirmed, surgery to remove the appendix is required. Prophylactic antibiotics will be given before surgery in case the appendix ruptures.

Treatment

To treat a patient with suspected appendicitis, establish IV access, administer analgesics and antiemetics, and transport the patient to the hospital in a comfortable position.

Mesenteric Ischemia

Pathophysiology

Mesenteric ischemia is caused by an occlusion of the mesenteric artery or vein. Symptoms typically include an acute onset of nausea, vomiting, diarrhea, and severe midabdominal pain that appears to be out of proportion to abdominal tenderness and physical findings. The condition is more common in older adult patients and in those with a history of myocardial infarction, arrhythmia, valvular heart disease, or peripheral vascular disease. Use of oral contraceptives, hypercoagulability, aortic dissection, and trauma can also precipitate an ischemic event. It is a rare but serious condition, with a mortality rate of between 60% and 100%.

Signs and Symptoms

Depending on the exact cause of the abdominal pain, it may have a gradual or sudden onset. The location of the pain tends to be ill defined and is severe. Nausea, vomiting, and diarrhea are also common. Blood may be present in the stool.

Differential Diagnosis

The disease is difficult to diagnose. Its cardinal presentation includes severe abdominal pain with normal abdominal examination results. A thorough history is needed. No laboratory studies are specifically diagnostic, although elevated serum lactate can be a clue. Abnormal radiologic findings are a late sign. You should suspect mesenteric ischemia in patients with other risk factors and no other cause for the abdominal pain.

Treatment

Mesenteric ischemia can progress to infarction if not identified early and may result in gangrenous bowel, perforation, and death. Treatment for these patients requires rapid transport. Monitor the patients closely, checking vital signs for evidence of sepsis. If shock is present, fluid resuscitation should be initiated. Analgesics may be indicated. In-hospital treatment will include imaging studies (angiogram and computed tomography angiography) and antibiotics. Depending on the cause, surgery or vasodilators will be used.

Intestinal Obstruction

Pathophysiology

Intestinal obstruction is an emergent event in which stool, a foreign body, or a mechanical process obstructs passage of intestinal contents. Mounting pressure in the intestine diminishes blood flow, leading to septicemia and intestinal necrosis. The mortality rate rises dramatically as shock develops. Patients with a history of bowel obstruction, abdominal surgery, recent abdominal illness, cancer, radiation, chemotherapy, or hernia are at greater risk of experiencing an intestinal obstruction.

Signs and Symptoms

Patients with intestinal obstruction have nausea, vomiting, and abdominal pain. In addition, they may be unable to pass flatus (bowel gas) and may have constipation and a distended abdomen. The natural peristalsis of the intestines continues despite the obstruction, causing intermittent pain the patient may describe as being crampy or feeling like a knot. Mechanical causes of small-bowel obstruction are intussusception, adhesions, polyps, volvulus, and tumors. Gastric **volvulus**, a condition in which the stomach rotates more than 180 degrees, is a rare event that has been documented in only 400 cases in the United States. This twisting seals the stomach on both ends, blocking the flow of blood and the passage of fluid and food. The condition is characterized by an acute onset of abdominal pain, severe vomiting, and shock. The patient is likely to die in the absence of timely intervention.

Intussusception occurs when a portion of the bowel telescopes into an adjacent portion of the intestine, thereby occluding passage of intestinal contents and diminishing blood flow to the area. Intussusception accounts for 7% of all intestinal obstructions. The condition is more common in children than among adults. About 80% of intussusceptions in adults occur in the small intestine.

Large-bowel obstruction is less common than small-bowel obstruction because of the greater diameter of the colon. When such an obstruction does develop, it is usually caused by cancer, fecal impaction, ulcerative colitis, volvulus, diverticulitis, or intussusception.

Any abdominal complaint should prompt you to ask about appetite and bowel regimen as you gather the patient's history.

In a patient with an obstruction, auscultation of the bowel will reveal high-pitched or absent sounds. The sounds can be difficult to hear because sound may be referred from one portion of the abdomen to the other, so be sure to auscultate each quadrant for several minutes. Percussion may reveal a hollow sound. Palpation may provoke the pain, and a distended, firm abdomen indicates a severe obstruction.

Differential Diagnosis

It is impossible to make a definitive diagnosis of intestinal obstruction in the field, but you can still treat the patient if you suspect the condition.

Treatment

Begin treatment by addressing any life threats. Then establish IV access and administer medications for nausea and pain per local protocol. Give nothing by mouth, because the patient may need to undergo immediate surgery. Transport the patient in a comfortable position.

In the ED, a CT scan or both flat and upright radiographs of the abdomen and chest will be taken to confirm the obstruction. A complete blood count and electrolyte analysis will be performed. An elevated white blood cell count may indicate ischemia and impending bowel necrosis. A nasogastric tube may be placed to remove excess pressure pending surgical intervention.

Abdominal Compartment Syndrome

Pathophysiology

Abdominal compartment syndrome is caused by intra-abdominal hypertension and is a critical presentation for patients with abdominal discomfort.

Signs and Symptoms

The patient may have a tense, tender, distended abdomen, respiratory distress, metabolic acidosis, declining urine output, and dwindling cardiac output. The drop in cardiac output occurs as the pressure builds up in the abdomen, restricting venous return to the heart.

The condition is more common among trauma patients, but it may be seen in medical patients as well. Because these signs and symptoms are often associated with other critical events such as hypovolemia, compartment syndrome may be missed. Awareness is essential. You can worsen the condition by placing equipment on a patient's abdomen during transport.

Differential Diagnosis

The differential diagnosis may include appendicitis, congestive heart failure, mesenteric ischemia, and urinary obstruction.

Treatment

Treatment in the field for this condition is limited to loosening restrictive clothing, avoiding excessive fluid administration, and possibly administering diuretics. In the ED, the abdomen may be decompressed by removing fluid.

Acute Gastroenteritis

Pathophysiology

Acute gastroenteritis, the second leading cause of illness in the United States, is characterized by watery diarrhea, nausea and vomiting, mild abdominal pain, and low-grade fever. Many viruses cause acute gastroenteritis. These agents typically enter the body via the fecal–oral route through contaminated food or water. The norovirus is responsible for most cases of acute viral gastroenteritis in adults, whereas rotavirus causes the same condition in children. Various parasites may be contracted by swimming in water contaminated with them. Viral gastroenteritis is easily transmissible and can cause large outbreaks, which are usually sporadic and tend to flourish in the winter months.

Signs and Symptoms

Depending on the organism involved, patients may begin to experience GI upset and diarrhea in as little as several hours or days after contact with the contaminated food or water. The disease can run its course in 2 to 3 days or continue for several weeks.

Patients can experience various types of diarrhea—large dumping type or frequent small liquid stools. The diarrhea can contain blood and/or pus, and it may have a foul odor or be odorless. Abdominal cramping is frequent as hyperperistalsis continues. Nausea and vomiting, fever, and anorexia are also present.

If the diarrhea continues, dehydration and hemodynamic instability will result. As the volume of fluid loss increases, the likelihood of potassium and sodium imbalance also increases. Watch for changes in level of consciousness and other profound signs of shock, which clearly indicate a critical volume loss.

Differential Diagnosis

The possible diagnoses include appendicitis and food poisoning.

Treatment

Treatment is symptomatic and consists of administering antiemetics and providing IV fluid replacement.

Sepsis

Abdominal pain is not a typical presentation of sepsis, but some patients do have nausea and vomiting. Sepsis is discussed further in Chapter 4 relative to shock.

Abdominal Disorders Associated with Liver Disease

Jaundice

The presence of excessive (unconjugated) serum bilirubin in the bloodstream that gives the skin, mucous membranes, and eyes a distinct yellow color is called jaundice. Jaundice is often associated with liver disease, such as hepatitis or liver cancer, and causes fatigue, fever, anorexia, and confusion. Bilirubin, to be eliminated from the body, must be conjugated by the liver. As the excess unconjugated bilirubin crosses the blood–brain barrier, encephalopathy and death can occur. Jaundice is often associated with premature infants, but it can be present in persons any age.

Signs and Symptoms

Patients with jaundice may show no symptoms or a wide variety of symptoms, depending on the underlying cause, from mild symptoms to life-threatening symptoms. Patients with acute illness may have a fever, chills, abdominal pain, and flulike symptoms. Patient history may include recent trauma, blood transfusion, viral illness, chronic alcohol use, acetaminophen overdose, hepatitis, pregnancy, malignancy, or encephalopathy. Weight loss and pruritus are also common. Physical examination may reveal abdominal pain with palpation in the right upper quadrant, an enlarged liver, and ascites.

Differential Diagnosis

During the early stages of liver disease, patients may be diagnosed with influenza or gastroenteritis. In-hospital diagnostic tests include CT or ultrasound and laboratory studies such as a complete blood count, serum bilirubin, alkaline phosphatase, prothrombin time/partial thromboplastin time (PT/PTT), serum amylase, ammonia level, a pregnancy test, and a toxicology screening.

Treatment

The treatment for liver disease is mainly supportive. Follow general management guidelines for patients with GI problems.

Hepatitis

Pathophysiology

Hepatitis simply means an inflammation of the liver. Despite its simple name, the etiology of hepatitis is often complex. Causes include viral, bacterial, fungal, and parasitic infections, exposure to toxic substances, adverse drug reactions, and immunologic disorders.

Alcohol is one of the toxic substances that can cause severe liver disease and hepatitis, since the liver is responsible for degrading alcohol. Chronic alcohol abuse leads to liver disease, malnutrition, accumulation of toxic metabolites, and enzyme alteration. The interaction of these mechanisms is thought to cause hepatitis, although researchers do not yet understand precisely how.

Viruses are among the most frequent causes of hepatitis. Viral hepatitis is classified as type A, type B, or type C. Although the incidence of all types is declining, these infectious diseases still pose a threat. The progression of hepatitis leads to fulminant hepatic failure.

Hepatitis A Hepatitis A virus (HAV) is typically spread from person to person through the fecal–oral route. It thrives in areas with poor sanitation, particularly in unsanitary cooking facilities. HAV exposure is widespread. In fact, in some regions of the world, 100% of the population has been exposed. In the United States, the rate of exposure is as high as 50%. However, very few of those who have been exposed have actually become ill. A vaccination can be given to prevent HAV. HAV is not a chronic illness.

Hepatitis B In infected people, hepatitis B virus (HBV) can be found in most bodily secretions, including saliva, semen, stool, tears, urine, and vaginal secretions. The virus is usually spread through exposure to infected blood or by sexual activity. The highest rates, then, are among IV drug users and men who have sex with men. Historically, blood transfusions were a frequent cause of HBV, but careful screening of blood products has virtually eliminated the risk of exposure. Unlike with HAV, once infected with HBV, a person is always a carrier and can always transmit the disease. A vaccine for HBV is also available.

Hepatitis C Hepatitis C is commonplace in the United States and is linked to blood transfusions. Other possible causes are unsafe needle-sharing practices and exposure of healthcare workers to the blood of infected patients. The cause of infection is not found in 40% to 57% of cases.

Fulminant Hepatic Failure **Fulminant hepatic failure** sets in when hepatitis progresses to hepatic necrosis (death of the liver cells). Extensive hepatic necrosis is irreversible and can be treated only with a liver transplant. Hepatitis B and C are most often responsible, but drug toxicity (acetaminophen overdose) and metabolic disorders can also be the cause. Liver function test results will be elevated.

Signs and Symptoms

The symptoms of hepatitis vary but tend to be nonspecific. They include malaise, fever, and anorexia, followed by nausea and vomiting, abdominal pain, diarrhea, and jaundice later in the course of the disease. The disease is typically asymptomatic until it evolves into alcoholic hepatitis, at which time signs and symptoms may include nausea and vomiting, abdominal pain, tachycardia, fever, ascites, and orthostatic hypotension. Classic symptoms of fulminant hepatic failure include anorexia, vomiting, jaundice, abdominal pain, and asterixis, or "flapping." The mechanism causing asterixis is unknown. To test for it, ask the patient to extend the arms, flex the wrists, and spread the fingers, and then observe for flapping.

Differential Diagnosis

The possible differential diagnoses include peptic ulcer disease, gallstones, cholecystitis, and small-bowel obstruction.

Treatment

Treatment is merely supportive. In the case of acetaminophen overdose, if the patient is seen soon after ingestion, an antidote of *N*-acetylcysteine can be given with excellent results. Time of ingestion of the acetaminophen is key to determining whether the patient meets treatment criteria. First, support the patient's airway, breathing, and circulation. Then establish IV access, and administer antiemetics and pain medication as necessary.

Abdominal Disorders Associated with Inflammatory Conditions

Irritable Bowel Syndrome

Pathophysiology

Irritable bowel syndrome is a chronic disorder that affects 10% to 15% of the U.S. population. Although not life threatening, it causes abdominal pain, diarrhea, constipation, and nausea that can greatly impair the quality of life. Because lab findings and radiologic studies are normal in patients with irritable bowel syndrome, the disorder was originally thought to be psychiatric. Current physiologic research, however, suggests that the condition is due to an error of gut motility and sensation. The condition does arise more often in persons with a history of depression or anxiety and worsens when the person is under stress. The condition also appears to be predominant among women.

Signs and Symptoms

Irritable bowel syndrome is a chronic condition. Prehospital presentations will typically involve a flare-up of the condition. Patients may be initially seen with abdominal pain or discomfort. This pain is relieved by a bowel movement. When the pain starts, there is usually a change in the frequency and consistency of bowel movements. Patients may experience diarrhea, constipation, and bloating.

Differential Diagnosis

The differential diagnosis must include a coexisting psychiatric disorder. Severe depression may be noted. Other possible diagnoses include food allergies, gastroenteritis, endometriosis, and mesenteric ischemia.

Treatment

Treatment is mainly supportive. Assess the patient's mood and thoughts. Be compassionate. Consider whether the patient is severely depressed. If depression and/or suicide are noted, treat those accordingly. Analgesia may be needed. A confirmed diagnosis may indicate dietary modification and behavioral therapy and supportive care.

Diverticular Disease

Diverticular disease is characterized by small, saclike appendages called *diverticula* that form when the lining of the colon herniates through the mucosal wall. Diverticular disease was first described as recently as the 20th century and is thought to be attributable to a lack of fiber in the modern diet. Researchers believe that the formation of smaller stools containing little fiber raises pressure in the colon, and small outpouchings form in weakened areas of the intestinal wall. The disease is far more likely to appear in those older than 50 than among younger adults. The condition of having diverticula is referred to as diverticulosis.

Signs and Symptoms

Diverticulosis is often asymptomatic. When the disorder does generate symptoms, they include abdominal bloating, crampy pain, and changes in bowel habits. Diverticulitis sets in when the diverticula become infected, precipitating bleeding, persistent left lower quadrant pain, diffuse tenderness, vomiting, and abdominal distention. Patients can either have diarrhea or constipation.

Differential Diagnosis

The differential diagnosis may include appendicitis, bowel obstruction, mesenteric ischemia, and inflammatory bowel disease.

Treatment

Treatment is mainly focused on making the patient comfortable. Potential complications include bowel perforation and consequent sepsis. The patient should be monitored closely to ensure severe infection is not present. Patients may need large amounts of fluids and/or vasopressors to maintain blood pressure. In-hospital treatment will include antibiotics, allowing the GI tract to rest by giving the patient a liquid diet, and possibly surgery. Patients with severe diverticulitis may require surgical colectomy or abscess drainage.

Cholecystitis and Biliary Tract Disorders

Pathophysiology

Biliary tract disorders are a group of conditions that involve inflammation of the gallbladder. Cholangitis and cholelithiasis are diseases that affect the gallbladder, a structure that produces bile to aid digestion of fats and fat-soluble nutrients. Cholangitis is an inflammation of the bile duct. In cholelithiasis, an elevated level of cholesterol that cannot be converted by bile acids leads to the formation of gallstones. This condition is more prevalent among older adults and women and in people with morbid obesity, those who have lost weight rapidly, those with a familial predisposition to the disorder, and those who have taken certain drugs. Cholecystitis is a complete obstruction of the bile duct caused by gallstones, a stricture, or a malignancy.

Signs and Symptoms

Gallstones are asymptomatic in some people. In others, they provoke severe pain in the right upper quadrant, sometimes referred to the right shoulder, accompanied by nausea and vomiting. This pain, called *biliary colic*, is typically cyclic and tends to be aggravated by eating fatty foods. Murphy's sign may also be present and can be elicited by pressing firmly upward into the right upper quadrant and asking the patient to take a deep breath. Arrest of inspiration because of pain is a positive finding.

Signs and symptoms of cholecystitis include persistent right upper quadrant pain, nausea, vomiting, and fever. The condition will be treated urgently with antibiotics and cholecystectomy (gallbladder removal).

Cholangitis has the same symptoms as cholecystitis, but with jaundice. Sepsis will develop if the condition is left untreated.

Differential Diagnosis

Differential diagnoses include appendicitis, mesenteric ischemia, abdominal aortic aneurysm, and peptic ulcer disease.

Treatment

Prehospital treatment is directed at making the patient comfortable. Biliary colic can be treated with outpatient elective cholecystectomy. Treatment of cholangitis centers on maintaining hemodynamic stability, controlling pain and nausea, administering antibiotics, and decompressing the biliary tract.

Ulcerative Colitis

Pathophysiology

Ulcerative colitis is caused by inflammation of the colon. The inflammation is generalized and does not occur in patches, as in Crohn's disease. It is unclear what causes the chronic inflammation, though genetics, stress, and autoimmunity have been speculated. In this condition, the inflammation causes a thinning of the wall of the intestine, resulting in a weakened dilated rectum. The damaged lining of the colon is prone to infections by bacteria and bleeding.

Signs and Symptoms

The onset of the condition is usually gradual, with bloody diarrhea, hematochezia, and mild to severe abdominal pain. Other signs and symptoms can be joint pain and skin lesions. These effects lend credence to the idea of an autoimmune component to the disease. Patients can also experience fever, fatigue, and loss of appetite from infection.

Differential Diagnosis

Differential diagnoses may include gastroenteritis, Crohn's disease, and irritable bowel syndrome.

Treatment

Treatment of patients with ulcerative colitis is mainly supportive. Determine the degree of hemodynamic instability. Look for signs of shock. If the diarrhea and bleeding have caused sufficient volume loss to make the patient's condition unstable, administer fluids to return the patient to a near-normal volume balance. Patients are often treated with long-term prednisone or other immunosuppressive therapy. Complications include intra-abdominal abscess and fistula formation.

Crohn's Disease

Pathophysiology

Crohn's disease is similar to ulcerative colitis; however, the entire GI tract can be involved. The main part of the GI tract that tends to be involved is the ileum, which is the last portion of the small intestine before it joins the small intestine. There are several theories as to the cause, though no definitive cause has been identified. Regardless of the cause, the result is a series of attacks by the immune system on the GI tract. This activity of white blood cells damages all layers and a portion of the GI tract involved. The result is most often a scarred, narrowed, stiff, and weakened portion of the small intestine. This patch of damage is found among areas of intestine that are normal. This narrowing can cause bowel obstruction.

Signs and Symptoms

Of interest with Crohn's disease and colitis is the presence of signs and symptoms outside the GI system. This evidence helps support the theory that an autoimmune component is operating within the disease. Patients with Crohn's disease experience chronic abdominal pain, often in the lower right area. This pain corresponds to the location of the ileum. Rectal bleeding, weight loss, diarrhea, arthritis, skin problems, and fever may also be present. Bleeding tends to be in small amounts over a long period of time. Acute, severe hemorrhage is rare, but chronic bleeding resulting in anemia and hypotension does occur. Patients can have episodes of mild to severe signs and symptoms.

Differential Diagnosis

The distinction between Crohn's disease and ulcerative colitis is hard to make. Laboratory studies and imaging studies may help narrow down the diagnosis.

Treatment

Patients may require volume resuscitation if diarrhea and chronic hemorrhage are occurring. Control of nausea and pain are commonly required.

Neurologic Causes of Abdominal Disorders

A broad range of mechanisms not directly related to a GI diagnosis can cause nausea and vomiting. These mechanisms include neurologic complaints such as migraines, tumors, and increased intracranial pressure. If such a diagnosis is suspected, you should perform a more in-depth neurologic assessment. Table 6-10 outlines neurologic causes of abdominal discomfort in patients. In addition, Chapter 5 contains detailed information on neurologic complaints.

Intracerebral Bleeding

Although intracerebral bleeding does not cause abdominal pain, you should consider it when nausea and vomiting are present. In cases of acute onset of nausea and vomiting, you should undertake further assessment to confirm or eliminate this diagnosis. A history of recent head trauma, hemiparesis, hemiplegia, and difficulty speaking or swallowing, especially when accompanied by risk factors such as hypertension or advanced age, increases the likelihood of intracerebral bleeding. See Chapter 5 for more information.

Meningitis

Meningitis is a bacterial, viral, or fungal infection of the meninges of the brain. Although meningitis is not a GI disorder, you should consider this diagnosis when the patient has nausea or vomiting. Bacterial meningitis has a 25% to 50% mortality rate, is highly contagious, and requires aggressive antibiotic treatment. Viral meningitis calls for supportive care. It is critical to wear personal protective equipment, including a mask, because it is virtually impossible to know in the prehospital setting which type of meningitis a patient might have. See Chapter 5 for more information.

Vertigo

Vertigo is dizziness associated with a variety of conditions, trauma, infection, and intracranial bleeding, to name several. Although vertigo is not an abdominal illness, it can cause nausea and vomiting and may be peripheral or central. For peripheral vertigo (e.g., labyrinthitis, benign paroxysmal positional vertigo, vestibular neuronitis), provide supportive care. If the patient has other neurologic symptoms such as headache or confusion, you should suspect intracranial bleeding. See Chapter 5 for more information about vertigo.

Table 6-10 Neurologic Causes of Abdominal Discomfort			
	Description	**Symptoms**	**Treatment**
Migraine	Recurrent headache, sometimes accompanied by an aura Lasts 3–72 hours	Unilateral or bilateral throbbing or sharp headache Photophobia Nausea and vomiting	Provide supportive care. Dim the ambulance lights. Establish IV access. Administer antiemetics. Apply ice or heat packs.
Central nervous system tumor	Primary tumor: begins in the brain Secondary tumor: spreads from another cancerous site More common among people over age 65, in those who have had radiation to the head, and in those who smoke or are HIV positive	Recurrent, severe headaches Nausea and vomiting Dizziness and lack of coordination Vision alterations Seizures	Provide supportive care to reduce nausea and vomiting, ease pain, and prevent or control seizures.
Increased intracranial pressure	Can be caused by obstruction or by increase of cerebrospinal fluid in ventricles	Headache Photophobia Nausea and vomiting Seizures	Provide comfort care. Position the patient lying flat. Administer antiemetics and antiseizure medications.

Cardiopulmonary Causes of Abdominal Disorders

When abdominal discomfort is accompanied by respiratory distress, you must consider cardiopulmonary diagnoses. Frequent signs and symptoms of an acute myocardial infarction, for example, may include abdominal or epigastric pain and nausea and/or vomiting. Pulmonary embolism and pneumonia are other possible causes of abdominal pain with shortness of breath. Consider obtaining a 12-lead ECG if you suspect the patient's signs and symptoms have a cardiopulmonary cause.

Abdominal Aortic Aneurysm

Abdominal aortic aneurysm is an enlargement of part of the aorta caused by a weakness in the vascular wall. These bulges in the arterial wall typically begin small and become larger over the course of several months to years. Most such aneurysms do not rupture, leak, or dissect. Less than half of patients with an abdominal aortic aneurysm exhibit the classic triad of symptoms: hypotension, abdominal or back pain, and a pulsatile abdominal mass. Be sure to consider this diagnosis in patients with syncope or any one of the triad of symptoms.

Because of the large size of the aorta, rupture causes massive blood loss, and survival depends primarily on the body's ability to spontaneously contain the bleeding. Any patient suspected of having a ruptured abdominal aortic aneurysm should be treated as a critical patient. Fluid resuscitation may be necessary. Consider immediate transport to the operating room if the patient has a known ruptured aneurysm. If the patient is older than 50 and is complaining of abdominal or back pain, an abdominal aneurysm should be considered, even if hypotension or a pulsatile mass are not present. Consider bedside sonography as the first evaluative tool, followed by CT if necessary. A stable patient may undergo CT, because a sonogram cannot always detect retroperitoneal leakage or rupture. Remember that even with a patient in stable condition, deterioration can happen suddenly at any time. Even patients who have had a repair are at risk for an aneurysm rupture. See Chapter 3 for more information on aortic aneurysm.

Acute Coronary Syndrome

Myocardial infarction can be accompanied by midepigastric pain and nausea that cause it to mimic an abdominal complaint such as peptic ulcer disease or gastritis. Since it may be difficult to distinguish between GI and cardiac causes, assess the patient for acute coronary syndrome and initiate care as appropriate. Review Chapter 3 for the diagnosis and treatment of acute coronary syndrome and myocardial infarction.

Pulmonary Embolism

As with acute coronary syndrome, pulmonary embolism should be suspected in patients who have upper abdominal pain. A pulmonary embolism is a life-threatening condition that occurs when a thrombus (a blood clot, cholesterol plaque, or air bubble) travels through the bloodstream and becomes lodged in a pulmonary artery. The area of the lung perfused by that portion of the pulmonary artery no longer receives oxygenated blood, causing pain and shortness of breath.

You should suspect pulmonary embolism in patients with hip or long-bone fractures, people who are sedentary or have recently taken a long flight or car trip, those who smoke, use oral contraceptives, have a history of deep vein thrombosis or cancer, and women who are pregnant or were recently pregnant. See Chapter 2 for more information about pulmonary embolism.

Budd-Chiari Syndrome

Budd-Chiari syndrome is an extremely rare cardiovascular disorder resulting from occlusion of the major hepatic veins or inferior vena cava. The venous thrombosis that characterizes this syndrome can be due to hematologic disease, coagulopathy, pregnancy, use of oral contraceptives, abdominal trauma, or a congenital disorder. Signs and symptoms include acute or chronic fulminant liver failure, emergent abdominal pain, hepatomegaly, ascites, and jaundice. Diagnosis is usually made by ultrasound. The treatment selected depends on the cause of the occlusion, but anticoagulants and supportive therapy are typically given.

Lobar Pneumonia

Lobar pneumonia causes upper abdominal pain in some patients. The pain tends to be more focal than in bronchopneumonia, which causes inflammation of the entire lung. Lobar pneumonia is usually accompanied by a fever, chest pain, and respiratory distress. Chapter 2 addresses pneumonia at greater length.

Genitourinary Causes of Abdominal Disorders

Placenta Abruptio

Pathophysiology

During the second half of pregnancy, about 4% of women have vaginal bleeding. Bleeding during the second trimester signals imminent fetal distress and should be considered an emergency. Placenta abruptio, the premature separation of the placenta from the uterine wall, is responsible for about 30% of all cases of bleeding during the second half of pregnancy. Trauma, maternal hypertension, or preeclampsia typically precipitates abruption. Other risk factors include patients younger than 20, advanced maternal age, multiparity or a history of smoking, prior miscarriage, prior placenta abruption, or cocaine use.

Signs and Symptoms

Placenta abruption should be considered in patients with vaginal bleeding, contractions, uterine or abdominal tenderness, and a decrease in fetal movement. The majority (80%) of patients with placenta abruptio report vaginal bleeding. The blood is usually dark. With small abruptions, bleeding may not be noted until delivery. The volume of blood loss can vary from minimal to life threatening. The condition of these patients can progress from stable to unstable in a short period of time. Fetal distress or death occurs in about 15% of patients.

Differential Diagnosis

Possible diagnoses include appendicitis, placenta previa, preeclampsia, preterm labor, and ectopic pregnancy.

Treatment

Assessment should include evaluation of vaginal bleeding, contractions, and uterine tenderness and assessment of fundal height and fetal heart tones. Fetal heart tones may vary from absent to fetal bradycardia to decelerations. Short-term variability may be decreased as well if the fetus is compromised. Vaginal exams should not be performed until an ultrasound can be completed to rule out placenta previa. Management is based on the severity of the blood loss. The following may be indicated: oxygen, fluid support with two large-bore IVs, blood administration, and administering Rh globulin if the patient is Rh negative.

Placenta Previa

Pathophysiology

In some pregnancies, the placenta becomes implanted over the cervical os (opening). This anomaly is one of the leading causes of vaginal bleeding in the second and third trimesters. It may be identified early in the pregnancy but may resolve as the uterus expands. The patient is at risk of significant bleeding, however, if the condition does not resolve and the placenta completely occludes the cervix. Ultrasound is used to localize the placenta. Advanced maternal age, multiparity, and a history of smoking and prior cesarean section predispose a woman to placenta previa.

Signs and Symptoms

The patient will usually present with bright red bleeding. The bleeding is usually painless, but some patients (20%) will have uterine irritability as well. Many patients have an initial episode of bleeding that spontaneously stops and then have additional episodes of bleeding later in the pregnancy.

Differential Diagnosis

Possible diagnoses include placenta abruptio, disseminated intravascular coagulopathy, and preterm labor.

Treatment

In addition to monitoring the patient's bleeding, monitor the patient for signs and symptoms of shock, uterine tone (usually soft and nontender), and fetal heart tones. Do not perform vaginal or rectal examinations. Speculum exam can trigger hemorrhage if the condition is present. Monitor for disseminated intravascular coagulopathy, as maternal deaths with placenta previa are associated with blood loss or disseminated intravascular coagulopathy. Care is directed at supporting the patient's hemodynamic status to include oxygen, two large-bore IVs, fluids, and administration of blood as needed.

Preeclampsia/HELLP

Pathophysiology

Preeclampsia with HELLP syndrome (*H* indicates hemolysis; *EL*, elevated liver enzymes; *LP*, low platelet count) is a not-uncommon, life-threatening complication of pregnancy thought to be a variant or complication of preeclampsia. Preeclampsia, which occurs in 6% to 8% of pregnancies, is characterized by hypertension and protein in the urine. The risk of preeclampsia is higher among women younger than age 20 and in those with first or multifetal pregnancies, gestational diabetes, obesity, or a family history of gestational hypertension. Gestational hypertension typically resolves within 6 weeks postpartum. HELLP and preeclampsia usually occur during the last trimester of pregnancy or soon after delivery.

HELLP syndrome is considered by some authorities to be a severe and rare form of preeclampsia; others suggest that it may be a syndrome of its own. The precise cause of HELLP syndrome has not been established. HELLP is a multisystem disease that results in vasospasm, thrombi formation, and coagulation issues. It is often misdiagnosed or found later in the course of the syndrome, so your awareness of the signs and symptoms is vitally important. HELLP syndrome usually occurs antepartum, but it may also present during the postpartum period (approximately one-third of cases appear postpartum). Left untreated, HELLP syndrome can lead to maternal end-organ failure as well as fetal demise.

Signs and Symptoms

Right upper quadrant pain, midepigastric pain, nausea and vomiting, and visual disturbances are the chief symptoms of preeclampsia. Patients should also be monitored for hyperreflexia or clonus. Seizures occur in eclampsia.

Most patients with HELLP syndrome complain of feeling generally unwell or fatigued, abdominal pain—especially in the upper quadrant—nausea, vomiting, and headache. The key to identification is a low platelet count. An elevated D-dimer may also help identify HELLP syndrome.

Differential Diagnosis

The diagnosis of preeclampsia may be difficult in the field, especially if no previous blood pressure readings are available. You will need to rely on a thorough history and examination to refine the diagnosis.

Treatment

Prehospital treatment is supportive and aimed at blood pressure control, fluid replacement, blood product replacement, and monitoring for disseminated intravascular coagulopathy development. Pharmacologic interventions may include corticosteroids (for fetal lung development), magnesium sulfate, Apresoline (hydralazine), or labetalol (to address hypertension). Delivery may have to be induced to protect both the fetus and mother. Transport the pregnant patient on her left side to prevent the gravid uterus from compressing the vena cava.

Ectopic Pregnancy

Pathophysiology

Ectopic pregnancy, implantation of the fertilized ovum (egg) outside of the uterus, is a life-threatening condition. The characteristic site of implantation in an ectopic pregnancy is the fallopian tube, but the ovum may also implant in the abdominal cavity or elsewhere. If the fertilized ovum implants in the fallopian tube, the tube will begin to stretch as the embryo divides, causing pain and bleeding. The bleeding may be internal or vaginal.

Risk factors for ectopic pregnancy include scarring or inflammation of the pelvis from previous surgeries or ectopic pregnancies, pelvic inflammatory disease, tubal ligation, and placement of an intrauterine device. Because symptoms become apparent within 5 to 10 weeks of implantation, many women are not yet aware that they are pregnant.

Signs and Symptoms

Consider ectopic pregnancy in any woman of childbearing age who has vaginal bleeding with or without abdominal pain. Especially after an ectopic rupture, the bleeding can be severe, placing the patient at risk of shock.

Differential Diagnosis

Possible diagnoses include appendicitis, placenta previa, and complications from an abortion.

Treatment

Your initial goals for the patient will be to ensure that the airway and breathing are secure and to establish IV access. In the ED, a urine or serum pregnancy test can be obtained to establish whether the patient is pregnant. If a pregnancy is confirmed, a quantitative beta-hCG (human chorionic gonadotropin) should be obtained to help determine the stage of the pregnancy. The level of beta-hCG rises as the pregnancy progresses through the early stages. The next step will be transvaginal ultrasound to determine whether the pregnancy has been established in the uterus or in an extrauterine location. If the latter is confirmed, surgical intervention will be required.

Hyperemesis

Hyperemesis occurs early in pregnancy, usually in the first trimester, and can result in dehydration and fluid and electrolyte imbalance. It is defined by weight loss, starvation metabolism, and prolonged ketosis. Once other causes of vomiting are ruled out, management includes fluid therapy, electrolyte replacement, and antiemetics.

Pyelonephritis

Pyelonephritis is a bacterial infection of the kidneys. Pyelonephritis can be acute or chronic, and it is most often due to the ascent of bacteria from the bladder up the ureters to infect the kidneys. Symptoms include flank (side) pain, fever, shaking chills, sometimes foul-smelling urine, frequent and urgent need to urinate, and general malaise. Tenderness is elicited by gently tapping over the kidney with a fist (percussion). Diagnosis is made via urinalysis, which reveals white blood cells and bacteria in the urine. Usually there is also an increase in circulating white cells in the blood. Treatment involves IV fluids, antipyretics, pain medications, and use of appropriate antibiotics.

Renal Failure

Pathophysiology

Renal failure is typically classified as acute or chronic. In acute renal failure, the kidneys suddenly stop working, and waste products quickly begin to accumulate. If the condition is not corrected, it will progress to chronic renal failure.

Acute Renal Failure Acute renal failure has three phases: oliguric, diuretic, and recovery. These phases are summarized in Table 6-11. Oliguric acute renal failure can be due to one of three causes: prerenal failure, intrinsic renal failure, or postrenal failure. In prerenal failure, the kidney responds to inadequate perfusion by retaining fluids, which retards the glomerular filtration rate and encourages the reabsorption of sodium and water. This process is usually reversible if caught within 24 hours of onset.

Intrinsic acute renal failure is commonly caused by autoimmune disease, chronic uncontrolled hypertension, or diabetes mellitus. Heavy metals, poisons, and nephrotoxic medications may also be responsible for intrinsic acute renal failure. Under certain conditions, a heat emergency or crush injury may lead to rhabdomyolysis, in which myoglobin released from damaged muscles obstructs the tubular portion of the nephrons, causing permanent damage if not caught early. Myoglobin in the urine turns it tea colored, and this may be an early clue.

Postrenal failure occurs when urine flow is obstructed, causing a backflow of urine into the ureters and kidneys and causing the kidneys to dilate. This process disrupts kidney function, ultimately causing necrosis. If the backflow is not resolved, chronic renal failure may be the result.

Chronic Renal Failure Chronic renal failure is the permanent loss of renal function. The threshold for such metabolic disruption is reached when 80% of the estimated 1 million nephrons in the kidney are damaged or destroyed. At that point, dialysis or a kidney transplant is required for survival. In caring for the patient with chronic renal failure, you must know how the disease is typically managed and be aware of the complications associated with the disease and its treatment, especially dialysis.

Table 6-11 Phases of Acute Renal Failure

Phase	Description and Characteristics	Treatment
Oliguric phase	Usually lasts 10–20 days, with urine output decreasing by 50–400 mL/day Protein spill Hyponatremia Hyperkalemia Metabolic acidosis	Monitor ECG for peaked T waves and a widened QRS (hyperkalemia). Order a laboratory potassium study, since a lethal level may exist. Be prepared to administer sodium bicarbonate and calcium until dialysis can be initiated. CHF may also develop, so monitor for signs of left- and right-sided heart failure.
Diuretic phase	Occurs when urine output exceeds 500 mL in 24 hours Causes sodium and potassium loss in the urine May cause hypovolemia, since the patient may lose up to 3,000 mL in 24 hours through diuresis	Monitor for electrolyte disturbances and signs of hypovolemia. Be prepared to administer fluids and electrolytes to replace as much as 75% of the previous day's volume loss. Be prepared to treat GI bleeding and respiratory failure.
Recovery phase	May last weeks to months	Prevent fluid overload. Closely monitor electrolyte and fluid balance.

CHF, Congestive heart failure; ECG, electrocardiogram; GI, gastrointestinal.

Signs and Symptoms

A patient with renal complaints may have changes in urinary habits, edema, rash/itching, nausea, vomiting, dyspnea, chest discomfort, or acute coronary syndrome. It is important to remember that many renal patients have diabetes, so any coronary symptoms may be masked or silent. Initially patients with kidney failure may have no symptoms.

Differential Diagnosis

Kidney disease can have a variety of presentations, including urinary obstruction and coronary symptoms, depending on the stage of disease and the cause. The diagnosis of kidney failure is made by laboratory tests that measure serum urea nitrogen, creatinine, and the glomerular filtration rate, and radiologic studies.

Treatment

Patients with renal disease often have nausea and vomiting. Assessment to identify any life-threatening symptoms should be performed immediately. Warning signals include altered LOC, signs of congestive heart failure, dysrhythmia, and electrolyte imbalance.

If you are called to treat a patient in acute renal failure, you must know how to identify the most serious complications of acute renal failure: pulmonary edema and hyperkalemia. Aggressive treatment of the cause of acute renal failure—hemorrhage, sepsis, congestive heart failure, or shock of any kind—is the best way to stop prerenal acute renal failure in the field. If not managed properly, prerenal failure will progress to chronic renal failure, in which the renal tissue itself is damaged.

Patients with chronic renal failure will be some of the most challenging patients you will encounter. These patients usually have multiple medical problems, many of which are unique to chronic renal failure and end stage renal disease. Medical history is often extensive, with many comorbidities. It is impossible to cover all the presentations you may see in these patients. In chronic renal failure, fluid imbalances may lead to hypertension, pulmonary edema, or hypotension. Vascular overload caused by retention of fluid and sodium may be responsible for hypertension or congestive heart failure. Be cautious administering fluids, and in patients with hypertension, consider giving non–potassium-sparing diuretics, ACE inhibitors, or peripheral vasodilators.

Some myths and misconceptions regarding patients in renal failure are as follows:

- *Fluid administration.* Fluids should not be withheld from a renal failure patient in need of fluid resuscitation, but consult with medical control before initiating aggressive fluid resuscitation. Hypovolemic or hypotensive patients should receive a fluid bolus when indicated. Be careful to limit fluids in patients who do not need fluids. Typically, IV access is difficult to obtain in patients with renal failure. If IV access is indicated, it should not be deferred simply because a patient is in renal failure.
- *Diuretic administration.* Some end-stage renal failure patients continue to have some degree of residual kidney function. These patients may retain up to 20% of normal renal function, so a patient who presents in pulmonary edema may respond to a large dose of a loop diuretic like furosemide (Lasix). Patients will be able to tell you whether they still make urine, which will indicate whether diuretics will be effective in increasing urine output. Patients in renal failure often require large doses of diuretics, so consult medical control if necessary. In addition to decreasing fluid volume through increased renal excretion, furosemide causes venodilation and has a secondary therapeutic effect in fluid overload.
- *Morphine administration.* Pain is undertreated in 75% of the renal failure population, and yet pain medication administration in renal patients is extremely controversial. Codeine, meperidine (Demerol), propoxyphene (Darvon), and morphine are renally excreted. The metabolites build up in patients with chronic kidney disease and can cause neurotoxicity. According to the World Health Organization, the preferred pain medication is fentanyl. It has been proven safe and effective in patients with chronic kidney disease. Hydromorphone (Dilaudid) may also be used but with caution. The World Health Organization recommends that codeine, meperidine, propoxyphene, and morphine not be used. Other opinions are that in the emergency setting (i.e., pulmonary edema, acute myocardial infarction), it is safe to administer morphine. When in doubt, always consult with your medical control physician.

When you are assessing and evaluating the dialysis patient, the following information that may be crucial to your treatment.

- All dialysis patients require special consideration regarding any medication because of their altered pharmacokinetic and pharmacodynamic issues and increased potential for adverse reactions. They are at high risk for medication-related problems.
- Be sure to place a 12-lead ECG and initiate cardiac monitoring. If you suspect myocardial infarction or if the patient has premature ventricular contractions, administer oxygen. Fluids and antianginal medications may be indicated. Administration of antiarrhythmics may also be required. Consult medical control when administering medications to renal patients because of the complexity of their fluid and electrolyte imbalances and the potential for multisystem involvement.
- Do not overlook the possibility of hyperkalemia, which is a life threat. It can develop rapidly in the renal patient, and weakness may be the only sign or symptom present. Patients may remain asymptomatic until a fatal arrhythmia occurs. Cardiac monitoring and early lab work will help you identify this complication in time to treat it. If you suspect hyperkalemia, calcium, insulin, albuterol, furosemide, and Kayexalate (sodium polystyrene) should be administered. Calcium gluconate protects the myocardium, insulin and albuterol shift potassium into the cells, furosemide increases renal excretion of potassium, and Kayexalate removes potassium from the gut. If acidosis is

present, sodium bicarbonate may be used as well. Further discussion of hyperkalemia is found in Chapter 7. Acidosis stemming from an electrolyte imbalance, hypoperfusion, or diabetic complications may be identified if the patient exhibits an altered LOC, Kussmaul's respiration, or abnormal arterial blood gas levels. Management may include support of ventilation, fluid administration, and perhaps administration of sodium bicarbonate to address the electrolyte imbalance.

- Anticoagulant administration during dialysis may cause hemorrhage. This bleeding is complicated by anemia caused by dwindling erythropoietin secretion, which reduces red cell production. You should have a high index of suspicion for bleeding if the patient has shortness of breath or angina. Blood loss may be obvious, as in trauma to a vascular access site, or not so obvious, as in a patient with occult blood loss through GI bleeding. Prehospital priorities should be to control bleeding, ensure adequate oxygenation, and provide fluid support.
- Sudden onset of dyspnea, respiratory distress, chest pain, cyanosis, and hypotension indicates an air embolism. If this clinical picture becomes evident during dialysis, administer high-flow oxygen, and position the patient on his or her left side. Maintain IV access, and be prepared to support blood pressure. Consider placing the patient in a modified Trendelenburg position. This position is used to trap air in the right ventricle.
- Disequilibrium syndrome is a neurologic problem patients sometimes experience during or immediately after hemodialysis. Researchers believe the syndrome is caused by cerebral edema that develops when the serum urea nitrogen is lowered too quickly. In mild cases, the patient may complain of headache, restlessness, nausea, muscle twitching, and fatigue. In severe cases, signs and symptoms include hypertension, confusion, seizures, and coma. The event can be fatal. In most cases, however, the episode is self-limiting and will resolve over a few hours. If the patient does have a seizure, consider administering anticonvulsant medications. Prevention is the priority in this patients. Disequilibrium syndrome can be prevented by slowing the rate at which urea is removed from the body during hemodialysis.

In-hospital laboratory tests that indicate renal function include serum urea nitrogen and serum creatinine. If either level is elevated, the patient should be evaluated for renal insufficiency or failure. The normal ratio of serum urea nitrogen to creatinine is less than 20:1. A ratio of greater than 20:1 suggests a prerenal cause of the failure. A ratio of less than 20:1 indicates intrinsic renal failure.

Kidney Stones
Pathophysiology

Kidney stones, or renal calculi, form as a result of metabolic abnormalities, primarily calcium buildup. Those at greater risk are men, individuals with a family history of kidney stones, those who abuse laxatives, and patients with primary hyperparathyroidism, Crohn's disease, renal tubular acidosis, or recurrent urinary tract infection.

Although complete renal obstruction by kidney stones is an anomaly, it is possible and can precipitate renal failure. The size and location of the stone determines its ability to pass through the ureter.

Signs and Symptoms

Patients typically have constant dull flank pain that radiates to the abdomen, punctuated by bouts of sharp, colicky pain during hyperperistalsis of the smooth muscle of the ureter. Nausea, vomiting, and hematuria may be present. Fever indicates an infection but is an infrequent finding.

Differential Diagnosis

The differential diagnosis may include appendicitis, gallstones, inflammatory bowel disease, bowel obstruction, and abdominal aortic aneurysm.

Treatment

Prehospital treatment is supportive. Transport the patient in a position of comfort, establish IV access, and administer pain medications and antiemetics. At the hospital, a urinalysis will be ordered to look for blood in the urine. Serum urea nitrogen and creatinine levels will be checked, and CT or ultrasound studies will be performed.

Endocrine Causes of Abdominal Disorders
Diabetic Ketoacidosis

Diabetic ketoacidosis is a life-threatening complication of diabetes. It is often characterized by nausea, vomiting, and abdominal pain in addition to polyuria, polydipsia, hyperglycemia, polyphagia, and metabolic acidosis. Although it is possible for diabetic ketoacidosis to develop in people with type 2 diabetes, especially in the presence of an infection, the condition is far more characteristic of type 1 diabetes. More information is available in Chapter 7. Additional endocrine causes of abdominal discomfort are addressed in Chapter 7 as well.

Special Considerations
Home Medical Devices

As medical technology advances, prehospital medical providers are encountering in the home environment a wider variety of medical devices used by patients with abdominal disorders. The devices that you are most likely to see are as follows.

- *Nasogastric and nasointestinal feeding tubes.* Nasogastric and nasointestinal feeding tubes are typically small-diameter, flexible tubes that travel from the nose to the stomach or intestines. They are used for food intake or fluid administration in patients who cannot consume sufficient amounts of food or water by mouth, and they are used for medication infusion. Patients who use such devices might include those with a history of cancer, gastric bypass surgery, or stroke. Many complications can occur, including:

  - The tube can become displaced, causing the patient to aspirate fluid into the lungs. A dislodged tube can actually go into the lungs. Suspect either of these if the patient begins coughing or choking, is unable to speak, or air bubbles appear when the proximal end of the tube is placed in water.

  - The walls of the tube are typically thin and can easily develop a small leak.

  - An occlusion can form if the tube is not irrigated sufficiently after food or medication administration.

  - If any abnormalities occur, use of the tube should be discontinued.

- *Transabdominal feeding tubes.* Transabdominal feeding tubes are tubes placed surgically to provide a route for direct feeding into the stomach (gastrostomy tube; **Figures 6-7** and **6-8**), jejunum (jejunostomy tube), or both (gastrojejunostomy tube). They are used when food, fluid, or medication must be administered for a longer term than would be suitable for a nasally placed tube.

  Transabdominal feeding tubes are often used in patients who have difficulty swallowing, esophageal atresia, esophageal burns or strictures, chronic malabsorption, or severe failure to thrive. Potential complications include:

  - The stoma site can become infected. Look for drainage at the site and redness and inflammation of the surrounding skin.

  - Leakage from the stoma can occur if the tube is too small.

  - The feeding tube can become occluded or dislodged.

  - The patient can develop peritonitis or gastric or colonic perforation.

    If any abnormalities are apparent, feedings should be discontinued.

- *Bowel ostomy.* A bowel ostomy is a surgically created opening to eliminate waste from the bowel. It can be placed temporarily or permanently in patients with congenital bowel abnormalities, cancer, severe Crohn's disease, ulcerative colitis, or abdominal trauma. Any portion of the intestine can be rerouted through the abdominal wall. If the intestinal opening is closer to the stomach in the ileum, the patient is likely to have diarrhea, since stools cannot be formed. A bag placed over

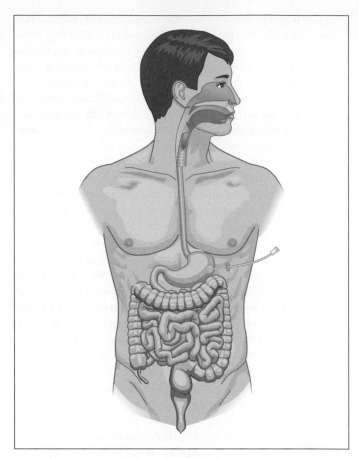

Figure 6-7 A gastrostomy tube is surgically placed into the stomach through the abdominal wall.
© Nucleus Medical Media/Visuals Unlimited/Corbis

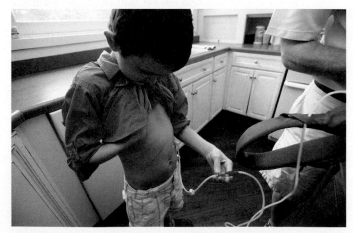

Figure 6-8 Gastrostomy button.
© Sara Caldwell/ZUMA Press/Corbis

the ostomy to collect waste must be emptied regularly to minimize tissue degradation caused by prolonged contact with stool.

- *Hemodialysis access devices.* Hemodialysis is the process of passing the patient's blood through a machine called a *dialyzer* to remove waste products and stabilize the patient's fluid and electrolyte balance. Multiple sites and devices are used to gain vascular access so the blood can be cleaned and returned to the body during dialysis. These include:

- A shunt is a temporary synthetic connection between an artery and a vein.
- A fistula is a permanent surgical connection between an artery and a vein.
- A catheter placed in the subclavian artery may also be used to gain vascular access.
- A button-shaped port (Hemasite) may be placed at the entry site.

  Assess for a thrill or bruit to verify the patency of a shunt or fistula, which is usually found in the arm but may be located in the leg. It's important not to take blood pressure in the extremities when a shunt or fistula is in place.

- *Peritoneal dialysis access devices.* A peritoneal dialysis access device is a catheter that allows fluids to be infused into and then drained out of the abdomen. This process removes waste products and temporarily stabilizes the electrolyte and fluid balance.

Older Adult Patients

Caring for the older adult population presents special challenges for prehospital providers. Because of diminishing cardiac and pulmonary reserves, altered gastric motility, and inadequate nutrition, older adult patients may become ill more quickly and be more vulnerable to conditions such as abdominal aortic aneurysm, ischemic colitis, pancreatitis, cholecystitis, and large-bowel obstruction.

Many abdominal complaints that become more common with advanced age have ambiguous symptoms. In fact, in diagnosing abdominal pain in patients over age 50, the rate of accuracy is less than 50%. The rate drops to less than 30% in patients over age 80. Further confounding the diagnosis is the fact that many medications frequently prescribed to older adults can mask signs of critical illness. Finally, obtaining a reliable and complete history may be complicated by memory deficits, dementia, hearing impairment, or anxiety.

Bariatric Patients

Morbid obesity is defined as having a body mass index of 40 or higher or, alternatively, being 100 pounds or more overweight. This condition has become more prevalent in the United States. Abdominal assessments in these patients can be very challenging. Surgical options are available to facilitate weight loss in patients with morbid obesity. Restrictive procedures shrink the size of the stomach or the bowel circumference. Gastric banding, for example, reduces the amount of food the patient can eat by restricting the size of the opening from the esophagus to the stomach. These bands are sometimes adjustable, allowing the bariatric surgeon to enlarge or reduce the capacity of the stomach as indicated. Another option is gastric bypass surgery, in which food is diverted around the stomach and upper small bowel through a pouch about the size of an egg. Unlike gastric banding, this procedure is not reversible.

The problems clinicians should be concerned with in bariatric patients are dependent on when the procedures were performed. As with all surgeries, both procedures carry the risk of complications, including infection, bleeding, abdominal pain, abdominal hernia, and lower-extremity deep vein thrombosis secondary to inactivity during recovery from surgery. Potential complications specific to patients who have had bariatric surgery include nausea, vomiting, diarrhea, electrolyte imbalance, and malnutrition, especially if the patient does not take vitamins as advised. These complications are ongoing and not only associated with the surgery itself.

Obstetric Patients

When you assess any woman of childbearing age for an abdominal complaint, you should assume she is pregnant until proven otherwise. Many complications of pregnancy can be mistaken for abdominal complaints, and abdominal complaints can be exacerbated by pregnancy. Keep in mind that medications administered to treat abdominal symptoms may be harmful to the fetus.

While caring for a pregnant patient, you must recognize that the survival of two patients depends on maintaining adequate perfusion. As the fetus grows, it places increasing pressure on the internal organs, diaphragm, and venae cava. Because of the boost in cardiac output and expansion of intravascular volume during pregnancy, signs of hypoperfusion may be delayed. During the second half of pregnancy, you should position the patient carefully to avoid triggering hypotension by putting pressure on the venae cava. Tilt or wedge the patient on her left side, and transport. Consider transport to a facility that cares for high-risk obstetric patients as appropriate.

Putting It All Together

Assessment of the patient with abdominal discomfort begins with the initial observation to determine whether the patient is sick or not sick. Let this initial impression tell you whether to intervene immediately or proceed to a more detailed assessment. Assess the patient for critical or emergent diagnoses first, and then consider less menacing conditions. The rule of thumb is to consider the more common or likely diagnosis and work toward the less common. To confirm or rule out conditions that make up your differential diagnosis, use tools such as SAMPLER, OPQRST, physical examination findings, and lab results. If the patient becomes unstable, support of airway, breathing, and circulation always takes precedence. Once the patient has been stabilized, return to your assessment. Because the possible causes of abdominal discomfort are so numerous, it is important to recognize that you may not be able to make a definitive diagnosis in the field. Offering supportive care, managing signs and symptoms, and providing quick transport is the best strategy for many patients with abdominal discomfort.

SCENARIO SOLUTION

- There are many possible causes of this patient's abdominal pain. She is still of childbearing age so it's possible she has a gynecologic problem such as ectopic pregnancy. She's the right age for cholecystitis. If she's a frequent drinker, she could have pancreatitis. It's also possible she's having a sickle cell crisis, or she could have an ulcer.
- To narrow your differential diagnosis, you'll need to complete a past history as well as the history of the present illness. Perform a physical examination of her abdomen.

- Assess her oxygen saturation. Consider obtaining a 12-lead ECG. Palpate for tenderness, masses, guarding, or pulsatile mass.
- The patient has signs of impending shock. You should administer oxygen. Prepare to suction her airway if she vomits again. Establish vascular access, and deliver IV fluids. Consider medication for nausea or pain if her blood pressure improves. Transport her to the closest appropriate hospital for further diagnostic tests and definitive intervention.

Summary

- The causes of abdominal discomfort are innumerable and may seem overwhelming when you try to make a diagnosis.
- Identify life threats first and then progress toward making a diagnosis as time and the patient's condition allow.
- Patient presentation, history, physical examination, and lab results will be the keys to arriving at an accurate diagnosis of abdominal discomfort.
- The abdomen contains multiple systems, each of which—alone or in combination—may be responsible for abdominal discomfort.
- Abdominal discomfort may be associated with other cardinal symptoms, such as nausea and vomiting, constipation, diarrhea, GI bleeding, jaundice, and vaginal bleeding. Taking into account these cardinal symptoms/chief complaints may assist pinpointing a diagnosis.
- Making a diagnosis should not take precedence over intervention in a patient with abdominal discomfort.

KEY TERMS

antiemetic   A substance that prevents or alleviates nausea and vomiting.

fulminant hepatic failure   A rare condition that occurs when hepatitis progresses to hepatic necrosis (death of the liver cells); classic symptoms include anorexia, vomiting, jaundice, abdominal pain, and asterixis (flapping tremor).

gastrointestinal (GI)   Pertaining to the organs of the GI tract. The GI tract links the organs involved in consumption, processing, and elimination of nutrients. It begins at the mouth, moves to the esophagus, travels through the chest cavity into the abdomen, and terminates in the pelvic girdle at the rectum.

gastroparesis   A medical condition consisting of a paresis (partial paralysis) of the stomach, resulting in food remaining in the stomach for an abnormally long time.

hematemesis   Vomiting of bright red blood, indicating upper GI bleeding.

hematochezia   Passage of red blood through the rectum.

intussusception   Prolapse of one segment of the bowel into the lumen of another segment. This kind of intestinal obstruction may involve segments of the small intestine, colon, or terminal ileum and cecum.

melena   Abnormal black, tarry stool that has a distinctive odor and contains digested blood.

referred pain   Pain felt at a site different from that of an injured or diseased organ or body part.

somatic (parietal) pain   Generally well-localized pain caused by an irritation of the nerve fibers in the parietal peritoneum or other deep tissues (e.g., musculoskeletal system). Physical findings include sharp, discrete, localized

KEY TERMS (CONTINUED)

© HunThomas/ShutterStock, Inc.

pain accompanied by tenderness to palpation, guarding of the affected area, and rebound tenderness.

visceral pain Poorly localized pain that occurs when the walls of the hollow organs are stretched, thereby activating the stretch receptors. This kind of pain is characterized by a deep, persistent ache ranging from mild to intolerable and commonly described as cramping, burning, and gnawing.

viscus (*pl.* viscera) The internal organs enclosed within a body cavity, including the abdominal, thoracic, pelvic, and endocrine organs.

volvulus A condition in which the stomach rotates more than 180 degrees; this twisting seals the stomach on both ends, blocking the flow of blood and the passage of fluid and food. The condition is characterized by an acute onset of abdominal pain, severe vomiting, and shock.

BIBLIOGRAPHY

© HunThomas/ShutterStock, Inc.

Aehlert B: *Paramedic practice today: Above and beyond*, St. Louis, MO, 2009, Mosby.

American Academy of Orthopaedic Surgeons: *Nancy Caroline's emergency care in the streets*, ed 7. Burlington, MA, 2013, Jones & Bartlett Learning.

Anemia in chronic kidney disease. kidney.niddk.nih.gov

Carale J, Azer A, Mekaroonkamol P: *Portal hypertension*. http://emedicine.medscape.com/article/175248-overview

Becker S, Dietrich TR, McDevitt MJ, et al.: *Advanced skills: Providing expert care for the acutely ill*, Springhouse, PA, 1994, Springhouse.

Bucurescu G: *Uremic encephalopathy*. http://www.medscapecrm.com/article/1135651-overview

Chronic renal failure. May 2001. www.nephrologychannel.com/crf/index.shtml

Dean M: Opioids in renal failure and dialysis patients, *J Pain Symptom Manage*. 28:497–504, 2004.

Deering SH: Abruptio placentae. http://emedicine.medscape.com/article/252810-overview, updated September 29, 2014.

Gould BE: *Pathophysiology for health care professionals*, ed 3, Philadelphia, PA, 2006, Saunders.

Hamilton GC: *Emergency medicine: An approach to clinical problem-solving*, ed 2, Philadelphia, PA, 2003, Saunders.

Haram K, Svendsen E, Abildgaard U: The HELLP syndrome: clinical issues and management: a review. Feb 26;9:8. doi: 10.1186/1471-2393-9-8, 2009.

Holander-Rodriguez JC, Calvert JF Jr: Hyperkalemia, *Am Fam Physician*. 73:283–290, 2006.

Holleran RS: *Air and surface patient transport: Principles and practice*, ed 3, St. Louis, MO, 2003, Mosby.

Johnson LR, Byrne JH: *Essential medical physiology*, ed 3, Amsterdam, Boston, 2003, Elsevier Academic Press.

Kidney failure. www.mayoclinic.com/healty/kidney failure/ds00280

Ko P, Yoon Y: *Placenta previa*. http://emedicine.medscape.com/article/796182-overview, updated March 23, 2015.

Krause R: Dialysis complications of chronic renal failure. http://emedicine.medscape.com/article/777957-media, updated April 16, 2013.

Lehne RA: *Pharmacology for nursing care*, ed 6, St. Louis, MO, 2007, Saunders.

McCance KL, Huether SE: *Pathophysiology: The biologic basis for disease in adults and children*, ed 6, St. Louis, MO, 2009, Mosby.

Mosby: *Mosby's dictionary of medicine, nursing & health professions*, ed 8, St. Louis, MO, 2009, Mosby.

Padden MO: HELLP syndrome: Recognition and perinatal management, *Am Fam Physician*. 30:829–836, 1999.

Paula R: Abdominal *compartment syndrome: Differential diagnosis & workup*. Updated February 23, 2009. http://emedicine.medscape.com/article/829008-diagnosis

Pitts SR, Niska RW, Xu J, et al: *National hospital ambulatory medical care survey: 2006 emergency department summary*, National health statistics reports No. 7, Hyattsville, MD, 2008, National Center for Health Statistics.

Rosen P, Marx JA, Hockberger RS, et al: *Rosen's emergency medicine: Concepts and clinical practice*, ed 6, St. Louis, MO, 2006, Mosby.

Sanders M: *Mosby's paramedic textbook*, rev ed 3, St. Louis, MO, 2007, Mosby.

Silen W, Cope Z: *Cope's early diagnosis of the acute abdomen*, Oxford, 2000, Oxford University Press.

Song L-M, Wong KS: *Mallory-Weiss tear*. Updated April 16, 2008. http://emedicine.medscape.com/article/187134-overview

Taylor MB: *Gastrointestinal emergencies*, ed 2, Baltimore, 1997, Williams & Wilkins.

Wagner J, McKinney WP, Carpenter JL: Does this patient have appendicitis? *JAMA*. 276:1589, 1996.

Wakim-Fleming J: Liver disease in pregnancy. In: Carey WD, ed. *Cleveland clinic: current clinical medicine* 2010. ed 2, Philadelphia, PA, 2010, Elsevier Saunders.

Wingfield WE: ACE SAT: *The aeromedical certification examinations self-assessment test*, 2008, The ResQ Shop Publishers.

CHAPTER REVIEW QUESTIONS

1. A 33-year-old man has right lower quadrant abdominal pain and vomiting. Five minutes after you administer a dose of ondansetron, he vomits forcefully. His vital signs are now include a blood pressure of 102/72 mm Hg; a pulse rate of 52 beats/min, and respirations of 20 breaths/min. The alteration in his vital signs is likely related to:
    a. Cardiac conduction defect
    b. Fluid loss
    c. Medication side effects
    d. Vagal stimulation

2. Your patient is complaining of a cramping pain around her umbilical area that won't let up. This is most suggestive of disease involving the:
    a. Appendix
    b. Gallbladder
    c. Liver
    d. Ovary

3. A 43-year-old man with diffuse abdominal pain and vomiting has a yellowish discoloration of his sclera. This indicates he has excess serum:
    a. Amylase
    b. Bilirubin
    c. Fibrinogen
    d. Protein

4. A 42-year-old man complains of a gnawing, severe pain in the epigastric area that radiates to his back. His vital signs include a temperature of 102°F, a blood pressure of 94/68 mm Hg, a pulse rate of 128 beats/min, and respirations of 24 breaths/min. Your highest priority intervention would be to administer:
    a. Metoclopramide, 5 mg IV
    b. Morphine, 2 mg IV
    c. Normal saline, 250 mL bolus
    d. Thiamine, 100 mg IV

5. A 22-year-old woman at a restaurant is complaining of abdominal pain and diarrhea. Her skin is flushed, and she feels faint. Her vital signs include a blood pressure of 98/50 mm Hg, a pulse rate of 124 beats/min, and respirations of 24 breaths/min. Which finding in her SAMPLER history is most likely to guide your differential diagnosis for this patient?
    a. Medical history includes endometriosis.
    b. Home medicines include Tegretol (carbamazepine) and Keppra (levetiracetam).
    c. Illness began about 10 minutes after eating.
    d. She had a normal menstrual period 3 weeks ago.

6. A 45-year-old woman complains of right upper quadrant abdominal pain. To help confirm your differential diagnosis if you suspect cholecystitis you should:
    a. Ask her to take a deep breath as you press upward into her right upper quadrant.
    b. Auscultate her bowel sounds.
    c. Percuss her abdomen.
    d. Tap her heel.

7. An 18-year-old, 35-kg adolescent female is vomiting copious amounts of bright red blood. The most likely diagnosis would be:
    a. Crohn's disease
    b. Esophageal varices
    c. Mallory-Weiss syndrome
    d. Peptic ulcer disease

8. An 88-year-old woman complains of nausea, vomiting, and constipation. Her abdomen is tender to palpation and appears distended. Her lungs are clear, and her vital signs include a blood pressure of 104/76 mm Hg, a pulse of 120 beats/min, and respirations of 20 breaths/min. An appropriate action would be to:
    a. Administer sodium bicarbonate, 1 mEq/kg IV.
    b. Ask her to contact her personal physician in the morning.
    c. Infuse normal saline at 250 mL/h.
    d. Suggest an enema to relieve the pressure of her stool.

9. A 45-year-old man complains of severe epigastric pain radiating to his back. He has vomited several times. His history is significant for alcohol abuse and hypertension. You suspect an inflammatory condition of a gastric accessory organ. To confirm your differential diagnosis on physical exam you should assess for:
    a. Blood in the stool
    b. Psoas sign
    c. Grey Turner sign
    d. Pain when the leg is extended

10. When you are assessing your patient's medication history, which would indicate the patient may have a preexisting ulcer?
    a. Atropine
    b. Diphenhydramine
    c. Famotidine
    d. Tegretol

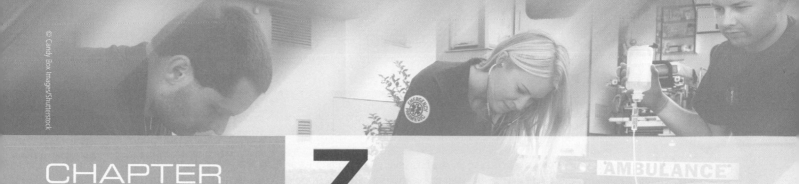

CHAPTER 7

Endocrine and Metabolic Disorders

This chapter will give you a fundamental understanding of endocrine and metabolic disorders. You will learn to integrate your knowledge of anatomy, physiology, and pathophysiology with the Advanced Medical Life Support (AMLS) assessment pathway in order to formulate differential diagnoses for life-threatening, critical/emergent, and nonemergent conditions. You will also learn how to implement and adapt management strategies for a variety of endocrine and metabolic disorders in prehospital and hospital settings.

LEARNING OBJECTIVES

At the conclusion of this chapter, you will be able to:

- Describe the anatomy, physiology, and pathophysiology of common endocrine disorders.

- Outline primary, secondary, and ongoing assessment strategies for the patient with an endocrine disorder using the AMLS assessment pathway.

- Identify the cardinal presentations/chief complaints of a broad range of endocrine disorders.

- List and be able to recognize the signs and symptoms of acid–base imbalances, electrolyte derangements, and endocrine disorders.

- Formulate provisional diagnoses on the basis of assessment findings for a variety of endocrine disorders.

- List the causes, diagnostic techniques, and treatment strategies for diseases of glucose metabolism and thyroid, parathyroid, and adrenal disorders.

- Use clinical reasoning skills to formulate and refine a differential diagnosis on the basis of a systematic, thorough secondary survey of a patient with an endocrine disorder.

- Implement effective treatment plans consistent with your assessment findings, and determine whether to continue the treatment on the basis of your ongoing assessment.

- Describe the pathophysiologic processes responsible for electrolyte and acid–base derangements, explain their causes, and discuss common modalities used to treat them.

- Compare and contrast normal and abnormal electrocardiogram (ECG) findings in the patient with an electrolyte derangement.

SCENARIO

You are caring for a 58-year-old woman who tells you she has severe fatigue and weakness. She has a history of type 2 diabetes, polymyalgia rheumatica, hypertension, and heart failure. Her medications include metformin, prednisone, lisinopril, furosemide, and digoxin. Her vital signs include a blood pressure of 88/52 mm Hg; pulse rate, 58 beats/min; and respirations, 20 breaths/min.

- Which differential diagnoses are you considering based on the information you have now?
- Which additional information will you need to narrow your differential diagnosis?
- What are your initial treatment priorities as you continue your patient care?

The endocrine system regulates metabolic processes of the body. The primary functions of the endocrine glands include the following:

- Regulating metabolism
- Regulating reproduction
- Controlling the balance of extracellular fluid and electrolytes (sodium, potassium, calcium, and phosphates)
- Maintaining an optimal internal environment such as regulation of blood glucose levels
- Stimulating growth and development during childhood and adolescence

Performing an assessment of a patient's endocrine system is challenging because the locations of the majority of these glands (with the exceptions of the thyroid gland and testes) make it impossible to inspect, palpate, percuss, or auscultate. It is also difficult to assess this system because of the different effects the hormones have on various systems throughout the body. Assessment of endocrine function depends on gathering data and recognizing the underlying pattern of an endocrine disorder.

Anatomy and Physiology

Glands are organs that manufacture and secrete chemical substances. Glands may be endocrine or exocrine. Exocrine glands secrete chemicals to the outer surface of the body (i.e., sweat and tears) or into a body cavity (i.e., saliva and pancreatic digestive enzymes). Endocrine glands secrete chemical hormones into the bloodstream. These chemicals travel to and act upon various tissues, where they signal and affect target cells that have appropriate receptors. They then act on these cells to cause a specific cell function. The network of endocrine glands that secrete hormones throughout the body is collectively referred to as the endocrine system.

The major components of the endocrine system include the pituitary gland, thyroid gland, parathyroid glands, adrenal glands, pancreas (both an endocrine and exocrine gland), and the reproductive organs (ovaries in women and testes in men) (**Figure 7-1**). Hormones released by these glands regulate homeostasis, reproduction, growth, development, and metabolism by transmitting messages directly to receptors located on their respective target organs. A complex system of feedback loops work together to maintain balanced levels of all hormones. Levels of hormone secretion may be regulated by either positive or negative feedback mechanisms. Increased levels of a particular hormone will inhibit secretion, and decreased levels of a particular hormone will stimulate secretion. The pituitary gland (**Figure 7-2**) is often referred to as the *master gland* because its secretions orchestrate the activity of other endocrine glands. The hypothalamus, which is located directly on top of the pituitary gland, is the part of the brain responsible for monitoring body conditions and maintaining homeostasis in the body. The hypothalamus contains several control centers for body functions and emotions. It is the primary link between the endocrine system and the nervous system.

To illustrate the interdependent nature of endocrine gland function and the feedback loops that work to maintain homeostasis, the complex regulation of the thyroid gland should be examined. The thyroid gland is located in the anterior part of the neck at the level between the fifth cervical and first thoracic vertebrae below the larynx (voice box). It is located beneath the rigid cartilage palpable in the anterior part of the neck. Its two lobes straddle the midline, joined by a narrow isthmus. Histologically, it's composed of secretory cells, follicular cells, and C cells (parafollicular cells). Hormones secreted by the thyroid (triiodothyronine [T_3] and thyroxine [T_4]) affect many tissues and organs in the human body, including the heart, musculoskeletal and nervous systems, and adipose tissue. Thyrotropin-releasing hormone (TRH), secreted by the hypothalamus, causes the release of thyroid-stimulating hormone (TSH, or thyrotropin) from the pituitary. The TSH then travels to and activates receptors in the thyroid gland, activating a biochemical cascade that results in the secretion of T_4 and T_3 by follicular cells in the thyroid gland. T_3 and T_4 travel through the bloodstream to affect many tissues but also inhibit synthesis of TRH in the hypothalamus, closing the feedback loop. Like many substances in the body,

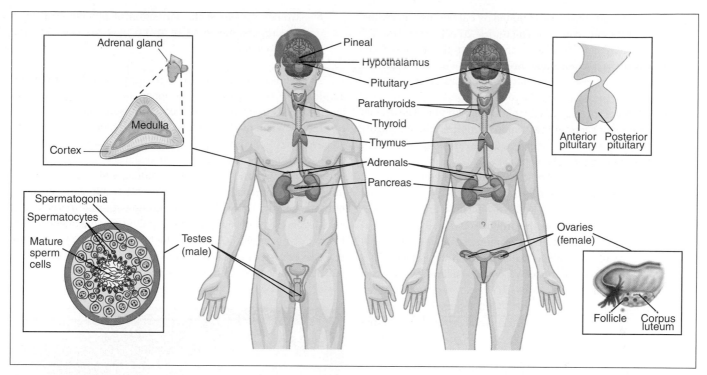

Figure 7-1 The endocrine system uses the various glands within the system to deliver chemical messages to organ systems throughout the body.

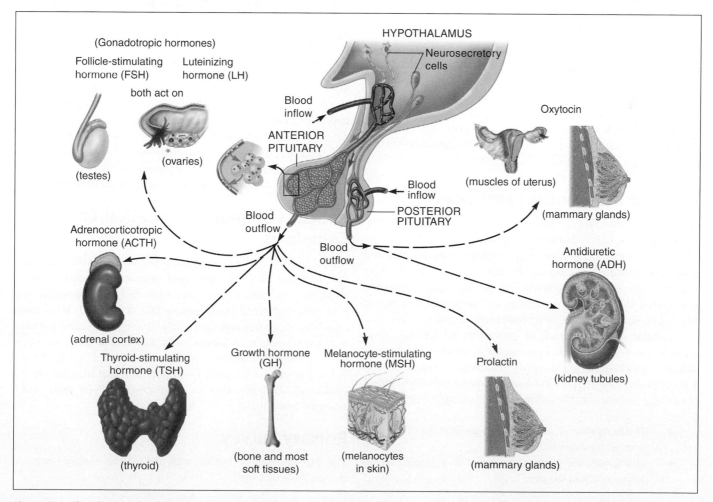

Figure 7-2 The pituitary gland secretes hormones from its two regions: the anterior pituitary lobe and the posterior pituitary lobe.

thyroid hormones will be largely bound by carrier proteins while circulating in the bloodstream. The terms "free T_3" and "free T_4" refer to thyroid hormones that are in circulation but not protein bound. Only these free hormones are able to act on target tissues. TSH secretion can also be inhibited by factors such as stress, glucocorticoids, and warmth. There is a second, less numerous type of cell in the thyroid called a parafollicular cell. These cells are responsible for secreting calcitonin hormone, which controls calcium metabolism. Calcitonin regulation depends on serum level, rather than on a feedback process.

The parathyroid glands lie posterior to the thyroid gland and comprise three types of cells, each of which has a particular function. Chief cells are responsible for producing parathyroid hormone (PTH), which stimulates the production of active vitamin D in the kidneys, encourages the reabsorption of calcium by the renal tubules, and inhibits phosphate reabsorption in the kidneys. PTH also liberates calcium from bone to increase calcium levels. A low calcium concentration stimulates PTH secretion, whereas an increase in calcium inhibits the production and liberation of PTH.

At the apex of each kidney is a triangular adrenal gland about 1.5 inches tall and 3 inches long. These two glands lie retroperitoneal and lateral to the inferior vena cava and abdominal aorta. Their venous and arterial blood supply is derived from upper and lower branches of the inferior vena cava and aorta, respectively. The cortex, or surface, of each adrenal gland secretes glucocorticoids such as cortisol, mineralocorticoids such as aldosterone, and supplemental sex hormones. The medulla, or body, of each adrenal gland produces epinephrine and norepinephrine.

The hypothalamus secretes corticotropin-releasing factor (CRF), stimulating the pituitary to produce adrenocorticotropin hormone (ACTH) and melanocyte-stimulating hormone (MSH). The adrenal gland reacts to ACTH by producing cortisol and aldosterone. Once a sufficient amount of cortisol has been produced by the adrenal glands, the hypothalamus automatically inhibits the production of ACTH and MSH.

Glucose Metabolism and Control

Glucose is a vital fuel for key metabolic processes in organs, especially those controlled by the central nervous system (CNS). The CNS is particularly dependent on glucose metabolism and relatively intolerant to changes in blood glucose levels. This explains why, for example, acute episodes of hypoglycemia are manifested as mental status changes, and persistent episodes of hypoglycemia can lead to irreversible brain damage.

Cellular survival depends on preserving a balanced serum glucose concentration. Under normal circumstances, the body is able to maintain serum glucose in the relatively tight range of 70 to 150 mg/dL (3.9 to 8.3 mmol/L) before and after meals. This control essentially derives from the following three metabolic processes:

- *GI absorption*: direct intestinal absorption of glucose through the intestine
- *Glycogenolysis*: glucose produced as glycogen breakdown occurs in the liver

- *Gluconeogenesis*: the formation of new glucose from precursors including pyruvate, glycerol, lactate, and amino acids

A complex interaction of hormones, neural (autonomic) and humoral (circulating or hormonal) factors, and regulatory mediators ensures maintenance of a normal serum glucose concentration. When the level of glucose in the blood is insufficient, glucagon is released from alpha cells in the pancreas to increase glucose production through gluconeogenesis. Glucagon release can also be triggered by exercise, trauma, and infection. These mechanisms increase glucose levels within minutes but do so only transiently. Epinephrine and norepinephrine increase glucose levels even more rapidly by enabling gluconeogenesis and hepatic glycogenolysis. Insulin, which is secreted by the pancreatic islet cells, is essential for efficient cellular glucose utilization and also drives glucose into the cells.

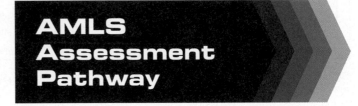

AMLS Assessment Pathway

▼ Initial Observations

Scene Safety Considerations

Make sure that all potential hazards are addressed and follow standard precautions. Your observation of the scene can give you important clues about the patient's underlying illness. Look for medications on the top of dressers, inside the refrigerator (for insulin), and inside the medicine cabinet in the bathroom. Take note of any insulin pumps or other medical devices that may be present. Bring any medication bottles to the hospital with the patient.

Patient Cardinal Presentation/Chief Complaint

Investigate the patient's cardinal presentation/chief complaint. Consider the patient's signs and symptoms. Remember that endocrine disorders present with signs and symptoms that indicate hormone secretion or production is affected. With many endocrine disorders and altered metabolic functioning, patients may experience restlessness, agitation, and a short attention span. In patients who have an altered mental status, check for a medical identification bracelet or necklace that may list known conditions. Patients who are unresponsive need their ABCs assessed immediately.

Primary Survey

The primary survey begins with the ABCs. Manage any life threats immediately.

Level of Consciousness

A patient who is experiencing an endocrine emergency will often be in serious distress. The patient's position may give you an indication of the severity of the condition. The patient who is unresponsive is in a critical state and may be experiencing an endocrine crisis such as hypoglycemia or hyperglycemia.

Airway and Breathing

Patients with endocrine emergencies may present with a variety of breathing levels. You should immediately assess the patient's effort of breathing. Increased work of breathing, abnormal respiratory rate, and hypoxia may all be indications that oxygen administration is necessary, such as with a nasal cannula or nonre-breathing mask. Be alert for abnormal respiratory patterns such as Kussmaul's respirations, which are often present in patients experiencing a diabetic ketoacidosis event. It is one of the body's compensatory mechanisms to "blow off" excess acid that is produced in this condition by increasing both respiratory rate and volume (a respiratory compensation to a metabolic acidosis).

Circulation/Perfusion

Assess the patient's skin color, moisture, and temperature, and obtain the patient's blood pressure. A patient with pale, cool, moist skin may be in shock or have hypoglycemia, whereas a patient with hot, dry skin may have a fever or hyperglycemia. A patient in hypoglycemic crisis will have a rapid, weak pulse. Because endocrine emergencies may affect the body's compensating systems, IV administration or blood component replenishment may be necessary. As always, follow your local protocols.

▼ First Impression

The difficult part of assessing patients with endocrine emergencies is that their problems tend to affect many organ systems and the seriousness of their presentations varies greatly. Many of the patients will have had their conditions for some time and may already be receiving treatment from their primary doctor or a specialist. These patients or their family members will likely share with you that there is a history of an endocrine problem. This information, along with the common signs and symptoms associated with each endocrine emergency described in this chapter, should help you determine possible causes of the current problem and generate an initial differential diagnosis.

▼ Detailed Assessment

History Taking

Collecting a complete history is critical to identifying endocrine emergencies. In diabetic emergencies in particular, the family history can give you pertinent information. Learning that other family members have a history of diabetes is a major clue and will help you in your differential diagnosis.

OPQRST and SAMPLER

The OPQRST and SAMPLER mnemonics should be used to obtain the patient's complete history using a systematic approach. Look for any signs that may assist you in confirming the patient's reported symptoms. Additional symptoms that may occur include polyphagia, polyuria, and polydipsia in patients with undiagnosed or poorly managed diabetes. Tachycardias, premature ventricular contractions (PVCs), premature atrial contractions (PACs), and other atrial dysrhythmias may all occur with hyperthyroidism and thyrotoxicosis.

It is possible that your patient's condition has been diagnosed prior to your arrival. In that case, the patient may have a significant amount of health-related information to provide you. Document all medications the patient is currently taking and whether the patient has been compliant with the regimen. Medications often provide another clue to the patient's condition.

Ask females of childbearing age about their last menstrual period because some patients with hypothyroidism may have a history of light or absent periods. A history of gestational diabetes is also important as it increases the risk of diabetes developing in a woman following her pregnancy.

Secondary Survey

Start your examination by noting the patient's appearance and the position in which he or she is found. Seizure activity and decorticate or decerebrate posturing should also be noted. If present, both are signs of serious illness.

Your physical examination should be geared toward identifying as many atypical findings as possible. Unless the patient had an endocrine emergency that caused some sort of trauma, a focused trauma assessment is usually not necessary. As always, a full-body exam should be completed after any life threats are managed.

When you check the patient's vital signs, look for the combination of hypertension and bradycardia, which suggests increased intracranial pressure.

Your secondary survey will reveal finer abnormalities that will help you determine your treatment. For example, if the patient's skin is cold and clammy, this may signal shock or severe hypoglycemia, as from an insulin reaction and the body's response to catecholamine release. Cold, dry skin may indicate an overdose of sedative drugs or alcohol intoxication. Hot, dry skin suggests hyperglycemia, fever, or possibly heat stroke. The goals of the secondary survey are twofold. First, you want to determine your patient's level of consciousness with precision so that later assessments can readily reveal whether the patient's condition is improving or deteriorating. Second, if your patient is in a coma, you need to look for clues to determine the cause.

Diagnostics

In patients with diabetes, obtain blood specimens early on, because any administration of prehospital dextrose or other medications will significantly change the chemical makeup of subsequent blood samples. An IV with 0.9% normal saline should be administered to patients with an altered mental status. Immediately assess the patient's blood glucose level and begin treatment if the reading is less than 60 mg/dL and the patient has a change in mental status. Give 12.5 g to 25 g of dextrose; this dose will reverse most cases of hypoglycemia.

▼ Refine the Differential Diagnosis

The components of the primary and secondary survey will help you refine your differential diagnosis and determine the severity of the patient's condition. Manage any life threats as they appear during the assessment process. Remember that most diseases or conditions, including endocrine disorders, are caused by more than one factor. The specific conditions described later will provide an approach for helping you determine the differential diagnosis and recognize key findings.

▼ Ongoing Management

Remember than an important aspect of patient care is to address the patient's emotional needs. Endocrine disorders can be stressful conditions for patients to manage. Always be empathetic and responsive to the patient's needs. Recheck vital signs and level of consciousness frequently in unstable patients and at least every 15 minutes in stable patients. Every patient should have at least two sets of vital signs documented.

Parathyroid, Thyroid, and Adrenal Gland Disorders

Hypoparathyroidism

Hypoparathyroidism is a rare condition characterized by low serum levels of PTH or resistance to its action. Congenital, autoimmune, and acquired diseases are among its many causes. Regardless of etiology, the hallmark of the condition is hypocalcemia, which will be discussed later.

Pathophysiology

The most common cause of acquired hypoparathyroidism is iatrogenic damage or inadvertent removal of the glands during thyroidectomy. Damage (during neck dissection, for example) can be transitory or permanent.

Signs and Symptoms

Patients with acute hypoparathyroidism report muscle spasm, paresthesia, and tetany. The patient may even have seizures. These signs and symptoms are directly due to hypocalcemia.

Differential Diagnosis

In the prehospital setting, no laboratory studies are immediately available to confirm hypoparathyroidism, so you must have a high index of suspicion on the basis of history and physical examination findings. Recent anterior neck surgery is a risk factor for iatrogenic hypoparathyroidism.

You should be familiar with Trousseau's sign (**Figure 7-3**) and Chvostek's sign (**Figure 7-4**), both of which will help you detect muscular irritability caused by hypocalcemia. To obtain a positive Trousseau's sign, place a blood pressure cuff around the arm, inflate it 30 mm Hg above systolic blood pressure, and hold

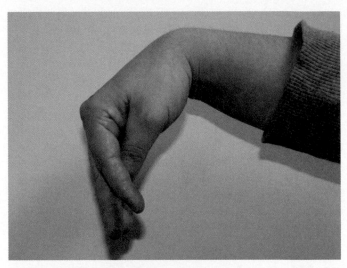

Figure 7-3 Trousseau's sign.
© Jones & Bartlett Learning. Photography by Carolyn Arcabascio.

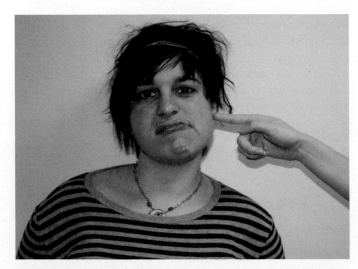

Figure 7-4 Chvostek's sign.
© Jones & Bartlett Learning. Photography by Carolyn Arcabascio.

it in place for 3 minutes. This will induce spasm of the muscles of the hand and forearm. The wrist and metacarpophalangeal joints flex, the distal and proximal interphalangeal joints extend, and the fingers adduct. You can elicit a positive Chvostek's sign by tapping the facial nerve against the mandibular bone just anterior to the ear, which produces a spasm of the facial muscles. This sign, however, is not as sensitive as Trousseau's sign.

Another tool available is the electrocardiogram (ECG). In patients with hypocalcemia, the QT interval is prolonged (**Figure 7-5**).

Treatment

As in any emergent condition, you must assess and stabilize the patient's airway, breathing/ventilation, and hemodynamic status. Obtain intravenous (IV) access and provide supportive treatment. If the patient is having seizures, administer benzodiazepines. When you have a strong clinical suspicion or laboratory analysis confirms hypocalcemia, the patient may be given IV calcium. In emergent situations, administer calcium chloride or calcium gluconate, 0.5- to 1-g IV bolus. In nonemergent situations, administer 100 to 300 mg of calcium diluted in 150 mL of 5% dextrose in water (D$_5$W) solution over 10 minutes.

Hyperthyroidism

Hyperactivity of the thyroid gland, or hyperthyroidism, is a common ailment that results in a hypermetabolic state called **thyrotoxicosis**. Contrast this with **thyroid storm**, which is a more rare complication of hyperthyroidism that occurs in only 1% to 2% of patients, but it is a life-threatening condition characterized by hemodynamic instability, altered mental status, gastrointestinal (GI) dysfunction, and fever.

Pathophysiology

Graves' disease, also known as *diffuse toxic goiter*, is the most common form of hyperthyroidism. It is an autoimmune disorder in which antibodies that mimic the role of TSH produce an increase in secretion of thyroid hormones. This condition most often occurs in women of middle age, but it can occur at any age and can also affect men. Other causes of hyperthyroidism include acute intoxication with exogenous thyroid hormones, and (less commonly) as a result of drugs with high iodine loads such as amiodarone or iodinated IV contrast, which may precipitate sudden release of excess thyroid hormones in susceptible individuals. In cases of autoimmune destruction of the gland, there may be a temporary hyperthyroidism preceding the more chronic hypothyroidism.

Thyroid storm occurs when the body is stressed by a diabetic emergency, an adverse drug reaction, or some serious challenge. You should suspect thyroid storm if the patient experienced cardiac decompensation after taking amiodarone, an antiarrhythmic agent rich in iodine. Other triggers of thyroid storm are summarized in Table 7-1.

Signs and Symptoms

The characteristic clinical presentation of a patient with hyperthyroidism includes apprehension, agitation, edginess, heart

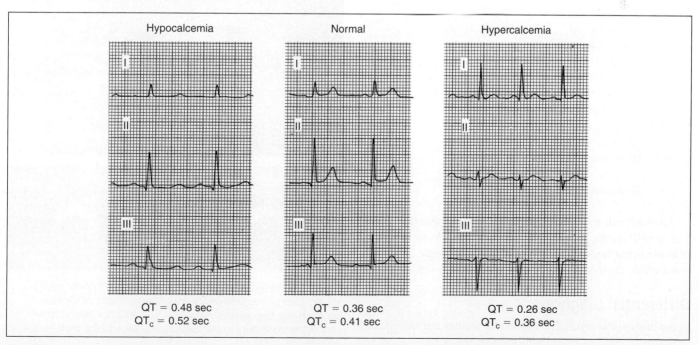

Hypocalcemia	Normal	Hypercalcemia
QT = 0.48 sec	QT = 0.36 sec	QT = 0.26 sec
QT$_c$ = 0.52 sec	QT$_c$ = 0.41 sec	QT$_c$ = 0.36 sec

Figure 7-5 Hypocalcemia prolongs the QT interval by stretching out the ST segment. Hypercalcemia decreases the QT interval by shortening the ST segment so that the T wave seems to take off directly from the end of the QRS complex.

From Goldberger A: *Clinical electrocardiography: a simplified approach,* ed 7, St. Louis, MO, 2006, Mosby.

Table 7-1 Triggers of Thyroid Storm

Medical Triggers	Endocrine Triggers	Pharmacologic Triggers
Infectious disease	Hypoglycemia	Iodine therapy
Cardiac ischemia	Diabetic ketoacidosis	Amiodarone ingestion
Serious burns	Nonketotic hyperosmolar state	Administration of contrast medium
Thromboembolism		Drug interactions
Major surgery		
Trauma		

palpitations, and weight loss of as much as 40 pounds over a few months. Heat intolerance and increased sweating caused by this hypermetabolic state are frequent symptoms.

A complete physical exam will reveal signs and symptoms of thyrotoxicosis, including the exophthalmos that is characteristic of the condition (**Figure 7-6**). Other signs and symptoms of hyperthyroidism include the following:

- Shortness of breath
- Disorientation
- Abdominal pain
- Diarrhea
- Chest pain
- Enlarged thyroid gland (palpable goiter)
- High-output cardiac failure
- Fever
- Drug interactions
- Altered mental status
- Jaundice
- Weakness

Apathetic thyrotoxicosis is a rare form of thyrotoxicosis seen only in older adults. In this condition, the characteristic symptoms of hyperthyroidism are absent. The patient is lethargic, has an apathetic affect, develops a goiter, and experiences weight loss.

Differential Diagnosis

In the prehospital setting, no laboratory studies are immediately available to confirm hyperthyroidism or thyroid storm, so you must have a high index of suspicion on the basis of history and physical examination findings. You can begin to stabilize the patient and initiate early treatment on the strength of clinical judgment alone.

In the hospital, the most rapid and useful test for hyperthyroidism is TSH serum level; if it is low and the patient has clinical signs and symptoms of hyperthyroidism, the test is essentially diagnostic. To confirm this presumptive diagnosis, the levels of the actual thyroid hormones, usually T_4 and T_3, may be obtained. Imaging studies and biopsy can help determine the specific cause of the disorder.

As part of the differential diagnosis, consider stroke, diabetic emergencies, congestive heart failure (CHF), toxic ingestion (particularly ingestion of a sympathomimetic agent), and sepsis.

Treatment

The key to providing optimal patient care is to differentiate among the various hypermetabolic states induced by thyroid disorders. These include subacute (chronic) hyperthyroidism, acute severe hyperthyroidism, and its most critical complication, thyroid storm. When you are caring for a patient with chronic hyperthyroidism, the patient generally requires only supportive care and early management of symptoms. If severe hyperthyroidism or thyroid storm is detected, it is imperative to stabilize the patient's condition. As in any acute emergency, begin with the ABCs. Be alert to the fact that patients experiencing acute severe

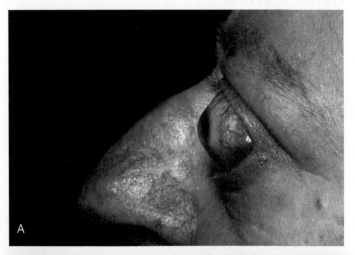

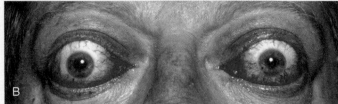

Figure 7-6 Person with hyperthyroidism (A and B). Wide-eyed, staring gaze caused by overactivity of the sympathetic nervous system is one feature of this disorder. The accumulation of loose connective tissue behind the eyeballs also adds to the protuberant appearance of the eyes.

A © Science Photo Library; B © SPL/Custom Medical Stock Photo, Inc hyperthyroidism or thyroid storm may exhibit altered mental status progressing to coma.

The patient with thyroid storm often has moderate to severe dehydration because of excessive diarrhea and sweating. For aggressive hydration, establish two peripheral IV lines early in the course of treatment. Although aggressive hydration is indicated, care must be taken to avoid inducing acute pulmonary edema, as these patients may experience cardiac instability.

A patient with hyperthyroidism is prone to arrhythmias such as sinus tachycardia, atrial fibrillation, atrial flutter, and premature ventricular contractions. For this reason, you should begin continuous cardiac monitoring as soon as you suspect this diagnosis.

Patients with thyroid storm may have fever associated with the pathophysiologic process itself or with an infection that precipitated the thyroid storm. Assess body temperature and treat hyperpyrexia in thyroid storm with acetaminophen. *Do not* use aspirin because it is associated with decreased protein binding of thyroid hormones and correspondingly increased levels of unbound or free T_3 and T_4, which will exacerbate symptoms.

The goals of pharmacologic treatment in the prehospital setting are to block the peripheral adrenergic hyperactivity the thyroid hormones elicit (tachycardia, fever, anxiety, and tremors) and to inhibit the conversion of T_4 to T_3 in peripheral tissues. Both objectives can be achieved by administering beta-blockers. The drug of choice is propranolol, given 1 mg IV every 10 minutes up to a total of 10 mg IV or until symptoms have resolved. Propranolol is contraindicated in patients with bronchial asthma, chronic obstructive pulmonary disease (COPD), atrioventricular blocks, hypersensitivity, and severe heart failure. A patient with thyroid storm and concomitant heart failure most likely has a high-output cardiac failure. This is not considered a contraindication to the use of propranolol unless he or she also has significant cardiomyopathy with systolic dysfunction. Adjunctive corticosteroid therapy—either hydrocortisone, 100 mg IV, or dexamethasone, 10 mg IV—may be given to slow the conversion of T_4 to T_3.

Hypothyroidism

Hypothyroidism is an endocrine dysfunction characterized by decreased or absent secretion of thyroid hormones. Its incidence in the United States is 4.6% to 5.8%, but half of those with the condition are asymptomatic. Hypothyroidism is most common among white adult women between the ages of 40 and 50. It is highly associated with autoimmune conditions.

Pathophysiology

Defective thyroid hormone secretion is classified as either primary or secondary hypothyroidism. The causes of each are summarized in Table 7-2. Primary hypothyroidism involves direct thyroid injury caused by an autoimmune disorder or an

Table 7-2 Causes of Hypothyroidism	
Primary	**Secondary**
Autoimmune hypothyroidism	Sarcoid infiltration
Hereditary hypothyroidism	Pituitary mass
Radiation therapy	
Iodine deficiency	
Use of lithium	
Use of antithyroid medications	
Idiopathic	

adverse drug reaction. Patients who have had surgical thyroidectomy or radioablation therapy (using radiation to decrease the amount of functional glandular tissue) for a hyperthyroid state may have resultant hypothyroidism. In secondary hypothyroidism, damage to the hypothalamus or pituitary gland results in decreased stimulation of the thyroid gland (specifically, a decline in the production and release of TSH). Many complications result from clinical hypothyroidism, including hypoxia, hypothermia, hypoglycemia, sepsis, and narcosis.

Signs and Symptoms

Hypothyroidism has a deleterious effect on many body systems, including the integumentary, metabolic, nervous, and cardiovascular systems. The skin of a patient with this condition is cool, dry, and yellow. The patient typically has thinning of the eyebrows, coarse hair and skin, marked intolerance to cold temperatures, and neurologic changes such as altered mental status, ataxia, and delayed relaxation of deep tendon reflexes. When hypothyroidism becomes chronic and extreme, it may evolve into a life-threatening condition called **myxedema** coma (**Figure 7-7**), characterized by hypotension, bradycardia, hypoglycemia, and low serum sodium (hyponatremia). Precipitants of myxedema coma include the following:

- Lung infection
- Cold exposure
- Heart failure
- Stroke
- Gastrointestinal bleeding
- Trauma
- Stress
- Hypoxia
- Electrolytic disturbances
- Low serum glucose levels

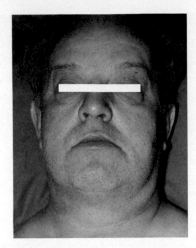

Figure 7-7 Localized accumulations of mucinous material in the neck of a hypothyroid patient.

Differential Diagnosis

In the prehospital setting, no laboratory studies are immediately available to confirm hypothyroidism or myxedema coma. History and physical examination findings will suggest the diagnosis. Stabilization and early treatment must be initiated solely on the basis of clinical judgment.

In the hospital, TSH levels will be greater than 10 µU/mL or (10 mU/L). In addition, a free thyroxine (FT$_4$) study may be ordered to evaluate abnormal protein levels that may in turn affect the level of T$_4$. A T$_4$ level below 0.8 ng/dL (10 pmol/L) indicates that the thyroid gland is not producing adequate levels of the hormone. Ultrasound imaging can be performed to reveal the size, shape, and position of the thyroid gland and to identify cysts or tumors that may contribute to thyroid dysfunction.

Treatment

You should be able to differentiate among the various hypometabolic states induced by thyroid disorders: hypothyroidism, severe hypothyroidism, and its most critical complication, myxedema coma. Patients with hypothyroidism require supportive care and early management of symptoms. You must have a high index of suspicion for this disorder. If severe hypothyroidism or myxedema coma is detected in the prehospital environment, it is imperative to stabilize the patient's condition and provide transport immediately to a facility with adequate resources to provide definitive treatment.

As in any acute emergency, begin with the ABCs. Patients with hypothyroidism, similar to those with acute hyperthyroidism and thyroid storm, may show evidence of altered mental status or be comatose. Airway management and ventilatory support may be needed. Particular attention must be paid to assessing the patient for heart failure. Initiate a peripheral IV line early during prehospital management to support conservative hydration.

If the patient has altered mental status, determine the serum glucose level. If the value is less than 60 mg/dL (3.3 mmol/L), administer IV dextrose.

The hypothyroid patient is prone to experiencing heart arrhythmias, especially bradycardia, so begin continuous cardiac monitoring as soon as possible. Be aware, however, that standard treatments for bradycardia may be ineffective until thyroid hormone has been replaced.

A patient suffering from myxedema coma may be hypothermic as a result of the pathophysiologic process itself or because of an infection. Always assess body temperature, and treat hypothermia with blankets and other warming techniques. Rapidly transport the patient to a well-equipped hospital facility for definitive treatment, which may include L-triiodothyronine, 0.25 mcg IV; hydrocortisone, 100 mg IV every 8 hours; and subsequent daily oral replacement therapy if the condition proves irreversible.

Chronic Adrenal Insufficiency

Adrenal insufficiency, the failure of the adrenal cortex to produce a sufficient amount of cortisol, is classified as primary, secondary, or tertiary, depending on whether the cortex is damaged directly or indirectly. Primary adrenal insufficiency, known as **Addison's disease**, is a metabolic and endocrine ailment caused by a direct insult to, or malfunction of, the adrenal cortex. It is a chronic disease with a protracted onset. Almost any condition that directly harms the adrenal cortex can cause primary adrenal insufficiency, including autoimmune disorders, adrenal hemorrhage, and infectious diseases such as acquired immunodeficiency syndrome (AIDS), tuberculosis, and meningococcemia.

Pathophysiology

As noted previously, the adrenal cortex produces the corticosteroid hormones aldosterone and cortisol. Aldosterone is responsible for keeping serum levels of sodium and potassium in balance. When the body experiences any stress—trauma, infection, cardiac ischemia, or a severe illness, to name a few—the adrenal glands may become unable to produce sufficient amounts of corticosteroid hormones to supply the body's demands, triggering an acute exacerbation of Addison's disease.

In secondary adrenal insufficiency, although the cortex itself is intact, it fails to receive a signal to produce cortisol because the pituitary gland fails to release adrenocorticotropin hormone (ACTH), which normally stimulates the adrenal cortex—thus the adrenal insufficiency is one step removed. Tertiary (third-level) adrenal insufficiency, in which the pituitary's failure to release ACTH stems from a disorder of the hypothalamus, is even less direct.

In primary adrenal insufficiency, patients may develop hyperpigmentation of the skin due to overproduction of melanocyte-stimulating hormone (MSH). This overproduction results from the fact that MSH and ACTH are produced from the same precursor protein (pro-opiomelanocortin) in the pituitary. MSH stimulates melanocytes in the skin to produce the skin pigment melanin. Secondary and tertiary adrenal insufficiency are not associated with hyperpigmentation of the skin because they involve low levels of MSH rather than high levels.

Signs and Symptoms

The clinical presentation of a patient with Addison's disease is consistent with the endocrine and electrolyte disorders brought on by the disease. The patient will have chronic fatigue and weakness, loss of appetite and consequent weight loss, and hyperpigmentation of the skin and mucous membranes due to the excess MSH production (**Figure 7-8**). The patient will have electrolyte disturbances associated with hyponatremia, hyperkalemia, and hypotension and might also have GI disturbances such as abdominal pain, nausea, vomiting, and diarrhea.

Differential Diagnosis

Diagnostic tools for chronic adrenal insufficiency are not available in the prehospital setting. It's important that you ask the patient for any old diagnostic laboratory reports that might be readily available. Past abnormal electrolyte findings that correlate with the patient's current clinical presentation, such as metabolic acidosis, hyponatremia, hyperkalemia, and hypoglycemia, should raise a red flag. Definitive diagnosis of this condition is made by measuring the patient's baseline serum cortisol level and then conducting stimulation testing, in which synthetic ACTH (called *cosyntropin*) is administered. If the cortisol level fails to rise shortly afterward, the patient can be diagnosed as having primary adrenal insufficiency.

Treatment

The prehospital management of an acute exacerbation of Addison's disease, known as an "addisonian crisis," is limited to supportive care. If the patient has tachycardia and hypotension, administer a 20-mL/kg fluid bolus of normal saline solution. Continual reevaluation of the patient's hemodynamic state, early administration of hydrocortisone (100 to 300 mg IV, or as dictated by local EMS protocol and medical control orders) to supplement the failing adrenal function, and rapid transport to the emergency department (ED) are paramount

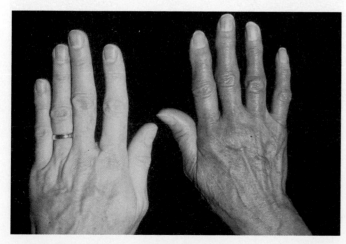

Figure 7-8 The hand of a patient with Addison's disease (right) compared with the hand of a healthy person (left).

in treating this condition. Provide correction of hypoglycemia, as well as symptomatic medical treatment of nausea and vomiting.

In the hospital, diagnostic testing will be carried out to identify electrolyte abnormalities such as hyponatremia and hyperkalemia. Elevated hematocrit levels are common. Management includes correction of electrolyte abnormalities, restoration of metabolic balance (e.g., by replacing glucocorticoids), and volume replacement for hypovolemia.

Acute Adrenal Insufficiency

Acute adrenal insufficiency is a condition in which the body's need for glucocorticoids and mineralocorticoids exceeds the delivery of these hormones by the adrenal glands. The most common cause is abrupt discontinuation of pharmacologic steroid therapy after prolonged use. It can also occur when such a patient fails to receive an adjusted dosage during times of stress, such as during illness or after major surgery or trauma.

Pathophysiology

Like chronic adrenal insufficiency, acute insufficiency is classified as primary, secondary, or tertiary, depending on the dysfunctional endocrine gland. *Primary adrenal insufficiency* refers to dysfunction of the adrenal glands, *secondary adrenal insufficiency* refers to dysfunction of the pituitary gland, and *tertiary insufficiency* is linked to hypothalamic dysfunction.

Signs and Symptoms

The clinical picture of acute adrenal insufficiency will include nausea, vomiting, dehydration, abdominal pain, and weakness. Historical clues, such as tan skin on a patient who denies sun exposure, may indicate chronic adrenal insufficiency. Ask the patient about recent medication changes that may have precipitated the symptoms. When adrenal insufficiency is accompanied by hypotension, the condition is called **adrenal crisis** and constitutes a true life-threatening emergency.

Differential Diagnosis

The diagnosis of this condition in the prehospital setting can be challenging. The definitive confirmatory laboratory test is not available in the field, and the presentation of acute adrenal insufficiency can easily be confused with more common conditions such as GI disorders. As the EMS provider, you have to use your available tools to find indirect evidence of an adrenal disorder. Assess for hypoglycemia with a glucometer, and look for evidence of hyperkalemia on the ECG. Assess for signs and symptoms of other abnormalities such as anemia, hyponatremia, and metabolic acidosis.

Vital signs can also provide key clues. For example, hypotension that's poorly responsive to administration of IV fluids is seen in adrenal crisis. Confirmation of the disorder can be performed in the ED, using the cosyntropin stimulation test.

Treatment

As with any life-threatening emergency, first evaluate the patient's ability to maintain his or her airway, breathing, and circulation. For hypotension, immediate resuscitation with normal saline is warranted. Administer dextrose if hypoglycemia is present. Address a deficit of glucocorticoids with hydrocortisone, 100 to 300 mg IV, which must be ordered under medical direction in some systems. If a cosyntropin stimulation test is to be performed at a later time, dexamethasone, 4 mg IV, is preferable to hydrocortisone because hydrocortisone can create a false-positive test result. Rapidly transport the patient to the ED for definitive treatment.

Hyperadrenalism

Hyperadrenalism, or Cushing's syndrome, is the clinical condition caused by long-standing exposure to excessive circulating serum levels of glucocorticoids, particularly cortisol, as a result of overproduction in the adrenal cortex. It is more common in women, especially those aged 20 to 50. Cushing's syndrome can be brought on by an adrenal gland or pituitary tumor or by long-term corticosteroid use.

Pathophysiology

Regardless of the cause, excess cortisol causes characteristic changes in many body systems. Metabolism of carbohydrate, protein, and fat is disturbed, such that the blood glucose level rises. Protein synthesis is impaired so that body proteins are broken down, which leads to loss of muscle fibers and muscle weakness. Bones become weaker and more susceptible to fracture.

Signs and Symptoms

Patients with Cushing's syndrome have a distinct appearance characterized by obesity, a moon face (**Figure 7-9**), and other cardinal features. Signs and symptoms that tend to accompany this disorder include the following:

- Chronic weakness
- Increased body and facial hair
- Full, puffy face
- Fatty "buffalo hump" at the back of the neck
- Central body obesity
- Purple striae on the abdomen, buttocks, breasts, or arms
- Atrophied proximal muscles
- Thin, fragile skin
- Amenorrhea
- Decreased fertility or diminished sex drive
- Diabetes mellitus
- Hypertension

Differential Diagnosis

Definitive diagnostic testing for Cushing's syndrome is not available in the prehospital setting. Ask the patient for any old diagnostic laboratory reports that might be readily available as a part of recent discharge paperwork. Past abnormal electrolyte findings that correlate with the patient's current clinical presentation, such as metabolic alkalosis, hypernatremia, hypokalemia, and hyperglycemia, should raise suspicion for the disease.

Treatment

Patients with Cushing's syndrome often have chronic or subacute symptoms. Management is guided by the clinical presentation. Affected patients may have fluid retention or, because of

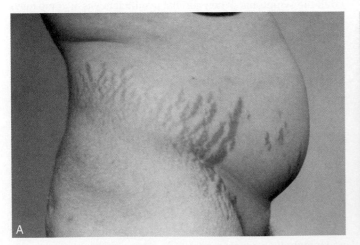
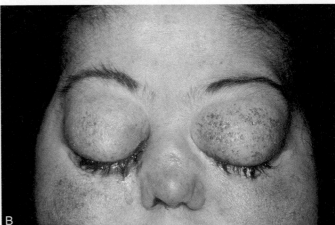

Figure 7-9 Patient with Cushing's syndrome **A.** Central obesity. **B.** "Moon faces."
© BIOPHOTO ASSOCIATES/Science Source/Getty Images.

the osmotic diuresis brought on by hyperglycemia, may be dehydrated. Thus fluid replacement should be dictated by volume status. Hypertension does not require specific therapy unless it has caused end-organ dysfunction or symptoms (e.g., CHF, cardiac ischemia, encephalopathy, acute renal failure). If such a condition is present, administer antihypertensive treatment. Monitor vital signs, mental status, and cardiac rhythm closely.

Glucose Metabolic Disorders

Metabolic emergencies represent true diagnostic and management challenges for basic life support (BLS) providers because so few diagnostic tools are available in the prehospital setting. Many metabolic conditions are associated with nonspecific symptoms, causing a potential delay in treatment. The following sections discuss some of the fundamental clinical principles to consider in order to promptly arrive at a diagnosis and begin appropriate treatment.

Diabetes Mellitus

Diabetes mellitus is the most common endocrine disorder and refers to a group of conditions characterized by hyperglycemia (high blood glucose levels) resulting from defects in insulin production, insulin action, or both. Glucose is a vital energy source for the body, but insulin is required for glucose to travel into the cell, where it can be used. Insulin acts like a key to unlock the cell membrane and allow the glucose to enter.

Pathophysiology

Clinically, diabetes manifests as a high level of blood glucose and unbalanced lipid and carbohydrate metabolism. Untreated diabetes results in hyperglycemia. A random plasma glucose level > 200 mg/dL (> 11.1 mmol/L) or a fasting serum glucose > 140 mg/dL (> 7.7 mmol/L) meets the threshold for a diagnosis of diabetes. The percentage of glycated hemoglobin (also called glycosylated hemoglobin or Hb_{A1c}) is often used as a measure of a patient's diabetes control because the percentage correlates to the average blood glucose levels over a 3-month period. Chronically poor glucose control tends to cause microvascular problems in multiple organ systems, including the heart, kidneys, eyes, and neurologic system. Patients with diabetes should be considered at high risk for coronary disease and complications from infections.

Hypoglycemia among people with diabetes is the result of inadvertent overdose of insulin or (less commonly) oral hypoglycemic agents. Because glucose levels must be maintained within a narrow range, diabetes is a difficult disease to control, and diabetic emergencies account for between 3% and 4% of EMS calls, most of which are for hypoglycemia, and 10% to 12% of which are for acute and chronic medical problems associated with hyperglycemia. Rarely, diabetic medications may be employed in intentional overdoses, underscoring the need for blood glucose measurement in all patients with altered mental status of unknown etiology. On the other end of the spectrum, uncomplicated hyperglycemia, diabetic ketoacidosis, and hyperosmolar hyperglycemic nonketotic coma (HHNC) can occur.

Signs and Symptoms

Current classification of diabetes is based upon the underlying pathologic process related to insulin production and insulin resistance. The three main categories are as follows:

- *Type 1 diabetes mellitus*: characterized by being unable to produce any insulin due to pancreatic β-cell destruction. This type of diabetes is typically diagnosed during childhood or adolescence and accounts for 5% to 10% of all cases of diabetes mellitus. Patients with type 1 diabetes usually require daily insulin administration to stay alive.
- *Type 2 diabetes mellitus*: characterized by progressive cellular insulin resistance and a gradual failure of pancreatic β-cell insulin production. Type 2 diabetes accounts for 90% to 95% of all diagnoses of diabetes, is most common among older adults, and is associated with physical inactivity and obesity. It is common for patients with type 2 diabetes to remain asymptomatic for years before they begin to show signs and symptoms. Type 2 diabetes is often treated initially with oral hypoglycemic medications but may eventually require insulin therapy to maintain adequate glucose control. There has been a significant rise in the number of pediatric patients who are being diagnosed with type 2 diabetes. Increasing rates of childhood obesity and decreasing levels of physical exercise appear to be contributing factors.
- *Gestational diabetes*: characterized by glucose intolerance that can occur among pregnant women. It typically has the same clinical presentation as type 2 diabetes. Patients usually have hyperglycemia but no acidosis. Gestational diabetes predisposes women to developing type 2 diabetes.

The classic clinical manifestations of diabetes mellitus are referred to as the three *P*s: polyuria, polydipsia, and polyphagia. As the levels of glucose increase in the bloodstream, the kidneys' ability to reabsorb glucose may be overwhelmed, causing a "spilling" of glucose in the urine and an osmotic diuresis. Normally glucose is not found in the urine, so the presence of any glucose in the urine is an abnormal finding. Weight loss, thirst, blurred vision, and fatigue may also be present.

Differential Diagnosis

Hyperglycemia secondary to other causes may include hormonal tumors, pharmacologic agents, liver disease, and muscle disorders. Diagnostic procedures for diabetes are complex and include a thorough history, physical exam, urinalysis, and blood analysis.

Treatment

Using a glucometer to quantify serum glucose at the patient's side has become a standard of care in modern EMS practice. In the past, dextrose was given empirically to all patients with altered mental status without first quantifying serum glucose. Later, researchers found that few patients benefited from such an approach. A glucometer gives rapid bedside glucose results, and its use in the prehospital setting has been found to be safe and accurate. Ideally, you should measure glucose using capillary blood samples, not venous blood obtained during placement of an IV line, because the latter can produce inaccurate readings. Many glucose strips are required to be stored in temperature-controlled, airtight compartments in the ambulance to ensure their accuracy and reliability.

Hypoglycemia

Hypoglycemia, a frequent complication of diabetes, is the most common endocrine emergency. **Hypoglycemia** is defined as a blood glucose level < 60 mg/dL (3.3 mmol/L). Keep in mind that individual responses to blood glucose levels vary, and the levels discussed here represent averages. Generally, as the plasma glucose level falls below 60 mg/dL (3.3 mmol/L), the following sequence of events occurs in quick succession:

- First, the body decreases insulin secretion in an effort to arrest the decline in blood glucose levels.
- Next, there is an increase in the secretion of counterregulatory hormones, primarily epinephrine and norepinephrine.
- Finally, signs and symptoms, including impaired cognition, become apparent. Once the glucose level falls below 50 mg/dL (2.8 mmol/L), significant mental status changes occur.

Untreated hypoglycemia is associated with significant morbidity and mortality. To decrease these risks, you should be able recognize the signs and symptoms and be prepared to initiate treatment quickly and effectively.

Pathophysiology

Hypoglycemia in persons with insulin-dependent diabetes often is the result of having taken too much insulin, too little food, or both. The tissues of the central nervous system (including the brain), unlike other tissues that can usually metabolize fat or protein in addition to sugar, depend entirely on glucose as their source of energy. If the level of glucose in the blood drops dramatically, the brain is literally starved. Triggers of hypoglycemia are given in Table 7-3.

Table 7-3 Triggers of Hypoglycemia

Decreased Food Intake	Volume Depletion
Exogenous insulin administration (factitious hypoglycemia)	Kidney disease
Medications - Oral hypoglycemic agents - Beta-blockers - Antimalarial drugs	Liver disease
Alcohol abuse	Pancreatic tumors

Aggressive treatment of hyperglycemia
 - Diabetic ketoacidosis
 - Nonketotic hyperosmolar state
 - Uncontrolled blood glucose levels
 - Administration of excessive doses of therapeutic insulin
	Endocrinopathy
	 - Thyroid disease
	   □ Hypothyroidism
	   □ Hyperthyroidism
	 - Adrenal disease
	   □ Addison's disease

Malnutrition	
Medication adjustments	
Insulin pump failure	
Sepsis	

Hypoglycemia in patients who have no history of diabetes is called *fasting* or *postprandial hypoglycemia*. Fasting hypoglycemia is usually the result of an imbalance between glucose utilization and production. Postprandial hypoglycemia is characterized by alimentary hyperinsulinism and is commonly seen in patients who have undergone gastric surgery. A number of conditions may elicit fasting hypoglycemia. Among the most common are severe liver disease, pancreatic tumors (such as insulinomas), enzyme defects, drug overdoses (for example, insulin, sulfonylureas), and severe infection. The clinical characteristics are similar to those of diabetic hypoglycemia.

Signs and Symptoms

Clinical manifestations of hypoglycemia usually evolve rapidly. The patient will seek treatment for a myriad of signs and symptoms directly related to the release of endogenous stress hormones, including diaphoresis, tachycardia, tremors, and pale, cold, clammy skin. If hypoglycemia is not treated, an altered mental status and generalized seizures may develop in the patient. It is important to check the serum glucose in every patient who is having an active seizure to rule out hypoglycemia. While the definition of hypoglycemia is a blood glucose level < 70 mg/dL, the absolute level at which signs and symptoms appear may be altered by the patient's medical history, age, sex, and overall health. For example, an older adult with a complex medical history may have signs of severe hypoglycemia at a glucose level above 50 mg/dL (> 2.8 mmol/L). A young adult, however, may have signs of severe hypoglycemia at a level well below 50 mg/dL (< 2.8 mmol/L).

Most clinical manifestations of hypoglycemia are generated by secretion of counterregulatory hormones (e.g., epinephrine), which are secreted in response to a low glucose concentration. Signs and symptoms may include the following:

- Sweating
- Tremors
- Nervousness
- Tachycardia
- Altered level of consciousness (LOC) or behavior
- Seizures
- Coma

You must consider that the patient may be taking a medication, such as a beta-blocker, whose effects initially mask signs of hypoglycemia. Such patients can rapidly lose consciousness or begin having a seizure in the absence of any early symptoms of hypoglycemia.

Differential Diagnosis

Differential diagnoses may include Addison's disease, anxiety disorders, cardiogenic shock, adrenal crisis, and insulin resistance. A comprehensive history and physical exam that is suspicious for hypoglycemia can be confirmed with a serum glucose test. As part of the initial evaluation, obtain a complete set of vital signs.

Treatment

Pharmaceutical management of diabetes emphasizes tight plasma glucose control, which means getting the blood glucose level as close to normal (nondiabetic) as you safely can, using subcutaneous insulin injections, oral antihyperglycemics, or a combination of both. This tight control helps to decrease the risks for long-term complications such as renal failure and heart disease. However, patients on such medications are at increased risk of hypoglycemic episodes. To prevent further complications, such as seizures or permanent brain damage, begin providing glucose immediately when symptomatically hypoglycemic. The simplest option is to give oral glucose in the form of a small snack, a sugar-containing beverage, or a sugar gel. This option should always be considered in awake and alert patients who are able to swallow. For patients who have altered mentation or cannot safely swallow due to risk of aspiration, administration of 50 mL of $D_{50}W$ has been the standard, but such a high concentration of glucose can have serious complications if extravasation or infiltration

occurs. Recently, EMS has begun to embrace the use of $D_{10}W$. Studies have found no difference in the amount of time necessary for a hypoglycemic patient to regain consciousness when the two solutions are compared. When patients are given $D_{10}W$, they may receive a considerably smaller amount of glucose while achieving the same therapeutic response and are less likely to have a high glucose level after treatment.

If quick IV access proves difficult, intramuscular (IM) administration of glucagon can be an effective alternative. Glucagon may not work, however, in patients with chronic illness who have depleted glycogen stores (e.g., those with alcoholism and chronic liver disease). Recovery time with glucagon is significantly longer than with IV dextrose, and glucagon may cause side effects such as nausea and vomiting. If it is used, the standard dose is 1 to 2 mg IM.

Management of hypoglycemia in nondiabetic patients is similar to management of the condition in patients with diabetes. However, hypoglycemia in nondiabetic patients may recur, especially in patients with drug overdose. Such patients may require more than one dose of dextrose or even a continuous infusion.

Patients may wish to refuse transportation to the hospital after successful treatment of hypoglycemia by EMS. While there is some literature supporting this practice, extreme care must be taken when the patient is taking any long-acting antihyperglycemic medications (insulin or oral medications) due to the risk of recurrent hypoglycemia. Additionally, a careful search for the cause of the hypoglycemic episode should be undertaken. Some patients may have an obvious cause such as change in medication regimen or lack of oral intake that can be addressed. Unexplained episodes of hypoglycemia may be the first manifestation of other conditions that are increasing the body's metabolic needs (i.e., infection, trauma).

Diabetic Ketoacidosis

Diabetic ketoacidosis (DKA) is characterized by a plasma glucose concentration > 350 mg/dL (> 19.4 mmol/L), ketone production, a serum bicarbonate level < 15 mEq/L, and anion gap metabolic acidosis. The mortality rate for DKA ranges from 9% to 14%. DKA is an acute endocrine emergency in which insulin deficiency and an excessive glucagon level combine to create a hyperglycemic, acidotic, volume-depleted state. The condition is often associated with electrolyte imbalances.

Pathophysiology

DKA may be elicited by certain metabolic stressors such as infection, myocardial infarction, trauma, and sometimes pregnancy. The common trigger among these conditions is often the interruption of the insulin regimen of a person with diabetes. Lack of insulin prevents glucose from entering cells, and consequently, the cells become starved of glucose for cellular metabolism and turn to other sources of energy such as fat. As a result, glucose begins to accumulate in the bloodstream.

Overflow of glucose into the renal tubules draws water, sodium, potassium, magnesium, and other ions into the urine, creating a significant osmotic diuresis. This diuresis, combined with vomiting, produces volume depletion, electrolyte imbalances, and, consequently, shock. These osmotic changes are largely responsible for the declining mental status of a patient with DKA and are particularly dangerous in children. The clinical hallmark of DKA is metabolic acidosis, which is discussed later. Physiologically, the body attempts to compensate and eliminate acids by breathing faster and deeper (Kussmaul's respiration) and trying to use more bicarbonate. Acidosis encourages the shift of potassium into the bloodstream, where it is lost in the osmotic diuresis occurring in the kidneys. This process results in a pseudohyperkalemia or initially high blood level that rapidly changes to hypokalemia with the treatment of DKA.

Signs and Symptoms

Patients with DKA are dehydrated and will appear ill. They usually report polydipsia, polyphagia, and polyuria. Patients with severe DKA will exhibit altered mental status during the initial examination. Tachycardia, rapid breathing, and orthostatic changes are likely to be present. Additionally, $ETCO_2$ will be low, reflecting the metabolic acidosis present in DKA. The signs and symptoms include the following:

- Nausea and vomiting
- Abdominal pain (especially common in children)
- Tachypnea/hyperpnea
- Fruity breath odor
- Fatigue and weakness
- Increased diuresis
- Altered LOC
- Orthostatic hypotension
- Cardiac dysrhythmia
- Seizures
- Hemodynamic shock in severe cases

Differential Diagnosis

Several conditions bear a clinical resemblance to DKA and distinguishing among them may be difficult in the field without the diagnostic testing used in hospitals. Conditions that produce acidosis like sepsis—for example—may mimic DKA. Prolonged fasting in a third-trimester pregnant patient or nursing mother who is not eating properly can also resemble DKA. People who abuse alcohol may have a fruity breath odor and a rapid respiratory rate due to alcoholic ketoacidosis. Remember that rapid breathing should raise your suspicion that the body is trying to compensate for metabolic acidosis. It is critical to check the patient's blood glucose level to try to narrow the differential diagnosis.

Make sure to perform a 12-lead ECG if you suspect DKA. The information it provides could change your management strategy (e.g., if the ECG reveals a myocardial infarction). In addition, electrolyte abnormalities often accompany diabetic emergencies, and a 12-lead ECG could reveal worrisome anomalies. Although there are many conditions that can present similarly to DKA, initial treatments steps are often the same.

Treatment

Patients with severe DKA look critically ill and require immediate treatment. A patient with an altered LOC may be actively vomiting, putting him or her at risk of aspiration. In such cases, consider early intubation to protect the airway. Remember that patients with DKA breathe rapidly to compensate for their metabolic acidosis. Therefore, if you intubate such a patient, you must maintain hyperventilation to prevent deterioration of acid–base status. Initiate aggressive fluid resuscitation using 0.9% normal saline administered through two peripheral lines. Adult patients with DKA usually require 3 to 6 L of fluid during initial resuscitation. Children may have similar fluid deficits but must be managed much more cautiously to prevent severe complications resulting from rapid electrolyte shifts. Monitor patients in DKA closely because their condition can decompensate rapidly. Patients with a history of heart failure can easily go into fluid overload; therefore be cautious when administering IV fluids. Consider underlying causes of DKA, such as myocardial infarction, and provide appropriate treatment.

Insulin therapy is a mainstay of treatment for DKA along with fluid resuscitation and electrolyte correction. Generally, however, insulin is not administered in the prehospital setting. EMS services that transport patients on insulin infusions (i.e., interfacility services) should have a protocol in place to guide management of such patients during transport. You must be able to recognize potential and common side effects of continuous insulin therapy. High-dose insulin is associated with iatrogenic hypoglycemia and hypokalemia, for example. This is caused by a shift of glucose and potassium into the cells after insulin administration. Although patients with DKA initially appear to be hyperkalemic, this is only due to a temporary shift of potassium out of the cells into the bloodstream caused by the acidosis. They typically have a total-body deficiency in potassium. Abnormal potassium levels can result in life-threatening cardiac arrhythmias, so you should confirm the patient's most recent potassium level before transport.

Key treatment considerations for patients with DKA or HHNC include the following:

- If the patient is intubated, maintain hyperventilation to prevent worsening of acidosis.
- Provide fluid rehydration. You may need to rapidly administer 1 to 2 liters of normal saline. Monitor glucose levels regularly because fluid resuscitation will decrease glucose levels.
- Evaluate the ECG for signs of hyperkalemia (peaked T waves, widened QRS complex, loss of P waves, bradycardia, or sign wave morphology), and treat accordingly.

- In pediatric patients, administer initial fluid resuscitation of 20 mL/kg. Additional fluids should be administered only with expert consultation or direction from on-line medical control.

For extended critical care transports, consider the following treatment:

- Change the IV solution to D_5W in 0.45% normal saline when glucose levels fall below 300 mg/dL (< 16.6 mmol/L).
- Correct electrolytes when indicated, using the following guidelines:
  - *Potassium.* If the potassium level is low, first ensure that the patient's renal functioning is adequate, and then add 20 to 40 mEq/L of potassium chloride for each liter of fluid administered.
  - *Magnesium.* If the magnesium level is low, correct the level with 1 to 2 g of magnesium sulfate in the first 2 liters of fluid administered.
  - *Acidosis.* If the pH falls below 7, correct it by adding 44 to 88 mEq/L of sodium bicarbonate to the first liter of IV fluid administered.
  - *Complications.* Be aware of the potential complications of insulin infusions, such as hypokalemia and hypoglycemia.
- Remember, constant monitoring is essential. Treat underlying causes if possible, and transport the patient to a hospital with ICU capabilities.

An important consideration in DKA treatment relates to fluid administration in pediatric patients. Rapid shifts in fluid and electrolyte balances cause potentially fatal cerebral edema in a small percentage of children with DKA. Although there is still no definitive answer as to the specific risk factors for development of cerebral edema, consensus guidelines recommend a measured approach to fluid resuscitation in pediatric DKA. While these patients are most certainly volume depleted, they are rarely in hypovolemic shock, and the initial bolus should not exceed 10 to 20 mL/kg over 1 to 2 hours unless there is hemodynamic instability.

Complications of Treatment of DKA The treatment of diabetic ketoacidosis is difficult and complex, requiring the participation of a multidisciplinary group of medical professionals. Even then, complications may develop in patients. Five major complications increase morbidity and mortality in DKA:

- *Hypokalemia:* can occur as a result of inadequate potassium replacement during treatment because aggressive insulin treatment shifts potassium into the cells.
- *Hypoglycemia:* can be attributed to aggressive treatment and failure to closely observe glucose. It is important to begin administering a 5% dextrose in water (D_5W) solution when glucose levels fall below 300 mg/dL.
- *Fluid overload:* can be caused by aggressive fluid resuscitation in patients with congestive heart failure.

- *Alkalosis:* can be caused by overly aggressive treatment with bicarbonate. Alkalosis can further complicate electrolyte imbalances, specifically by increasing potassium requirements as potassium is displaced into body cells.
- *Cerebral edema:* the most feared complication of DKA treatment. It occurs as a result of rapid osmolar shifts. Cerebral edema generally appears 6–10 hours after the initiation of therapy and carries a mortality rate of 90%. You should suspect this complication in a patient who becomes comatose after acidosis is reversed during treatment of DKA.

Hyperosmolar Hyperglycemic Nonketotic Coma

Hyperosmolar hyperglycemic nonketotic coma (HHNC) is a serious diabetic emergency, carrying a mortality rate of 10% to 50%. You may not be able to differentiate DKA from HHNC in the field, but you should suspect it based on the patient's history, extremely elevated glucose, and absence of low ETCO$_2$. HHNC is more common in patients with type 2 diabetes mellitus and is triggered by the same stressors that cause DKA. The condition is characterized by the following:

- Elevated plasma glucose concentration, often greater than 600 mg/dL (> 33.3 mmol/L)
- Absent ketone production
- Increased serum osmolality, usually > 315 mOsm/kg

HHNC is associated with significant dehydration and a decline in mental status. Occasionally it progresses to full coma. In contrast to DKA, acidosis and ketosis are usually absent, so ETCO$_2$ will not be decreased. It is important to realize that other factors such as underlying sepsis or respiratory dysfunction may still alter the ETCO$_2$.

Pathophysiology

The pathophysiology of HHNC is complex but similar to that of DKA. The condition does not usually develop suddenly but evolves over a period of several days. The time frame varies, depending on the patient's overall health. HHNC usually occurs in older adults and in patients debilitated by comorbid conditions. As in DKA, the hallmark is decreased insulin action, which triggers a volley of counterregulatory mechanisms that increase serum glucose. Once insulin function decreases, gluconeogenesis (the body's internal manufacture of glucose), glycogenolysis (the release of glucose stored as glycogen), and decreased glucose uptake in the periphery begin to dominate. Hyperglycemia then pulls fluid into the extracellular space, triggering osmotic diuresis, which in turn causes hypotension and volume deficit. Patients are initially able to maintain intravascular volume with constant fluid intake, but the diuresis eventually overtakes the system. Keep in mind that other conditions such as sepsis may be causing further volume depletion. Common causes of HHNC include the following:

- Trauma
- Drugs
- Myocardial infarction
- Cushing's syndrome
- Sepsis
- Cerebrovascular accident (stroke)
- Dialysis
- CNS insult (e.g., subdural hematoma)
- Hemorrhage
- Pregnancy

Signs and Symptoms

Patients with HHNC are usually acutely ill, with marked volume depletion, nausea, vomiting, abdominal pain, tachypnea, and tachycardia. It is common for these patients to have a 25% fluid deficit. In addition, they may have focal neurologic deficits and seizures or signs of stroke. Signs and symptoms of HHNC include the following:

- Fever
- Dehydration
- Vomiting and abdominal pain
- Hypotension
- Tachycardia
- Rapid breathing
- Thirst, polyuria or oliguria, polydipsia
- Focal seizures
- Altered LOC
- Focal neurologic deficits

Differential Diagnosis

Many conditions have signs and symptoms similar to those of DKA (see earlier discussion) and HHNC. In most cases, your initial intervention will be similar for all of these possible illnesses, but be alert for time-sensitive underlying conditions that can cause DKA and HHNC, such as myocardial infarction and sepsis.

To differentiate HHNC from DKA, remember that the former is usually accompanied by a more profound decrease in mental status. Additionally, ETCO$_2$ may help distinguish the presence or lack of a metabolic acidosis. Signs and symptoms of HHNC can be confusing because they may be similar to those of hypoglycemia. If blood glucose cannot be rapidly evaluated, hypoglycemia must be assumed until proved otherwise. The administration of dextrose could minimally worsen glucose levels in HHNC, but it can be lifesaving in a patient with hypoglycemia.

Treatment

The initial management of a patient with HHNC is the same as that of a patient with DKA. Take immediate steps to stabilize the

airway, breathing, and circulation. The patient may have significant volume depletion; begin IV fluid resuscitation immediately. The initial fluid of choice is 0.9% normal saline. Early boluses may be necessary to stabilize the patient hemodynamically. Use caution, however, when the patient has comorbidities such as CHF. Remember that fluid administration alone will correct much of the hyperglycemia. DKA management controversies apply to HHNC as well. For example, rapid correction of serum osmolality can predispose patients—especially children—to the development of cerebral edema.

Acid–Base Disorders

As previously discussed, endocrine disorders involve the body's overproduction or underproduction of certain hormones. In comparison, acid–base disorders affect the body's ability to process certain nutrients and vitamins.

Acid–Base Balance

The body requires a delicate balance, or homeostasis, to function optimally. Fluid, electrolytes, and pH all play critical roles in maintaining homeostasis. Acid–base stability is crucial to sustain life and maintain health. Acid–base balance is achieved through a variety of buffer systems and compensatory mechanisms. Body fluids, the kidneys, and the lungs play a pivotal role in maintaining this balance. Acid–base balance is measured by examining pH (the concentration of hydrogen) and is associated with a narrow safety margin (serum pH is 7.35–7.45). Acid–base balances can vary in severity based on the degree of pH change. A pH below 7.35 constitutes acidosis. In contrast, a pH level above 7.45 constitutes alkalosis. These pH derangements are classified according to their primary cause as either metabolic or respiratory. Death can occur if serum pH levels fall below 6.8 or rise above 7.8. Changes can occur because of various conditions including infections, organ failure, or trauma. In many cases the acid–base fluctuations can cause more negative effects than the causative condition; therefore, the resulting acid–base imbalance is often corrected before treating the underlying condition.

Two body systems can compensate for pH imbalances—the renal and respiratory systems. If the cause of the imbalance originates within one of those systems, the other system will have to be the primary compensatory mechanism. The system will not be able to resolve its own problem. Thus, if the problem originates in the lungs, the kidneys will manage it. If the problem originates outside the lungs, the lungs will manage it.

Buffers

Buffers are the chemicals that combine with an acid or base to resist changes in pH. Buffering is an immediate reaction to counteract pH variations until longer-term compensation is established. The body has four major buffer mechanisms—the bicarbonate–carbonic acid system, the phosphate system, the hemoglobin system, and the protein system.

Respiratory Regulation

The respiratory system manages pH deviations by changing the amount of expired carbon dioxide (acid excretion). Speeding up respirations will lead to excretion of more carbon dioxide, thereby decreasing acidity. Slowing down respirations will lead to excretion of less carbon dioxide, increasing acidity. Chemoreceptors that sense pH changes trigger this change in breathing pattern. The only way the lungs can remove acids is through the elimination of carbon dioxide from carbonic acid—the lungs cannot remove other acids. The respiratory system is also a mechanism that can respond quickly to pH imbalances, but its quick action is short lived. The respiratory system reaches its maximum compensatory response in 12 to 24 hours, but it can maintain the changes in breathing pattern for only a limited time before becoming fatigued.

Renal Regulation

The renal system is the slowest mechanism to react to pH changes, taking hours to days to achieve its buffering effect, but it is the longest lasting. The kidneys respond by changing the excretion or retention of hydrogen (acid) or bicarbonate (base). The renal system acts to balance pH levels by permanently removing hydrogen from the body. Additionally, the kidneys can reabsorb acids or bases and produce bicarbonate to correct pH imbalances.

Compensation

To maintain homeostasis, the body will take actions to compensate for the pH changes. The body never overcompensates; the pH is adjusted so that it remains just within the normal range. The cause of the imbalance often determines the compensatory change. For example, if pH is becoming more acidic because of lung disease that limits gas exchange (e.g., emphysema), the renal system will kick in to compensate for the problem by releasing more bicarbonate and excreting more hydrogen. If a lung disease is increasing carbon dioxide excretion (e.g., hyperventilation), which will increase pH, the kidneys will compensate by decreasing bicarbonate production and hydrogen excretion. In contrast, if the problem originates outside the lungs, the lungs can compensate for it. For example, if a condition increases the loss of an acid (e.g., vomiting), the lungs will decrease the rate and depth of respirations to retain more carbon dioxide. If a condition increases the loss of a base (e.g., diarrhea), the lungs will increase the rate and depth of respirations to excrete more carbon dioxide. If the kidneys and lungs cannot compensate to restore the pH levels to normal range, cellular activities are affected, leading to disease states. Various mathematical formulas exist to calculate expected levels of compensatory responses and help determine if a condition is acute or chronic.

Respiratory Acidosis

Respiratory acidosis is one of the most common acid–base problems encountered in the prehospital setting. Respiratory acidosis is characterized by a decline in pH as a result of CO_2 retention. Hypoventilation is the classic example of a clinical problem that leads to CO_2 retention. Respiratory acidosis may be classified as acute or chronic. The only way to distinguish between these states is to determine whether the body has begun to retain bicarbonate to compensate for the acidosis. During the acute phase, the serum bicarbonate level is normal. Once the body begins to retain bicarbonate, it has made the transition to chronic status.

Pathophysiology

Any disorders that result in hypoventilation (e.g., primary pulmonary problems, airway obstruction, illnesses that depress the respiratory drive) will cause respiratory acidosis. Precipitants of respiratory acidosis are summarized in Table 7-4.

Table 7-4 **Precipitants of Respiratory Acidosis**	
Acute	**Chronic**
Pharmacologic CNS Depression	*Lung Disease*
■ Narcotics ■ Benzodiazepines ■ Alcohol abuse ■ Gamma-hydroxybutyrate (GHB) toxicity	■ Chronic bronchitis ■ COPD ■ Pulmonary fibrosis
Lung Disease	*Neuromuscular Diseases*
■ Interstitial edema ■ Pneumonia	■ Muscular dystrophy ■ Myasthenia gravis
Airway Problems	*Obesity*
■ Foreign body ■ Aspiration ■ Bronchospasm ■ Apnea	■ Sleep apnea
Hypoventilation	
■ Pneumothorax ■ Flail chest ■ Myasthenia gravis ■ Guillain-Barré syndrome ■ Primary CNS disorders ■ Brain injury	

CNS, central nervous system; *COPD*, chronic obstructive pulmonary disease.

Signs and Symptoms

You may encounter different clinical scenarios, depending on the severity of the primary problems. Common signs and symptoms include weakness, breathing difficulty, and altered LOC. Noting the LOC is critical when evaluating a patient with suspected respiratory acidosis because it may indicate the severity of the process and signal the need for advanced airway management. For example, in a patient with COPD who has a diminished mental status, a high level of CO_2 is most likely responsible for the altered LOC. Such a patient has a higher risk of complications such as aspiration and therefore requires more aggressive intervention.

Differential Diagnosis

Many conditions can cause hypoventilation and/or impair gas exchange, resulting in respiratory acidosis (see Table 7-4).

Treatment

Standard monitoring equipment should be used according to your provider level, including an ECG monitor, Spo_2, and $ETCO_2$. The $ETCO_2$ measurement is an approximate measure of $Paco_2$, and is generally felt to be accurate to within 5–10 mm Hg. After your initial evaluation and stabilization of the patient's airway, breathing, and circulation (ABCs), therapy should focus on correcting minute ventilation to decrease CO_2 levels and thereby correct the acidosis. Depending on the etiology, you can accomplish this either by assisting ventilation or by providing pharmacologic intervention. Ventilatory assistance can range from airway positioning to bag-mask ventilation with nasopharyngeal airway or oropharyngeal airway, continuous positive airway pressure (CPAP) or bilevel positive airway pressure (BiPAP), or endotracheal intubation with ventilator support. Pharmacologic intervention, such as naloxone administration, can reverse respiratory depression in patients whose hypoventilation can be attributed to the toxic effects of opiate overdose. Albuterol, ipratropium, and other medications may improve hypoventilation in patients with COPD.

All hypoxic patients should be treated with supplemental oxygen. Patients with chronically elevated CO_2 levels (i.e., patients with COPD who chronically retain CO_2) may have switched from relying on the normal hypercarbic respiratory drive to relying on the hypoxic drive and must be monitored for decreased respiratory effort when supplemental oxygen is administered. See Chapter 2 for a discussion of the hypercarbic and hypoxic drives.

Respiratory Alkalosis

An increase in ventilation per minute is the cause of respiratory alkalosis, characterized by a decreased $Paco_2$ level and increased pH. The only way to differentiate between acute and chronic respiratory alkalosis is to measure serum bicarbonate. A patient with acute respiratory alkalosis will have a normal serum bicarbonate level. A patient with chronic respiratory alkalosis, however, will have a decrease in serum bicarbonate level.

Pathophysiology

Respiratory alkalosis is usually seen as a secondary compensatory mechanism to a primary metabolic problem, but it can be a primary derangement as well. Some causes of primary respiratory alkalosis include aspirin overdose, anxiety reaction, and pulmonary embolism. On occasion, it may be a normal physiologic response. The classic example is alkalemia of pregnancy, in which the pH is 7.46 to 7.5. This condition is primarily respiratory in origin and is characterized by a Pco_2 of 31 to 35 mm Hg. Precipitants of respiratory alkalosis are given in Table 7-5.

Table 7-5 **Precipitants of Respiratory Alkalosis**
Pulmonary
• Pulmonary embolism • Pneumonia (bacterial or viral) • Acute pulmonary edema • Atelectasis • Assisted hyperventilation
Infections
• Septicemia
Drug Induced
• Vasopressors • Thyroxine • Aspirin or caffeine toxicity
Hypoxia
• Ventilation-perfusion mismatch • Altitude changes • Severe anemia
Hyperventilation
• Hysteria/anxiety • Psychogenic disorders • Central nervous system tumor • Stroke
Metabolic and Electrolyte Disturbances
• Hepatic insufficiency • Encephalopathy • Hyponatremia

Signs and Symptoms

The patient's clinical presentation depends on whether the respiratory alkalosis is chronic or acute. Most signs and symptoms are nonspecific and are related to peripheral or CNS complaints such as paresthesia of the face or lips, lightheadedness, dizziness, and muscular pain or cramps.

Differential Diagnosis

A diagnosis of respiratory alkalosis may not be obvious because some of its signs and symptoms are almost identical to those of certain electrolyte emergencies such as hypocalcemia. A thorough history and physical exam will yield clues to the underlying cause of the respiratory alkalosis, which may guide your management strategies. Be careful not to overlook life-threatening toxicologic causes such as aspirin overdose.

Treatment

Administer oxygen to patients with hypoxemia without delay, and take steps to stabilize and support the airway, breathing, and circulation. For hyperventilation caused by anxiety, use coaching techniques to calm the patient. Instruct him or her to use pursed-lip breathing. To avoid precipitating hypoxia, do not use a paper bag or a nonrebreathing mask without oxygen attached.

Metabolic Acidosis

Metabolic acidosis is caused by a deficiency of bicarbonate ion (base) and an excess of hydrogen ion (acid). In the acute state, the body's physiologic response is to hyperventilate and compensate by reducing Pa_{CO_2}. This is sometimes referred to as "blowing off CO_2." Chronic status is reached when the renal system begins to reabsorb bicarbonate in an effort to compensate for the metabolic acidosis.

Pathophysiology

Metabolic acidosis is generated by three mechanisms: decreased renal excretion of acids, increased production or ingestion of acids, and loss of buffering mechanisms in the body.

Signs and Symptoms

The clinical manifestations of metabolic acidosis are directly related to the severity of the metabolic problem. Most patients have nausea, vomiting, abdominal pain, a rapid and deep respiratory pattern (Kussmaul's respiration), and in more severe cases, altered LOC and shock.

Differential Diagnosis

Metabolic acidosis is classified as either non–anion-gap acidosis or anion-gap acidosis. The anion gap is calculated using the following formula:

$$AG = Na^+ - (Cl^- + HCO_3^-)$$

This information gives the provider an estimate of unmeasured anions in the plasma. An anion gap of 12 to 15 is considered normal. An elevated gap points to conditions that may cause acidosis. The mnemonic CAT MUDPILES can help you remember the precipitants of high anion-gap metabolic acidosis. The mnemonic F-USED CARS will help bring to mind the causes of normal-anion-gap metabolic acidosis.

Providers may not have access to the laboratory information necessary to calculate the anion gap. Management decisions, therefore, are often made on the basis of sound clinical judgment, a thorough history, and physical exam findings. A specialty-care transport provider conducting a hospital transfer may have laboratory values for calculating the anion gap and can adjust the differential diagnosis accordingly. Capnometry can also provide key information. A patient with tachypnea and a low P_{CO_2} should be suspected to have metabolic acidosis or a primary respiratory alkalosis, as previously discussed.

When patients present with clinical signs of acidosis, the following five conditions must be considered:

- *Diabetic ketoacidosis.* As discussed earlier in the chapter, DKA is caused by inadequate use of insulin as a result of poor compliance or increased need. Patients with diabetes sometimes require higher insulin doses during periods of infection, after trauma, or in other circumstances that increase metabolic demand. DKA sets in when glucose utilization is impaired and fatty acids are metabolized, causing the formation of ketone bodies that generate hydrogen ions. If more acids are produced than the body's buffering system is able to tolerate, acidosis ensues.
- *Renal failure.* The kidneys are vital in maintaining an optimal acid–base balance. Most patients with renal failure have uremia because the kidneys are unable to secrete acid by-products. The renal tubules have the primary responsibility for eliminating hydrogen ions. This function is directly related to the filtration rate of the kidneys, known as the glomerular filtration rate (GFR). Any pathology that alters this process will increase the concentration of hydrogen ions, especially in the form of hydrogen sulfate (HSO_4) and HPO, increasing the anion gap. Patients with chronic renal failure will have some degree of anion gap acidosis, but the gap rarely exceeds 25. Patients with acute renal failure, however, more often have hyperchloremic non–anion-gap acidosis.

CAT MUDPILES

Mnemonic for Precipitants of High-Anion-Gap
Metabolic Acidosis

C   Carbon monoxide or cyanide intoxication

A   Alcohol intoxication or alcoholic ketoacidosis

T   Toluene exposure

M   Methanol exposure

U   Uremia

D   Diabetic ketoacidosis

P   Paraldehyde ingestion

I   Isoniazid or iron intoxication

L   Lactic acidosis

E   Ethylene glycol intoxication

S   Salicylate (ASA) intoxication

ASA, Acetylsalicylic acid.

F-USED CARS

Mnemonic for Precipitants of Normal-Anion-Gap
Metabolic Acidosis

F   Fistulae, pancreatic

U   Ureteroenteric conduits

S   Saline administration (0.9% normal saline)

E   Endocrine dysfunction

D   Diarrhea

C   Carbonic anhydrase inhibitor ingestion

A   Arginine, lysine (parenteral nutrition)

R   Renal tubular acidosis

S   Spironolactone (diuretic) ingestion

■ *Lactic acidosis.* Lactic acid is largely generated when a significant number of cells in the body are inadequately perfused. Hypoperfusion shifts the cellular metabolism from aerobic (with oxygen) to anaerobic (without oxygen). Anaerobic metabolism produces lactic acid as its most important end product. This reaction occurs in time-sensitive medical conditions associated with hypoperfusion (e.g., sepsis, ischemia, extreme physical exertion states, prolonged seizures, circulatory shock). Lactic acidosis occurs when lactic acid accumulates in larger amounts than the body can buffer.

■ *Toxin ingestion.* Toxic metabolites that cause metabolic acidosis may be a by-product of ingestion of toxins such as acetylsalicylic acid (ASA), ethylene glycol, methanol, and isoniazid. Patients with toxin-induced metabolic acidosis show some degree of respiratory compensation. The toxin must be identified as soon as possible because an antidote may be available to prevent further adverse effects.

■ *Alcohol ketoacidosis.* This is caused by abrupt cessation of intake after a prolonged period of ingesting a considerable amount of alcohol. The main problem—accumulation of keto acids—is precipitated by dehydration, hormone imbalance, and chronic malnutrition. Although the condition is similar in presentation to DKA, blood glucose levels are normal or low. Patients with alcohol ketoacidosis often have mixed acid–base disorders associated with the vomiting that accompanies alcohol withdrawal.

Treatment

Most patients with metabolic acidosis will require a significant amount of volume resuscitation. Rapidly establish intravascular access to replenish volume status. Support the airway, breathing, and circulation with oxygen as appropriate, and ensure adequate ventilation. In patients with history of renal failure or CHF, use caution to avoid causing pulmonary edema when administering IV fluids. If the patient needs ventilator support, be sure to maintain hyperventilation. Patients with metabolic acidosis are hyperventilating as a respiratory compensatory mechanism, and if they are sedated or paralyzed for intubation, metabolic acidosis will worsen. Initiate adjunct treatments on the basis of primary etiology. For example, patients with high-anion-gap metabolic acidosis due to DKA can be started on insulin.

The use of sodium bicarbonate may be necessary for certain conditions that elicit acute metabolic acidosis, but administration of bicarbonate can be fraught with complications, including hypocalcemia, volume overload, CNS acidosis, hypokalemia, and impaired oxygen delivery. Despite the controversy that surrounds its use, rapid administration of sodium bicarbonate may be useful in treating certain life-threatening conditions. Providers use arterial blood gas and plasma electrolyte values to guide the decision of whether to administer bicarbonate. Although it is unlikely that such information will be available in the prehospital setting, administering bicarbonate is warranted in the following circumstances:

- Cardiac arrest caused by acidosis associated with hyperkalemia
- Overdose with tricyclic antidepressants (ECG shows QRS complex widening > 0.10 sec)
- Hyperkalemia (presumptive diagnosis made on the basis of history and ECG findings)

Metabolic Alkalosis

Metabolic alkalosis is produced by illnesses that raise the level of serum bicarbonate or reduce the level of hydrogen in the body, such as those that cause volume, potassium, and chloride loss.

Pathophysiology

Metabolic alkalosis occurs by one of two mechanisms: either the body retains bicarbonate in response to hydrogen and chloride loss, or renal impairment precludes the excretion of bicarbonate. Table 7-6 provides a list of specific conditions that may precipitate metabolic alkalosis.

Signs and Symptoms

Common signs and symptoms in patients affected by metabolic alkalosis are anorexia, nausea, vomiting, confusion, hypotension, paresthesia, and weakness. A thorough assessment may reveal the use of antacids (e.g., sodium and calcium bicarbonates), loop diuretics such as thiazide, and corticosteroids. Underlying medical illnesses such as Cushing's syndrome and renal disease are common.

Table 7-6 **Precipitants of Metabolic Alkalosis**	
Normal Saline-Responsive Metabolic Alkalosis	**Normal Saline-Unresponsive Metabolic Alkalosis**
Volume depletion - Vomiting - Nasogastric suction - Diuretic use - Low chloride ingestion	Mineralocorticoid excess
	Exogenous ingestions - Chewing tobacco - Licorice
	Primary aldosteronism
	Cushing's syndrome
	Bartter syndrome

The patient will present with slow, shallow respirations. ECG changes with depressed T waves that merge with P waves indicate hypocalcemia and hypokalemia. Hypotension is also present. Many patients present with muscle twitching and loss of reflexes and numbness and tingling in the extremities; a thorough neurologic exam should be performed. Arterial blood gas analysis reveals a blood pH above 7.45 and an elevated Hco_3^-. If respiratory compensation is occurring, the $Paco_2$ level may be above 45 mm Hg.

Differential Diagnosis

To make a definitive diagnosis of metabolic alkalosis, you need to know the serum bicarbonate level and the arterial CO_2 level. A rise in the serum bicarbonate level may be a renal compensatory response to chronic respiratory acidosis. This information can be obtained only by blood gas testing.

Treatment

Management of metabolic alkalosis is directed toward correcting the underlying cause. A comprehensive history and physical exam are vital. Administration of IV fluids is essential if the primary cause is volume depletion. Isotonic solutions are the fluids of choice. Hypokalemia may need to be corrected with potassium replacement.

Mixed Disorders

Patients often have mixed acid–base disturbances, the diagnosis of which may be difficult even for an experienced emergency physician or intensivist. Mixed disturbances are identified on the basis of clinical history combined with blood gas analysis. Your initial clinical impression of whether the patient is sick or not sick is especially important. As always, take any immediate steps necessary to support airway, breathing, and circulation.

Electrolyte Disturbances

Electrolyte imbalances are common findings in patients with medical emergencies. A healthy electrolyte balance is fundamental to carrying out cellular functions. Electrolyte disturbances generally cannot be diagnosed on the basis of clinical examination alone, but a thorough history and exam may point to a likely diagnosis. Severe electrolyte disturbances can be fatal. Most patients have only nonspecific chief complaints until life-threatening manifestations appear. In the following section, the most important electrolyte problems you are likely to encounter in the field are discussed.

Hyponatremia

Sodium is the most important electrolyte in maintaining water balance in the body. As the principal cation in the extracellular fluid, sodium together with chloride and bicarbonate regulates osmotic forces (the flow of water in and out of cells). Water balance is maintained by hormonal regulation controlled by the brain and kidneys.

Hyponatremia is defined as a serum sodium concentration below 135 mEq/L. To guide management, hyponatremia is classified into the following three categories, depending on volume status:

- Hypervolemic hyponatremia occurs when an excessive amount of water is retained relative to the amount of sodium. The condition classically occurs in a patient with an edematous condition such as CHF. It may also occur in patients who have excessive water intake such as with psychogenic polydipsia or when large amounts of water are ingested intentionally over a short period of time.
- Hypovolemic hyponatremia is caused by the loss of water and sodium, with a higher degree of sodium loss relative to the amount of water loss. Common precipitants include vomiting, diarrhea, GI problems, nasogastric tubes, and third-spacing of fluids. Third-spacing (movement of intravascular and intracellular water into interstitial spaces) is a phenomenon that may occur in patients with burns, pancreatitis, and sepsis and in those who take certain medications such as diuretics.
- Euvolemic hyponatremia occurs when the serum osmolality is low despite the presence of concentrated urine.

Signs and Symptoms

The clinical presentation of hyponatremia depends on how quickly the sodium concentration declines. Patients who experience a rapid drop in serum sodium level often begin to show symptoms around 125–130 mEq/L; however, a patient with chronic hyponatremia may tolerate a level below 120 mEq/L without symptoms.

Most signs and symptoms of hyponatremia are related to CNS manifestations, such as agitation, hallucinations, weakness, lethargy, and seizures. Abdominal pain, cramps, and headache may also occur. Patients with severe hyponatremia appear to be very ill and may have seizures or exhibit an altered mental status.

Athletic events such as marathons and triathlons can precipitate exercise-induced hyponatremia. Although the mechanisms that cause this phenomenon are not completely understood, persistent increased vasopressin levels and a decrease in glomerular function in sweat-induced dehydration may be implicated. Exercise-induced hyponatremia can cause loss of coordination, pulmonary edema, and changes in intracranial pressure that result in seizure and coma.

Patients with very high glucose levels (or excessive lipids or proteins in the blood) will exhibit pseudohyponatremia with a measured sodium level that appears quite low. This low sodium measurement must be corrected using a formula to ascertain the true sodium level.

Differential Diagnosis

The differential diagnosis of hyponatremia as well as the identification of the underlying cause is often complex and may be a difficult task even for specialists in the hospital. In the prehospital environment the history and exam should help guide you to consideration of hyponatremia.

Treatment

On the basis of history and physical exam, try to determine if the patient may be suffering from hyponatremia and the most likely cause. Patients who are hemodynamically unstable should have fluid resuscitation initiated with 0.9% normal saline. All fluids, however, particularly in patients who are hemodynamically stable, should be administered with extreme caution in patients with hyponatremia. Until a serum sodium level is known and a total body water deficit has been calculated, aggressive hydration runs the risk of correcting the sodium too quickly and leading to severe complications.

You will rarely have serum sodium measurements to guide management in the prehospital environment, although point-of-care testing is available in some circumstances. As a general rule, hyponatremia should be corrected extremely slowly. The recommended rate of correction is no faster than 1 to 2 mEq/L per hour. The exception to this rule is patients with severe neurologic symptoms such as altered mental status or seizures. In these patients, a rapid correction may be needed to alleviate the symptoms. This may be done with a 100-mL bolus of 3% sodium chloride (hypertonic saline). Hypertonic saline should never be administered without direct supervision of medical control. Correcting the sodium level too aggressively (either with normal saline or hypertonic saline) can cause severe neurologic complications as a result of osmotic demyelination.

Hypokalemia

Potassium is responsible for the following vital functions in the body:

- Maintaining a normal electrical and osmotic gradient in all cells
- Facilitating neuronal transmission and cardiac impulse conduction
- Serving as a buffering mechanism in the cell membranes to help maintain acid–base homeostasis

Normal serum potassium levels range from 3.5 to 5 mEq/L but do not accurately reflect total body stores of the cation because most potassium is stored within cells. Hypokalemia is an abnormally low serum level of potassium, usually < 3.5 mEq/L. Hypokalemia is fairly common and usually occurs secondary to decreased intake or increased excretion.

Signs and Symptoms

Hypokalemia often manifests with no signs or symptoms initially. As it progresses and the potassium level falls below 2.5 mEq/L, signs and symptoms of hypokalemia become apparent in multiple organ systems, including the neurologic, GI, and cardiovascular systems. Common symptoms include weakness, nausea, vomiting, lethargy, confusion, and paresthesia of the extremities.

A patient with severe hypokalemia (< 2 mEq/L) will appear to be very ill and may also have cardiac dysrhythmias and muscular paralysis. Frequent cardiovascular manifestations include palpitations, low blood pressure, and cardiac electrical disturbances such as heart blocks, premature ventricular contractions, and supraventricular tachycardia. Fatal types of dysrhythmia, such as ventricular fibrillation and asystole, can also occur (**Figure 7-10**).

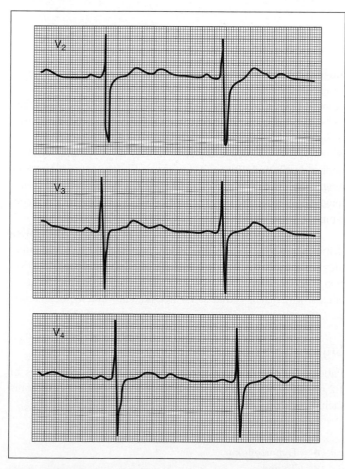

Figure 7-10 Electrocardiographic manifestations of hypokalemia. Serum potassium concentration was 2.2 mEq/L. ST segment is prolonged, primarily because of a U wave following the T wave, and T wave is flattened.

This article was published in Cecil's textbook of medicine, ed 23, Goldman L, Ausiello D, Copyright Saunders 2007.

Differential Diagnosis

Signs of hypokalemia apparent on a 12-lead ECG include flattened T waves, U waves, and ST-segment depression. Clinical manifestations of hypokalemia are similar to those of hyperkalemia.

Treatment

Treatment of hypokalemia may require IV fluids for dehydration. Oral potassium replacement (20 to 40 mEq per dose) is preferred over IV administration because of the potential side effects of IV potassium. Patients who are unable to take oral replacement or are critically ill will require IV potassium administered at a rate of 10 to 20 mEq per hour. Critically ill patients (those with respiratory muscle weakness) can receive higher doses, but they should be given through a central venous catheter. Overly rapid infusion of IV potassium can result in cardiac arrest. A common complaint during IV administration is burning at the site of infusion, which you can usually resolve by slowing the rate of infusion. Hyperkalemia is a complication of potassium administration, which is especially likely in patients with kidney disease. It is therefore critical to know the patient's renal function status before you administer potassium.

Hyperkalemia

Hyperkalemia, a level of serum potassium > 5.5 mEq/L, is an electrolyte disorder that can be caused by ingestion of potassium supplements, acute or chronic renal failure, blood transfusion, sepsis, Addison's disease, acidosis, and crush syndrome (from rhabdomyolysis).

Signs and Symptoms

Hyperkalemia manifests primarily as neurologic and cardiovascular dysfunction. The patient may have generalized weakness, muscle cramps, tetany, paralysis, or cardiac palpitations or arrhythmias.

Differential Diagnosis

In the prehospital setting, the only diagnostic study available to guide you toward a diagnosis of hyperkalemia is the ECG, which can help you determine whether the patient has an associated arrhythmia. Classically, the first change detected on the ECG of a patient with hyperkalemia is the development of peaked T waves. As serum potassium continues to increase, P waves disappear, and the QRS complex widens. If hyperkalemia is not corrected, the ECG will progress to bradycardia and then terminate in a sine wave pattern or asystole.

Treatment

Assess and treat the underlying cause of hyperkalemia, institute rapid and appropriate treatment, and transport the patient to a hospital facility. Treatment of hyperkalemia has the following three goals:

- *Cellular membrane stabilization and decreased cardiac irritability.* Maintain the patient on a cardiac monitor at all times. If the patient has signs of hyperkalemia on ECG, hypotension, or arrhythmias, administer 5 mL of 10% solution of calcium chloride. In many systems, this may require consultation with online medical control unless the patient is already in cardiac arrest.
- *Potassium shift into cells.* Sodium bicarbonate, 44 mEq/L IV, may be administered to drive potassium into cells and out of the serum. Nebulized albuterol, 5 to 20 mg, will lower the serum potassium level by shifting potassium into cells. The combined administration of 10 units of insulin and IV dextrose similarly produces a shift of potassium into the cells.
- *Elimination of potassium from the body.* To help eliminate potassium from the body, the use of exchange resins is common practice although supported by limited data. An oral dose of 20 g sodium polystyrene sulfonate can be used. Be careful when using exchange resins in a cardiac patient, however, since they can produce fluid overload.

Hypocalcemia

As previously discussed in the section on hypoparathyroidism, calcium is essential for a number of body functions, including muscular contraction, neuronal transmission, hormone secretion, organ growth, and immunologic and hematologic response. Most calcium in an adult is stored as a mineral component of bone. Hypocalcemia occurs when ionized calcium levels fall below 4 mEq/L. This condition occurs as a result of increased losses or decreased intake of calcium.

Signs and Symptoms

Patients with symptomatic hypocalcemia may have seizures, hypotension, tetany, or cardiac dysrhythmias.

Differential Diagnosis

In addition to the signs and symptoms, two signs may be present—Trousseau's and Chvostek's signs—to help you narrow down the possible diagnosis.

Treatment

Treatment of hypocalcemia is guided principally by laboratory results, but when hypocalcemia is presumed to be the cause of the patient's symptoms, it may be reasonable to begin empirical treatment. Parenteral calcium is the primary treatment in patients with symptomatic hypocalcemia. Use one of the following two options:

- 10 mL 10% calcium chloride, which contains 360 mg elemental calcium
- 10 mL 10% calcium gluconate, which contains 93 mg elemental calcium

In an adult patient, the recommended dose is 100 to 300 mg elemental calcium. In a pediatric patient, administer 0.5 to 1 mL/kg of a 10% calcium gluconate solution over 5 minutes. To avoid significant side effects, dilution in normal saline or D_5W is highly recommended. Care must be taken to ensure the peripheral catheter is working properly before administering calcium because extravasation may cause tissue necrosis. Calcium administration will increase the serum concentration of calcium for only a short period of time, so you may need to give repeated doses, especially during a long transport or interfacility transfer.

Patients whose signs and symptoms persist after adequate treatment may have concomitant electrolyte problems such as hypomagnesemia.

Hypomagnesemia

Magnesium is the second most abundant intracellular bivalent cation in the human body. It is a cofactor in the activation of numerous enzymatic reactions. Its physiologic effects on the CNS are similar to those of calcium. Magnesium is distributed throughout the body in a unique way. Half of the total amount of magnesium (2,000 mEq/L) is stored as a mineral component of bone, and 40% to 50% is intracellular. Only 1% to 2% of magnesium in the body is in extracellular fluid; thus the serum magnesium level is a poor reflection of the body's total magnesium content.

Hypomagnesemia is one of the most common electrolyte disturbances you will see in clinical practice. It often accompanies conditions that involve malnutrition, alcoholism, dehydration, diarrhea, kidney disease, diuresis, or starvation and tends to coexist with diseases that cause hypokalemia and hypocalcemia.

Signs and Symptoms

Patients usually become symptomatic at magnesium levels of 1.2 mg/dL (0.06 mmol/L) or less. Common signs and symptoms include the following:

- Tremors
- Hyperreflexia
- Tetany
- Nausea or vomiting
- Altered mental status and confusion
- Seizures
- Cardiac dysrhythmias, including torsades des pointes, polymorphic ventricular tachycardia, and cardiac arrest

Treatment

Take immediate steps to maintain the airway, breathing, and circulation. It is reasonable to start magnesium replacement therapy when you suspect a diagnosis of hypomagnesemia. In patients with no history of renal problems, administer a dose of 2 g of 50% magnesium sulfate. It must be given with normal saline or dextrose, ideally administered over 30 to 60 minutes per gram. However, in a patient with severe signs and symptoms, including dysrhythmias, you may need to give a rapid infusion over the course of 5 or 10 minutes. Do not give magnesium sulfate as a bolus because this been associated with severe side effects, including bradycardia, heart block, and hypotension.

Rhabdomyolysis

Rhabdomyolysis is a breakdown of muscle tissue that causes myoglobin to be released into the bloodstream, causing kidney damage. This muscle injury usually results from prolonged periods of immobilization, certain metabolic insults, or pressure or crush force on the tissue. Patients such as those who have experienced an opioid overdose, a person pinned under an industrial machine, or an elderly person who has spent several hours on the floor after falling may all suffer from rhabdomyolysis. Regardless of the particular insult to the tissue, the end result in each of these cases is the release of intracellular contents as the individual muscle cells rupture and die. Myoglobin, one of the main proteins found in skeletal muscle cells, travels to the kidneys and causes injury and even renal failure. Electrolytes that are normally sequestered within the cell may also be released, resulting in metabolic disturbances that are only exacerbated by the concurrent renal injury. In extreme cases, patients may have massive hyperkalemia resulting in fatal cardiac arrhythmias.

Pathophysiology

Rather than being a primary problem, rhabdomyolysis occurs as a consequence of another insult. Common precipitants of rhabdomyolysis include the following:

- Metabolic problems
- Heatstroke and other severe heat-related emergencies
- Trauma
- Crush injuries
- Drugs of abuse
- Toxic ingestion/overdose
- Infections (rarely)
- Electrolyte abnormalities

Dysfunction of the Na^+/K^+-ATPase pump allows uncontrolled calcium influx into skeletal muscle cells. The increased intracellular calcium content leads to cellular necrosis and release of myoglobin, potassium, and intracellular enzymes, such as creatinine phosphokinase. Once myoglobin enters the plasma, it is filtered and excreted through the kidneys. An excess of myoglobin can be directly toxic to the renal tubules or can obstruct them, especially if the patient is hypovolemic or acidotic as a result of the primary problem. If not treated aggressively with IV fluids, rhabdomyolysis can cause severe kidney damage and renal failure.

Signs and Symptoms

Patients with rhabdomyolysis report diffuse or localized weakness and muscle pain. Once the process of rhabdomyolysis has begun, patients may have dark-colored urine. If the patient develops hyperkalemia, the aforementioned signs and symptoms may also occur.

Differential Diagnosis

Rhabdomyolysis is diagnosed in the ED by noting myoglobinuria (the presence of myoglobin, a protein released in muscle breakdown in the urine) and an elevated creatine kinase level in the blood. However, you should suspect this diagnosis on the basis of a comprehensive history (including that of the primary condition) and physical exam findings. The patient may not have rhabdomyolysis initially, but an emergent condition may induce the condition later. A thorough physical exam is the key to identifying potential causes. For example, you may discover dark or even cola-colored urine, which is a strong indicator of the presence of rhabdomyolysis.

Treatment

Aggressive fluid hydration is crucial. IV fluids should be given (taking care to avoid hypothermia) in an effort to mitigate the complications of rhabdomyolysis. In addition to routine medical care, consider the following:

- Aggressive saline infusion early, especially in patients with trauma or crush injuries. Saline infusion is vital in the treatment of rhabdomyolysis.
- Titration of saline infusions to obtain a urine output of 200 to 300 mL/h. Be aware of potential electrolyte complications (such as hyperkalemia with hypocalcemia) that may elicit malignant cardiac dysrhythmias. If they occur, you must treat them aggressively.
- Administration of mannitol for osmotic diuresis.
- Initiation of a bicarbonate infusion to begin alkalinizing the urine if you already know the patient's primary diagnosis (e.g., when carrying out an interfacility transfer).

Putting It All Together

Patients with endocrine and metabolic disorders can be some of the most challenging problems a healthcare provider faces. Similarities and differences in the chief complaint/cardinal presentation are sometimes subtle, and your ability to determine the underlying diagnosis can be obscured, delaying appropriate interventions. Using the AMLS assessment pathway will assist you in obtaining a comprehensive history and focused physical exam. The assessment-based approach supports putting

your knowledge of anatomy, physiology, and pathophysiology to work to figure out both the common and uncommon causes of these diverse disease processes. The use of pattern recognition can help you compare your patient's clinical presentation to the chief complaint and formulate a working diagnosis. Becoming proficient in analyzing and synthesizing information to safely, efficiently, and effectively care for these patients will be well worth the effort it takes. Your contributions as an EMS team member are always a vital link in helping improve patient outcomes.

SCENARIO SOLUTION

© HunThomas/ShutterStock, Inc.

- Differential diagnoses may include an electrolyte imbalance such as hypokalemia or hypernatremia, metabolic alkalosis (related to Cushing's syndrome) or metabolic acidosis (related to treatment with metformin), hyperglycemia or hypoglycemia, digoxin toxicity, sepsis, or heart failure.
- To narrow your differential diagnosis, you'll need to complete the history of past and present illness. Perform a physical examination that includes assessment for dehydration, assessment of heart and breath sounds, and

mental status. Diagnostic testing should include blood glucose, ECG monitoring and 12-lead ECG, Sao_2, $ETCO_2$, and blood chemistry if available.

- The patient has signs that may indicate shock, infection, or electrolyte imbalance. Signs of shock may be masked by prednisone treatment, and the presence of digoxin will prevent the increase in heart rate to compensate for shock. Administer oxygen, establish vascular access, and administer IV fluids. Continue to monitor the ECG, and transport the patient to the closest appropriate hospital.

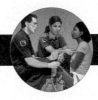

Summary

- The endocrine system is responsible for hormone regulation, including homeostasis, reproduction, growth, development, and metabolism, and is composed of the pituitary, thyroid, parathyroid, and adrenal glands, as well as the pancreas, ovaries, and testes.
- Hormones stimulate growth and development throughout the body, regulate the flow of water in and out of cells, help muscles contract, control blood pressure and appetite, modulate the sleep cycle, and influence many other functions.
- Endocrine glands are interdependent on one another.
- Parathyroid glands are composed of three types of cells and are responsible for producing parathyroid hormone (PTH), detecting changes in extracellular calcium concentration, and inhibiting calcitonin secretion.
- Hypoparathyroidism is characterized by low serum levels of PTH, with the hallmark of this condition being hypocalcemia.
- The thyroid gland is composed of secretory cells, follicular cells, and C cells.
- Hyperthyroidism can result in thyrotoxicosis and, potentially, thyroid storm.
- The adrenal gland secretes glucocorticoids, mineralocorticoids, and supplemental sex hormones.
- Addison's disease, or primary adrenal insufficiency, is a metabolic and endocrine ailment caused by direct insult to or malfunction of the adrenal cortex.
- Acute adrenal insufficiency is a condition in which the body's need for glucocorticoids and mineralocorticoids exceeds the delivery of these hormones by the adrenal glands.
- Hyperadrenalism, or Cushing's syndrome, is caused by long-standing exposure to excessive circulating serum levels of glucocorticoids, particularly cortisol, as a result of overproduction in the adrenal cortex.
- Glucose is a vital fuel for key metabolic processes in organs, especially those in the central nervous system (CNS).

Summary (CONTINUED)

- Cellular survival depends on preserving a balanced serum glucose concentration.
- Diabetes is the most common endocrine disorder, and hypoglycemia, a frequent complication of the treatment of diabetes, is thus the most common endocrine emergency.
- Diabetes mellitus is characterized by defective insulin production or utilization, a high level of blood glucose, and unbalanced lipid and carbohydrate metabolism. Left untreated, diabetes results in hyperglycemia.
- Hypoglycemia among diabetics is the result of a disruption in the delicate balance between the interdependent factors of exogenously administered insulin, glucose metabolism, and glucose intake.
- Hypoglycemia may occur in patients taking only oral hypoglycemic agents, but should alert the healthcare provider to the potential presence of an underlying pathophysiologic state such as new-onset renal failure.
- Type 1 diabetes is characterized by pancreatic beta cell destruction, which renders the body incapable of producing the insulin necessary to carry out cell metabolism.
- Type 2 diabetes is characterized by cellular insulin resistance and a gradual failure of pancreatic insulin production.
- Gestational diabetes is a form of glucose intolerance that can occur in pregnant women.
- Healthy cellular function is directly related to a precise acid–base balance in the body, with the kidneys and lungs maintaining this balance, which is measured by pH.
- Hypoglycemia results in a decrease in insulin secretion and secretion of counterregulatory hormones such as epinephrine. Symptoms include impaired cognition. If untreated, hypoglycemia can lead to significant morbidity and mortality.
- Hypoglycemia in nondiabetic patients is characterized by alimentary hyperinsulinism, commonly seen in patients who have undergone gastric surgery or as the result of an imbalance between glucose utilization and production.
- Diabetic ketoacidosis is an acute endocrine emergency in which insulin deficiency and an excessive glucagon level combine to create a hyperglycemic, acidotic, volume-depleted state.
- Hyperosmolar hyperglycemic nonketotic coma (HHNC) is a serious diabetic emergency, carrying a mortality rate of 10% to 50%.
- Respiratory acidosis is characterized by a decline in pH as a result of CO_2 retention. An increase in ventilation per minute is the cause of respiratory alkalosis, which is characterized by a decreased Pa_{CO_2} and increased pH.
- Metabolic acidosis is caused by the accumulation of acids in excess of the body's buffering capabilities. The most common serious causes of metabolic acidosis are diabetic ketoacidosis, renal failure, lactic acidosis, toxic ingestion, and alcoholic ketoacidosis.
- Metabolic alkalosis is produced by illnesses that raise the level of serum bicarbonate or reduce the level of hydrogen in the body, such as those that cause volume, potassium, and chloride loss.
- A healthy electrolyte balance is fundamental to carrying out cellular functions; electrolyte imbalances include hyponatremia, hypokalemia, hyperkalemia, hypocalcemia, and hypomagnesemia.
- Rhabdomyolysis is a skeletal muscle injury characterized by release of cellular contents, specifically myoglobin, potentially leading to acute renal failure and hyperkalemia.

KEY TERMS

Addison's disease An endocrine disease caused by a deficiency of corticosteroid hormones produced by the adrenal cortex. The disease is characterized by nausea, vomiting, abdominal pain, and tanning of the skin.

adrenal crisis An endocrine emergency caused by a deficiency of corticosteroid hormones produced by the adrenal cortex. The disease is characterized by nausea, vomiting, abdominal pain, hypotension, hyperkalemia, and hyponatremia.

KEY TERMS (CONTINUED)

diabetic ketoacidosis (DKA)   An acute endocrine emergency caused by a lack of insulin. The condition is characterized by an elevated blood glucose level, ketone production, metabolic acidosis, dehydration, nausea, vomiting, abdominal pain, and tachypnea.

hyperosmolar hyperglycemic nonketotic coma (HHNC)   An endocrine emergency characterized by a high plasma glucose concentration, absent ketone production, and increased serum osmolality (> 315 mOsm/kg). The syndrome causes severe dehydration, nausea, vomiting, abdominal pain, and tachypnea.

hypoglycemia   A plasma glucose concentration of less than 70 mg/dL. This condition is often associated with signs and symptoms such as sweating, cold skin, tachycardia, and altered mental status.

myxedema   Severe hypothyroidism associated with cold intolerance, weight gain, weakness, and declining mental status.

thyroid storm   An endocrine emergency characterized by hyperfunction of the thyroid gland. This disorder is associated with fever, tachycardia, nervousness, altered mental status, and hemodynamic instability.

thyrotoxicosis   A condition of elevated thyroid hormone levels, which often leads to signs and symptoms of tachycardia, tremor, weight loss, and high-output heart failure.

BIBLIOGRAPHY

American Academy of Orthopaedic Surgeons: *Nancy Caroline's emergency care in the streets*, ed 7. Burlington, MA, 2013, Jones & Bartlett Learning.

Hamilton GC, Sanders AB, Strange GR: *Emergency medicine*, ed 2. St. Louis, MO, 2003, Saunders.

Kumar G, Sng BL, Kumar S: Correlation of capillary and venous blood glucometry with laboratory determination. *Prehosp Emerg Care*. 8(4):378, 2004.

Marx JA, Hockberger RS, Walls RM: *Rosen's emergency medicine*, ed 7. St. Louis, MO, 2009, Mosby.

Mistovich JJ, Krost WS, Limmer DD: Beyond the basics: Endocrine emergencies. *EMS Mag*. 36(10):123–127, 2007.

Mistovich JJ, Krost WS, Limmer DD: Beyond the basics: Endocrine emergencies, Part II. *EMS Mag*. 36(11):66–69, 2007.

Pagan KD, Pagana TJ: *Mosby's manual of diagnostic and laboratory tests*, ed 4. St. Louis, MO, 2010, Mosby.

Sanders MJ: *Mosby's paramedic textbook*, ed 3. St. Louis, MO, 2005, Mosby.

Story L: *Pathophysiology: A practical approach*, ed 2. Burlington, MA, 2015, Jones & Bartlett Learning.

U.S. Department of Transportation National Highway Traffic Safety Administration: *EMT-paramedic national standard curriculum*. Washington, DC, 1998, The Department.

U.S. Department of Transportation National Highway Traffic Safety Administration: *National EMS education standards*, Draft 3.0. Washington, DC, 2008, The Department.

CHAPTER REVIEW QUESTIONS

1. Your patient complains of discomfort in his hand as you inflate the cuff to assess the blood pressure. You note flexion of the wrist and adduction of his fingers. Which endocrine disorder do you suspect?
   a. Addison's disease
   b. Cushing's syndrome
   c. Hypoparathyroidism
   d. Myxedema

2. A 47-year-old woman is anxious and complaining of heart palpitations. She reports a recent diagnosis of "thyroid problems." On exam you note exophthalmos. Her vital signs include a blood pressure of 108/72 mm Hg; pulse rate, 128 beats/min; and respirations, 20 breaths/min. Interventions should include administration of:
   a. Amiodarone
   b. Aspirin
   c. Intravenous fluids
   d. Methylprednisolone

CHAPTER REVIEW QUESTIONS
(CONTINUED)

3. Which assessment finding(s) should you anticipate in a patient who has myxedema?
   a. Chvostek's sign
   b. Dry, yellow skin
   c. Exophthalmos
   d. Hyperactive reflexes

4. Which treatment should you anticipate in a patient with a history of Addison's disease who has the following vital signs: a blood pressure of 94/58 mm Hg; pulse, 124 beats/min; respirations, 20 breaths/min?
   a. Blood products
   b. Catecholamines
   c. Potassium
   d. Hydrocortisone

5. Which finding should you anticipate on the physical examination of a patient with Cushing's syndrome?
   a. Blood glucose, 180 mg/dL (10 mmol/L)
   b. Blood pressure, 94/54 mm Hg
   c. Heart rate, 50 bpm
   d. Thin face and body profile

6. When serum glucose levels drop below 70 mg/dL (3.9 mmol/L), which of the following occurs?
   a. Epinephrine secretion increases.
   b. Glucagon secretion decreases.
   c. Growth hormone secretion increases.
   d. Insulin production increases.

7. A 22-year-old man complains of a 2-day history of abdominal pain. His skin is flushed, and he has a fruity odor on his breath. Assessment reveals a blood pressure of 106/54 mm Hg; pulse rate, 128 beats/min; respirations, 28 breaths/min; and glucose level, 568 mg/dL. Your highest-priority intervention would be to:
   a. Administer glucagon IM.
   b. Perform endotracheal intubation.
   c. Infuse normal saline rapid IV.
   d. Perform a 12-lead electrocardiogram.

8. Which patient would be an appropriate candidate for immediate intravenous administration of sodium bicarbonate?
   a. A 22-year-old who is unresponsive after a heroin overdose with respirations of 8 breaths/min
   b. A 22-year-old with anxiety, a racing heart rate, and tachypnea
   c. A 34-year-old with nausea, vomiting, and diarrhea of 4 days' duration, who has shallow respirations and mild confusion
   d. A 45-year-old who initially complained of chest pain and is now in cardiac arrest and unresponsive to treatment

9. A 72-year-old complains of a headache and being depressed, intermittent twitching in the facial muscles, and general weakness over the past 2 weeks. She has a medical history of hypoparathyroidism. The ECG reveals a prolonged QT segment. During transport she has a seizure. Which electrolyte imbalance is most likely?
   a. Hypocalcemia
   b. Hyperkalemia
   c. Hypercalcemia
   d. Hyponatremia

10. A 10-year-old boy presents with lethargy. His vital signs include a blood pressure of 106/70 mm Hg; pulse rate, 140 beats/min; respirations, 32 breaths/min; oxygen saturation, 98%; and temperature, 99.0°F (37.2°C). Which of the following is most consistent with a diagnosis of DKA?
    a. Glucose 406 mg/dL; $ETCO_2$, 40 mm Hg
    b. Glucose 806 mg/dL; $ETCO_2$, 60 mm Hg
    c. Glucose 806 mg/dL; $ETCO_2$, 35 mm Hg
    d. Glucose, 406 mg/dL; $ETCO_2$, 25 mm Hg

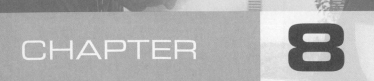

CHAPTER 8

Infectious Diseases

As a healthcare provider, you come into daily contact with patients who have a wide range of illnesses and infections. Patients may or may not know they have a communicable disease, may have an altered level of consciousness that prevents disclosure, or may choose not to reveal such information to you. This chapter will give you more expertise in recognizing and understanding the nature and communicability of infectious diseases. Safe practice and standard precautions will be reviewed, as will the signs, symptoms, and treatment of a number of infectious diseases.

LEARNING OBJECTIVES

At the conclusion of this chapter, you will be able to:

- Define specific terminology associated with infectious diseases.

- Explain how healthcare providers and the general public are protected from communicable and infectious diseases through regulations developed by federal, state, and various local governmental agencies.

- Outline primary, secondary, and ongoing assessment strategies for the patient with an infectious disease using the AMLS assessment pathway.

- Identify the links in the chain of infection, and describe how bacteria, fungi, parasites, and viruses cause disease.

- Explain how an exposure to a pathogen may evolve into an infection, and describe how each body system responds.

- Identify and discuss the epidemiology, pathophysiology, methods of transmission, clinical

manifestations, and treatment and prevention protocols and strategies for common infectious diseases, blood-borne diseases, enteric (intestinal) diseases, sexually transmitted diseases, parasites, zoonotic (animal-borne) diseases, vector-borne diseases, infection with multidrug-resistant organisms, communicable diseases of childhood, and emerging diseases.

- Explain the rationale for the various types of personal protective equipment, and describe proper disinfection of patient care equipment.

- Describe the healthcare provider's responsibilities in prevention of communicable and infectious diseases and maintaining patients' confidentiality.

- Formulate provisional diagnoses on the basis of assessment findings for a variety of infectious diseases.

- Identify and analyze your local protocol for reporting and documenting a communicable disease.

SCENARIO

© HunThomas/ShutterStock, Inc.

Paramedics arrive at a local hotel to find a 54-year-old woman seeking care for abdominal pain, vomiting, and diarrhea. She is found lying on the bed in a fetal position holding her abdomen. She tells you she is in town for a conference. She has a history of asthma and uses an inhaler when she has an attack. She has been vomiting for about 6 hours. She is pale and tells you she gets dizzy when she stands up. While you are present, she sits up and has projectile vomiting. You do not note any blood in the vomit. Her vital signs include a blood pressure of 102/54 mm Hg; pulse rate, 118 beats/min; and respirations, 24 breaths/min. Her Spo$_2$ is 97% on room air, with a temperature of 99.6°F (37.5°C).

- On the basis of the information you have now, what differential diagnoses are you considering?
- What additional historical and physical exam information will you need to narrow your differential diagnosis?
- What are your initial treatment priorities as you continue your patient care?
- How can you decrease your risk of acquiring infection if you are exposed to blood or bodily fluids during your care of this patient?

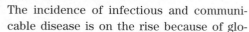

The incidence of infectious and communicable disease is on the rise because of globalization and the reemergence of diseases once thought to have been eradicated. Healthcare providers must maintain awareness of the risks of disease transmission when assessing patients and their environment. When responding to an emergency call, EMS typically arrives to an uncontrolled environment. Transmission of a communicable disease is more likely in situations where people live in close proximity to each other. Providers may not be aware the patient has an infectious disease, so it is crucial to perform a risk assessment any time providers care for patients.

Cautiousness, however, must be tempered by the obligation to give the best possible care to all who request it. Having a fundamental knowledge of disease processes, understanding the communicability of infectious organisms, and observing standard precautions will allow providers to administer care without undue concern about the transmission of infectious disease.

Infectious and Communicable Diseases

Infectious diseases are illnesses caused by pathogenic organisms such as bacteria, viruses, fungi, and parasites. Most infectious diseases, such as the common cold, are not life threatening. **Communicable diseases** are a subset of infectious diseases made up of illnesses that can be transmitted from person to

person. Communicable diseases pose a threat to the healthcare provider. Not all infectious diseases are communicable. A case of human-to-human transmission has never been documented. Infectious diseases are spread from person to person by several specific mechanisms:

- *Contact transmission.* Direct contact with an infected person may be brief, such as touching a patient. Most cases of the common cold are thought to be transmitted through casual direct contact. Venereal diseases, such as syphilis and gonorrhea, are transmitted principally by direct sexual contact. Direct contact also includes puncture by a contaminated needle or other sharp instrument or by transfusion of contaminated blood products from one patient to another.

    Indirect contact occurs by touching or handling an infected object or by coming into contact with a person who is contaminated with pathogens from a person or his or her excretions. When indirect transmission occurs, the organism survives for at least a brief period of time outside the human host.

- *Droplet transmission.* Droplet transmission of a communicable disease occurs when the droplets of an infected person, which can travel only 3 to 6 feet, are spread during close person-to-person contact: kissing, hugging, or otherwise touching someone, sharing eating or drinking utensils, or talking to someone within a 3-foot radius. In contrast to airborne transmission, the particles passed by droplet transmission are larger and do not travel as far. The heavy particles do not become aerosolized, so they can't hang suspended in the air for any appreciable length of time. Exposure to a disease communicable by droplet transmission is defined as direct contact with a patient's oronasal secretions, which may occur, for example, during unprotected mouth-to-mouth ventilation, suctioning, or spraying of secretions with no facial protection during intubation.

- *Airborne transmission.* A common transmission of communicable pulmonary diseases occurs during inhalation of airborne pathogens. This vapor of infectious particles can remain suspended in the air for long periods and can drift to new locations far from their source. Patients with compromised immune systems and those living and working in densely populated areas are at risk of acquiring these types of diseases. Healthcare providers must maintain a vigilant awareness of the potential risk of these types of diseases and ensure appropriate personal protective equipment (PPE) and work in well ventilated areas.
- *Vector transmission.* A vector is an organism that harbors pathogens that are harmless to the organism but cause disease to a human host. For example, a mosquito infected with West Nile virus that bites a susceptible person may transmit the disease.

Infection control always centers on early recognition through proficient assessment. Healthcare providers must strike a careful balance between caring for patients and limiting the spread of infectious agents to others, including themselves, other healthcare workers, and the public. When patients with communicable diseases are being treated, always consider the impact of the disease process not only on the infected patient but also on the community. The risk of transmission can be limited by taking the following simple precautions:

- Receive immunizations/vaccinations.
- Use PPE consistent with the signs and symptoms of infectious disease.
- Pursue postexposure medical reporting and follow-up.
- Gain a broad comprehension of typical disease progression and recommended supportive management of the conditions for which patients seek care.

Infectious Agents

Bacteria

Bacteria are single-celled microorganisms that live in water, inside the human body, in organic matter, and on inorganic surfaces (fomites). Antibiotics are effective against most bacterial infections. Aerobic bacteria, such as those that cause tuberculosis and plague, can survive only in the presence of oxygen. Anaerobic bacteria, however, such as *Clostridium* strains, which cause botulism and tetanus, carry out their cellular functions without oxygen.

Most bacteria are surprisingly fastidious, requiring specific conditions in order to grow, reproduce, and flourish. Certain bacteria, for example, must be confined to a narrow temperature range and must be supplied with particular nutrients to survive.

Viruses

Viruses, one of the smallest disease agents, must grow and multiply inside the living cells of a host. Viruses can cause minor illnesses, such as the common cold, or grave diseases, including acquired immunodeficiency syndrome (AIDS) and smallpox.

Only supportive care is required to treat most viral illnesses. In general, viruses are not vulnerable to antibiotics. Antiviral drugs have been formulated, and many more vaccines are being developed to prevent lethal viral infections or to moderate the severity of symptoms and reduce the length of illness.

Fungi

Fungi are plantlike microorganisms, most of which are not pathogenic. Yeast, mold, mildew, and mushrooms are types of fungi. Those of particular importance to humans and the illnesses they cause are as follows:

- Dermatophytes (skin infections such as tinea corporis, also called *ringworm*)
- *Aspergillus* spp. (pulmonary aspergillosis and infections of the external ear, sinuses, and subcutaneous tissue)
- *Blastomyces dermatitidis* (blastomycosis, which causes abscesses of skin and subcutaneous tissue)
- *Histoplasma capsulatum* (histoplasmosis)
- *Candida* spp. (vaginal candidiasis and oral candidiasis, also called *thrush*)

Antifungal agents have been developed to treat most of these infections.

Parasites

Parasites are a common cause of disease where sanitation is poor, generally in developing countries, although cases are still found in developed countries. Unlike viruses, parasites are living organisms. Like viruses, however, they must have a living host in order to survive and reproduce. Parasites live in or on the host and feed on it or consume some of the host's supply of nutrients at the host's expense.

Depending on the parasite, irritation and infection can be topical or systemic. Treatment is focused on agents that will relieve the irritating symptoms as well as eradicate developing eggs and live parasites. Antihistamines may be prescribed to relieve urticaria. Insecticides, acetylcholinesterase inhibitors, ovicidals, and pediculicides can be effective.

Stages of the Infectious Process

Disease progression varies greatly depending on the pathogen dose (the number of organisms present), the **virulence** of the organism, and the susceptibility of the host. Several conditions must be met for infection to occur.

A key concept in infection control is that exposure to a pathogen is not tantamount to infection. It simply means that the pathogen entered the host. Whether infection occurs depends on the factors previously described. Postexposure prophylaxis can also decrease likelihood of infection, although hepatitis C is one exception to this rule.

Communicable diseases have stages, or periods, that identify the components of the infectious process: the latent period, incubation period, communicability period, and disease period (Table 8-1).

Latent Period

The latent period begins when the pathogen enters the body by evading the host's outermost layers of defense, such as skin or acidic mucous secretions. During this period, the infection is not communicable, and the person exhibits no symptoms. This period may be protracted, lasting for months or years, or it may be as brief as a single day. This latent period is not the same as a latent infection or a latent disease. A latent infection is an inactive yet communicable infection that may become symptomatic at some future time. A disease is said to be latent when signs and symptoms wane between flare-ups. The herpes virus family is an example of a pathogen that often enters a period of latency. During this stage, symptoms disappear; they reappear when the pathogen is reactivated.

Incubation Period

The incubation period is the interval between exposure to the pathogen and the onset of symptoms. Like the length of the latent stage, the length of the incubation period varies from one organism to another, ranging from hours to years. The difference is that during the incubation period, the pathogen reproduces in the host, mobilizing the body's immune system to produce specific disease antibodies. At this point, seroconversion may occur, which means that the antibodies reach a detectable level, and the infected person's blood begins to test positive for exposure to the pathogen. After infection, a window may occur during which no disease-specific antibodies can be detected in the blood.

Communicability Period

A period of communicability follows the latent stage. This stage lasts as long as the agent remains in the body and can be spread to other people. This period varies in length and is dependent on the virulence, number of organisms that are transmitted, mode of transportation, and the host's resistance. The age and general health status of the individual prior to exposure affects the susceptibility and risk factors of contracting the infectious disease.

Disease Period

A period of disease follows the incubation period. Its duration depends on the particular pathogen. This stage may be symptom free or may produce obvious symptoms such as skin lesions or a cough. The body may eventually be able destroy the pathogen and thus eliminate the disease. Some tenacious pathogens, however, cannot be removed from their new surroundings despite the immune system's best efforts to do so. They may lie dormant for a while, causing a latent infection, but pathogens such as HIV and herpesviruses remain in the body indefinitely once an infection has occurred.

Public Health and Safety Regulations

The public health and safety system is responsible for ensuring the general health of the population by means of education, disease reduction and surveillance, sanitation, and pollution control. An important segment of public health is **epidemiology**,

Table 8-1 **Components of the Infectious Process**		
Stage	**Begins**	**Ends**
Latent period	With invasion	When the agent can be shed
Incubation period	With invasion	When the disease process begins
Communicability period	When the latent period ends	Continues as long as the agent is present and can spread to others
Disease period	Follows incubation period	Variable duration

the branch of medicine concerned with studying the causes, distribution, and control of disease in a population. Applied epidemiology also helps public health officials prevent or identify and control trends in the spread of infectious diseases.

Protecting public health is a multifaceted process consisting of:

- Instituting preventive measures, such as establishing immunization programs
- Overseeing health-related environmental matters, such as ensuring clean food, air, and water
- Pursuing educational initiatives, such as smoking cessation and obesity reduction programs

Agencies

At the local level, agencies including fire departments, EMS providers and agencies, health departments, healthcare facilities, and laboratories are the first line of defense in disease surveillance, outbreak identification, and pandemic planning. Local agencies also support efforts to reduce the incidence and prevent the spread of infectious diseases by collecting and sharing data related to illness and injury; organizing it according to geographical region, race, age, sexual orientation, and ethnicity; and implementing priority initiatives.

At the international level, the United Nations World Health Organization (WHO) coordinates worldwide disease prevention efforts for members of the United Nations by providing leadership on global health issues and technical and logistical support for health research. WHO also establishes evidence-based standards related to health trends. Many countries have their own agencies that monitor the incidence of infectious diseases and provide standards of care. Regional and local agencies may be involved as well. In the United States, the Centers for Disease Control and Prevention provides these guidelines along with other agencies such as the Department of and Human Services and the Department of Labor's Occupational Safety and Health Administration (OSHA).

U.S.-Specific Requirements

In the United States, public health and safety initiatives at the national level are executed primarily by the Department of Health and Human Services. The following agencies operate under its auspices:

- The Centers for Disease Control and Prevention (CDC) in Atlanta, Georgia, is the chief agency responsible for tracking and preventing morbidity and mortality associated with infectious disease. It's the most visible epidemiologic agency in the international medical community. The CDC monitors national infectious disease data and distributes this information to all healthcare providers and to the community through the Internet (www.cdc.gov) and in publications such as *Morbidity and Mortality Weekly Report (MMWR)* and *Emerging Infectious Diseases*.
- The Office of the Surgeon General oversees the U.S. Public Health Service and spearheads risk reduction activities, such as promoting childhood immunization, ensuring public preparedness for bioterrorist attacks, and addressing disparities in rates of infectious disease and access to treatment among various racial, ethnic, and socioeconomic patient population groups.
- The Food and Drug Administration (FDA) is responsible for ensuring the safety of prescription and over-the-counter drugs and medical devices, including those associated with transmission of infectious disease, such as indwelling catheters.

In addition, The Department of Homeland Security's Federal Emergency Management Agency works with the CDC, the Office of the Surgeon General, and other agencies to coordinate emergency preparedness for hurricanes, earthquakes, and other natural disasters that foster outbreaks of a variety of diseases. Infectious diseases are associated with floodwater, sewer line breaks, and crowded living conditions in shelters.

Standards, Guidelines, and Statutes

The Department of Labor's Occupational Safety and Health Administration (OSHA) oversees compliance, enforcement, inspection, tracking, and reporting related to infection control practice in the workplace. This agency establishes guidelines for preventing transmission of airborne and **blood-borne pathogens** and develops postexposure protocols for use in occupational settings. OSHA standard 1910.120 specifies the PPE that must be available in given occupational settings and dictates how employees must be educated on its use to protect themselves from the hazards they are likely to encounter during the normal course of their work.

One of the OSHA regulations most important to healthcare workers is 29 CFR 1910.1030, which is intended to reduce the number of **exposure incidents**, defined as the transmission of blood-borne pathogens through **parenteral** contact with blood or other potentially infectious materials and the eyes, mouth, or other mucous membranes or nonintact skin during the performance of an employee's duties.

The Ryan White Care Act, passed by the U.S. Congress in 1990 and reappropriated in September 2009, constitutes Part G of the law. It contains a provision requiring that each emergency response agency has a designated infection control officer who is notified in the event of an exposure. The designated infection control officer acts as a liaison between the exposed employee and the medical facility to ensure proper notification, testing, and reporting of results.

Immunization Schedule

A recommended immunization schedule can be obtained from the CDC.

OSHA Bloodborne Pathogens Standard

Prevention efforts in the healthcare setting are now subject to OSHA's Bloodborne Pathogens Standard (which has retained use of the term *universal precautions*).

Since 1991, when OSHA first issued its Bloodborne Pathogens Standard to protect healthcare personnel from blood exposure, the focus of regulatory and legislative activity has been on implementing such control measures, including removing sharps hazards by developing and using engineering controls. The federal Needlestick Safety and Prevention Act, signed into law in November 2000, authorized OSHA to revise its Bloodborne Pathogens Standard to require more explicitly the use of safety-engineered sharps devices.

After a needlestick exposure, your risk of infection depends on the pathogen involved, your immune status, the severity of the needlestick injury, the amount of circulating virus in the source patient, and the availability and use of appropriate postexposure prophylaxis. Since 1991, each fire/rescue department has been required to formulate a comprehensive plan to address these issues. Exposure control plans are summarized in Table 8-2.

Needlesticks

The passage of the Needlestick Safety and Prevention Act of 2000 prompted the development of many engineering controls, including self-capping intravenous (IV) catheter needles, needleless IV tubing, resheathing scalpels, and safety syringes for medication administration. OSHA requires that sharps and other disposal containers be easily accessible at their sites of use.

Equipment Cleaning

Decontaminate infected equipment according to the CDC guidelines.

OSHA requires that healthcare providers be given education and training on syphilis and that this disease be part of any postexposure evaluation and medical follow-up.

Special Considerations

Patients with methicillin-resistant *Staphylococcus aureus* (MRSA) and vancomycin-resistant *Enterococcus* (VRE) may be protected by the Americans with Disabilities Act, so it is important to exercise sensitivity with the use of unnecessary PPE, which may be considered discriminatory.

Department members are to be updated annually on new information about diseases, technology, equipment modifications, department exposure rates, and number of infectious disease transmissions and tuberculosis (TB) contacts during the previous year. This information serves to place risk in a proper perspective. Risk of disease transmission is present, but the risk is low when proper protective measures are followed by healthcare providers. OSHA has framed such risk-reduction and education requirements as a right-to-know issue.

Infection Control

Standard Precautions

Transmission of blood-borne viruses occurs through exposure incidents. The prevention of such incidents involves **standard precautions** (formerly called *universal precautions*) for routine patient care.

In addition to using PPE, safe work practices can help to protect mucous membranes and nonintact skin from exposure. These include keeping gloved and ungloved hands that may be **contaminated** from touching your mouth, nose, eyes, or face, and positioning patients to direct sprays and splatter away from your face. Carefully selecting and gathering PPE before direct patient contact will help you avoid the need to make PPE adjustments, reduce the likelihood of face or mucous membrane contamination during use, and reduce the possibility of contaminating gloves before you have contact with the patient. In areas where the need for resuscitation is unpredictable, mouthpieces,

---

Table 8-2 Elements of an Agency Exposure Control Plan

- Policy for health maintenance and surveillance
- Appointment of a designated infection control officer to serve as a liaison between the agency and healthcare facilities
- Identification of work functions when a risk of exposure to pathogens exists
- Policy for use of PPE and availability of PPE to healthcare workers
- Procedure for identifying and evaluating exposures and a strategy for postexposure counseling, medical care, and documentation (as required by the Ryan White Emergency Response Notification Act, Part G)
- Effective plan for decontaminating personnel and for disinfecting and storing equipment
- Education regarding disease transmission, cleaning and disinfection procedures, use of PPE, and the purpose of immunization
- Steps for complying with medical waste regulations
- Strategy for compliance monitoring
- Record keeping policies and procedures

pocket resuscitation masks with one-way valves, and other ventilation devices provide an alternative to mouth-to-mouth ventilation, preventing exposure of your nose and mouth to the patient's oral and respiratory secretions during the procedure.

Preventing Sharps Injuries

Sharps injuries have been associated with transmission of hepatitis B and C viruses (HBV, HCV) and HIV to healthcare personnel. The prevention of sharps injuries has always been an essential element of standard precautions. Needles and other sharp devices must be handled in a way that will prevent injury to the user and to others who may encounter the device during or after the procedure.

Needle-Safe Devices

Historically, most needlesticks have occurred during recapping procedures. To address this issue the development of many engineering controls, including self-capping IV catheter needles, needleless IV tubing, resheathing scalpels, and safety syringes for medication administration has occurred. Keeping sharps and other disposal containers readily available is recommended.

Responsibilities of Healthcare Providers

Employers are required to establish specific policies and procedures to protect personnel during the course of their duties. However, employees and volunteers play a role in protecting themselves as well. Employee self-protection responsibilities include the following:

- Giving full consideration to participation in vaccination/immunization programs
- Attending required education and training programs
- Using PPE properly
- Promptly reporting exposures
- Complying with all aspects of the department's exposure control plan

Hand Washing

The best means of preventing transmission of infectious agents remains the most basic one: effective hand washing. Because no barrier is 100% effective, hands should be washed before and after caring for each patient and after removing gloves. Alcohol-based antimicrobial products may be used when no gross contamination is visible or when conventional soap and water are not available.

Personal Protective Equipment

Protective barriers offer a second line of defense to block entry of pathogens. These barriers include gloves, gowns, masks and other protective eyewear, sharps containers, and engineering controls that limit needlesticks. Gloves reduce contamination of hands but do not prevent penetrating injuries by needles or other sharp objects. Gowns prevent saturation of clothing and contact of skin with body fluids during procedures and patient care. Masks, face shields, and other protective eyewear reduce the likelihood of contamination of mucous membranes of the eyes, nose, and mouth.

PPE selection should be task specific. For example, gloves are not required for giving intramuscular or subcutaneous injections. Table 8-3 shows the PPE necessary to perform various tasks when caring for a patient infected with HIV or HBV. Local protocols, policies, and procedures should be followed.

Cleaning and Decontamination Procedures

Decontaminate infected equipment according to the WHO guidelines and in keeping with local requirements. **Decontamination** of equipment should be performed only in marked, designated areas. Each area should have an appropriate ventilation system and adequate drainage. Providers should always wear gloves, a cover gown if their uniform might become contaminated, and protective eyewear or a full face mask if blood or other potentially infectious materials might be splashed when decontaminating equipment.

Begin decontamination by removing gross dirt and debris with soap and a copious amount of water. Then disinfect as appropriate. It is important to follow the manufacturer's recommendations for each piece of equipment so as not to void the warranty.

Postexposure Procedures

In the event you experience an exposure to a communicable or infectious disease while on duty, report the occurrence without delay to your supervisor per protocol. Many agencies and institutions have designated personnel to recommend immediate and follow-up testing and evaluation.

Patient care should continue as appropriate. Hand washing and proper disposal of contaminated items should continue.

Epidemics and Pandemics

An **epidemic** is a disease outbreak in which many people in a community or region become infected with the same disease, either because the disease has been brought into the community by an outside source, such as an infected traveler, or because a pathogen (in this case, a bacterium or virus) has mutated in a way that either has enabled it to evade the immune system or has made it more virulent. Some epidemics occur when an entirely new disease emerges, as occurred with HIV and severe acute respiratory syndrome (SARS). Others begin when a new version of an old disease reemerges, as was the case with influenza A strains H1N1 and H5N1.

A **pandemic,** such as the devastating 1918 influenza pandemic, is an epidemic that sweeps the globe, reaching all seven

Table 8-3 Examples of Recommended Personal Protective Equipment for Protection of Workers Against HIV* and HBV Transmission in Prehospital Settings

Task or Activity	Disposable Gloves	Gown	Mask	Protective Eyewear
Bleeding control with spurting blood	Yes	Yes	Yes	Yes
Bleeding control with minimal bleeding	Yes	No	No	No
Emergency childbirth	Yes	Yes	Yes, if splashing is likely	Yes, if splashing is likely
Blood drawing	At certain times†	No	No	No
Starting an intravenous (IV) line	Yes	No	No	No
Endotracheal intubation, esophageal obturator use	Yes	No	No, unless splashing is likely	No, unless splashing is likely
Oral/nasal suctioning, manually cleaning airway	Yes¶	No	No, unless splashing is likely	No, unless splashing is likely
Handling and cleaning instruments with microbial contamination	Yes	No, unless soiling is likely	No	No
Measuring blood pressure	No	No	No	No
Measuring temperature	No	No	No	No
Giving an injection	No	No	No	No

*The examples provided in this table are based on application of universal precautions, commonly referred to as standard precautions. Universal precautions are intended to supplement rather than replace recommendations for routine infectious control, such as hand washing and using gloves to prevent gross microbial contamination of hands (e.g., contact with urine or feces).

†In performing tasks where you can reasonably anticipate hand contact with blood or other potentially infectious materials, you must wear gloves.

§While not clearly necessary to prevent HIV or HBV transmission unless blood is present, gloves are recommended to prevent transmission of other agents (e.g., herpes simplex).

Data from the Department of Health and Human Services (NIOSH), Centers for Disease Control and Prevention, Guidelines for Prevention of Transmission of HIV and HBV to Health Care and Public-Safety Workers, *Morbid Mortal Weekly Rep (MMWR)*, Vol 38, No. S-6, June 23, 1989. http://wonder.cdc.gov/wonder/prevguid/p0000114/p0000114.asp

continents. As might be expected, a pandemic usually results in a high death toll. As with an epidemic, a pandemic may arise from an old disease, such as smallpox or the bubonic plague, or from the development of a new disease or a new form of an old disease.

If the source of the pandemic is a virulent new pathogen or a new form of a pernicious old pathogen, very few people if any will have antibodies that make them resistant to the disease. Consequently, the rates of illness and death may be catastrophic unless effective prevention strategies are rapidly developed and implemented. Although immunization is often an effective prevention strategy, developing a vaccine and ensuring its safety and efficacy in humans is a protracted process. The purpose of a vaccination is to induce a long-lasting protective immune response to prevent disease in a healthy individual receiving the vaccine. A recommended immunization schedule can be obtained from the World Health Organization. Evolving technology has begun to compress the amount of time necessary to develop, manufacture, and distribute new vaccines.

AMLS Assessment Pathway

▼ Initial Observations

The AMLS assessment process for a patient suspected of having an infectious disease rests on a thorough, comprehensive, efficient approach to diagnosing and managing associated medical emergencies.

Scene Safety Considerations

In assessing any patient, providers must maintain a keen awareness of the risk for transmission of an infectious disease, not only from patient to provider but also from provider to patient. Standard precautions must be followed to minimize the risk of disease transmission through selection of proper PPE and other infection control strategies.

Patient Cardinal Presentation/Chief Complaint

As you begin to assess the patient and the scene and situation, note the character and severity of the patient's signs and symptoms as clues to the possible presence of an infectious process. Typical chief complaints include fever, nausea, rash, pleuritic chest pain, and difficulty breathing. It is essential to be able to recognize the cardinal presentation/chief complaint of a wide variety of infectious diseases and to know how they are most effectively treated or prevented. In the following sections, this can be accomplished by exploring signs and symptoms, with diagnostic studies, and

assessment and management strategies for the infectious diseases likely to be encountered most often in the prehospital setting.

Primary Survey

At the start of the primary survey, perform a risk assessment for possible exposure and take the appropriate standard precautions. Then the provider must ensure that the patient has a patent airway, efficient work of breathing, and adequate perfusion.

Evaluate the quality and regularity of the patient's pulse and the color, temperature, and moisture of the skin. Assess the patient's alertness using the AVPU mnemonic. Determine whether his or her condition is urgent or emergent, and identify and manage promptly any diagnoses of immediate concern. Initiate early treatment on the basis of these initial findings.

▼ First Impression

Identify how sick the patient appears to be. Focus on addressing any life-threatening conditions. Generate differential diagnoses based on the cardinal presentation/chief complain with a focus on life-threatening presentations and the most common presentations.

▼ Detailed Assessment

History Taking

The differential diagnosis and subsequent working diagnosis should be refined based on the following:

- Incident and past medical history taken using the OPQRST and SAMPLER mnemonics
- A focused physical examination
- Interpretation of diagnostic findings

OPQRST and SAMPLER

The OPQRST mnemonic will help you elaborate on the patient's chief complaint. Be sure to obtain a SAMPLER history, paying particular attention to medications the patient is currently taking, the events leading up to today's problem, recent infections or exposures, the events leading up to the current problem, and whether the patient has recently traveled. Risk factors such as a compromised immune system, age, multiple medical problems, or indwelling devices should also be taken into consideration during this component of the history collection.

Secondary Survey

The secondary survey of a patient suspected of having an infectious disease should be approached much like that of any other medical patient. Vital signs should be obtained to determine the overall stability of the patient. Perform a full-body head-to-toe examination, as detailed in Chapter 1, to evaluate the workings of specific body organ systems.

Diagnostics

Clinical reasoning and the patient's response to treatment should guide you in determining laboratory or radiographic diagnostic tools that can confirm or rule out potential infectious disease processes in order to arrive at a definitive diagnosis.

▼ Refine the Differential Diagnosis

As you perform your reassessment, you will continually work to rule in or rule out certain conditions from your differential diagnosis list. Keep an open mind as you gather all your patient information and modify your differential diagnosis based on new findings.

▼ Ongoing Management

Continue to monitor the patient's condition. Obtain another complete set of vital signs, and compare them with the expected outcomes from your therapies. Document all of your findings with each reassessment so that your medical record is accurate and complete for handoff at the emergency department. Remember it is key to report suspicion of infection or sepsis to the receiving facility so that precious time is not lost should antibiotics or other treatments for infectious diseases be needed.

The Chain of Infection

Infection involves a chain of events through which the communicable disease spreads. Microorganisms that ordinarily reside in the human body without causing disease are part of the body's normal flora and constitute one layer of the host's defenses. Normal flora help keep the host disease free by creating environmental conditions inhospitable to pathogens, which are disease-causing microorganisms that rely on a host to supply their nutritional needs. The state of balance maintained by normal flora, in which conditions are favorable to the host and unfavorable to pathogens, is known as "homeostasis."

Reservoir/Host

Pathogens may live and reproduce on and within humans, animal hosts, or other organic substances. Once infected, the human host may show clinical signs of illness or may become an asymptomatic carrier who has no knowledge of the infection but is nevertheless capable of transmitting the pathogen to another person. The life cycle of the pathogen depends on several factors: demographics of the host (e.g., age), genetic factors, temperature, and the efficacy of any therapeutic measures taken once the infection has been recognized.

Portal of Exit

A portal of exit is necessary if a pathogenic agent is to leave one host to invade another. The organism may exit the body by a single portal or several, such as the genitourinary tract, intestinal tract, oral cavity, respiratory tract, or an open lesion.

Transmission

Direct or indirect transmission may occur through the portal of exit and the portal of entry. Modes of direct and indirect transmission and examples of each are listed in Table 8-4.

Table 8-4 Modes of Transmission of Infectious Diseases

Mode	Examples of How Contact Might Occur	Selected Infectious Diseases Transmitted by This Mode
Direct Transmission		
Touching an infected person	Shaking hands Wrestling	Influenza, chickenpox Scabies
Oral transmission	Kissing or drinking after an infected person	Mumps, pertussis, infectious mononucleosis, herpes simplex virus type 1
Droplet transmission	Source coughs or sneezes, and new host inhales airborne mucus particles	Rubeola, mumps, pertussis, chickenpox, respiratory syncytial virus, SARS, bacterial meningitis, H1N1 influenza
Fecal contamination	Contact with feces at a daycare center	Viral meningitis, CMV
Sexual contact	Having intercourse without a condom	HIV, herpes simplex virus type 2, gonorrhea, CMV, syphilis, HPV

(continues)

Mode	Examples of How Contact Might Occur	Selected Infectious Diseases Transmitted by This Mode
Table 8-4 Modes of Transmission of Infectious Diseases (*continued*)		
Indirect Transmission		
Food	Consumption of raw shellfish	Hepatitis A
Water	Drinking from a contaminated municipal water supply	*Escherichia coli*
Biological matter	Needle sharing, needlestick injuries, tattooing, and body piercing	HIV, hepatitis B, hepatitis C
	Touching an infected surface such as a bed rail	Rubeola, respiratory syncytial virus, HA-MRSA
	Contact with fomites such as towels and linens	Scabies
	Healthcare provider who has had contact with an infected patient touches another patient without washing his or her hands	*Clostridium difficile*
Soil/ground surfaces	Puncture wound Contact of nonintact skin with field turf	Tetanus CA-MRSA
Air	Cleaning a basement or barn that contains infected rodent feces	Hantavirus

CA-MRSA, Community-acquired methicillin-resistant *Staphylococcus aureus*; CMV, cytomegalovirus; HA-MRSA, hospital-acquired methicillin-resistant *Staphylococcus aureus*; HIV, human immunodeficiency virus; HPV, human papillomavirus; SARS, severe acute respiratory syndrome coronavirus.

Portal of Entry

The portal of entry is the site at which the pathogenic agent enters a new host. The organism may be ingested, inhaled, or injected through the skin, or it may cross a mucous membrane, the placenta, or nonintact skin. The amount of time it takes for the infectious process to begin in a new host after the pathogen enters varies with the organism and the host's susceptibility. In fact, exposure to an infectious agent usually does not produce illness in a healthy person, since the immune system is able to destroy it before it can multiply to cause an infection. The duration of exposure and the quantity of pathogens required to produce infection in the host differ for each pathogen.

Host Susceptibility

For an organism to produce illness, the host must be susceptible to infection by the pathogen—that is, he or she must be in an unhealthy or weakened state. If the host is healthy, the immune system subdues the pathogen and protects the host

from infection (**Figure 8-1**). However, certain factors can impair the host's ability to do so. These factors are summarized in **Table 8-5**.

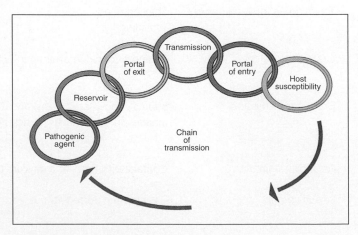

Figure 8-1 Chain of transmission for infection. The chain must be intact for an infection to be transmitted to another host. Transmission can be controlled by breaking any link in the chain.

Table 8-5 Factors That Increase Host Susceptibility to Infection

- *Age.* The very young and the very old are more at risk of contracting an infectious disease.
- *Use of drugs.* Taking immunosuppressive medications, steroids, or other drugs may affect immune response.
- *Malnutrition/Obesity.* Poor nutrition weakens the immune system. Obesity is often associated with multiple chronic disease processes and places patients at risk for infection due to a compromised immune system.
- *Chronic disease.* Chronic disease, such as diabetes and heart disease, gradually saps the body of its ability to defend itself.
- *Shock/trauma.* When a person is in shock or has been injured, body defenses are mobilized to restore organ function and to recover from injury, leaving him or her in a weak position to fight infection.
- *Smoking.* Use of tobacco products has been shown to impair the body's immune response.

Natural Defenses of the Body

The body is equipped with an arsenal of defenses that inhibit pathogen invasion. The arrival of a pathogen through a portal of entry touches off a complex cascade of immune system responses.

First, a nonspecific inflammatory response occurs; it involves migration of neutrophils and release of inflammatory substances in an effort to contain and inactivate the pathogen. Then a more specific response is initiated in which T lymphocytes develop receptors for a specific antigen on the pathogen. This allows the T cells to attach to and ingest the pathogen. B lymphocytes are activated and begin to produce **antibodies** (free-floating proteins) that have an affinity for the specific antigen as well. These circulating antibodies then bind to the antigen on the pathogen, either rendering the pathogen ineffective or allowing other body defenses to inactivate or destroy it. An antigen might be a component of a pathogen such as a virus, parasite, dust mite, or a blood product transfused into the body. The **antigen** is a molecule the immune system does not recognize as its own. The immune system sometimes reacts to components within the body, known as "self-antigens," but the immune system is activated primarily in response to exogenous antigens—that is, those introduced into the body from an external source. The immune system's capacity to distinguish between self and other is essential. Without it, the body would indiscriminately lay siege to its own cells.

Some cloned B cells become memory cells, which generate specific antibodies quickly in the event of a reexposure. This reaction supports immunity to certain diseases by zeroing in on specific antigens and disabling them when they make a reappearance.

The human body has many other nonspecific protective mechanisms, such as the skin, mucus, and cilia, that trap organisms (**Figure 8-2**). Acidic secretions, such as those in the

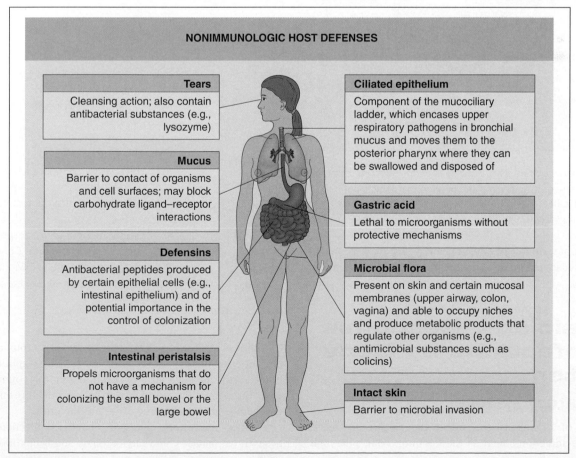

NONIMMUNOLOGIC HOST DEFENSES

Tears
Cleansing action; also contain antibacterial substances (e.g., lysozyme)

Mucus
Barrier to contact of organisms and cell surfaces; may block carbohydrate ligand–receptor interactions

Defensins
Antibacterial peptides produced by certain epithelial cells (e.g., intestinal epithelium) and of potential importance in the control of colonization

Intestinal peristalsis
Propels microorganisms that do not have a mechanism for colonizing the small bowel or the large bowel

Ciliated epithelium
Component of the mucociliary ladder, which encases upper respiratory pathogens in bronchial mucus and moves them to the posterior pharynx where they can be swallowed and disposed of

Gastric acid
Lethal to microorganisms without protective mechanisms

Microbial flora
Present on skin and certain mucosal membranes (upper airway, colon, vagina) and able to occupy niches and produce metabolic products that regulate other organisms (e.g., antimicrobial substances such as colicins)

Intact skin
Barrier to microbial invasion

Figure 8-2 The body has a number of defense mechanisms to prevent infection.

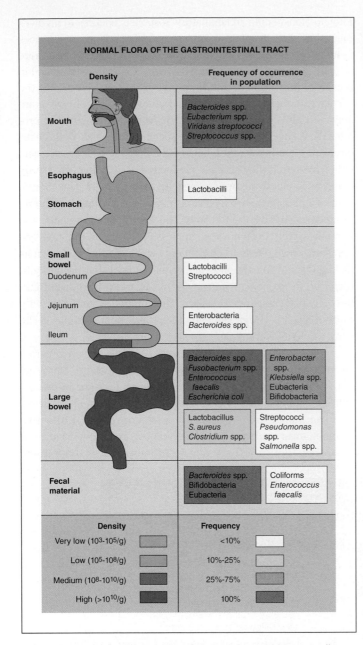

Figure 8-3 The gastrointestinal and genitourinary tracts normally have extensive bacterial (normal flora) living in them that help these body systems perform their functions and prevent infection.

intestinal tract, inhibit organism growth (**Figure 8-3**). Several body systems also have mechanisms that affect immunity (**Table 8-6**).

Physiologic Response to Infections by Body System

Respiratory System

A variety of organisms can infect the respiratory system. Respiratory infections such as the common cold, pharyngitis, tonsillitis, sinusitis, laryngitis, epiglottitis, and croup are principal causes of illness in the United States. Acute respiratory infections are the leading cause of death in children younger than 5 years throughout the world. Nevertheless, a healthy human body is generally able to stay free of serious infection.

Upper respiratory illnesses comprise infections of the nose, throat, sinuses, and larynx. Signs and symptoms of upper

Table 8-6 The Role of Body Systems in Immunity

System	Role
Integumentary system	The immune system's first line of defense is intact skin. Organisms are unable to pass through intact skin, and the normal secretions of the skin are bactericidal, killing off many would-be invaders. Nonintact skin, on the other hand, serves as a portal of entry for pathogens.
Ocular system	The conjunctiva are protected in two ways. First, blinking sweeps away pathogens before they can enter the eye. Second, tear film dilutes the concentration of organisms present.
Respiratory system	Built-in protections in the lungs include moist mucous membranes and cilia that trap organisms that enter during inhalation. Then the cough reflex expels the pathogens from the body.
Gastrointestinal tract	Gastric acids and juices, along with helpful microorganisms that live in the GI tract, serve as another line of defense. Phagocytes assist in the ingestion and digestion of bacteria.
Genitourinary system	The genitourinary system is protected by a thick layer of cells and by the acidic secretions of the mucous membranes that line the genitourinary tract.
Immunologic system	Chemical properties of the immune system include properdin, a protein that acts with the complement system to protect against viruses and bacteria. The viricidal protein, interferon, is stimulated when viruses are present in tissue cells. Leukocytes initiate a nonspecific inflammatory response, then T and B lymphocytes generate cellular and humoral response specific to the invading organism.

respiratory infection include sore throat, fever, chills, nasal drainage, and painful swallowing or speaking. One of the most common reasons for seeking medical care is pharyngitis, an inflammatory syndrome of the oropharynx, often localized to the lymphatic tissue and producing swelling of the tonsils, fever, and occasional secondary otitis media from blockage of the pharyngotympanic tube.

Lower respiratory infections, including pneumonia, often require antibiotic therapy. For patients with compromised immune function, respiratory infections may exacerbate underlying pulmonary conditions and progress to significant infection. Management should focus on supporting ventilation and hydration and on preventing spread of the pathogen.

Cardiovascular System

Significant increases in pulse rate may occur as infection sets in and body temperature rises. Fever increases metabolic needs, necessitating more oxygen and nutrients to carry out physiologic functions. Hypotension may also occur because of dehydration, vasodilation, or both, as happens with septic shock. In rare cases, infection of the heart valves (endocarditis) may lower cardiac output, resulting in cardiogenic shock.

Identify and aggressively treat hypotension promptly. The treatment you select depends on its etiology. If the patient's lungs are clear and you suspect hypovolemia due to dehydration, vomiting, or diarrhea, aggressive use of IV fluids may be indicated.

Most patients with bacterial endocarditis have one of three predisposing factors: rheumatic or congenital heart disease, a history of endocarditis, or IV drug use. The most common site of infection in endocarditis is the mitral valve. Patients often have tachycardia, tachypnea, hyperthermia or hypothermia, and in severe cases, profound hypotension. Release of inflammatory mediators causes vasodilation and hyperdynamic cardiovascular effects. The patient will appear flushed, with warm extremities and adequate capillary refill. Prevention of septic shock and/or cardiogenic shock is an emergent care priority.

Depending on the type and virulence of the infectious organism, the general course of treatment is aggressive antibiotic therapy. In cases where the infection has damaged heart valves, surgical intervention to replace the valves may be necessary.

Neurologic System

Neurologic infections can be caused by either viruses or bacteria, and their severity ranges from virtually innocuous to life threatening. Symptoms of central nervous system (CNS) viral infections can be mild and self-limiting, as seen in the mumps, or they can cause significant brain tissue injury, as in encephalopathies that accompany rabies and herpes simplex virus. Brain tissue injury may cause permanent neurologic deficits, therefore early diagnosis and management are essential if the patient is to have a favorable outcome.

Genitourinary System

Indwelling catheters are a major source of infection, especially among older adults. Decreased renal function, loss of muscle strength for urination, bladder obstruction, and lack of sphincter control are factors that often necessitate placement of an indwelling catheter. You should suspect infection when the patient has fever, chills, dysuria, back pain, difficulty voiding, an unusual color or odor of urine, or hematuria.

Integumentary System

The skin serves as a barrier to pathogens, ultraviolet radiation, and loss of body fluids. It also helps regulate body temperature and maintain an internal homeostatic environment.

Wounds such as burns and even IV punctures can predispose a person to skin infection by breaking the continuity of the skin structures and allowing a portal for infection. Local infection such as cellulitis is easily recognized and treated. Signs of infection include redness, tenderness, warmth, drainage, and induration. Infection also makes skin vulnerable to parasites such as scabies and lice, which can be diagnosed on the basis of a visual inspection and the patient's report of intense itching, especially at night.

Common Infectious Diseases

Meningitis

Meningitis is an inflammation of the membranes that cover the brain and spinal cord. Two types of meningitis are distinguished: viral and bacterial. Meningitis is a droplet-transmitted disease. The most common bacterial organisms associated with meningitis are *Neisseria meningitidis*, *Haemophilus influenzae* type b (Hib), and *Streptococcus pneumoniae*. Viral and bacterial meningitis occur worldwide. More than 90% of meningitis cases have a viral etiology. The highest incidence of viral meningitis is in the first year of life. Bacterial meningitis from Hib and *S. pneumoniae* can be prevented by vaccination. The incidence of bacterial meningitis has greatly diminished since immunization programs have been initiated.

The common bacterial organisms are discussed in detail as follows:

Neisseria meningitidis (Meningococcal Meningitis)

Neisseria meningitidis is a gram-negative organism that is part of the normal flora of the nasopharynx in many people. In certain circumstances, such as weakened host resistance, the bacteria enter the bloodstream and gain access to the CNS, including the meninges, causing meningococcal meningitis. Meningococcal meningitis is seasonal and tends to occur in the early spring and fall and occurs worldwide, especially in sub-Saharan Africa. Globally, meningococcal meningitis is fatal in 50% of the cases if it is untreated. Each year in the United States, 2,500 to 3,500 cases of *N. meningitidis* infection are diagnosed, 10% to 14% of which are fatal. Those at increased risk of contracting meningococcal meningitis include infants and young children, refugees living in crowded or unsanitary conditions, military recruits, college freshmen living in a dormitory for the first time, high school students, and the household contacts of those who have the illness.

Pathophysiology Transmission of meningococcal meningitis occurs by direct contact with droplets from the oronasal secretions of an infected person. This pathogen is not passed by airborne transmission. It has five primary serotypes: A, B, C, Y, and W-135. Types A and C appear primarily in Asia and Africa.

Signs and Symptoms The classic symptom of meningococcal meningitis is a petechial rash that rapidly develops into purpura, accompanied by high fever, headache, and meningismus (**Figure 8-4**). Leg pain, cold hands and feet, and pallor may indicate that the condition has progressed to septic shock. Neurologic symptoms of meningococcal meningitis, which can occur within 48 hours of the onset of the illness, include mental status changes, seizures, and coma. Ask the patient or his or her family about vaccination status. Check for evidence of an earlier infection, such as aches, rash, and flulike symptoms.

Differential Diagnosis Gram stain analysis of cerebrospinal fluid (CSF) is diagnostic and should be available in less than 30 minutes. A culture of CSF takes 24 to 72 hours.

Treatment Antibiotics are administered to patients infected with *N. meningitidis*. Third-generation cephalosporins, such as cefotaxime (Claforan) and ceftriaxone (Rocephin), are tried initially. Strains resistant to ciprofloxacin (Cipro and Ciloxan) have been documented in several states in the United States. Some strains of *Neisseria* are susceptible to penicillin G (Bicillin and Wycillin).

Prevention Vaccination is recommended for people in high-risk groups: children aged 2–18, first-year college students living in a dormitory, and military recruits. Postexposure treatment consists of either oral rifampin for 2 days or one dose of oral ciprofloxacin. Prophylaxis should be started within 24 hours of the exposure. The sub-Saharan African region known as the "meningitis belt" has seen a decrease in size and frequency of epidemics since vaccination has been initiated.

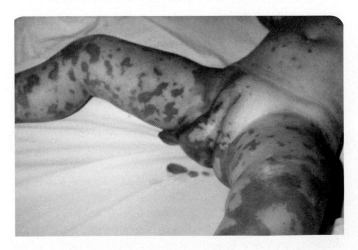

Figure 8-4 Purpura in a child with meningococcal sepsis.
Courtesy of Ronald Dieckmann, MD

Haemophilus influenzae Type B Meningitis

H. influenzae appears to be an exclusively human pathogen. In infants and young children, Hib causes bacteremia, pneumonia, acute bacterial meningitis, and sometimes cellulitis, osteomyelitis, epiglottitis, and joint infections. Before 1985 when a vaccine became available, 1 in 200 children was believed to have had Hib meningitis by 2 months of age. The worldwide incidence of Hib was 2 million cases annually, resulting in 300,000 deaths. As of 2013, immunization programs are now available in 189 countries. Countries with Hib immunization have had a significant decrease in incidence and mortality.

Pathophysiology The incubation period for Hib meningitis is unknown, but it may be about 2 to 4 days.

Signs and Symptoms The signs and symptoms of Hib meningitis are similar to those of other types of meningitis as follows:

- Fever
- Severe headache
- Irritability and crying (common in babies and young children)
- Bulging fontanelles
- Stiff neck (not as common in babies and young children)
- Photophobia (not as common in infants and young children)
- Tiredness, drowsiness, or difficulty waking up
- Vomiting
- Refusing food and drink
- Convulsions or seizures
- Loss of consciousness

Hib epiglottitis, a dangerous infection that may accompany meningitis, causes noisy, labored breathing and is often misdiagnosed as croup in children between the ages of 6 and 8 years. Up to 50% of patients who have meningitis may have long-term neurologic involvement.

Differential Diagnosis Laboratory confirmation of Hib meningitis is made by isolating the organism in a culture of blood or CSF.

Treatment Support oxygenation and administer IV drugs to control seizure activity or treat shock if present. Antibiotics should be administered intravenously as early as possible.

Prevention Children are immunized against Hib in a series, beginning at 2 months of age. Doses are given at 2, 4, and 6 months, followed by another dose at age 12 to 15 months, depending on the vaccine used. When you are treating a child suspected of having bacterial meningitis, use good hand-washing practices. No postexposure treatment is needed or recommended for adults.

Streptococcus pneumoniae (Pneumococcal Meningitis)

Streptococcus pneumoniae (often called *pneumococcus*) is a bacterium that can be cultured from the nasopharynx of most healthy people. The presence of pneumococcus in the nasopharynx is referred to as *carriage*. Most people have been carriers of *S. pneumoniae* at some point in their lives. Carriage is more common in young children and generally causes no illness.

Worldwide, *S. pneumoniae* is the most common cause of bacterial meningitis, community-acquired pneumonia, bacteremia, and otitis media. More than 90 serotypes of *S. pneumoniae* have been identified. Globally, in 2000, an estimated 14.5 million incidences of serious pneumococcal disease occurred in children younger than 5 years, resulting in about 826,000 deaths. Certain populations in the United States, including Alaska Natives, have high rates of pneumococcal disease.

Pathophysiology *S. pneumoniae* is an exclusively human pathogen spread from person to person by respiratory droplet transmission. Carriers of *S. pneumoniae*, while generally healthy themselves, often infect others. *S. pneumoniae* sometimes causes disease by spreading from the nasopharynx of a colonized person to other parts of the body, such as the middle ear (otitis media), nasal sinuses (sinusitis), and lungs. Meningitis is the result when the bacteria colonize the brain and spinal cord. If the bacteria reach the bloodstream, bacteremia may result.

Signs and Symptoms Signs and symptoms of pneumococcal meningitis may include difficulty breathing, abnormal breath sounds, fever, irritability, and ear infection.

Differential Diagnosis Sensitive, rapid diagnostic tests are not available for most types of pneumococcal infection, although a new urinary antigen test may be useful in adults. Sputum culture can be performed, but a Gram stain is the quickest way to diagnosis the infection.

Treatment Penicillins, cephalosporin, and macrolides (e.g., azithromycin) are the first-choice antibiotics for treating pneumococcal infection, but many strains of pneumococcal bacteria resist commonly prescribed antibiotics.

Prevention When you are treating a patient suspected of having pneumococcal meningitis, place a mask on the patient or wear a surgical mask. Observe standard precautions, including good hand-washing practices. At this time, three pneumococcal conjugate vaccines are marketed internationally. These vaccinations are indicated to prevent pneumococcal disease that may present as meningitis, pneumonia, or septicemia. These vaccines cover 7, 10, and 13 serotypes (PCV7, 10, and 13) and an unconjugated polysaccharide vaccine covers 23 serotypes (PPV23). The 23-valent vaccine is primarily designed for use in older children and adults who are at high risk for pneumococcal disease. It is not licensed for use in children younger than 2 years. The polyvalent pneumococcal polysaccharide (PPS) vaccine used today for older children and adults is 23 valent—that is, it is effective against 23 types of pneumococci. Consequently, it protects against 85% to 90% of the strains of pneumococcus that cause serious infection. Adults aged 65 and older and those younger than 65 who have a chronic illness should receive the PPS 23-valent (PPSV23) vaccine.

For infants, the pneumococcal conjugate 7-valent (PCV7) vaccine (Prevnar) is given as a series of four vaccinations at 2, 4, 6, and 12 to 15 months of age.

The viral form of meningitis is described in detail in the following sections.

Pathophysiology Viral meningitis is a common and relatively mild illness spread by direct contact with infected feces or nose and throat secretions. The incubation period is 2 to 10 days. The virus spreads most rapidly among young children and among those in group living situations. It usually strikes in the summer and early autumn. High schools and colleges are common sites of seasonal outbreaks. Most children and adults recover completely from viral meningitis within 10 to 14 days. Anyone can contract the disease, but most people older than age 40 have developed immunity to it.

Signs and Symptoms Signs and symptoms include the sudden onset of a headache, sensitivity to light, fever, stiff neck, and vomiting. Some strains of viral meningitis cause a rash, which may cover most of the body or just the arms and legs. The rash is red and mostly flat, although it may be raised in some areas. It is not the same as the rash seen in meningococcal meningitis, which is characterized by small, bright-red pinpoint spots covering most of the body.

The clinical presentation of viral meningitis can seem benign. Patients typically have fever, headache, and nausea and vomiting. Photophobia and nuchal rigidity are less common and are not definitive signs of CNS infection. Alterations in mentation indicate the need for emergent intervention and stabilization. You must identify increased intracranial pressure and signs of seizure activity early in the assessment process. Monitor the patient continually for seizures, disseminated intravascular coagulation, arrhythmias, and increased intracranial pressure.

Differential Diagnosis A recent history of travel may point to a specific cause. Patients who have headaches that worsen when they lean forward, sneeze, or cough may have increased intracranial pressure.

A thorough neurologic exam, including cranial nerves, is also performed. Bacteria that form neurotoxins, such as *Staphylococcus* and *Streptococcus*, can cause changes in mentation similar to those observed in patients with viral meningitis, so they must be included in your differential diagnosis. In addition, inflammation of the meninges can also be caused by fungi such as *Candida albicans* and *Cryptococcus neoformans* and by tumors and subarachnoid hemorrhage.

Blood and CSF cultures must be drawn to distinguish viral from bacterial or fungal causes. A cloudy appearance of the CSF indicates an increased white blood cell (WBC) count. The presence of a large concentration of WBCs in the CSF points to bacterial meningitis or a cerebral abscess. Gram stain analysis can identify the causative organism and allow antibiotic therapy to be targeted more precisely.

Before a spinal tap is performed, the plasma glucose level is determined. This level is a diagnostic clue because when the number of bacteria in the CSF cells rises, more glucose is utilized during cell metabolism. A low CSF glucose level (< 60% mg/dL [< 3.3 mmol/L] of blood glucose) suggests meningitis. In addition, diagnostic studies such as an electroencephalogram, computed tomography scan, or magnetic resonance imaging study may provide valuable diagnostic information about potentially serious complications.

Treatment Identifying underlying treatable causes of the meningitis improves outcomes. The earlier you can pinpoint such conditions, the sooner effective management strategies can be initiated. Stabilizing airway, breathing, and circulation and obtaining a thorough history and conducting a physical exam are the keys to identifying any latent disease process that may be causing the meningitis.

Antimicrobial medications such as antibiotics, antifungals, and antivirals usually offer definitive treatment. Supportive therapy includes ensuring adequate hydration and administering antipyretics and analgesics. If seizure activity is present, initiate anticonvulsant therapy. Observe local protocol regarding notifying the public health department in order to assist in early identification of any uptick in the incidence of meningitis in the area. In severe cases, the patient may require rehabilitation and physical therapy during recovery from the illness.

Prevention Prevention through vaccination is the ideal way to prevent meningitis. Follow standard precautions, including practicing scrupulous hand hygiene. Use proper PPE when treating a patient suspected of having viral meningitis.

Tuberculosis

Tuberculosis (TB) is caused by the bacterium *Mycobacterium tuberculosis*. TB has plagued humankind for centuries and remains a second leading cause of death from an infectious agent throughout the world. Historically, the incidence of the disease has surged every 30 or 40 years. In 2013, 1.5 million people died of TB and 9 million became ill with the disease. WHO has published a plan, the Stop TB Global Strategy, to reduce the worldwide incidence of TB. TB rates are highest in Africa and Southeast Asia. Between 1990 and 2013, the TB death rate dropped 45%.

In discussing the illness, a distinction must be made between TB infection and TB disease. *TB infection* or latent TB means only that exposure to TB has occurred. The exposed person does not have active disease, and it may never develop. Nearly one-third of the world's population is estimated to have latent TB. People with TB infection do not pose a threat to others. Depending on the exposure, nature of infection, and drug-resistant profile, individuals may be prescribed one medication, such as isoniazid or multidrug regimens, such as isoniazid and rifampin. *TB disease* refers to active TB illness verified by laboratory testing and a positive chest radiograph. Patients with active TB disease will be prescribed several medications. Individuals with compromised immune symptoms are at highest risk for the development of active TB.

Drug-resistant tuberculosis includes the following types:

- *Multidrug-resistant tuberculosis.* Multidrug-resistant tuberculosis (MDR-TB) was first identified in the United States in 1985, and it continues to occur in small numbers. In MDR-TB, *M. tuberculosis* is resistant to two of the first-line oral medications used to treat the illness. MDR-TB is a treatable disease because many other oral medications, including isoniazid and rifampin, are effective against the bacterium. MDR-TB is no more easily communicable than non–drug-resistant TB.

Resistance to medications used to treat TB is either primary or acquired. Acquired resistance is more common and occurs in patients who have undergone prior TB treatment. These are called *retreatment cases*. Primary resistance occurs when a patient is resistant to medications used to treat TB without having had any previous exposure to them.

In 2013, an estimated 480,000 people developed MDR-TB. Greater than 50% of these cases were in India, China, and the Russian Federation.

In an effort to reduce the incidence of MDR-TB, the United States and WHO are instituting direct observed therapy, a strategy intended to ensure full compliance with drug therapy. In this instance, the healthcare provider watches the patient ingest the medication. In some cases, the patient may be required to come to a clinic on a daily basis for drug administration. In assisted living environments, providers witness and document ingestion of the medications. In the United States, this program is overseen by local public health departments.

- *Extensively drug-resistant TB (XDR-TB).* In 2006, another emerging global problem was identified in KwaZulu-Natal, South Africa. In extensively drug-resistant TB (XDR-TB), *M. tuberculosis* is resistant to isoniazid, rifampin, and at least three of the six main classes of second-line drugs (aminoglycosides, polypeptides, fluoroquinolones, thioamides, cycloserine, and para-aminosalicylic acid).

XDR-TB is not more communicable than TB or MDR-TB, and it is treatable in this country. XDR-TB is seen in immunocompromised hosts, especially patients who are HIV positive, and carries nearly a 100% mortality rate in those patients because of the lack of treatment options. The prevalence of XDR-TB is lower than that of MDR-TB, but for the first time, XDR-TB is being reported by WHO. The majority of the countries in the world have reported at least one case of XCR-TB as of 2011.

Pathophysiology

Tuberculosis is not a highly contagious disease. Transmission occurs by passage of airborne particles when a person with active, untreated disease coughs. In general, such exposure occurs among people who have continuous intimate exposure to the infected individual, chiefly those living in the same household. For the healthcare provider working in the field, such intense exposure is likely to occur only if mouth-to-mouth ventilation is given to a patient with active untreated TB. Ten percent of people no longer have communicable disease after 2 days of treatment with new medications. The rest of the patients are no longer communicable after 14 days of treatment even though they continue taking medication for 12 months. The incubation period for TB is 4 to 12 weeks. There are three types of TB: atypical and extrapulmonary (TB of the bone, kidney, or lymph glands, for example), which are not communicable, and typical, which is communicable.

Signs and Symptoms

Signs and symptoms of TB disease (including the drug-resistant types) include a persistent cough for 2 to 3 weeks, night sweats, headache, weight loss, hemoptysis, and chest pain. If the patient has signs and symptoms of TB, ask about a history of TB treatment and check the patient's breath sounds. Oxygen administration may be necessary. Place a surgical mask on the patient for transport. Check the patient's medications; if the patient has been receiving treatment, the infection may no longer be communicable.

Differential Diagnosis

The Mantoux skin test is the most common screening done to determine exposure to TB. Induration of less than 5 mm is regarded as negative to exposure. Sputum cultures and chest radiographs are indicated if the test is positive.

TB testing for healthcare providers depends on risk assessment in the workplace. If a given place of employment has not had contact with three or more patients with active untreated TB during the previous year, annual testing is to be discontinued. Testing is then carried out only on newly hired employees and in healthcare providers known to have been exposed to TB. However, in emergency care settings, annual testing is often mandated.

Treatment

Patients with TB may need supplemental oxygen when oxygen saturation levels are diminished and there are signs of dyspnea. Initial treatment with antimycobacterial drugs such as isoniazid and rifampin are indicated. Patient isolation should be implemented for infectious patients. It is estimated 37 million lives have been saved between 2000 and 2013 by TB diagnosis and treatment.

Prevention

Place a surgical mask on the patient. If one is not available or the patient cannot be masked, mask yourself. During transport, an N95 respirator may be worn but is not required, since vehicles have rapid air exchange systems and exhaust fans, and transport times are generally short. If preventive measures were not taken, exposure to the provider may have occurred. Given that the incubation period for TB is 4 to 12 weeks, a provider who suspects he or she has been exposed to TB should assess the need for baseline testing and then be retested in 8 to 10 weeks.

No special cleaning methods or solutions are required, and no airing of the vehicle is necessary after transporting a patient suspected of having active TB.

Pneumonia

Each year more than 60,000 people in the United States die of pneumonia, which is an inflammation of the lungs. The disease is discussed in detail in Chapter 2. The cause of pneumonia may be bacteria, viruses, fungi, or other organisms. More than 50 types of pneumonia have been identified, ranging from mild to life-threatening. Cases caused by *Staphylococcus* or *Streptococcus* may be communicable and would be transmitted via respiratory secretions. Any risk of exposure may be reduced by placing a mask on the patient or yourself.

A severe form of pneumonia, severe acute respiratory syndrome coronavirus (SARS-CoV), had a brief and puzzling history. It was first identified in 2003. From its point of origin somewhere in China, an outbreak of this new virus swept through Asia and quickly made its way around the world. The virus vanished, however, almost as quickly as it had appeared. Panicky predictions of global calamity failed to materialize, and not a single case of SARS has been reported since 2003.

During its brief appearance, the disease was spread through close person-to-person contact by means of large-particle respiratory droplets. The virus was also spread by contact with contaminated surfaces.

Respiratory Syncytial Virus

Respiratory syncytial virus (RSV) is the leading cause of lower respiratory tract infections in infants, older people, and immunocompromised people. Although RSV is also covered in Chapter 2, its importance merits further discussion here. The virus spreads in the hospital environment and in the community. In the community setting, outbreaks generally occur in the late fall, winter, and early spring. In countries near the equator, the virus is present year-round. Globally, 30 million children younger than 5 years present each year with new acute lower respiratory infection due to RSV. Severe RSV results in more than 3.4 million hospitalizations each year. Information suggests the majority of deaths associated with RSV (> 90%) occur in low- and middle-income countries.

Most healthy adults recover from respiratory syncytial virus infection in 1 to 2 weeks. In the United States, RSV is the most common cause of bronchiolitis (inflammation of the small airways in the lungs) and pneumonia in children younger than 1 year.

Pathophysiology

Transmission of respiratory syncytial virus occurs by airborne droplets or by contact with contaminated surfaces. The portal of entry is usually the eyes, nose, or mouth. Respiratory syncytial virus is a large-particle virus that travels only about 3 feet. It may have a limited range, but it compensates by surviving well on fomites; for example, virus can be cultured more than 5 hours after it has transferred to an impervious surface such as a bed rail. The virus has an incubation period of 2 to 8 days.

Signs and Symptoms

Symptoms of respiratory syncytial virus include fever, sneezing, wheezing, cough, decreased appetite, and nasal congestion. Hypoxemia and apnea are common in infants with respiratory syncytial virus and constitute the primary reason for hospitalization. Patients suspected of having RSV should be assessed for a history of exposure to the virus with an evaluation of ventilation and breath sounds.

Differential Diagnosis

Testing is usually used during the respiratory syncytial virus season to help diagnose the illness in patients who have moderate to severe symptoms and lower respiratory tract involvement. Testing is ordered primarily on infants between ages 6 months and 2 years, elderly patients, and those with compromised immune systems, such as those with preexisting lung disease and recipients of organ transplants.

Treatment

Respiratory syncytial virus immune globulin intravenous is an FDA-approved treatment for prevention of lower respiratory tract infections in infants at high risk of contracting respiratory syncytial virus. Treatment is limited to the administration of beta-agonists, and supportive care may include administering oxygen, hydrating the patient, and providing suctioning, ventilation assistance, or intubation as necessary.

Prevention

Prevention requires following standard precautions, including frequent hand washing and cleaning contaminated surfaces.

Mononucleosis

Mononucleosis ("mono") is caused by the herpesvirus Epstein-Barr virus. Epstein-Barr virus is also suspected of causing a disease called *chronic fatigue syndrome*, which produces similar signs and symptoms, but the etiology of the syndrome has not been well established. The Epstein-Barr virus grows in the epithelium of the oropharynx and sheds into saliva, which explains why it is often referred to as the *kissing disease*.

Pathophysiology

Transmission occurs by direct contact with the saliva of an infected person. Cases of transmission have also been linked to transfusion of contaminated blood or blood products. The incubation period is 4 to 6 weeks. The period of communicability is prolonged, and pharyngeal shedding may persist for a year or more after infection.

Signs and Symptoms

Signs and symptoms include a sore throat, fever, pharyngeal secretions, and swollen lymph glands, with or without malaise, anorexia, headache, muscle pain, and an enlarged liver and spleen.

Differential Diagnosis

For patients with classic symptoms, a positive heterophile antibody test (monospot) is diagnostic, but this test may not become positive until the second or third week of illness. If the test is negative, and infectious mononucleosis strongly suspected, specific antibody testing for Epstein-Barr virus can be performed. DNA testing for Epstein-Barr virus is also available.

Treatment

Treatment is supportive in most cases. Antiviral agents may be prescribed for patients with compromised immune systems.

Prevention

When providers have the potential for direct contact with a patient's oral secretions, standard precautions should be followed, including the use of gloves and good hand-washing techniques. No special cleaning solution is required or recommended after transporting a patient suspected of having mononucleosis. No postexposure treatment is needed or recommended.

Influenza

Influenza (flu) viruses cause acute respiratory illnesses generally presenting as winter epidemics. In the United States, the flu causes approximately 36,000 deaths per year.

The H1N1 virus is a resurgence of an influenza A virus, with the highest concentration of cases occurring in Mexico. The illness spread from this suspected point of origin and was declared a pandemic by WHO in May 2009. However, WHO qualified this declaration by noting that the H1N1 pandemic has not been particularly severe. In fact, H1N1 has acted much like a normal seasonal flu virus, except that children, young adults, and pregnant women, rather than older adults, have been most vulnerable to the illness.

Pathophysiology

H1N1 is a large-particle virus passed by the droplet route. The incubation period is 1 to 7 days, and the illness is thought to be transmissible for up to 24 hours after fever has subsided.

Signs and Symptoms

Signs and symptoms initially resemble those of a regular seasonal flu, except that the patient also has diarrhea. Severe signs and symptoms include the following:

- In Children
  - Respiratory distress
  - Fever with rash
  - Low fluid intake
  - Bluish skin color
  - Irritability
  - Drowsiness and lethargy

- In Adults
  - Shortness of breath
  - Chest pain or pressure

- Dizziness
- Confusion
- Persistent vomiting

These signs and symptoms could lead to respiratory distress and the need for ventilatory assistance.

Differential Diagnosis

Specific serologic testing is used to determine infection. A rapid influenza diagnostic test may be ordered to detect the novel influenza A (H1N1).

Treatment

Treatment is supportive unless the patient shows signs of respiratory distress, in which case ventilation assistance may be needed. Be sure to obtain a travel history for all patients who have respiratory difficulties. Hospitalized patients will receive antiviral drug treatment (Tamiflu [oseltamivir] or Relenza [zanamivir]).

Prevention

If possible, place a surgical mask on the patient. If the patient is unable to tolerate a mask, you should wear one yourself. Currently, scientific data do not support the use of N95 respirators for droplet-transmitted infectious diseases. WHO guidelines for H1N1 patient care do not call for such equipment. Immunization is the key to slowing the spread of H1N1. Postexposure treatment with antivirals is not indicated.

Blood-Borne Diseases
Human Immunodeficiency Virus Infection and Acquired Immunodeficiency Syndrome

HIV, the virus that causes AIDS, was first identified in a human specimen in 1959. HIV is a double-stranded RNA **retrovirus** that attacks the immune system, which reduces the ability to fight off infection. Persons are generally considered able to transmit the HIV virus once they have tested HIV positive. However, some people who are HIV positive cannot transmit the virus because they have inherited a mutated gene (CCR5) that protects them either from developing active disease or from transmitting the virus. Such patients, called *nonprogressors*, make up about 10% of the HIV-positive Caucasian population and an unknown percentage of the nonwhite HIV-positive population. People exposed to HIV who have not inherited this mutation may develop AIDS.

Pathophysiology

A healthy person has 500 to 1,500 CD4 cells/mm³; CD4 cells are also called *T-helper cells*. These specialized lymphocytes are an important component of the body's cellular immune system.

A person's CD4 count is reduced during the first 6 weeks after HIV infection because of uncontrolled replication of the virus, called the *initial phase* of the disease process. The flulike condition associated with it is sometimes referred to as *acute retroviral syndrome*. This phase is followed by mobilization of a cellular and humoral response to the presence of the HIV virus. If the infection is left untreated, the number of CD4 cells declines. Seroconversion, meaning that antibodies can be detected in the blood, occurs, usually within the first 3 months following exposure.

AIDS is the end-stage disease process caused by HIV. A patient with AIDS is extremely vulnerable to numerous opportunistic infections that would not affect a person with an intact immune system. The incubation period of AIDS spans the time between documented infection (that is, becoming HIV positive) and development of end-stage disease, which is determined by the CD4 cell count and the presence of opportunistic infections.

Signs and Symptoms

HIV infection affects the entire body system—cardiovascular, respiratory, and musculoskeletal. Signs and symptoms of HIV/AIDS are summarized in Table 8-7.

Differential Diagnosis

Patients with HIV infection may be asymptomatic. In symptomatic patients, it should be differentiated from similar diseases that cause *fever*, fatigue (mononucleosis), and acute viral hepatitis. Consider a diagnosis of AIDS in all patients presenting with symptoms of *immunodeficiency* or opportunistic infections.

Treatment

Antiretroviral agents halt replication of the HIV virus and prevent damage to the immune system. These drugs are so effective that, during treatment, many individuals begin to test negative for the virus in their circulating blood. People who are HIV positive live as active members of their communities, participating fully in work and other aspects of normal life. Antiretroviral treatment, once started, must continue for the remainder of the patient's life. Every missed dose increases the risk that the drugs will become ineffective.

Antiretroviral drugs include Ziagen (abacavir), Videx (didanosine), Emtriva (emtricitabine), Epivir (lamivudine), Zerit (stavudine), and AZT (zidovudine). They may be prescribed individually, but combination medications pack two or three agents into a single pill. These compound agents include Combivir (lamivudine and zidovudine), Trizivir (abacavir sulfate, lamivudine, and zidovudine), Epzicom (abacavir and lamivudine), and Truvada (emtricitabine and tenofovir). Laboratory testing of viral load and CD4 cell count is essential in gauging how well the patient is responding to drug treatment.

Adverse drug reactions associated with antiretroviral agents may include headache, diarrhea, nausea, hypersensitivity reaction, and peripheral neuropathy (nerve damage). Because many of these symptoms are also symptoms of HIV disease itself, it

Table 8-7 Selected Signs and Symptoms of HIV/AIDS

General

- Enlarged lymph nodes, liver, spleen
- Vision loss, which may indicate cytomegalovirus infection of the retina
- Muscle wasting
- Weight loss

Neurologic

- Encephalopathy
- Peripheral neuropathy
- Increased intracranial pressure
- Behavioral changes
- Rapid eye movements
- Tremors or seizures

Respiratory

- Low oxygen saturation
- Signs of pneumonia, such as:
  - Difficulty breathing
  - Rapid respiration
  - Persistent cough
  - Chest pain
  - Coughing up blood

Cardiovascular

- Chest pain
- Pale, ashen skin

Integumentary

- Purplish lesions (Kaposi's sarcoma; **Figure 8-5**)
- Thrush (candidiasis of the mouth)
- Herpes lesions

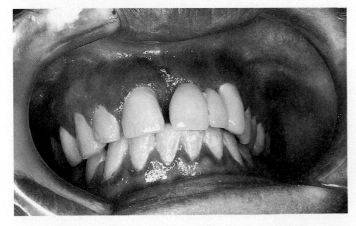

Figure 8-5 An HIV-infected patient with Kaposi's sarcoma.
© Scott Camazine/Alamy.

is important to assess when they began relative to the start of antiretroviral therapy.

Prevention

HIV cannot survive outside the human host. Transmission occurs primarily during sexual contact or inoculation of infected blood directly into the bloodstream of an uninfected person, as occurs when IV drug users share needles. To protect yourself from HIV infection, use gloves when you are in contact with a patient's nonintact skin, mucous membranes, blood, or other potentially infectious materials. Use needle-safe devices and wear eye, nose, and mouth protection when you intubate a patient or suction the airway.

Routine use of a mask is not necessary. Good hand washing, however, is an important part of risk reduction. If an exposure to a patient's blood occurs, the medical facility must perform rapid HIV testing on the source patient. Such testing produces results in less than 1 hour. Rapid testing is accurate, identifying proteins present during the beginning of the life cycle of the HIV virus.

The use of postexposure rapid HIV testing is encouraged (in the United States it is enforced by OSHA). If the source patient tests negative for HIV, no testing of the exposed provider is needed or recommended. If the source patient tests positive, the provider may be offered antiretroviral drugs as a preventive measure. However, because these agents have substantial side effects, such treatment is given only to patients who meet certain risk criteria. The exposed provider should be counseled regarding the risks and benefits of the treatment.

Hepatitis B Virus Infection

Hepatitis B is a global problem. It is estimated by the World Health Organization that 240 million people are infected with chronic hepatitis B. Transmission of hepatitis B virus (HBV) occurs primarily through exposure to blood and blood products, sexual contact, or perinatal exposure. Risk activities for HBV infection include IV drug use and multiple sexual contacts.

Pathophysiology

Needles, including those used for tattooing and acupuncture, and occasionally other objects, such as shared razors, have been implicated in the transmission of HBV. It is particularly common in IV drug users who share needles.

Limited data suggest that the HBV can survive outside the body in the medium of dried blood for as long as 7 days. The incubation period varies widely, from 30 to 200 days. The communicable period starts weeks before the first symptoms appear and may persist for years in chronic carriers. An estimated 2% to 10% of all HBV-infected people will become chronic carriers.

Signs and Symptoms

Signs and symptoms of HBV infection occur in two phases. During the first phase, the patient has flulike symptoms including fever, nausea, diarrhea, and abdominal pain. A large amount of virus is present in circulating blood. During the second phase, the patient's skin and eyes become jaundiced (**Figure 8-6**), the stools become whitish, and the urine becomes almost brown. The viral load drops, and antibodies appear in the blood. About 10% of those with HBV infection will become chronically infected, and the disease may progress to liver failure or liver cancer.

For both stages of infection, assessment is primarily visual but also depends on taking a thorough history. Ask the patient when symptoms began and the character and location of any pain.

Differential Diagnosis

Laboratory markers for HBV infection (HBcAg and HBeAg) may be present for 2 to 7 weeks before symptoms appear. The appearance of symptoms coincides with a rise in levels of alanine aminotransferase, bilirubin, and aspartate aminotransferase. These markers will decrease over about the next 6 months.

Treatment

Pharmacologic treatment is available for patients with chronic infection. Check the patient's medication list for interferon drugs, which may cause flulike symptoms, depression, and anxiety. Other drugs used for treatment, such as adefovir and tenofovir, may cause kidney dysfunction.

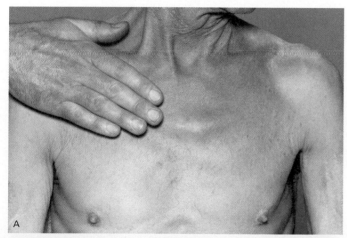

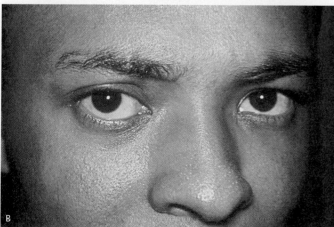

Figure 8-6 Signs of HBV infection. **A**. Jaundice. **B**. Scleral icterus.

A © SPL/Photo Researchers, Inc.; B Courtesy of Dr. Thomas F. Sellers/Emory University/CDC.

Prevention

Providers can protect themselves from HBV infection by following standard precautions when they must be in contact with blood or blood-tinged fluids. However, HBV vaccination is the primary method of protection for all people in the United States, where immunization is universal. Since 1991, all newborns have been vaccinated within 12 hours of birth. As of 2000, all middle school, high school, and college students were required to have been vaccinated before enrolling in school. Most healthcare personnel have been vaccinated since 1982. Recommendations for preventing and controlling hepatitis B can be obtained from the World Health Organization. The risk for and incidence of HBV has declined precipitously in the United States. Vaccination confers lifetime protection from the illness, so no booster or routine titer testing is required or recommended.

Hepatitis C Virus Infection

Hepatitis C virus (HCV) is the most common chronic blood-borne infection and the leading cause of liver transplantation in the United States. The virus was first identified in 1988. Testing became available in 1992. HCV is a single-stranded RNA virus that infects an estimated 1.5% of the U.S. population and 3% of the world population. The incidence has declined by 80% in the United States since 1990.

Pathophysiology

HCV transmission occurs through injection of contaminated blood, chiefly among IV drug users who share needles, but occasionally in the following other ways:

- Tattooing or body piercing
- Needlestick injury
- Organ transplantation
- Transfusion of blood or blood products
- Sexual contact

Transmission though mucous membrane or nonintact skin exposure is rare. The virus cannot survive in the environment long enough to pose a risk for any means of transmission except via blood-borne contact. The incubation period is 6 or 7 weeks but appears to be shorter when exposure occurs through transfusion.

Signs and Symptoms

Early signs and symptoms of HCV infection are the same as those for HBV infection, including fatigue, abdominal pain, and hepatomegaly (an enlarged liver). Check for fever. Only 20% of patients with HCV infection experience symptoms associated with the second phase of hepatitis: jaundice, whitish stools, and dark urine. Chronic infection develops in about 20% of these patients, and 30% become carriers of the illness.

Differential Diagnosis

Laboratory testing has improved in recent years (**Figure 8-7**). The blood tests that are now available include tests that screen for antibodies to HCV such as enzyme immunoassay (EIA) and enhanced chemiluminescence immunoassay (CIA). Other tests include qualitative tests that are able to detect the presence or absence of the virus (HCV RNA polymerase chain reaction [PCR]). Quantitative tests such as HCV RNA PCR also are used to detect the amount (titer) of virus present. Anti-HCV screening can identify HCV infection 4 to 10 weeks after infection. At 6 months after exposure, anti-HCV can be detected in more than 97% of infected individuals. PCR is able to detect HCV RNA in the blood as early as 2 to 3 weeks after infection. False-positive results do occur, and occur more often when low-risk individuals are tested, so it is important to follow-up in order to identify the presence of current infection.

Treatment

People found to be infected with HCV receive a 24-week course of medication. The administration of interferon A, often in combination with antiviral drugs, is a consideration for treatment.

Prevention

You can reduce your risk of contracting HCV by following standard precautions, including good hand-washing practices, when in contact with a patient's blood or other potentially infectious materials. Promptly report any exposure so that the source patient can be tested. If the source patient tests positive for HCV, you should have the following done:

- Perform a baseline testing for anti-HCV for the source.
- Perform a baseline test for the person exposed to an HCV-positive source, which includes anti-HCV and ALT activity baseline testing and follow-up testing at 4 to 6 months. Testing for HCV RNA may be performed at 4 to 6 weeks if earlier diagnosis of HCV infection is desired.
- To confirm a diagnosis, perform supplemental anti-HCV testing of all anti-HCV results reported as positive by enzyme immunoassay.

Currently, no medication can be given for postexposure prophylaxis, and no HCV vaccine has been developed. If you test positive for HCV at 4 weeks after exposure, a course of pegylated

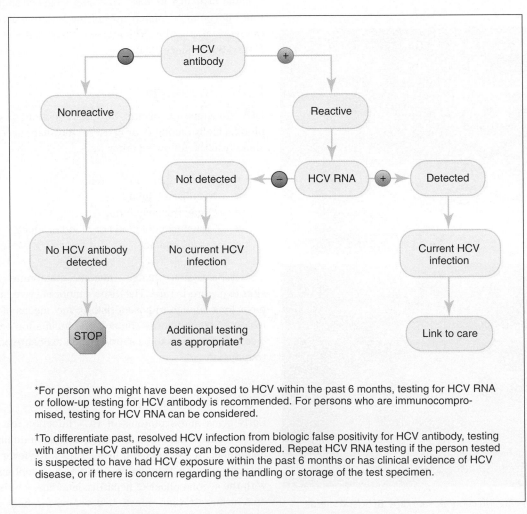

*For person who might have been exposed to HCV within the past 6 months, testing for HCV RNA or follow-up testing for HCV antibody is recommended. For persons who are immunocompromised, testing for HCV RNA can be considered.

†To differentiate past, resolved HCV infection from biologic false positivity for HCV antibody, testing with another HCV antibody assay can be considered. Repeat HCV RNA testing if the person tested is suspected to have had HCV exposure within the past 6 months or has clinical evidence of HCV disease, or if there is concern regarding the handling or storage of the test specimen.

Figure 8-7 Recommended testing sequence for identifying current hepatitis C virus infection.

interferon plus ribavirin (Pegasys) will clear the blood of the virus. Additional medications are currently being utilized, but according to the CDC, "the optimal treatment regimen and when it should be initiated remains uncertain."

Hepatitis D Virus Infection

Hepatitis D virus (HDV), or delta agent, was first identified in 1977. HDV requires that the host be infected with HBV for HDV infection to occur. Consequently, it is often referred to as a *parasite of HBV*. This virus is most often seen in IV drug users, but the HDV infection rate is decreasing in countries using the vaccination against HBV.

Pathophysiology

Transmission occurs by percutaneous exposure and, in addition, inefficient transmission occurs by sexual contact. The incubation period for this disease is 30 to 180 days. Blood is considered to be infectious during all phases of the illness.

Signs and Symptoms

Assess the patient for signs and symptoms of HBV infection, which include fever, abdominal pain, nausea, and vomiting. Often, behavioral factors such as anorexia can occur.

Differential Diagnosis

Serologic studies are done to evaluate the presence of the HDV antigen and HDV IgM antibody as a sign of active infection. The HDV has two properties, which are both hepatitis D antigens. These antigens are identified early in the infectious process and are involved in inhibiting the replication of the virus.

Treatment

Treatment consists of supportive care, because research does not support the use of antiviral medications for HDV.

Prevention

HDV can be prevented with vaccination against HBV. Always follow standard precautions, including good hand-washing practices, when in direct contact with a patient's blood or other potentially infectious materials.

Enteric (Intestinal) Diseases

Norovirus

Gastroenteritis may be caused by bacterial or viral pathogens, parasites, chemical toxins, allergies, or immune disorders. The inflammation may cause hemorrhage and erosion of the mucosal layers of the gastrointestinal (GI) tract, affecting absorption of water and nutrients.

What is typically called *acute gastroenteritis*, or a *stomach flu*, is a viral infection of the stomach and intestines, leading to abdominal cramping, vomiting, and diarrhea. Noroviruses are the most common cause of acute gastroenteritis, with strains causing symptoms for 1 to 3 days. The most important treatment is maintenance of hydration.

Norovirus is an international problem and is extremely contagious. Outbreaks are common in semiconfined communities such as schools, cruise ships, nursing homes, hospitals, hotels, and restaurants.

Pathophysiology

Norovirus, or Norwalk-like virus, also known as "winter vomiting disease," is caused by nonenveloped, single-stranded RNA viruses of the genus *Norovirus*. When *Norovirus* enters the body, it begins to multiply in the small intestines. The norovirus incubation period is 12–48 hours and can be transmitted from infected persons, contaminated food or water, or by touching contaminated surfaces. The virus can be shed for weeks after infection.

Signs and Symptoms

Patients will present with gastrointestinal complaints including abdominal pain, vomiting, projectile vomiting, diarrhea, and fever. Symptoms usually last 1 to 2 days, and then patients recover fully. Norovirus can be devastating for young children and the elderly.

Differential Diagnosis

A diagnosis is made by the patient's signs and symptoms, obtaining a thorough patient history, and culturing a stool sample.

Treatment

Care is supportive and aimed at oral or intravenous rehydration. Antimotility agents are not recommended in children younger than 3 years. In older children and adults, antimotility and antiemetic agents may be useful in rehydration. Antibiotics are not useful in treating gastroenteritis caused by Norovirus. Vaccines for norovirus are not available. Individuals can contract norovirus multiple times in their lifetime.

Prevention

Following standard precautions, including good hand-washing practices, can reduce the risk of contracting norovirus. Ensure that the water supply is safe and that appropriate facilities are available for disposal of feces. Rooms, vehicles, and equipment must be cleaned thoroughly per local protocols. The CDC indicates a high concentration of domestic bleach (5–25 tablespoons bleach per gallon of water) may be used for disinfection. Soiled articles of clothing should be washed at the maximum available cycle length and machine-dried at high heat. In semiclosed environments such as cruise ships, patients may be isolated to prevent spread of the disease.

Hepatitis A Virus Infection

Hepatitis A virus (HAV), known as "infectious hepatitis," is the most common type of hepatitis in the United States. HAV is a single-stranded RNA virus found in the feces of infected people. This virus replicates in the liver, but it usually does not directly damage the liver. Infection with HAV is often described as a benign disease because acquiring it provides lifelong immunity to it.

Infection rates in the United States have declined about 90% since a vaccine for HAV became available in 1995. In 2008, 2,585 cases were reported in the United States, the lowest rate ever reported in this country. HAV is present throughout the world, although the incidence is not well tracked.

Pathophysiology

Transmission of HAV occurs by the fecal–oral route. HAV colonizes the GI tract and is detectable in the blood 4 weeks before symptoms occur. The incubation period is 2 to 4 weeks. The communicable period starts toward the end of the incubation period and continues for a few days after the patient becomes jaundiced.

Signs and Symptoms

Patients with HAV may initially have malaise, fatigue, anorexia, nausea, vomiting, diarrhea, fever, or abdominal discomfort. Signs and symptoms during the second phase of the illness are the same as those for any type of hepatitis: jaundice, dark urine, and whitish stools.

Differential Diagnosis

To help refine your diagnosis, ask the patient about any recent travel outside the United States, and inquire about possible dietary intake of contaminated water or food, such as raw shellfish. Laboratory tests can detect the presence of anti-HAV and immunoglobulin M (IgM) antibodies within 3 weeks of exposure.

Treatment

Treatment is supportive and centers on providing good nutrition and administering IV fluids.

Prevention

Follow standard precautions, including good hand-washing practices, when you are in direct contact with a patient's stool. HAV vaccination is recommended for Federal Emergency Management Agency response team members who may work outside the United States, but not for any other healthcare provider groups.

Hepatitis E Virus Infection

Hepatitis E virus (HEV), which is often termed *enterically transmitted non-A, non-B hepatitis*, is a small RNA virus that multiplies in the liver cells and in peripheral blood mononuclear cells. Four genotypes have been identified—two involve human viruses and two are zoonotic. This virus is the leading cause of hepatitis in developing countries and elsewhere in the world, including Russia, South Asia, Africa, Mexico, and Central America.

Pathophysiology

HEV infection is strongly associated with floods and poor sanitation and hygiene and is extremely rare in the United States. Transmission usually occurs via the fecal–oral route by ingestion of contaminated water. In developing countries, rare cases of

transmission via blood transfusion have been documented; sexual transmission has also been documented.

The disease is not chronic, and the incubation period is 2 to 9 weeks. The communicability period is believed to be the same as that for HAV infection.

Signs and Symptoms

Signs and symptoms of HEV infection are the same as those for other forms of hepatitis.

Differential Diagnosis

When you are assessing a patient suspected of having HEV, begin by asking about country of origin and travel history. In low-prevalence areas, test for HEV-specific immunoglobulin M (IgM) to indicate infection.

Treatment

Evaluate the patient for abdominal pain or tenderness, fever, nausea, and malaise. Treatment of HEV is limited to supportive care.

Prevention

Observe standard precautions and use good hand-washing practices when you are in direct contact with a patient's stool.

Escherichia coli Infection

Although most strains of *Escherichia coli (E. coli)* are harmless, some strains cause food-borne illnesses. *E. coli* has been recognized as a major cause of colonization and infection in cattle, which can contaminate food. The first serious outbreak caused by the O157:H7 subtype occurred in a fast-food restaurant in Washington State in 1993. Epidemiologists estimate that this bacterium is the cause of more than 75,000 cases of illness each year, resulting in more than 3,000 hospital stays and 60 deaths. Illness occurs mostly in young children and in older adults. The disease is a problem worldwide, although it is not well tracked in developing countries and therefore data on incidence are limited.

Pathophysiology

E. coli is a gram-negative bacterium belonging to the Enterobacteriaceae family. More than 30 serotypes of *E. coli* have been identified. Of these, *E. coli* O157:H7 has been the most notable in recent years for being found in improperly cooked meat, municipal water supplies, milk, raw vegetables, unpasteurized apple cider, lettuce, and products contaminated by cattle waste. The organism has an incubation period of 1 to 9 days. The Shiga toxin–producing strain of *E. coli*—O157:H7—is one of the most potent toxins known to humans.

Signs and Symptoms

Infection with *E. coli* O157:H7 begins with abdominal pain and tenderness, myalgia, and headache. Vomiting may also occur, followed by hemorrhagic colitis, which causes visible blood in the stool. This stage may last 3 to 7 days and occurs mostly in people aged 65 or older. A grave complication of this illness is hemolytic uremic syndrome, a life-threatening condition that occurs in about 10% of those infected with *E. coli* O157:H7. As a result, hemolytic uremic syndrome is now recognized as the most common cause of acute kidney failure in infants and young children. Adolescents and adults are also susceptible, and older adults often succumb to the disease.

Differential Diagnosis

To refine your diagnosis, ask patients whether they might have eaten any uncooked or undercooked meat. Question the patient about the appearance of his or her stool. Watery, yellow-green, or bloody stool, or stool that contains pus is a clue to this illness. Check for signs of dehydration or shock. Diagnosis is made on the basis of a stool culture. Ninety percent of bloody stools culture positive for *E. coli* bacteria.

Treatment

Supportive treatment is offered because antibiotics have not been effective against the O157:H7 strain of *E. coli*. Transfusion may be indicated if the patient becomes severely anemic. Dialysis may be indicated for acute renal failure.

Prevention

The best prevention is education on hand washing, appropriate preparation of raw foods, the preparation of cooked foods, and proper storage of all foods. Standard precautions, including the use of gowns to protect clothing, are recommended. As always, follow thorough hand-washing practices. Rooms, vehicles, and care equipment must be cleaned thoroughly per local protocols.

Shigellosis

Shigellosis is a highly infectious acute bacterial enteritis that affects the large and small intestines. Only a small amount of bacteria—possibly as few as 10 to 100 organisms—is needed to cause infection. The disease is believed to be responsible for more than 600,000 deaths each year worldwide. Most infections and deaths occur in children younger than 10 years.

Pathophysiology

Shigella is a genus of gram-negative, non–spore-forming, rod-shaped bacteria closely related to *E. coli* and *Salmonella*. *Shigella* spp. are transmitted by the fecal–oral route. Failing to wash hands or not doing so properly after defecation is an easy way to spread this infection. The incubation period may be as brief as 12 hours but can extend to 96 hours. A person can harbor this disease for up to 4 weeks.

Signs and Symptoms

Shigella strains can produce three different enterotoxins, which have enterotoxic, cytotoxic, and neurotoxic effects. Patients infected with this illness have watery diarrhea, fever, vomiting, and cramps. Rehydration may be necessary. Convulsions are a

complication sometimes seen in young children. Illness lasts about 4 to 7 days. In mild infection, the only sign may be watery diarrhea. Other symptoms may include nausea, high fever, and abdominal tenderness and cramping.

Differential Diagnosis

Diagnosis is made by the patient's history, signs and symptoms, and culturing a stool sample.

Treatment

The patient will show improvement after 3 days of rehydration and antibiotic therapy.

Prevention

Following standard precautions, including good hand-washing practices, can reduce the risk of contracting shigellosis. Ensure that the water supply is safe and that appropriate facilities are available for disposal of feces. Chlorination of the water supply also reduces risk.

Sexually Transmitted Diseases

Gonorrhea

Gonorrhea is the second most commonly reported disease in the United States. Worldwide, more than 60 million cases are reported annually. Gonorrhea is caused by *Neisseria gonorrhoeae*, a spore-forming, gram-negative diplococcus bacterium.

Pathophysiology

Anorectal and oral gonorrhea are common. Perinatal transmission also occurs, but the primary mode of transmission is intimate sexual contact with an infected partner. The incubation period for *N. gonorrhoeae* ranges from 2 to 10 days. The infection is communicable for months if not treated. If treated, the disease is noncommunicable within hours.

Signs and Symptoms

Gonorrhea has a different clinical presentation in men than in women. In assessing a patient suspected of having gonorrhea, ask him or her about the presence of vaginal or urethral discharge or burning on urination.

Men In men, gonorrhea is localized to the penis (**Figure 8-8**). It causes discomfort and/or a thick white, yellow, or greenish discharge from the tip of the penis. Infection in men can spread to the prostate, seminal vesicles, testes, and bladder, perhaps leading to abscess, difficulty urinating, and swollen testicles.

Women More than 50% of women infected with gonorrhea have no symptoms, especially in the early stages of infection. Symptoms include burning or frequent urination, a yellowish vaginal discharge, redness and swelling of the genitals, and vaginal burning or itching. If untreated, gonorrhea can cause a severe

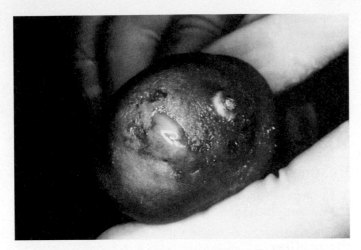

Figure 8-8 Male with a purulent penile discharge from gonorrhea and an overlying penile pyodermal lesion. Pyoderma involves the formation of a purulent skin lesion, as in this case located on the glans penis and overlying the sexually transmitted disease, gonorrhea.

Courtesy of Joe Miller/CDC.

pelvic infection, with inflammation of the fallopian tubes and ovaries. Gonorrheal infection of the fallopian tubes can lead, in turn, to a dangerous, painful infection of the pelvis known as "pelvic inflammatory disease." Pelvic inflammatory disease may cause a puslike discharge from the vagina. To assess for pelvic infection, evaluate the patient for abdominal pain or tenderness.

Differential Diagnosis

Diagnosis is made by testing drainage from the site. In men, a Gram stain of urethral drainage may also be performed to screen for the disease.

Treatment

In uncomplicated cases, oral cefixime (Suprax) is prescribed, or ceftriaxone (Rocephin) intramuscular is given in a single dose.

Prevention

Follow standard precautions, including good hand-washing practices, when in contact with drainage or lesions. No special cleaning is needed for vehicles or equipment. For patients, partner notification is essential. Educate patients about the disease and its prevention, including the use of condoms.

Syphilis

Syphilis is a worldwide problem. In 2008, WHO reported an estimated 36 million people are infected with syphilis at any one time. Internationally, the incidence of the disease has been increasing. The disease tends to strike young people aged 20 to 35, with an especially high prevalence in urban areas. In May 2006, the CDC published guidelines with the goal of eliminating syphilis in the United States by 2015, using evidence-based practices and targeted

surveillance activities. This goal has not been achieved, with the number of cases actually increasing by 10.9%. In 2013, 75% of the cases reported occurred in men who had sex with men. Many people infected with HIV or HCV are also infected with syphilis.

Pathophysiology

Syphilis is caused by the spiral-shaped bacterium *Treponema pallidum*. Because the disease progresses in three stages, infection is considered to be either acute or chronic. Transmission generally occurs by direct contact, such as sexual contact, with the draining primary lesion(s). Syphilis can also be transmitted across the placenta from an infected mother to her fetus. In some cases, transmission has occurred by blood transfusion. The incubation period of *T. pallidum* is 10 days to 3 months. The communicable period is variable and has not been well established.

Signs and Symptoms

Initial infection with syphilis produces a chancre, a painless ulcerative lesion of the skin or mucous membranes at the site of infection (**Figure 8-9**). The site of infection is usually the genital region,

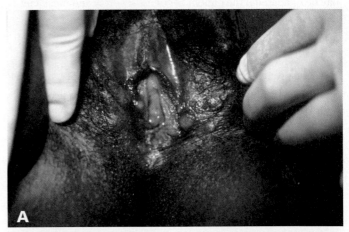

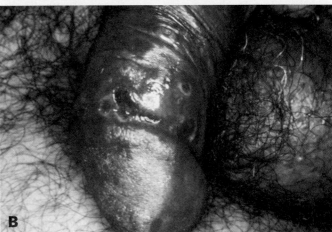

Figure 8-9 A chancre is a painless ulceration that arises at the site of syphilis infection, such as the rectum or genitals. **A.** It often appears on the vulva or vagina in women. **B.** It appears on the penis in men. This small round lesion heralds the primary stage of the disease.

A Dr. Ken Greer/Visuals Unlimited, Inc.; B © Dr. Gavin Hart/Dr. N. J. Fiumara/CDC.

so suspected syphilis may not be noted during routine physical assessment. Tertiary signs and symptoms of syphilis include:

- Rash
- Patchy hair loss
- Swollen lymph glands
- Cardiac, ophthalmic, auditory, or CNS complications
- Lesions of the tissues or bone

If signs and symptoms are observed, question the patient regarding high-risk sexual activities.

Differential Diagnosis

A diagnosis of syphilis is confirmed by performing a rapid plasma reagin test or the classic Venereal Disease Research Laboratory test.

Treatment

Routine treatment for syphilis includes administration of penicillin G. If the patient is pregnant, a second dose should be given 1 week later. If the patient is allergic to penicillin, give oral doxycycline or oral tetracycline, prescribed daily for 28 days.

Prevention

Observe standard precautions, including good hand-washing practices. No special cleaning precautions are needed or recommended. If you sustain a needlestick injury with a contaminated needle, follow exposure guidelines. The source patient should be tested if an actual exposure occurred. People who receive syphilis treatment must abstain from sexual contact with new partners until the lesions have healed completely. Sexual partners must be notified so they can be tested for the infection.

Genital Herpes

Genital herpes is a common illness produced by infection with the herpes simplex virus. The virus is further classified as type 1 or type 2. All sexually active persons are at risk for this infection. Cases of genital herpes do not have to be reported to the CDC, so data on incidence are not available.

Pathophysiology

Type 1 (HSV-1) is usually referred to as *oral herpes*, *cold sores*, or *fever blisters*. Herpes type 1 infection is usually activated from a dormant status by stress and febrile illness and causes a blister-like sore on the lips or inside the mouth. In children aged 6 months to 5 years, HSV-1 appears as herpes gingivostomatitis. This can be a serious infection accompanied by high fever, sore throat, and swollen lymph glands. In adolescents and young adults, the infection may present as herpes pharyngitis.

Genital herpes is a chronic recurrent illness produced by HSV type 2 (HSV-2). The disease is characterized by vesicular lesions. The incubation period for HSV-2 is 3 to 14 days. Genital herpes is a global problem.

Signs and Symptoms

In HSV-1, secretion of the virus in saliva has been noted to persist for up to 7 weeks following the appearance of a lesion. In HSV-2 in women, the vesicles may also appear on the vulva, legs, or buttocks. In men, lesions are most common on the penis, as well as around the anus in men who have sex with men. Lesions may also be present on the mouth as a result of oral sex. Genital herpes, if transmitted to a neonate during birth, is life threatening and may result in death of the neonate in up to 50% of the cases.

Differential Diagnosis

In assessing a patient suspected of having genital herpes, ask the patient about localized pain, burning, and tenderness, fever, and headache. Testing for HSV-2 is the same as for HSV-1—indirect immunofluorescent staining of a specimen obtained by swabbing a lesion.

Treatment

There is no cure for genital herpes. However, it can be treated with antiviral drugs, the most common of which is oral acyclovir (Zovirax), taken daily.

Prevention

Follow standard precautions and good hand-washing practices. Cover open wounds when providing patient care.

Counsel patients that transmission of genital herpes can be prevented by using condoms to prevent contact with viral particles on the genitals of an infected person.

Papillomaviruses

Worldwide, human papillomavirus (HPV) is the most common sexually transmitted infection in adults. Epidemiologists estimate, for example, that more than 80% of American women will have contracted at least one strain of HPV by age 50.

Papillomaviruses were first identified in the early 20th century, when it was shown that skin warts, or papillomas, are communicable from person to person. HPV has been identified as a precursor of cervical cancer. WHO recommends that young women be immunized against HPV to prevent cervical cancer and genital warts and to reduce the need for painful and costly treatment for cervical dysplasia, a precancerous condition often caused by HPV.

Pathophysiology

The papillomavirus genome is composed of genetically stable, double-stranded DNA. Papillomaviruses replicate almost exclusively in the outermost layers of the skin, as well as in some mucosal surfaces, such as on the inside of the cheek and on the vaginal walls.

Signs and Symptoms

HPV cannot be identified on visual inspection unless it is associated with genital warts. If no warts are present, pathologic examination must be done to confirm the presence of the virus.

Differential Diagnosis

To assess a patient suspected of having HPV, ask about sexual history and, if the patient is a woman, ask her whether she has been vaccinated against HPV. Papanicolaou (Pap) smears and HPV DNA testing are useful in identifying HPV in women, but no testing is available for men.

Treatment

Chemoprevention can be implemented to assist in stopping aggressive neoplastic cell growth. Interferon therapy can also be introduced. Cryosurgery (cold), laser (heat) surgery, and invasive surgery (e.g., hysterectomy) are appropriate interventions.

Prevention

Women Vaccination prevents infection with certain species of HPV associated with the development of cervical cancer, genital warts, and some less common cancers. Two HPV vaccines are currently available: Gardasil and Cervarix. These vaccines protect against two types of HPV that can cause cervical cancer (HPV-16 and HPV-18) and prevent some other genital cancers as well. Gardasil also protects against two of the HPV types that cause genital warts.
Men HPV also occurs in men and can result in genital warts and cancer. Men can be vaccinated as well to prevent HPV infection.

Parasites

Scabies

Scabies is caused by the parasitic mite *Sarcoptes scabiei*. A scabies "infection" is actually an infestation with the organism itself; the scabies mite is not a vector for transmission of other infectious agents.

Scabies is a problem worldwide and can have devastating effects if not treated, this is particularly true in developing countries. Scabies is most prevalent in hot tropical climates in locations where poverty and overcrowding exist. In 2010, it was estimated that in developing countries, the direct effects of scabies infestation on the skin alone resulted in an excess of 1.5 million years lived with disability and had indirect effects such as renal and cardiovascular complications. Scabies infestation can affect families and children, sexual partners, patients who have chronic illnesses or are hospitalized, and people who live in group homes or in close proximity to others.

Pathophysiology

Transmission of scabies occurs by direct skin-to-skin contact. It can also occur when an uninfected person has contact with fomites such as undergarments, towels, and linens. The incubation period for people with no previous exposure is 2 to 6 weeks. The disease is communicable until the mites and their eggs have been destroyed by treatment. If treated early, few complications exist. If the disease persists, skin infections leading to ulcers, sepsis, and cardiovascular and renal complications may occur.

Signs and Symptoms

Signs and symptoms of scabies infestation include nocturnal itching and the presence of a rash (**Figure 8-10**) in any of the following areas:

- Hands and interdigits
- Flexor aspects of the wrists
- Axillary folds
- Ankles or toes
- Genital area
- Buttocks
- Abdomen

Differential Diagnosis

Diagnosis is made by microscopic examination of the mite. Specimens are taken using a needle or scalpel to remove mites that have burrowed into the skin.

Treatment

Permethrin (Elimite) is a topical treatment for scabies. Reapplication may be required to treat the infestation effectively in children. Lindane (Kwell) lotion may be prescribed as a second-line treatment, but lindane toxicity has been reported with overuse.

Prevention

Prevention requires wearing gloves and following good handwashing practices. Cleaning of linens require only routine

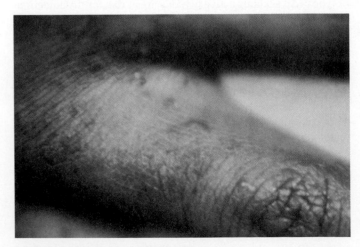

Figure 8-10 Rash produced by scabies.
Courtesy of CDC.

washing in hot water (10 min at 122°F [50°C]). Routine cleaning of rooms or vehicles after patient contact is sufficient. If providers are concerned they may have been exposed, follow routine notification guidelines. If a provider has been exposed, treatment will be indicated, and work restriction from patient care may be necessary. Treatment of the entire household may be indicated depending on living conditions and infestation. This is also true of institutional incidences.

Pediculosis (Lice)

Pediculus humanus capitis (head louse), *Pediculus humanus corporis* (body louse, clothes louse), and pubic lice, *Pthirus pubis* is a parasite that, like scabies, causes an infestation rather than a true infection. Each type of lice is different and typically infests different parts of the body. Lice are common in people who live in group homes, have poor hygiene, or have multiple sexual partners.

Pathophysiology

Transmission of lice occurs through physical contact. The incubation period is about 8 to 10 days after the eggs hatch. The lice are communicable until all mites and their eggs, including those in infested clothing, are destroyed by treatment. Humans are the only reservoir for lice. Body lice are known to transmit disease.

Signs and Symptoms

Signs and symptoms of lice include mild to severe itching and visible nits clinging to hair. Head lice infest the head and neck, body lice are found on the body, but usually lay their eggs on clothing, pubic lice are found on pubic, perianal, or perineal areas and may infest the eyelashes, eyebrows, axillae, scalp, and other hair-covered body areas.

Differential Diagnosis

Diagnosis of lice is made by a visual observation of nits (white eggs) attached to hair shafts.

Treatment

Manual removal of the nits and application of pediculicides is the treatment. Lindane shampoo (1%) is applied for 7 to 10 days to kill any hatching nymphs. These shampoos can be toxic if not used according to the directions, so for young children, a 1% permethrin cream rinse, such as Nix, is used. The cream kills both the lice and nits with one application.

Prevention

Prevention requires wearing gloves and practicing good hand-washing techniques. Routine cleaning of the room and vehicle after contact is sufficient. If an actual exposure occurred, treatment may be ordered with permethrin cream, and restriction from patient care may be indicated.

Zoonotic (Animal-Borne) Diseases

Rabies

The rabies virus is a bullet-shaped, single-stranded RNA virus that reaches the CNS by way of the peripheral nerves. The infection causes a progressive encephalomyelitis that is almost always fatal. In the United States, rabies is common in wild and domesticated animals—skunks, raccoons, bats, foxes, dogs, and cats. However, animal immunization programs have reduced the incidence of rabies and the number of deaths attributable to the disease to one or two per year. Hawaii is the only state whose animal population is free of rabies. Rabies is found on all continents except Antarctica, with the majority of deaths in Africa and Asia. In most instances, rabies occurs as a result of dog bites or scratches. Bats account for most cases in the Americas. Worldwide, most rabies deaths occur in countries with inadequate public health resources, limited access to preventive treatment, few diagnostic facilities, and virtually nonexistent rabies surveillance programs. Recently, numbers of rabies cases have been increasing in Africa, Asia, and Latin America.

Pathophysiology

Rabies is an acute viral infection of the CNS primarily affecting animals; however, it can be transmitted to humans through the virus-laden saliva of an infected animal. Transmission from person to person has never been documented. All animals found outside their natural habitat or behaving abnormally or aggressively should be presumed to be infected.

Signs and Symptoms

Two types of rabies may occur—furious and paralytic. In the furious form, victims have signs of hyperactivity, excited behavior, anxiety, confusion, hydrophobia, and sometimes aerophobia. One-third of the cases present as paralytic rabies. This form of the disease presents more gradually and is more prolonged. Muscles are become gradually paralyzed, moving out from the site of the bite or scratch. Coma develops, and death occurs. This form of rabies is often misdiagnosed, leading to the underreporting of the disease. Early symptoms are nonspecific, consisting of fever, headache, and general malaise. As the disease progresses, depending on the form, the person will present with neurologic symptoms, including insomnia, anxiety, confusion, slight or partial paralysis, excitation, hallucinations, agitation, hypersalivation, and difficulty swallowing. Contrary to popular belief, rabies does not make the infected person afraid of water. The patient will, however, be averse to drinking water, because doing so induces agonizing throat spasms. This condition is called *hydrophobia*, a term formerly synonymous with rabies itself. Death may occur within days of the onset of symptoms.

Differential Diagnosis

Humans are very susceptible to rabies virus infection after exposure to saliva in a bite or scratch from an infected animal. The lethality of the infection depends on several factors, including severity and location of the wound and the virulence of the strain. To refine your diagnosis, ask the patient about any recent history of contact with animals. Diagnosis is based on the patient's medical history, history of the exposure, and clinical presentation.

Treatment

Clean the wound area thoroughly, scrub for at least 15 minutes with soap and water, detergent, iodine, or a solution known to kill rabies. Begin rabies vaccination in accordance with current guidelines. Usually, a series of intramuscular injections is given starting on the day of injury or within 10 days, with follow-up injections on days 3, 7, 14, and 28. Rabies immunoglobulin is also given with first dose of vaccine. Dosage is determined on the basis of body weight.

Prevention

The incubation period of the rabies virus ranges from 9 to 30 days. In 1% of the cases incubation periods can be more than 1 year, with one possible case of 25 years. Vaccination of domestic animals is essential. When treating a patient suspected of having been exposed to rabies, observe standard precautions, including wearing gloves and using good hand hygiene. Rabies vaccination is available through public health programs. Criteria for administering this vaccine have changed because of reduced availability. Vaccination of healthcare providers as a preventive measure is not recommended.

Hantavirus

The *Hantavirus* genus of rodent-borne viruses is distributed worldwide and causes a group of related hantavirus diseases, including hantavirus pulmonary syndrome and hemorrhagic fever with renal syndrome. The virus is spread by the deer mouse, the white-footed mouse, and the cotton rat, as well as by garden-variety city rats.

Hantavirus occurs in Asia, western Russia, Europe, the United States, and South and Central America. Worldwide, approximately 150,000 to 200,000 cases are reported annually. The disease was first described in Korea in the early 1950s. There are two seasonal peaks for almost all outbreaks of hantavirus disease: a small outbreak appears in the spring, and a more substantial spike occurs in fall. Epidemiologists suspect that these upturns correspond with farming cycles and with seasonal increases in the infection rate of the rodents who carry the disease.

Pathophysiology

Transmission of hantavirus occurs by inhalation of aerosolized rodent waste. The virus is shed into the urine, feces, and saliva of chronically infected rodents. The incubation period is usually about 12 to 16 days, but it may be as few as 5 days or extend to 42 days. Although human-to-human transmission of hantavirus has been reported in Argentina and Chile, this disease is rarely transmitted from person to person, so there is no period of communicability.

Signs and Symptoms

Hemorrhagic fever with renal syndrome signs and symptoms begin with the sudden onset of fever, which lasts 3 to 8 days. The fever is accompanied by headache, abdominal pain, loss of appetite, and vomiting. Facial flushing is characteristic, and a petechial rash usually appears (generally limited to the axillae). Sudden and extreme albuminuria on about day 4 is a cardinal sign of severe hantavirus. The patient may also have ecchymosis and scleral injection (bloodshot eyes). Additional symptoms include hypotension, shock, respiratory distress or failure, and renal impairment or failure. The characteristic damage to the renal medulla is unique to hantaviruses. Hemorrhagic fever with renal syndrome has a mortality rate of up to 15%.

Hantavirus pulmonary syndrome is a febrile illness. It is characterized in the early phase by flulike symptoms including fever, myalgia, headache, cough, chills, muscle aches, abdominal pain, diarrhea, and malaise. In the later phase, 4–10 days after the initial onset, symptoms may include shortness of breath and tachypnea. The lungs fill with fluid and patients complain of chest tightness and a feeling of "suffocation." Ask the patient about exposure to mice or other rodent droppings if you observe symptoms consistent with hantavirus. Hantavirus pulmonary syndrome has a mortality rate of up to 50%.

Differential Diagnosis

The differential diagnosis for hantavirus pulmonary syndrome includes severe generalized pneumonia, interstitial pneumonia, and eosinophilic pneumonia. Diagnosis is confirmed by IgM antibody response or a rising IgG titer, or by polymerase chain reaction testing. Chest radiographs may reveal a diffuse interstitial infiltrate.

Treatment

No specific treatment is available other than supportive measures, including oxygen administration, monitoring of respiratory status, maintenance of fluid and electrolyte balances, and support of blood pressure.

Prevention

Follow standard precautions; hantavirus is not transmitted from person to person. Routine cleaning of the vehicle is sufficient. Public health officials will assess the need for cleaning out areas of rodent infestation.

Tetanus (Lockjaw)

According to the Centers for Disease Control and Prevention, during 2001-2008, a total of 233 cases and 26 deaths from tetanus were reported in the United States. Tetanus is more common in agricultural areas and in underdeveloped areas, where contact with animal waste is common and immunization is inadequate. Tetanus is a disease caused by the gram-positive anaerobic bacterium *Clostridium tetani*. Tetanus occurs worldwide and affects all age groups, with the highest prevalence found in neonates and young people. Tetanus is one of the target diseases of the WHO Expanded Program on Immunization. Overall, the annual incidence of tetanus is 500,000 to 1 million cases. About 60% of the cases occur in people older than 60. They are usually isolated to rural areas where contact with animal waste is common and immunization is inadequate. The tetanus bacillus is found in the intestines of horses and other animals and in contaminated soil. Some cases of tetanus have been linked to IV drug use.

Pathophysiology

Transmission of tetanus occurs when tetanus spores enter the body by way of a puncture wound contaminated with animal feces, street dust, or soil, by the injection of contaminated street drugs, or in neonates delivered at home where adequate sterile procedures are not available. Occasionally, cases have occurred postoperatively or after minor injuries that were left untreated. The incubation period is thought to be about 14 days from the exposure, but a period of as little as 3 days has been reported. A short incubation period is associated with a higher level of contamination. Tetanus is not transmitted person to person, so there is no period of communicability.

Signs and Symptoms

Signs and symptoms, a result of the neurotoxin released as the bacteria begin to grow, start at the site of the wound, followed by painful muscle contractions in the neck and trunk muscles. The most common initial sign is a spasm of the jaw preventing the person from opening the mouth, this is why tetanus is referred to as *lockjaw*. Another cardinal sign is abdominal spasms. Seizures, fever, sweating, high blood pressure, and tachycardia may also be present.

Differential Diagnosis

Diagnosis for tetanus is made on the basis of signs and symptoms; no laboratory testing for tetanus has been developed.

Treatment

The wound must be cleaned and surgically débrided. The antibiotic metronidazole (Flagyl) may be prescribed. Anyone infected with tetanus should be vaccinated against it, because having had the illness does not confer immunity to future infection with the bacterium. A decrease in the incidence of tetanus has occurred worldwide with the institution immunization programs.

Prevention

Wear gloves when handling any patient who has a draining wound. Prevention of tetanus requires vaccination during childhood and booster doses every 10 years. No special cleaning of the room or vehicle is necessary after caring for a patient with tetanus.

Vector-Borne Diseases

Lyme Disease

Lyme disease is the most common tick-borne disease in the United States. The number of reported cases has increased since 1982, when a national reporting system was established. Lyme disease is found worldwide, with most cases occurring in forested areas of Asia; northwestern, central, and eastern Europe; and regionally in the United States. Lyme disease is not caused by a virus but by a bacterium, the spirochete *Borrelia burgdorferi*. The disease occurs most often in children younger than 10 years and middle-aged adults.

Pathophysiology

Lyme disease is transmitted by the tick bite. Adult ticks are not as likely to transmit disease to humans because they prefer deer as hosts. The peak season is between June and August, with the incidence of the disease receding in early fall. The incubation period ranges from 3 to 32 days. The disease has no period of communicability because it is not transmitted person to person.

Signs and Symptoms

Lyme disease primarily affects the skin, heart, joints, and nervous system. Some patients are asymptomatic. The disease is usually divided into the following three stages:

1. *Early localized.* In the early localized stage, a round, slightly irregular red skin lesion called *erythema migrans* appears 3 to 32 days after the tick bite. This lesion is often described as a bull's-eye rash, because it consists of a central necrotic spot surrounded by an area of clearing, around which a dark-red ring appears, with lighter erythema around the periphery (**Figure 8-11**). The rash is more than 5 cm in diameter. It usually appears on the skin of the groin, thigh, or axilla and is easy to miss. The skin is warm to the touch and may be blistered or covered with a scab.

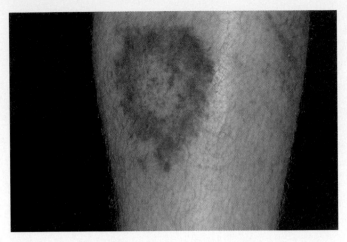

Figure 8-11 The bull's-eye rash of Lyme disease is most common in the area of the groin, thigh, or axilla.
© E. M. Singletary, MD. Used with permission.

2. *Early disseminated.* The second, early disseminated stage may develop within days. This stage is characterized by secondary lesions and flulike symptoms such as fever, chills, headache, malaise, and muscle pain. The patient may also have a nonproductive cough, sore throat, enlarged spleen, or enlarged lymph nodes. Men may have testicular swelling. Neurologic involvement occurs in 15% to 20% of untreated patients within 8 weeks. Cardiac involvement appears in about 10% of untreated patients.

3. *Late manifestations.* In the final phase of the illness, which may begin days or years after the second phase, arthritis occurs in about 60% of untreated patients. Intermittent joint pain lasting days or months occurs in about half of patients. Chronic neurologic symptoms are uncommon. In the United States, memory impairment, depressed mood, and severe fatigue are the most frequent symptoms.

Differential Diagnosis

Diagnosis for Lyme disease can be made by culturing the skin lesion for *B. burgdorferi.* More commonly, antibody titers are obtained. However, a thorough history and observation of the lesions and associated patient complaints are essential.

Treatment

The patient may receive oral doxycycline or amoxicillin for 10 to 21 days. Up to 20% of patients, predominantly with late diagnosis and having received antibiotic treatment, may have persistent or recurrent symptoms (referred to as *posttreatment Lyme disease syndrome*) that respond to oral antibiotic treatment as well. Patients who experience neurologic or cardiac forms of the disease may require intravenous treatment with drugs such as ceftriaxone or penicillin.

Prevention

As always, good hand washing is important, but Lyme disease is not transmitted person to person. Wear long sleeves and trousers when you must work in tick-infested areas. Repellents such as diethyltoluamide (DEET) can deter these insects, but such chemicals can be toxic and must be used judiciously, especially around young children. Postexposure treatment with antibiotics is not warranted or recommended.

West Nile Virus

West Nile virus is a *Flavivirus*—a genus of diseases—and is commonly found in Africa, Europe, the Middle East, North America, and West Asia. The disease derives its name from the place of its origin, along the Nile River. West Nile virus was first discovered in Uganda in the 1930s but made its first appearance in the Western Hemisphere when it was identified in New York City in 1999, marking the beginning of the largest outbreak of mosquito-to-borne illness in United States history. Other outbreaks of West Nile virus have been reported in Russia, Israel, and Romania. In most cases, the disease is mild and uneventful. In fact, about 80% of those infected are not aware that they have acquired the disease.

Pathophysiology

Transmission of West Nile virus occurs when a person is bitten by a mosquito carrying the virus. Only about 1% of mosquitoes are vectors for this pathogen. The disease is not transmitted from person to person. West Nile virus has been transmitted by donor blood, organ transplantation, and by needlestick injury among laboratory workers handling the virus. The incubation period is 2 to 14 days after the bite, during which time the virus multiplies in the lymph nodes before entering the bloodstream. Symptoms typically last 3 to 6 days.

Signs and Symptoms

About 80% of those infected with West Nile virus are asymptomatic. The remaining 20% have mild signs and symptoms such as fever, headache, body rash, and swollen lymph glands. About 1 in 150 will go on to have severe signs and symptoms develop, such as encephalitis and meningitis, which can lead to neurologic complications and death.

Differential Diagnosis

Keen observation of signs and symptoms is the key to making a preliminary diagnosis. Ask the patient about recent mosquito bites if cases have been reported in the area. Ask about risks for exposure, such as work and travel history. Observe the patient for severe signs and symptoms that suggest meningitis or encephalitis, such as loss of consciousness, confusion, stiff neck, and muscle weakness.

Laboratory diagnosis is accomplished by identification of West Nile virus–specific IgM antibodies through the testing of serum or CSF. Immunoassays for West Nile virus–specific IgM are available commercially and through state public health laboratories.

Treatment

Supportive treatment for the disease is offered. No prescribed treatment is available for West Nile virus.

Prevention

Use needle-safe device systems to avoid a contaminated sharps injury. No particular medical follow-up treatment is recommended if a needle exposure occurs. In addition, no special cleaning of the vehicle or equipment is needed or recommended after transporting a patient suspected of having West Nile virus.

The public can assist in controlling the spread of this infection by draining standing pools of water, using insect repellent, wearing long sleeves after dusk, and reporting dead birds to local authorities as birds are carriers of West Nile virus. These precautions will reduce reproduction capabilities and risk of exposure.

Rocky Mountain Spotted Fever

Rocky Mountain spotted fever is a tick-borne illness caused by *Rickettsia rickettsii*, a small bacterium that grows inside the cells of its hosts. The disease was first recognized in 1896, in the Snake River Valley of Idaho. It was originally given the foreboding name *black measles*. Rocky Mountain spotted fever has been a reportable disease in the United States since the 1920s. Despite its name, the disease can be found throughout most of the country, including the District of Columbia and states in the south Atlantic (Delaware, Maryland, Virginia, West Virginia, North Carolina, South Carolina, Georgia, and Florida), Pacific (Washington, Oregon, and California), and west south-central (Arkansas, Louisiana, Oklahoma, and Texas) regions. Worldwide, infection with *R. rickettsii* has been documented in Argentina, Brazil, Colombia, Costa Rica, Mexico, and Panama.

About two-thirds of Rocky Mountain spotted fever cases occur in children younger than 15 years, with a peak at ages 5 to 9. People who are often around dogs or who live close to wooded areas or patches of tall grass are also at increased risk of infection. American Indians have the highest incidence of Rocky Mountain spotted fever. Only about 60% of people diagnosed with Rocky Mountain spotted fever recall having had a tick bite.

Pathophysiology

More than 20 species are currently classified in the genus *Rickettsia*, but not all are known to cause disease in humans. The rickettsiae that cause spotted fever grow in the cytoplasm or in the nuclei of host cells. The organisms multiply, damaging or destroying those cells and causing blood to leak through tiny holes in vessel walls into adjacent tissues. This mechanism is responsible for the characteristic rash associated with the disease. The incubation period is 3 to 14 days after the tick bite. The illness is not transmissible from person to person.

Signs and Symptoms

Initial symptoms of Rocky Mountain spotted fever may include fever, nausea, vomiting, severe headache, muscle pain, and lack of appetite. A rash appears 2 to 5 days after the onset of fever (**Figure 8-12**). It often appears initially as a smattering of small, flat, pink, nonitchy spots (macules) on the wrists, forearms, and ankles.

Rocky Mountain spotted fever can be a life-threatening illness, because *R. rickettsii* infects the cells that line blood vessels throughout the body. Severe manifestations of this disease may involve the respiratory or renal system, the CNS, or the GI tract. Those with illness severe enough to require hospital care may have the following long-term effects:

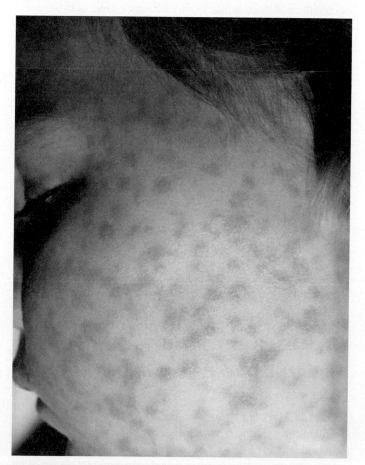

Figure 8-12 Late-acute stage of Rocky Mountain spotted fever.
© Robin Treadwell/Science Source.

- Partial paralysis of the lower extremities
- Gangrene requiring amputation of fingers, toes, arms, or legs
- Hearing loss
- Loss of bowel or bladder control
- Movement or language disorders

Differential Diagnosis

Diagnosis is often made on the basis of signs and symptoms, but indirect immunofluorescence assay can be used to detect IgG or IgM antibodies. Question any patient with a rash about possible tick bites. Check the patient for fever as well.

IgG antibodies are more specific and reliable, since other bacterial infections can also cause elevations in rickettsial IgM antibody titers.

Treatment

Doxycycline (100 mg every 12 hours for adults or 4 mg/kg of body weight per day in two divided doses for children under 100 lb [45 kg]) is the drug of choice for patients with Rocky Mountain spotted fever. Therapy is continued for at least 3 days after fever subsides and until there is unequivocal evidence of clinical improvement, generally for a minimum total course of 5 to 10 days. Severe or complicated disease may require a longer course of treatment.

Prevention

Good hand washing is essential for healthcare providers. Risk of contracting the disease can be limited by reducing your exposure to ticks. In those who are exposed to ticks, careful inspection and removal of crawling or attached ticks is a simple but important way of preventing disease.

When the presence of ticks is recognized, they should be removed. Ticks are easily removed with tweezers or forceps by identifying and grabbing the tick's mouth, very close to the person or animal's skin. The entire tick should be gently removed. In order to prevent further contamination, the body of the tick should not be squeezed. The area should be cleaned and an antiseptic applied.

Infection With Multidrug-Resistant Organisms

Methicillin-Resistant *Staphylococcus aureus*

Methicillin-resistant *Staphylococcus aureus* (MRSA), a global problem, has emerged as an organism that can be community acquired (CA), not just a healthcare-associated infection. MRSA infection usually affects several body systems and is resistant to multiple antibiotics, including nafcillin (Unipen), oxacillin (Bactocill and Prostaphlin), cephalosporins, erythromycins, and aminoglycosides.

Pathophysiology

HA-MRSA and CA-MRSA are caused by different organisms. CA-MRSA can be acquired from household pets, contaminated gym equipment, contact between field turf and nonintact skin, and improper hand washing or failure to wash hands. In 2011, a CDC study demonstrated that evidence of improved hand hygiene resulted in a decrease in hospital-acquired MRSA and in-hospital MRSA deaths.

Signs and Symptoms

A patient with MRSA may have fever, redness, localized pain, small red bumps, or deep abscesses that can affect bones, joints, heart valves, and the bloodstream. CA-MRSA has a different genetic makeup and is chiefly associated with soft-tissue infections such as abscesses and cellulitis. Abscesses are treated with incision and drainage and usually do not require antibiotics.

Differential Diagnosis

Diagnosis of MRSA is confirmed by Gram stain and/or culture. A rapid test for MRSA produces results in 2 hours. A culture takes 48 to 72 hours.

Treatment

Use gloves and follow meticulous hand-washing practices when in direct contact with draining wounds. No medical treatment is recommended after exposure to MRSA. Notify and document the event. Medications used for treating difficult MRSA infections include vancomycin (Vancocin), clindamycin (Cleocin), cotrimoxazole (Bactrim), quinupristin and dalfopristin injection (Synercid), and tigecycline (Tygacil).

Prevention

MRSA is a slow-growing bacterium and is easily destroyed by routine approved cleaning solutions. Clean the room, vehicle, and patient care equipment after each use. Shower after physical activity and clean exercise equipment before use. Cover open skin areas with a dressing.

Vancomycin-Resistant Enterococci

Enterococcus is a common organism that constitutes part of the normal flora of the GI tract, urinary tract, and genitourinary tract. This genus comprises more than 400 species, many of which are often resistant to antibiotics. A cagey organism, it flourishes equally well under conditions of scarce or abundant oxygen. When this organism becomes resistant to vancomycin (Vancocin), the primary drug used to treat *Enterococcus* infection, the patient is said to have vancomycin-resistant *Enterococcus* (VRE). This is primarily a hospital-acquired infection (HAI).

Pathophysiology

This organism may be found in patients with urinary tract or bloodstream infections. VRE has also been found in livestock waste and improperly prepared chicken. Those who work on farms or in processing plants are at higher risk of exposure. Patients identified with VRE outside the hospital setting often reside in nursing homes or spend time at hemodialysis centers. VRE can live on surfaces for long periods of time, so thorough cleaning of devices used in healthcare settings is important.

Transmission occurs by direct contact with contaminated surfaces or equipment, or by direct contact of an open cut or sore with a draining wound. This illness can be treated with a new synthetic antibiotic, linezolid (Zyvox), which belongs to a novel antibiotic class called *oxazolidinones*.

Signs and Symptoms

Signs and symptoms include wound infection, redness, tenderness, fever or chills, and urinary tract infection (indicated by an unusual urine color or odor and pain on urination).

Differential Diagnosis

To refine the diagnosis, ask the patient about his or her medical history, particularly any hospital stay for surgery and any prolonged antibiotic treatment. Diagnosis is made by culturing a wound, urine, blood, or stool.

Treatment

Antibiotic treatment is given using linezolid or another drug to which the organism demonstrates susceptibility on culture.

Prevention

Follow standard precautions, including wearing gloves and using good hand-washing techniques when you are in contact with wound drainage. A gown is needed only if wound drainage may come in contact with a provider's uniform. Clean all areas with which the patient had contact; no special cleaning solution is needed. Direct contact between an open wound and VRE-infected body fluids should be reported according to the organization exposure policy. An exposure report will need to be completed, but no postexposure medical treatment is indicated.

Clostridium difficile (Pseudomembranous Colitis)

Clostridium difficile (often called *C. diff*) is not a multidrug-resistant organism but is treated like one. Rates of *C. diff* infection in the United States have tripled since 2000, and mortality

has increased. Toxic variant strains are now widespread in North America and Europe.

This illness is the direct result of antibiotic therapy, which suppresses the normal flora in the GI tract and allows *C. diff* to predominate. Therefore, it is classified as an HAI but is also associated with outpatient antibiotic therapy. High-risk environments include acute and long-term facilities. An increase in incidence in pediatric patients that are immune compromised and peripartum women who have had cesarean sections has been reported. The highest incidence remains in the elderly population.

Pathophysiology

Clostridium difficile is a gram-negative, spore-forming anaerobic bacillus that produces two large toxins, A and B. Spore production causes heavy contamination of environmental surfaces. As a result, healthcare providers' unwashed hands are a major means of transmission of *C. diff*.

Signs and Symptoms

Patients with this illness have diarrhea that is not bloody but has a characteristic foul odor. Abdominal pain and cramping are present in about 22% of patients. If these signs are present, ask the patient about any recent hospital stays or antibiotic therapy.

Differential Diagnosis

To refine the diagnosis, check the odor of stool and assess for the presence of fever in the patient.

Diagnosis is made on the basis of a thorough history, focused physical exam, and the patient's chief complaint/cardinal presentation. In addition, an increased WBC count, a positive stool culture, and an enzyme immunoassay assist in identifying which toxin is present.

Treatment

Stopping any unnecessary antibiotic treatment may be enough to resolve the infection, but treatment with oral metronidazole (Flagyl) or vancomycin (Vancocin) for 10 days is usually required. In some cases, symptoms will return within 30 days, generally caused by the same strain of *C. diff*.

Prevention

Follow standard precautions, including good hand-washing practices with soap and vigorous rubbing. Use of just alcohol-based gels does not eradicate the spores. A chlorine-based solution must be used to clean equipment, since *C. diff* is a spore-forming organism. Avoiding the use of unnecessary antibiotics is essential and calls for a worldwide education program.

Communicable Diseases of Childhood

Immunizations have dramatically reduced the incidence of communicable diseases in children and adults, but they still occur. It's important to understand the clinical presentations of these diseases to implement appropriate PPE and interventions.

The measles, mumps, and rubella (MMR) and measles, mumps, rubella, and varicella (MMRV) vaccines use live, weakened viral strains to confer immunity to these three childhood diseases. First licensed as a combined vaccine in 1971, MMR contains the safest and most effective forms of each vaccine. Consideration for administration of the appropriate vaccine is determined by the patient's specific health history and underlying health factors. Vaccination is recommended for all healthcare providers who do not have proof of immunity. Vaccination is not, however, recommended for pregnant women, and women of childbearing age who are offered MMR vaccine must be counseled not to become pregnant for 3 months after being vaccinated.

Rubeola (Measles)

Rubeola is an illness caused by the measles virus, which can be found in an infected person's blood, urine, and pharyngeal secretions.

Pathophysiology

The rubeola virus resides in the mucus of the nose and throat of the infected person. When the person sneezes or coughs, droplets spray into the air. The virus remains active and contagious on infected surfaces for up to 2 hours. The illness lasts for about 9 days. It usually is passed directly or indirectly through contact with infected respiratory secretions. In severe cases, seizures may occur, or the illness may prove fatal. Serious complications are more common among children younger than 5 years and in adults older than 20.

Signs and Symptoms

One of the first signs of measles is often a high fever that develops about 10–12 days after exposure to the virus. A key sign of measles is the presence of Koplik spots (whitish-gray spots visible on the buccal mucosa). Other signs and symptoms of measles include diarrhea, conjunctivitis, cough, coryza (nasal congestion and discharge), and a blotchy red rash. Complications such as otitis media, pneumonia, myocarditis, and encephalitis occur in about 20% of reported measles cases.

Differential Diagnosis

Serologic testing for the measles virus and antigens is helpful for diagnosis and treatment. If an IgM blood test is positive, viral cultures are performed. IgM is the antibody first produced in an immune response.

Treatment

Treatment for measles is supportive with an emphasis placed on maintaining hydration and considering antibiotics for associated ear and eye infections or pneumonia should they occur. In developing countries, children should receive two doses of vitamin A supplements 24 hours apart. Vitamin A administration has been shown to decrease mortality from measles by 50%.

Prevention

If you are caring for a patient with rubeola and you have not been vaccinated or are not immune to rubeola, place a surgical mask on the patient. If you are unsure whether you are immune, a serologic blood test should be performed. If results indicate nonimmunity, consider being vaccinated.

Rubella

Rubella, or German measles, is also caused by a virus found in respiratory secretions. This illness lasts for about 3 days. Rubella contracted during pregnancy may cause miscarriage, premature birth, or a low-birth-weight infant. If rubella is passed from the mother to fetus during the first trimester of pregnancy, anomalies in fetal development can occur, including intellectual disability, deafness, and an increased risk of congenital heart disease and sepsis during the first 6 months of life. Collectively, these developmental anomalies are known as "congenital rubella syndrome."

Pathophysiology

Transmission occurs by direct contact with the nasopharyngeal secretions of the infected person—by droplet spread or by touching the patient or articles freshly contaminated with the patient's secretions. Rubella is highly contagious and can be transmitted from 4 days before the rash appears up to 4 days after the rash becomes evident.

Signs and Symptoms

Signs and symptoms of rubella include low-grade fever, rash, and swollen lymph glands behind the ears and at the base of the skull. Onset of symptoms is usually 2 to 3 weeks after exposure.

Differential Diagnosis

Serologic tests are performed to identify antibodies. Polymerase chain reaction identification is done to isolate the virus.

Treatment

Supportive care is central to the management of patients with rubella.

Prevention

Practice standard precautions. You can reduce your risk of contracting rubella by taking respiratory precautions such as placing a surgical mask on the patient, but vaccination is the key to risk reduction for healthcare personnel. As with measles, the only certain protection against rubella is immunity.

Mumps

Mumps is an acute, communicable, systemic illness caused by the mumps virus. It occurs most commonly in winter and spring. Anyone who has not been vaccinated is at risk for the disease.

Pathophysiology

The mumps virus is transmitted by droplet spread or direct contact with the saliva of an infected person. The virus has an incubation period of 12 to 26 days and a communicable period ranging from 1 week to 9 days after the onset of symptoms.

Signs and Symptoms

Mumps is characterized by swelling and tenderness of the parotid salivary glands, affecting one or both sides of the neck. The patient will also have a fever and may have been exposed to another person with mumps. When adults are infected, complications such as meningitis and orchitis (inflammation of one or both testicles) are more often seen. Rare complications include hydrocephalus, hearing loss, Guillain-Barré syndrome, pancreatitis, and myocarditis.

Differential Diagnosis

An assessment for parotid swelling should be performed to help determine whether the patient may have mumps. Serologic tests are not necessarily done for measles and mumps.

Treatment

Treatment is supportive and includes analgesic and antipyretic medications.

Prevention

Providers should take respiratory droplet precautions (place a surgical mask on the patient) when transporting a patient suspected of having mumps. Vaccination is the key to risk reduction among healthcare personnel.

Pertussis (Whooping Cough)

The gram-negative bacterium *Bordetella pertussis* is the organism that causes whooping cough. According to WHO, in 2013, 136,000 cases of pertussis occurred worldwide—this is a significant decrease from 50 million in 2005, with 89,000 deaths in 2008, attributable to the disease. About 84% of the global population is covered by immunization.

Pathophysiology

Pertussis has an insidious onset and is characterized by an irritating cough. The organism that causes pertussis can survive outside the respiratory tract for only a short period of time. When it does gain entry to the respiratory tract, it attaches to cilia, immobilizing them. The bacteria produce toxins that can cause systemic illness. The incubation period is 7 to 10 days, and transmission occurs by direct contact with oral or nasal secretions. The primary risk group is children and adolescents; however, a worrisome rise has been reported in the incidence of pertussis among adults. Complications include pneumonia, which is fairly common, seizures, and encephalitis, which are much more rare.

Signs and Symptoms

Signs and symptoms during the first stage of whooping cough, known as the "catarrhal phase," include fever, malaise, sneezing, and anorexia. This stage lasts several days. The second stage of the illness, the paroxysmal coughing phase, is the key to identifying the disease. The patient may have 50 or more episodes of spasmodic coughing per day. When each convulsive cough subsides, a whooping sound emerges. In very young patients, the coughing may be followed by episodes of apnea. Assess for vomiting, low oxygen saturation, convulsions, and coma. During the third stage, the convalescent phase, the coughing begins to subside, becoming less frequent and intense. The illness may last several weeks.

Differential Diagnosis

Laboratory testing for rising antibody titers is required to make a diagnosis.

Treatment

The treatment is primarily supportive. Close monitoring of respiratory status is indicated, and ventilation support should be initiated as needed. Treatment centers on antibiotic therapy, usually with erythromycin.

Prevention

A pertussis vaccine became available in 1940, and childhood vaccination remains the primary means of prevention and control. Take droplet precautions when caring for a patient suspected of having whooping cough. Place a surgical mask or an oxygen mask on the patient and follow standard precautions.

Vaccination may not provide lifetime immunity to pertussis as previously believed, so healthcare providers should receive a one-time booster dose of Tdap (tetanus, diphtheria, acellular pertussis). Report any exposure as soon as possible to receive a 14-day course of antibiotics.

Varicella-Zoster Virus Infection (Chickenpox)

Chickenpox is a highly contagious disease caused by the varicella-zoster virus (**Figure 8-13**), a member of the herpesvirus family. Chickenpox occurs worldwide, affecting people of all races, ages, and both sexes, but is more common in children younger than 10 years. An estimated 60 million cases occur worldwide each year. Chickenpox is often mild in children and more severe in adults. Varicella-zoster virus may result in chickenpox or shingles.

Once a person has had chickenpox, he or she is unlikely to contract the illness again because infection is thought to provide lifelong immunity in most people. Persons with a compromised immune system who are exposed to the virus are susceptible to the virus regardless of their medical history, and actions to either prevent or modify the course of the disease should be taken.

In some people, the virus is retained in the spinal dorsal nerve root ganglia after having chickenpox and reappears later in life as herpes zoster (shingles) infection (**Figure 8-14**). Reactivation of the virus may occur during a period of physical or emotional stress. The herpes zoster lesions drain live virus and are extraordinarily painful.

Pathophysiology

Transmission of this virus may occur in one of two ways: inhalation of airborne respiratory droplets or contact with drainage

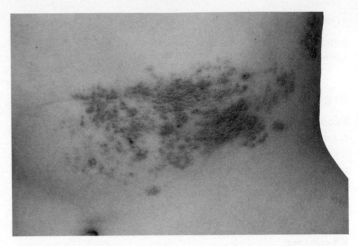

Figure 8-14 Herpes zoster (shingles).
© Franciscodiazpagador/iStock.

from vesicles. The portal of entry is usually the conjunctival or upper respiratory mucosa. The disease presents in stages. Viral replication takes place in regional lymph nodes 2 to 4 days after exposure, after which a primary viremia occurs (4 to 6 days after inoculation). The virus then replicates in the liver, spleen, and possibly in other organs. Secondary viremia occurs 14 to 16 days after initial exposure and is characterized by the spread of viral particles to the skin, which causes the typical vesicular rash. The rash initially appears on the covered areas of the body and spreads to the face, scalp, and sometimes the mucous membranes of the mouth or genitals. The shallow vesicles progress to become deeper pustules. As they heal, the lesions dry up and crust over, leaving scabs. The usual incubation period of varicella-zoster is 10 to 21 days. The patient is contagious for 1 to 2 days before the rash appears until all the lesions are dry and crusted.

Signs and Symptoms

Prodromal symptoms of chickenpox include fever, malaise, anorexia, and headache. Then blisters or a rash that itches develops.

Differential Diagnosis

Patients should be assessed for signs of superinfection, including impetigo, cellulitis, necrotizing fasciitis, and arthritis. Laboratory testing is generally not performed. Diagnosis is made on the basis of clinical presentation.

Treatment

Treatment for patients with chickenpox is symptomatic. Oral antihistamines or lotion can be prescribed to relieve itching. In children, fever should be reduced without the use of aspirin to avoid the risk of Reye syndrome. Fingernails should be trimmed to prevent skin excoriation from scratching. Antiviral

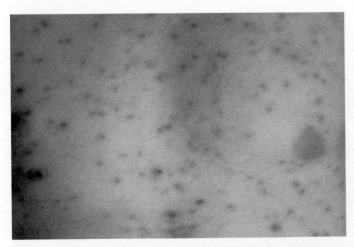

Figure 8-13 The distinctive rash produced by chickenpox is composed of small, blister-like vesicles that arise in clusters.
Courtesy of CDC.

medications and corticosteroids may be prescribed to shorten the duration of symptoms. Patients should be monitored for skin infections and pneumonia.

Prevention

Vaccination is the primary means of protection from varicella-zoster for both patients and healthcare providers. If possible, droplet precautions should be taken by placing a surgical mask on the patient. If the patient is unable to wear a mask, place one on yourself. Gloves should be worn when in direct contact with draining lesions. Routine cleaning of the vehicle, rooms or equipment is adequate, and no airing of the vehicle is needed. If an exposure occurs, follow up should occur, because postexposure medical treatment may be indicated. Providers who are vaccinated after exposure may be restricted from day 10 to day 28 after exposure. Studies have found that transmission to household members who have not had the disease is highly likely (90% infection incidence).

Vaccination can result in breakthrough varicella; infected patients are contagious. If varicella with more than 50 lesions develops in a person, that person is as contagious as an unvaccinated person. If fewer than 50 lesions develop, transmission is one-third as likely as an unvaccinated person.

Emerging Infectious Diseases

Chikungunya

Chikungunya was first identified in Tanzania in 1952. A mosquito-borne viral disease, it is an RNA virus belonging to the alphavirus genus of the family Togaviridae. *Chikungunya* is from a word in the Kimakonde language, meaning "to become contorted." It describes the stooped appearance patients often present with due to the joint pain (arthralgia) associated with the disease. Over 60 countries in Asia, Africa, Europe, and the Americas have reported incidences of Chikungunya.

Pathophysiology

The virus is transmitted from human to human through the bite of the mosquito. Onset is most often between 4 and 8 days, but may occur between 2 and 12 days.

Signs and Symptoms

Patients present with sudden onset of fever and joint pain that can be debilitating. Muscle pain, headache, joint swelling, nausea, fatigue, and rash may also be present. The majority of patients recover, and some may report ongoing joint pain. Neurologic, cardiac, and gastrointestinal complications may occur and have resulted in death, especially in the elderly. Chikungunya has been confused with Dengue fever.

Differential Diagnosis

Chikungunya diagnosis is generally identified by testing serum or plasma to detect virus, viral nucleic acid, or virus-specific immunoglobulin (Ig) M and neutralizing antibodies.

Treatment

Care is supportive and aimed at preventing dehydration and relieving pain. NSAIDs and acetaminophen can be administered to treat to reduce the pain.

Prevention

No special cleaning of the vehicle or equipment is needed or recommended after transporting a patient suspected of having Chikungunya. The public can assist in controlling the spread of this infection by draining standing pools of water, using insect repellent, and wearing long sleeves during the daytime as this disease is most commonly transmitted by mosquitos that bite during the daytime. These precautions will reduce reproduction capabilities and risk of exposure. Once infected, the patient's chance of being reinfected is not likely. Mosquitos can transmit the disease to others if the infected person is bitten during this time, so it is important for those individuals to avoid being bitten.

Viral Hemorrhagic Fevers

Viral hemorrhagic fevers include a group of illnesses that cause a severe multisystem syndrome that damages the body's vascular system and disrupts the body's ability to maintain homeostasis. The syndromes are caused by the *Arenaviridae*, Bunyaviridae, Filoviridae, and Flaviviridae viruses (Table 8-8).

Pathophysiology

Viruses are naturally carried by animals, rodents, and insects such as ticks and mosquitos. Humans become infected when exposed to the infected carrier, which can be by bites, contact with excrement, or during the butchering process. Some viruses can be spread by human to human contact and their bodily fluids. This is the case with Ebola and Lassa fever. In both of these cases, contaminated syringes have been responsible for the spread of the virus.

Signs and Symptoms

Signs and symptoms vary between viruses. Most of the illnesses present with a marked fever, fatigue, dizziness, muscle aches, weakness, and exhaustion. More severe cases present with petechiae, other bleeding under the skin or in internal organs, or bleeding from sites around the body including the mouth, nose and ears. Shock, neurological involvement, coma, delirium, and seizures may occur. In some cases renal failure is present.

Table 8-8 **Viruses That Cause Hemorrhagic Fevers**	
Virus	**Illness/Syndrome**
Arenaviridae	Lassa fever, Junin, and Machupo
Bunyaviridae	Crimean-Congo hemorrhagic fever, Rift Valley fever, Hantaan hemorrhagic fevers
Filoviridae	Ebola and Marburg
Flaviviridae	Yellow fever, dengue, Omsk hemorrhagic fever, Kyasanur Forest disease

Many of the syndromes listed in this table are associated with bleeding. In most cases, the bleeding is usually not life threatening. Some of the illnesses are life threatening, while others cause relatively mild illnesses. Although not the natural reservoir for these viruses, humans become infected when exposed. Humans can transmit the virus to other humans once infected. The carriers of some viruses such as Ebola and Marburg are unknown. Incidences of viral hemorrhagic fevers have occurred worldwide. Outbreaks where the virus is endemic have occurred, as well as instances of viruses being brought to new regions by individuals traveling from an area where an outbreak is present.

Differential Diagnosis

Awareness of possible exposure is key in identification. Lab tests have been developed to identify the various types of viruses. Great care should be taken with lab samples containing viruses due to the potential to infect the laboratory personnel.

Treatment

Care is supportive and aimed at preventing dehydration. An antiviral drug, ribavirin, has proven effective in treating some individuals with Lassa fever or hemorrhagic fever with renal syndrome. In patients with Argentine hemorrhagic fever, treatment with convalescent-phase plasma has been effective.

Prevention

The prevention of viral hemorrhagic fevers includes the following:

- *Vaccines.* Vaccines have been developed for yellow fever and Argentine hemorrhagic fever. Research is under way on vaccines for some of the other viral hemorrhagic fever illnesses, but none are available at this time so other actions to prevent spread of the disease should be taken.
- *Controlling rodent populations.* This is important because many of the viruses are carried by rodents. Actions should be taken to control rodent populations, to discourage rodents from entering homes and work places, and to safely clean up nests.
- *Arthropod control.* Actions to control tick and mosquito populations should be taken. In addition, people living in these areas should take actions to avoid being bitten by wearing proper clothing; using insect repellent; and using bed nets, window screens, and other barriers.
- *Person-to-person control.* Using personal hygiene and hand washing; avoiding contact with body fluids; avoiding close physical contact with infected individuals; using proper personal protective devices if handling of body fluids is required; and proper use, disinfection, and disposal of equipment used to care for infected individuals is required. Isolation of infected individuals should occur. Proper protection and decontamination of vehicles used to transport infected patients should be observed. Proper burial of deceased individuals should occur as well. Health care providers should follow the guidelines set forth by the World Health Organization. Patients should be questioned regarding travel to areas with recent outbreaks of the disease.

Chagas Disease (American Trypanosomiasis)

Chagas disease is a potentially life-threatening disease and is primarily found in Latin America, but has begun to expand to other countries as the population becomes more mobile. It is caused by exposure to the protozoan parasite *Trypanosoma cruzi*, which is secreted in the excrement of the triatomine bugs sometimes referred to as *kissing bugs*. Chagas disease is named after the Brazilian doctor, Carlos Ribeiro Justiniano Chagas, who discovered the disease in 1909.

Pathophysiology

The blood-sucking triatomine bugs carry the parasites and are found in the cracks of poorly constructed homes in rural or suburban areas. The bugs usually hide during the day and come out at night to feed on human blood. Typically, the disease is spread when the bug bites exposed skin such as the face and then defecates near the bite. Parasites enter the body when the person instinctively reaches up and smears the bug feces into the bite, the eyes, the mouth, or into any skin break.

Other methods of transmission include consumption of food contaminated with *T. cruzi*, blood transfusions from infected donors, transmission from an infected mother to the fetus or newborn during pregnancy or childbirth, organ transplants from infected donors, and accidents in laboratories.

Signs and Symptoms

Chagas disease occurs in two phases. In the acute phase, which lasts for about 2 months, the symptoms are absent or mild, even though a large number of parasites are circulating in the blood. Some of the first visible signs can be a skin lesion or a purplish swelling of the lids of one eye, fever, headache, enlarged lymph glands, pallor, muscle pain, difficulty in breathing, swelling, and abdominal or chest pain. In the second or chronic phase, the parasites primarily accumulate in the heart and digestive muscles. That is why up to 30% of patients suffer from cardiac disorders. An additional 10% will suffer digestive problems such as enlargement of the esophagus or colon. Neurologic or mixed presentations are possible. As the disease progresses, which may be years, sudden death or heart failure may occur due to the progressive destruction of the heart muscle and its nervous system.

Differential Diagnosis

In the early phase, diagnosis can be made by visualizing the parasite in a blood smear. In later phase of identification, it is more difficult and is based on patient history, signs and symptoms, and completing two serologic tests.

Treatment

Benznidazole and nifurtimox can be used to treat Chagas disease and kill the parasite. Treatment is 100% effective if the disease is caught early in the initial phase. Reinfected patients should be treated as should neonates. Treatment for adults in the chronic phase should be considered. Administration considerations include long-term administration requirements and the 40% incidence of adverse reactions. Pregnant women and people with kidney or liver failure should not take benznidazole and nifurtimox. In individuals with a history of neurologic or psychiatric disorders, nifurtimox is contraindicated. Special considerations for cardiac or digestive manifestations may be required.

Prevention

There is no vaccine for Chagas disease. Blood should be tested to prevent transmission from blood transfusions and organ donation. Spraying houses to control infestations should be completed. Proper handling, cleaning, and storage of food will prevent transmission. Screening of mothers and newborns to allow for appropriate intervention should be completed.

Special Populations
Older Adult Patients

Because of diminished functioning of the immune system as they age, the elderly are more vulnerable to infection than younger patients and suffer greater morbidity and a higher rate of mortality from infectious disease. Aging lowers primary antibody response and cellular immunity and increases susceptibility to infection and autoimmune disorders. The following factors increase the risk of infection among older adults:

- The frequent existence of comorbid conditions, such as diabetes and neurologic diseases
- The living conditions inherent to group living situations such as nursing care facilities
- The higher rate of hospitalization among this population, which significantly increases the risk of contracting a **hospital-acquired infection/healthcare-associated infection (HAI)** (formerly called **nosocomial infection**)
- An increased incidence of malnutrition, which directly impairs the immune response

Assessment of older adults with infections may be challenging because of the difficulty in taking a thorough, accurate history and the absence of fever in nearly half of older adults with bacterial infections. The older patient may not exhibit the typical signs and symptoms of infection because of difficulties regulating body temperature and a depressed immune system. Invasive instrumentation (e.g., IV therapy, tracheal intubation, Foley catheterization) is often associated with infection. The benefits should outweigh the risks of doing so. Pneumonia, urinary tract infections, and sepsis occur more often in older adult patients, and pneumonia is one of the leading causes of death and hospitalization in this patient population.

Bariatric Patients

Obesity was once associated with wealthy individuals and countries, but it is now a problem for people of all incomes and all countries. During an infection, the complications of obesity, such as hypertension, stroke, heart disease, and diabetes, can impact the immune system and exacerbate serious illness.

Patients Who Are Technology Dependent

Today many patients are cared for at home and are dependent on medical technology for their care, comfort, and survival. Care of such patients in the home setting is growing because of burdensome hospital costs, insurance limitations placed on length of hospital stay, and the goal of reducing risk of hospital-acquired infections. These patients' medical needs, most of which are attributable to neuromuscular and respiratory disorders, include mechanical ventilation, tracheostomy care, administration of IV medications, maintenance of feeding tubes, administration of oxygen, and wound care. Decubitus ulcers are more prevalent in patients who are immobile and have compromised immune systems and increase the patient's risk factors for acquiring an infection.

Patients in Hospice Care

Out-of-hospital end-of-life care is becoming an important option. Hospice care can be rendered in the patient's home or in a hospice care center. Vascular access devices, Foley catheters, and a compromised immune system from treatments such as chemotherapy diminish these patients' resistance to common viral and bacterial infections. Measures to reduce fever and control pain may be taken, and every effort will be made to promote the dying patient's comfort. When caring for such patients, you must consider the patient's and family's wishes with respect to advance directives for health care regarding resuscitation. Supportive care or comfort care is essential, especially for pain management.

Putting It All Together

Understanding the epidemiology and pathophysiology of a variety of infectious disease processes is essential in early identification of the cause of an illness. In addition, becoming aware of an abrupt increase in the incidence of patients with a similar cardinal presentation will help you and your public health colleagues pinpoint geographic trends that might need to be reported to the appropriate local, state, and federal authorities.

Identification of the patient's cardinal presentation or chief complaint, a thorough history, focused physical exam, and evaluation of diagnostic findings will help you recognize a communicable or infectious disease. Early recognition will support prevention of the spread of the disease by choosing the appropriate PPE early in patient contact. The healthcare team's assessment and early interventions are critical strategies in preventing transmission of infectious diseases. However, the healthcare environment is often unpredictable, and disease identification may not occur until after you have rendered care. Fortunately, research endeavors continue to make progress in identifying communicable and infectious diseases and developing new vaccines, medications, and treatment protocols.

SCENARIO SOLUTION

© HunThomas/ShutterStock, Inc.

1. Differential diagnoses may include viral hemorrhagic fever, norovirus, food poisoning, and appendicitis. You should consider associated dehydration and shock.

2. To narrow your differential diagnosis you will need to complete the patient's history of past and present illness. Assess her temperature. Asking about recent exposure to other individuals who are ill is key. You may also want to inquire about others with similar symptoms in the hotel. Recent travel to a country with an infectious disease outbreak (especially if you are considering viral hemorrhagic fever as a possible diagnosis) would provide essential information. Norovirus is common in settings such as cruise ships, hotels, schools, long-term care facilities, and hospitals.

3. The patient has signs of hypovolemia. Initiate an IV and titrate fluids based on your other physical findings. Transport the patient to the appropriate facility.

4. Use standard precautions with all patients. If you are exposed to blood or bloody body fluids, follow the same actions you would on any exposure. Report you exposure immediately to the healthcare provider at the receiving facility. Notify your infection control designated officer. Complete the necessary reports and follow up. This patient is high risk for Norovirus, which is extremely contagious. Good hand washing and cleaning any contaminated equipment are essential.

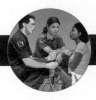

Summary

- Exposure to an infectious agent does not mean that a person has acquired the disease and can pass it on to others.
- PPE is a secondary barrier to the protection the body already offers.
- Vaccination is essential for risk reduction in the healthcare setting.

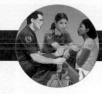

Summary (CONTINUED)

- PPE should be selected with an understanding of the mode of transmission of the diseases you expect to encounter.
- Meningitis is usually spread by inhalation of droplets and by direct contact with an infected person's respiratory or nasal secretions. Only exposure to meningococcal meningitis requires prophylactic antibiotics.
- Healthcare providers decrease the risk of exposure to infectious diseases by using standard precautions and thorough hand-washing techniques.
- Local and federal governmental agencies establish standards and guidelines to reduce the risk of infection for the healthcare provider and the communities in which they serve.
- Prevention of transmission of infectious diseases can result from an understanding of the pathophysiology, clinical manifestations, and treatment strategies for communicable and infectious diseases.

KEY TERMS

© HunThomas/ShutterStock, Inc.

antibodies Immunoglobulins produced by lymphocytes in response to bacteria, viruses, or other antigenic substances.

antigens Substances, usually proteins, that the body recognizes as foreign and that can evoke an immune response.

blood-borne pathogens Pathogenic microorganisms that are transmitted via human blood and cause disease in humans; examples include hepatitis B virus (HBV) and human immunodeficiency virus (HIV).

communicable diseases Any disease transmitted from one person or animal to another either directly, by contact with excreta or other discharges from the body; or indirectly, by means of substances or inanimate objects such as contaminated drinking glasses, toys, water, or by vectors such as flies, mosquitoes, ticks, or other insects.

contaminated A condition of being soiled, stained, touched, or otherwise exposed to harmful agents, making an object potentially unsafe for use as intended or without barrier techniques; for example, entry of infectious or toxic materials into a previously clean or sterile environment.

decontamination The process of removing foreign material such as blood, body fluids, or radioactivity; it does not eliminate microorganisms but is a necessary step preceding disinfection or sterilization.

epidemic A disease that affects a significantly large number of people at the same time and spreads rapidly through a demographic segment of the human population.

epidemiology The study of the determinants of disease events in populations.

exposure incident A state of being in the presence of or subjected to a force or influence (e.g., viral exposure, heat exposure).

hospital-acquired infection (HAI)/healthcare-associated infections An infection acquired from exposure to an infectious agent at a healthcare facility, defined as at least 72 hours after hospitalization.

infectious diseases Diseases caused by another living organism or virus, which may or may not be transmissible to another person.

nosocomial infection *See* hospital-acquired infection (HAI).

pandemic A disease occurring throughout the population of a large part of the world.

parenteral Pertaining to treatment other than through the digestive system.

retrovirus Any of a family of ribonucleic acid (RNA) viruses containing the enzyme, reverse transcriptase, in the virion; examples include human immunodeficiency virus (HIV1, HIV2) and human T-cell lymphotropic virus.

standard precautions Guidelines recommended by the Centers for Disease Control and Prevention for reducing the risk of transmission of blood-borne and other pathogens in hospitals. Standard precautions apply to (1) blood; (2) all body fluids, secretions, and excretions except sweat, regardless of whether or not they contain blood; (3) nonintact skin; and (4) mucous membranes.

virulence The power of a microorganism to produce disease.

BIBLIOGRAPHY

2007 Guideline for isolation precautions: Preventing transmission of infectious agents in healthcare settings. http://www.cdc.gov/hicpac/2007IP/2007isolationPrecautions.html

29 CFR 1910.1020 Medical records standard.

29 CFR 1910.1300 Bloodborne pathogens standard.

Aehlert B: *Paramedic practice today: Above and beyond*, St. Louis, MO, 2009, Mosby.

The AIDS Institute: *Where did HIV come from?* http://www.theaidsinstitute.org/education/aids-101/where-did-hiv-come-0.

Alter MJ, Kuhnert WL, Finelli L, et al: Guidelines for laboratory testing and result reporting of antibody to hepatitis C virus, *MMWR Recomm Rep.* 52(RR-3):1–13, 2003.

American Academy of Orthopaedic Surgeons: *Nancy Caroline's emergency care in the streets*, ed 7, Burlington, MA, 2013, Jones & Bartlett Learning.

American Academy of Pediatrics Committee on Infectious Diseases and Committee on Fetus and Newborn: Revised indications for the use of palivizumab and respiratory syncytial virus immune globulin intravenous for the prevention of respiratory syncytial virus infection, *Pediatrics.* 112(6 Pt 1):1442–1446, 2003.

Association for Professionals in Infection Control and Epidemiology, Inc: *APIC text of infection control and epidemiology*, Washington, DC, 2009, APIC.

CDC Division of Bacterial and Mycotic Diseases: *Streptococcus pneumoniae* disease prevention and control of meningococcal disease: Recommendations of the Advisory Committee on Immunization Practices (ACIP), *MMWR, Morb Mortal Wkly Rep*, May 27, 2005.

Centers for Disease Control and Prevention: *Chickenpox (varicella), clinical overview.* Updated August 22, 2013. http://www.cdc.gov/chickenpox/hcp/clinical-overview.html

Centers for Disease Control and Prevention: *Chikungunya virus.* Updated February 10, 2015. http://www.cdc.gov/chikungunya/

Centers for Disease Control and Prevention: *Controlling tuberculosis in the United States.* Published 2005. http://www.cdc.gov/mmwr/preview/mmwrhtml/rr5412a1.htm.

Centers for Disease Control and Prevention: *Fight the bite!* www.cdc.gov/ncidod/dvbid/westnile/index.htm.

Centers for Disease Control and Prevention: *Guidance on H1N1 influenza A.* www.cdc.gov/h1n1.

Centers for Disease Control and Prevention: *Immunization schedules.* http://www.cdc.gov/vaccines/schedules/

Centers for Disease Control and Prevention: *Guideline for hand hygiene in health-care settings: recommendations of the Healthcare Infection Control Practices Committee and the HICPAC/SHEA/APIC/IDSA Hand Hygiene Task Force.* 2002. http://www.cdc.gov/Handhygiene

Centers for Disease Control and Prevention: *Hantavirus.* Reviewed February 6, 2013. http://www.cdc.gov/hantavirus/hps/index.html

Centers for Disease Control and Prevention: *HPV and men—fact sheet.* Updated January 28, 2015. http://www.cdc.gov/std/hpv/stdfact-hpv-and-men.htm

Centers for Disease Control and Prevention: *HPV vaccination.* Updated July 31, 2015. http://www.cdc.gov/vaccines/vpd-vac/hpv/default.htm

Centers for Disease Control and Prevention: *Lyme disease.* Updated May 4, 2015. http://www.cdc.gov/lyme/

Centers for Disease Control and Prevention: *The national plan to eliminate syphilis from the United States.* May 2006. http://www.cdc.gov/stopsyphilis/SEEPlan2006.pdf

Centers for Disease Control and Prevention: *Parasites—American trypanosomiasis (also known as Chagas disease).* Updated July 19, 2013. http://www.cdc.gov/parasites/chagas/

Centers for Disease Control: *Parasites: Lice.* Updated September 24, 2013. http://www.cdc.gov/parasites/lice/

Centers for Disease Control and Prevention: *Rocky Mountain spotted fever (RMSF).* Updated November 21, 2013. http://www.cdc.gov/rmsf/

Centers for Disease Control and Prevention: *Syphilis & MSM (men who have sex with men)—CDC fact sheet.* Updated December 16, 2014. http://www.cdc.gov/std/syphilis/stdfact-msm-syphilis.htm

Centers for Disease Control and Prevention: *Tetanus.* Updated January 9, 2013. http://www.cdc.gov/tetanus/index.html

Centers for Disease Control and Prevention: *Rabies.* http://www.cdc.gov/rabies/

Centers for Disease Control and Prevention: *Special pathogens branch: Viral hemorrhagic fevers.* Reviewed June 19, 2013. http://www.cdc.gov/Ncidod/dvrd/spb/mnpages/dispages/vhf.htm

Centers for Disease Control and Prevention: *Updated U.S. public health service guidelines for the management of occupational exposures to HBC, HCV, and HIV, recommendations for postexposure prophylaxis.* 2005. http://www.cdc.gov/mmwr/preview/mmwrhtml/rr5011a1.htm

Centers for Disease Control and Prevention: *Viral hepatitis - hepatitis C information, hepatitis C FAQs for health professionals.* Updated May 31, 2015. http://www.cdc.gov/hepatitis/HCV/HCVfaq.htm#c2

Cohen J, Powderly WG: *Infectious diseases*, ed 2, St. Louis, MO, Mosby, 2004.

CPL 2-2.69, Enforcement procedures for the occupational exposure to bloodborne pathogens, Washinton, DC, Occupational Safety and Health Administration, November 27, 2001.

Cross JR, West KH: Clarifying HIPAA and disclosure of disease information, *JEMS.* August, 2007. http://www.jems.com/articles/2007/07/clarifying-hipaa-and-disclosur.html

Global tuberculosis control, WHO report. 2008. http://data.unaids.org/pub/Report/2008/who2008globaltbreport_en.pdf

Hall AJ, Lopman B: *Travelers' health, Norovirus.* Updated August 1, 2013. http://wwwnc.cdc.gov/travel/yellowbook/2014/chapter-3-infectious-diseases-related-to-travel/norovirus

Kretsinger K, Broder KR, Cortese MM, et al: Preventing tetanus, diphtheria, and pertussis among adults: Use of tetanus toxoid, reduced diphtheria toxoid, and acellular pertussis vaccine; Recommendations of the Advisory Committee on Immunization Practices (ACIP) and recommendation of ACIP, *MMWR Recomm Rep.* 55(RR-17):1–37, December 15, 2006.

Lessa FC, Gould CV, McDonald LC: Current status of *Clostridium difficile* infection epidemiology, *Clin Infect Dis.* 55(suppl 2):S65–S70, 2012. http://cid.oxfordjournals.org/content/55/suppl_2/S65.full

Mast EE, Weinbaum CM, Fiore AE, et al: A comprehensive immunization strategy to eliminate transmission of hepatitis B virus infection in the United States: Recommendations of the Advisory Committee on Immunization Practices (ACIP) part II; Immunization of adults, *MMWR Morb Mortal Wkly Rep.* 56(42):1114, 2007.

McCance KL, Huether SE: *Pathophysiology: The biologic basis for disease in adults and children*, ed 5, St. Louis, MO, 2006, Elsevier.

Meningitis Research Foundation: *Hib meningitis.* http://www.meningitis.org/disease-info/types-causes/hib-meningitis

Needlestick Prevention Act, public law 106-430, U.S. Congress, March 2000.

Recommended antimicrobial agents for treatment and postexposure prophylaxis of pertussis, *MMWR Recomm Rep.* 54(RR-14):1–16, 2005.

Respiratory protection for healthcare workers in the workplace against novel H1N1 influenza A: A letter report, Institute of Medicine, 2009. http://www.iom.edu/Reports/2009/Resp-ProtH1N1.aspx

Roome AJ, Hadler JL, Thomas AL, et al: Hepatitis C virus infection among firefighters, emergency medical technicians, and paramedics—selected locations, United States, 1991–2000, *MMWR Morb Mortal Wkly Rep.* 49(29):660–665, 2000.

Ryan White CARE Act, S. 1793, part G, §2695, notification of possible exposure to infectious diseases, September 30, 2009—reauthorization.

Sanders MJ: *Mosby's paramedic textbook*, ed 3 revised, St. Louis, MO, 2007, Mosby.

Shankar SK, Mahadevan A, Dias Sapico S, et al: Rabies viral encephalitis with proable (sic) 25-year incubation period! *Ann of Indian Acad Neurol.* 15(3):221–223, July–September 2012. http://www.ncbi.nlm.nih.gov/pmc/articles/PMC3424805/

Siegel JD, Rhinehart E, Jackson M, et al: *2007 guideline for isolation precautions: Preventing transmission of infectious agents in healthcare settings.* www.cdc.gov/ncidod/dhqp/pdf/guidelines/Isolation2007.pdf

Trends in tuberculosis—United States, 2008, *MMWR Morb Mortal Wkly Rep.* 58(10):249–253, 2009.

U.S. Department of Transportation National Highway Traffic Safety Administration: *EMT-paramedic national standard curriculum*, Washington, DC, 1998, The Department.

U.S. Department of Transportation National Highway Traffic Safety Administration: *National EMS education standards, draft 3.0*, Washington, DC, 2008, The Department.

West KH: *Infectious disease handbook for emergency care personnel*, ed 3, Cincinnati, OH, 2001, ACGIH.

Workowski KA, Berman SM: *Sexually transmitted diseases treatment guidelines, CDC.* 2006. http://www.cdc.gov/mmwr/preview/mmwrhtml/rr5511a1.htm

World Health Organization: *10 facts on obesity.* 2014. http://www.who.int/features/factfiles/obesity/en/

World Health Organization: *Global alert and response (GAR): Hepatitis C.* http://www.who.int/csr/disease/hepatitis/whocdscsrlyo2003/en/index4.html

World Health Organization: *Global incidence and prevalence of selected curable sexually transmitted infections, 2008*, Geneva, Switzerland, World Health Organization, 2012.

World Health Organization: *Immunizations, vaccines and biologicals: Pneumococcal disease.* Updated October 2011. http://www.who.int/immunization/topics/pneumococcal_disease/en/

World Health Organization: *Immunization, vaccines and biologicals: WHO Consultation on respiratory syncytial virus (RSV) vaccine development.* March 23–24, 2015. http://www.who.int/immunization/research/meetings_workshops/rsv_vaccine_development/en/

World Health Organization: *International travel and health: Hantavirus diseases.* http://www.who.int/ith/diseases/hantavirus/en/

World Health Organization: *International travel and health: Lyme borreliosis (Lyme disease)*, http://www.who.int/ith/diseases/lyme/en/

World Health Organization: *International travel and health: Mumps.* http://www.who.int/ith/diseases/mumps/en/

World Health Organization: *Measles, Fact sheet No 286.* Reviewed February 2015, http://www.who.int/mediacentre/factsheets/fs286/en/

World Health Organization: *Media centre: Chagas disease (American trypanosomiasis)*, Fact sheet 340. Updated March 2015. http://www.who.int/mediacentre/factsheets/fs340/en/

World Health Organization: *Media centre: Chikungunya*, Fact sheet 327. Updated May 2015. http://www.who.int/mediacentre/factsheets/fs327/en

World Health Organization: *Media centre: Immunization coverage*, Fact sheet 378. Reviewed April 2015. http://www.who.int/mediacentre/factsheets/fs378/en/

World Health Organization: *Media centre: Rabies*, Fact Sheet 99. Updated September 2014. http://www.who.int/mediacentre/factsheets/fs099/en/

World Health Organization: *Media centre: Tuberculosis*, Fact sheet 104. Reviewed March 2015. http://www.who.int/mediacentre/factsheets/fs104/en/

World Health Organization: *Media centre: West Nile virus*, Fact sheet 354. July 2011. http://www.who.int/mediacentre/factsheets/fs354/en/

World Health Organization: *Neglected tropical diseases: Scabies.* http://www.who.int/neglected_diseases/diseases/scabies/en/

World Health Organization: *Tetanus.* March 7, 2012. http://www.wpro.who.int/mediacentre/factsheets/fs_20120307_tetanus/en/

World Health Organization: *WHO launches guidelines for the treatment of persons with chronic hepatitis B infection.* 2012. http://www.who.int/hiv/en/

CHAPTER REVIEW QUESTIONS

1. Which of the following is an example of a pandemic?
   a. Three people are exposed to norovirus and two become ill.
   b. Thousands die or become ill from an influenza outbreak on all 7 continents.
   c. A child who was not immunized presents with a case of measles.
   d. Thousands die or become ill from an Ebola outbreak in a country.

2. You are treating a patient who has been diagnosed with *Mycobacterium* pulmonary tuberculosis. He has a persistent cough, night sweats, a headache, and chest pain. He has received an initial dose of isoniazid. He is in which stage of the communicable disease?
   a. Latent disease
   b. Incubation period
   a. Communicability period
   b. Disease period

3. What action can a provider take to decrease the chance of becoming infected when caring for patients with communicable diseases?
   a. Participate in vaccination/immunization programs
   b. Report exposures within 48 hours of the incident
   c. Keep gloves on at all times
   d. Wash hands before caring for patients

4. Antibodies are produced in response to exposure to?
   a. antigens
   b. defensins
   c. acids
   d. opsonins

5. Hepatitis C (HCV) is transmitted by which route?
   a. Airborne
   b. Droplet
   c. Oral–fecal
   d. Blood-borne

6. The best measures you can take to reduce your risk of acquiring meningococcal meningitis occupational exposure is to:
   a. Take care with sharps.
   b. Get immune globulin if you have an exposure.
   c. Take postexposure drugs as prescribed.
   d. Use standard precautions.

7. You are caring for a patient with *Clostridium difficile* (*C. diff*). Which actions should you take to clean after the event?
   a. Wash your hands with soap water and vigorous scrubbing.
   b. Air out the area and expose to light.
   c. Clean equipment/area with a nonchlorine bleach solution.
   d. Use an alcohol-based gel to clean your hands.

8. Which of the following can be prevented through vaccination?
   a. Shigellosis
   b. Pertussis
   c. *Escherichia coli*
   d. Lyme disease

9. Which of the following people with varicella-zoster (chickenpox) is no longer contagious?
   a. A 5-year-old with a fever 1 to 2 days before the rash appears.
   b. A 17-year-old with weeping vesicles and crusty dry lesions.
   c. A 14-year-old with lesions that are all crusted and dry.
   d. A 23-year-old who was immunized and now has a break-through rash.

10. Your adolescent patient presents with fever and abdominal cramps and is bent over due to the joint pain. Which infectious disease would you suspect?
    a. Chagas
    b. Dengue
    c. Chikungunya
    d. Ebola

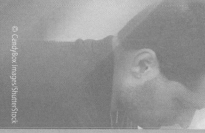

CHAPTER 9

Environmental-Related Disorders

In this chapter, illnesses and injuries related to cold, heat, and pressure are discussed. Unique to environmental emergencies are the conditions that directly cause harm or complicate treatment and transport considerations. Wind, rain, snow, temperature extremes, and humidity may all affect the body's ability to adapt to its environment. The AMLS assessment pathway will guide your decisions and help you recognize and effectively treat patients with environmental emergencies in various settings.

LEARNING OBJECTIVES

At the conclusion of this chapter, you will be able to:

- Describe the pathophysiology, assessment, and management of environmental emergencies.

- Formulate provisional diagnoses on the basis of assessment findings for various environmental-related disorders.

- Describe cold injuries and their underlying causes.

- Describe the process of providing emergency care to a person who has experienced an emergency related to cold using the AMLS assessment pathway.

- Describe the different forms of illnesses caused by heat exposure, including their signs and symptoms.

- Describe the process of providing emergency care to a person who has experienced an emergency related to heat using the AMLS assessment pathway.

- Define drowning, diving, and altitude emergencies and explain how they may be treated.

SCENARIO

You're caring for a 30-year-old man who fell through the ice while riding his snowmobile. He was able to walk home from the incident and wrap himself in a blanket. He was lying on the floor conscious and shivering when you arrived. His vital signs include a blood pressure of 80/40 mm Hg; pulse rate, 104 beats/min, weak and irregular; and respirations, 10 breaths/min, slow and shallow.

- How do you begin assessment of this patient?
- What clinical conditions and injuries might this patient be suffering from? What information do you need to determine which of these is present?
- What are your initial treatment priorities as you continue your patient care?

You may not expect to encounter environmental emergencies frequently in your practice environment, particularly if you are in an urban setting. However, environmental emergencies are more common than expected. Socioeconomic factors contribute to a surprisingly high number of environmental emergencies even in urban environments. For example, there were on average 1301 deaths annually in the United States from hypothermia during the years 1999–2011. Environmental emergencies (Table 9-1) include medical conditions caused or worsened by the weather, terrain, or unique atmospheric conditions present at high altitude or under water. Chapter 10 details the toxicology and treatment of envenomation.

Anatomy and Physiology

Temperature Regulation and Related Disorders

Most heat- and cold-related emergencies occur during seasonal exposure to significant temperature changes. You may associate such environmental emergencies with outdoor activities, but such problems are also common among special populations in urban areas, such as homeless patients who lack shelter and elderly people without proper environmental controls in their housing. Many medical conditions and medications impair the ability to regulate temperature and make people more susceptible to insults from changes in environmental temperature.

The process by which the body compensates for temperature changes is called **thermoregulation**. Normal body temperature has a diurnal fluctuation between 96.8°F and 99.5°F (36°C and 37.5°C), and the body uses both behavioral (avoidance of temperature discomfort) and physiologic mechanisms to maintain precise control within approximately 1 degree Fahrenheit of this range. Physiologic control is centered in the hypothalamus, which contains not only the control mechanisms (selecting a temperature set point like a thermostat) but also the sensory mechanisms necessary to detect temperature changes. The body responds to differences between the set point and actual temperature using both hormones and neural control to cause changes in heat production, dissipation, and retention. For example, sweating begins almost precisely at a skin temperature of 98.6°F (37°C) and increases quickly as skin temperature rises. Temperature measurements may be

Table 9-1 **Causes of Environmental Emergencies**	
Environmental Condition	**Resulting Disease States**
Cold	Hypothermia, nonfreezing injuries (immersion foot, frost nip), freezing injuries (frostbite)
Heat	Heat exhaustion, heatstroke, heat cramps, exercise-associated hyponatremia, heat-related syncope, and **neuroleptic malignant syndrome**
Pressure change	Diving related: **barotrauma**, decompression illness Altitude related: HACE, HAPE
Submersion	Near drowning, drowning

HACE, high-altitude cerebral edema; *HAPE*, high-altitude pulmonary edema.

obtained via the oral, axillary, forehead surface, tympanic, rectal, or esophageal routes using either a digital or analog thermometer. The core body temperature—the temperature in the part of the body comprising the heart, lungs, brain, and abdominal viscera—is considered the best representation of actual body temperature. Historically rectal temperature has been considered the best representation of core body temperature. However, because the rectal temperature lags behind actual core body temperature, intraesophageal temperature is considered the gold standard in many EMS systems, and some monitors are equipped to be able to obtain continuous esophageal temperatures.

If the body temperature falls below the set point determined in the hypothalamus, the body attempts to retain heat using a range of mechanisms, including:

- Vasoconstriction to decrease radiant heat loss from the skin
- Cessation of sweating
- Shivering to increase heat production in the muscles
- Secretion of norepinephrine, epinephrine, and thyroxine to increase heat production

If the body temperature rises above the set point determined in the hypothalamus, the body attempts to shed excess heat through vasodilation and sweating. Even when people are faced with extreme environmental heat, the heat production in the body from basal metabolic processes remains nearly constant.

In cases of infection, the temperature set point in the hypothalamus is adjusted temporarily to increase body temperature and make the body less hospitable to invading pathogens. This results in a transient increase in heat generation to achieve the new set point. As the body makes these adjustments, patients may be seen to shiver or have rigors during heat production and sweat to lose heat as the fever subsides. Many drugs and toxins may also alter this temperature set point, as reviewed in Chapter 10.

AMLS Assessment Pathway

▼ Initial Observations

Environmental conditions should be noted as you prepare for the problems your patient may have—wind chill, air temperature, and whether the conditions are wet or dry. Although your dispatch call may indicate a medical or trauma emergency, cold- or heat-related illness may be part of the picture. The environment,

especially when it is hot outside, may have an impact on your patient's illness. You must also remember to protect yourself from the cold and heat.

Scene Safety Considerations

On arrival, assess scene safety. Consider potential safety hazards, such as icy streets or extremely hot pavement. Cold weather may present special problems for you and your patients, especially if a hazard such as an avalanche exists. Use appropriate standard precautions and note the number of patients at the scene. Even in hot weather it may be more appropriate to wear long sleeves to help you from being splashed with blood and other body fluids. Identify whether you need additional help, such as a search and rescue team, and request assistance as soon as possible.

Patient Cardinal Presentation/Chief Complaint

In a cold emergency, the patient's cardinal presentation/chief complaint may be only that he or she is cold, or the cold may be a complication of an existing medical or trauma condition. The National Institutes of Health has initiated a public awareness campaign informing the public to watch for "umbles"—stumbles, mumbles, bumbles, and grumbles. These behaviors are good indicators of how the cold affects the cerebral and cognitive functioning of patients in the early stages of hypothermia.

In a heat emergency, the patient's cardinal presentation/chief complaint may indicate heat illness as the primary problem, or heat may be an aggravating factor in a medical or trauma condition. The patient may report specific signs and symptoms such as a decreased level of consciousness, muscle cramping, nausea, vomiting, and the absence of perspiration.

Primary Survey

Level of Consciousness

Evaluate the patient's mental status. The patient's level of consciousness diminishes as alterations in body temperature become more severe.

Airway and Breathing

Assess your patient's ABC and address any immediate life threats. With a suspected cold- or heat-related illness, your patient assessment should take into account the physiologic changes that occur. Remove the patient from the cold and into a warm ambulance or other controlled environment as soon as possible to minimize further heat loss. Provide warm, humidified oxygen if possible to help warm the patient from the inside out.

Be aware that nausea and vomiting may occur in heat-related illness and prepare the patient by placing the patient in a position that protects the airway. Breathing may be fast because of the body's core temperature. In unresponsive patients, you will need to insert an airway and provide bag-mask ventilations according to local protocol.

Circulation/Perfusion

Palpate the patient's pulse to assess circulation. Remember that patients suffering from hypothermia may have extreme bradycardia with as few as 1 or 2 beats per minute. Expect the patient's perfusion to be compromised with a cold emergency based on the severity of the cold the patient is experiencing. Similarly, a patient experiencing a heat emergency may become hemodynamically unstable.

If the patient's pulse rate is adequate, assess the patient for perfusion and bleeding. The patient's skin condition may provide clues to the primary problem and help distinguish the type of environmental condition the patient is suffering from.

Once all immediate life threats have been addressed, a more comprehensive exam may be done to uncover any injuries or information that may not have been uncovered during the primary survey.

▼ First Impression

After you have stabilized the patient and treated any life threats, form a general impression of the patient's status and develop a list of possible differential diagnoses. Order these into a differential diagnosis by classifying them as to severity (life threatening, critical, and non–life threatening) and by likelihood. Be sure to consider less obvious conditions as well as underlying conditions that may have contributed to the patient's cardinal presentation/chief complaint.

▼ Detailed Assessment

History Taking

It may be difficult to obtain the patient's history during an environmental emergency, but you should make an attempt. Find out how long the patient has been exposed to the cold or heat. You may need to talk with the patient's family members or bystanders to obtain the patient's history.

OPQRST and SAMPLER

The OPQRST and SAMPLER mnemonics should be used to obtain the patient's complete history using a systematic approach. If possible, find out whether your patient has any underlying medical conditions that could affect your treatment. Important information also includes the medications that your patient may be taking and the last oral intake. Find out what the patient was doing prior to the exposure to help you determine the cause of the problem. Remember that older people typically do not adjust well to heat—they perspire less, feel less thirsty in response to dehydration, and acclimatize more slowly. They are also more likely to have chronic conditions such as cardiovascular disease. Among young and healthy people, infants and young children are most vulnerable to heat stress when exposed to a hot environment.

Tailor your questions to help rule in and rule out conditions in your differential diagnosis.

Secondary Survey
Vital Signs

A patient's vital signs can be affected by cold or heat exposure. Vital signs are a good indicator of the severity of the condition. If the respirations are slow and shallow, low levels of oxygen in the body will be found. Low blood pressure and a slow pulse may indicate moderate to severe hypothermia. With heat exposure, your patient may be tachycardic and tachypneic. When heat-related illness becomes severe, the blood pressure begins to fall, and the patient may go into shock. Monitor the patient's vital signs closely.

Physical Exam

If time permits in the ambulance, the detailed assessment should focus on assessing any areas of the body that have been directly affected by cold exposure. Determine the degree of damage. Is the entire body involved, or have only parts been exposed to the cold? If the patient is shivering, heat is being produced. When shivering stops and the patient remains exposed to the cold, the injury is more severe. Particular attention should be paid to mental status and cardiovascular status.

With heat exposure, the physical exam should focus on the patient's metabolism, muscles, and cardiovascular system. Examine areas with muscle cramps. Continue to monitor the patient's mental status, skin temperature, and wetness. Perform a neurologic exam if time permits.

Diagnostics

A thermometer can be used to determine the patient's core body temperature. A low-temperature thermometer is required to take the temperature of a patient with hypothermia, generally done through the rectum or when available, the esophagus. Pulse oximetry readings are often inaccurate because of the lack of perfusion to the extremities. The ECG may show signs of hypothermia such as bradycardia or Osborne waves and electrolyte abnormalities.

▼ Refine the Differential Diagnosis

Use the information you gained during your secondary survey to refine your differential diagnosis. Remember that cold injuries, regardless of the severity of the exposure, require that you look for indicators of the underlying medical condition or trauma to enable you to provide the appropriate treatment.

If you are unsure about the cause of your patient's elevated temperature and suspect a heat-related illness, treat the patient for heatstroke and contact medical control if necessary to assist you in your treatment plan.

▼ Ongoing Management

All patients with cold injuries, even mild degrees of hypothermia, require immediate transport for evaluation and treatment. Handle the patient gently to avoid causing any pain or further injury to the skin. If the patient is alert and shivering, you may begin active rewarming by moving the patient into an area of warmth and using radiant heat to assist him or her to recover body temperature. Continue oxygen administration if applied during the primary survey, or consider administering oxygen.

If the patient has moderate or severe hypothermia, active rewarming should not be done because rewarming the patient too quickly may cause a fatal cardiac arrhythmia. Many regional and state protocols include passive rewarming using high indoor heat at a specialized facility.

Patients with heat-related illness need to be removed from the hot environment, if not already done earlier during the primary survey. Reassess your patient's condition by monitoring the vital signs at least every 5 minutes and note any deterioration. Avoid causing your patient to shiver during cooling because shivering generates more heat. Patients with heatstroke should be transported immediately during cooling.

Cold-Related Illness and Injury

Hypothermia related to wilderness cold exposure is considered primary hypothermia, whereas hypothermia related to socioeconomic or concurrent medical factors is considered secondary hypothermia. Cold-related illness includes injuries due to decreased temperature (for example, frostbite and hypothermia). Cold weather injuries can also occur when the weather is warmer when a person is wet as a result of water immersion. As a healthcare provider, you are also at risk if you work in a cold environment. If cold weather search and rescue operations are possible in the areas you serve, you need to receive specialized training to protect yourself and provide appropriate care.

Frostbite

Local cold injury sets in at extremely cold temperatures, usually below the freezing point. **Frostbite** is the formation of ice crystals within local tissue in exposed areas. It commonly occurs in distal extremities, particularly the toes and feet, but it can affect the upper extremities or other areas as well. Factors that can increase an individual's chance of a cold injury include central hypothermia, prolonged time of exposure, exposure to wind, wearing wet clothing, inactivity or immobility, alcohol consumption, and preexisting medical conditions and medications that result in decreased peripheral circulation. The areas of the body that are most at risk are the extremities and the nose, ears, and penis.

Frostbite injury can be divided into several clinical stages. **Frostnip** is the first and least severe manifestation of frostbite. For the purpose of management, frostbite is classified as either superficial or deep. However, like burns, frostbite has been classified into degrees of injury *after* rewarming, because most frostbite injuries initially appear similar (Table 9-2).

Pathophysiology

The pathophysiology of frostbite is complex and involves several stages of cold injury. The amount of tissue destruction is directly related to the extent of cold exposure. Systemic hypothermia predisposes to worse injury as the body is unable to oppose the cold temperatures at the extremities. The formation of ice crystals in vulnerable tissues touches off an inflammatory reaction that culminates in cellular death. The crystals tend to form in extracellular areas, altering the local electrolyte balance as the crystals draw water out of adjacent cells resulting in cellular dysfunction and death. If the affected areas continue to be exposed to cold, the crystals may grow, causing a local mechanical obstruction of blood vessels.

One of the most important concepts in the pathophysiology of frostbite is thawing. When a frozen tissue thaws, the supply of blood to local capillaries is temporarily restored. The blood

Table 9-2 Classification of Frostbite	
Degree	**Characteristics After Rewarming**
First	No blisters or erythema; numbness and tingling
Second	Clear blisters, edema, erythema
Third	Hemorrhagic blisters, subcutaneous involvement, dead skin, and tissue loss
Fourth	Full-thickness (bone and muscle) tissue loss, necrosis, and deformity

supply rapidly dwindles, however, as local arterioles and venules release small emboli, inducing hypoxia and thrombosis within the local vasculature. Starved of nutrients, local tissues begin to die, releasing further inflammatory substances and electrolytes. The process of thawing and refreezing, then, is more dangerous and damaging than the initial cold insult.

Signs and Symptoms

Frostbite can initially have a deceptively benign appearance, but it is important not to confuse frostbite with frostnip, a superficial cold insult. The patient may complain of clumsiness or heaviness in an extremity and will probably report coldness and numbness of the affected area, with pain and sensitivity to light touch. The patient may also report tingling, throbbing, and transient numbness that resolves fairly rapidly with rewarming. This is because nerves and blood vessels are most susceptible to cold injury. Complete anesthesia in a painful, cold extremity is a red flag for severe injury.

Your initial clinical examination will help you determine the extent and severity of frostbite, but it is important to note that it may take weeks or even months for the full extent of tissue damage to be visible. Frostbitten tissue will look white or blue-white, will be cool to the touch, and may be hard if still frozen. The skin may lack sensation. Signs and symptoms of superficial and deep frostbite are given in Table 9-3.

Treatment

Prehospital intervention is primarily limited to supporting vital functions and protecting affected extremities. Always search for and treat any systemic hypothermia or trauma first. If frostbite involves the lower extremities, do not allow the person to walk. Remove any jewelry or clothing that may compress the tissue, and remove wet or cold clothing. Apply constant warmth with blankets or towels. Friction or massage is ineffective and can damage injured tissue. The most effective therapy is rapid rewarming of the frozen area by immersion in warm water (104°F [40°C]). This treatment is not recommended, however, if there is *any* risk of refreezing. Transport the patient to an appropriate facility. Patients may require tetanus boosters, antibiotics, specialized wound care, and in some cases amputation.

Immersion Foot
Pathophysiology

Immersion foot, also known as "trench foot" or a "non-freezing cold injury," was most famously described in soldiers who spent many hours standing in the trenches during World War I. The condition results from prolonged periods of wetness of the feet, particularly in cool water. This prolonged cold, wet exposure is thought to result in vasoconstriction and ischemia of the tissues of the foot, which eventually leads to necrosis. Today this condition may be seen in builders, hikers, extreme-sports enthusiasts, security guards, campers, and aid-workers during natural disasters.

Signs and Symptoms

Immersion foot begins with local discomfort in the affected foot. A tingling or heavy sensation is sometimes described. The foot will be blotchy, cold, devitalized, and wrinkled appearing. The discomfort will increase with rewarming and the tissue will turn red. Blisters eventually form, and the skin may slough off.

Treatment

Prehospital management of immersion foot should be centered around removing the patient from the cold and wet conditions. Pain control may be needed. Longer term care involves strict hygiene, antibiotics if infection occurs, and keeping the feet warm and dry.

Systemic Hypothermia

Systemic **hypothermia**, defined as a core body temperature below 95°F (35°C), is a common environmental emergency. Hypothermia is caused by heat loss, decreased heat production, or a combination of the two. The condition can be attributed to a range of metabolic, traumatic, environmental, and infectious causes, but it occurs most often in patients who are exposed to cold environments. It is important to remember that in the presence of certain risk factors (prolonged time of exposure, exposure to wind, wearing wet clothing, inactivity or immobility, alcohol consumption), hypothermia can be precipitated at

Table 9-3 Comparison of Superficial and Deep Frostbite Initial Presentations	
Superficial Frostbite	**Deep Frostbite**
Numbness	Hemorrhagic blisters
Paresthesia (extreme pain during rewarming)	Diminished range of motion
Poor fine motor control (clumsiness)	Necrosis, gangrene
Pruritus	Cold, mottled, gray area (after rewarming)
Edema (usually after rewarming)	Immobile tissue (lost elasticity)
Coldness	

temperatures well above freezing. EMS providers must be able to recognize the signs and symptoms of systemic hypothermia.

Pathophysiology

Heat loss occurs via four mechanisms: radiation, conduction, evaporation, and convection. Anytime the body's heat production ability is overwhelmed by heat loss, the patient is at risk of hypothermia. The pathophysiology of hypothermia is complex and involves the cardiovascular, renal, neurologic, and respiratory systems. As the body's core temperature drops, each of these systems responds with the aim of preserving heat:

- *Vasoconstriction.* First, peripheral blood vessels constrict in an effort to shift more blood to vital organs. Later, in severe hypothermia, blood flow to entire organs such as the kidneys drops by up to 50%, threatening renal function and upsetting electrolyte balance.
- *Diuresis.* Vasoconstriction increases urinary output, a menacing development in a volume-depleted patient. Urinary output is up to 3.5 times higher if the patient is immersed in cold water. Alcohol consumption further increases diuresis.
- *Respiratory acidosis.* Respiratory rate decreases, followed by a drop in minute ventilation as a result of diminished metabolism. In severe hypothermia, CO_2 retention causes respiratory acidosis.

- *Tachycardia and bradycardia.* Sinus tachycardia predominates during the initial phases of hypothermia. Later, as hypothermia becomes more severe, bradycardia ensues as a result of diminished depolarization in the pacemaker cells. In this type of bradydysrhythmia, administration of atropine is often ineffective and is not needed because overall metabolism is diminished.
- *Atrial or ventricular fibrillation and asystole.* In mild to moderate hypothermia, atrial or ventricular dysrhythmias can develop as a result of conduction changes that decrease transmembrane resting potential. As hypothermia worsens, the risk of ventricular fibrillation and asystole increases.
- *Electrocardiographic anomalies.* Several unique electrocardiographic manifestations can point to a diagnosis of hypothermia. The classic Osborne (J) wave appears at the junction between the QRS complex and the ST segment (**Figure 9-1**). Osborne waves usually become evident at temperatures below 91.4°F (33°C). As the condition worsens, all intervals—particularly the QT interval—become prolonged. You may have trouble analyzing the ECG because of artifacts generated by the patient's shivering.

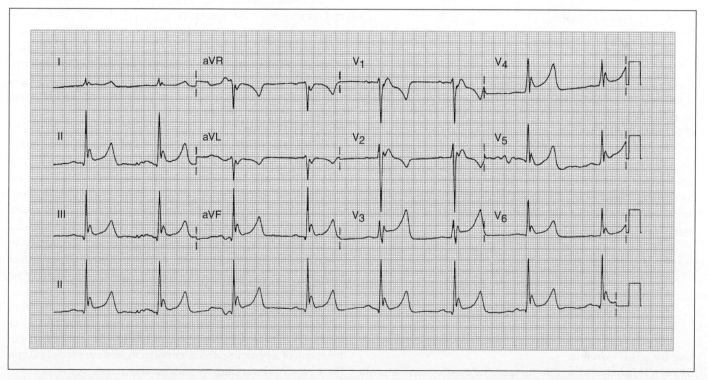

Figure 9-1 Systemic hypothermia is associated with distinctive bulging of the J point (very beginning of the ST segment). Prominent J waves (arrows) with hypothermia are referred to as Osborne waves.

Signs and Symptoms

EMS providers must maintain a high degree of suspicion for hypothermia. In some cases, when the patient has been exposed to the elements, the diagnosis is obvious. In other cases, the clinical findings may be subtle. Nonspecific symptoms—chills, nausea, hunger, vomiting, dyspnea, dizziness—may be early signs.

A rapid determination of accurate body temperature is often difficult in the prehospital environment. Normal household thermometers will not be able to accurately measure extreme low temperatures. Available methods such as tympanic, rectal, and esophageal all pose difficulties with accuracy and availability. Because of this, it is often necessary to diagnose systemic hypothermia in the prehospital environment based on history and presentation rather than discrete measurement. Systemic hypothermia is classified as mild, moderate, or severe based on temperature and the body's ability to rewarm itself. Certain clinical findings and core temperatures are characteristic of each stage, although signs and symptoms are variable, and the stages often overlap.

Mild Hypothermia In mild hypothermia (89.6°F to 95°F [32°C to 35°C]), most people will shiver vigorously. This can be accompanied by nonspecific symptoms such as dizziness, lethargy, nausea, and weakness. An increased metabolic rate occurs in this range as the body tries to produce more heat. More severe neurologic signs such as ataxia (uncoordinated movement) appear once a person's temperature drops to 91.4°F (33°C). Other signs include:

- Hyperventilation
- Tachypnea
- Tachycardia

In this stage, the body is generally able to rewarm itself if removed from the cold stress quickly and adequate energy reserves are still available.

Moderate Hypothermia As moderate hypothermia (82.4°F to 89.6°F [28°C to 32°C]) develops, clinical signs of deterioration become apparent. Breathing and heart rate slow, and mental status declines. At 89.6°F (32°C), the patient will become stuporous. As core temperature approaches 87.8°F (31°C), the patient will lose the shivering reflex. Other signs and symptoms of moderate hypothermia include:

- Poor judgment
- Atrial fibrillation
- Bradycardia, bradypnea
- Diuresis (increased urinary output)

In this stage, the body has very little if any ability to generate heat for self-rewarming.

Severe Hypothermia Life-threatening cardiovascular problems appear during severe hypothermia (68°F to 84°F [20°C to 28°C]). Hypotension and ventricular arrhythmias become apparent, and a J wave may be seen on the cardiac monitor. The patient is usually unconscious, with dilated and minimally responsive pupils. At this stage, the patient is near cardiac arrest and very susceptible to ventricular fibrillation from even minimal physical manipulation. In this stage the body has no ability to self-rewarm.

Differential Diagnosis

Other causes of hypothermia include metabolic disorders that are linked to a decreased basal metabolic rate and can be related to dysfunction of the thyroid, adrenal, or pituitary glands.

Treatment

Prehospital management must be guided by the severity of the hypothermia and by the methods available to rewarm the patient. The number one priority should be to stop further heat loss, usually by removing the patient from the cold environment. A patient in a cold, remote setting needs immediate evacuation to a warm environment. Rewarm the patient, prevent further heat loss, and avoid actions that may precipitate complications. For example, rough handling of a severely hypothermic patient can precipitate a cardiac arrhythmia.

Regardless of the severity of the hypothermia, you must focus on supporting airway, breathing, and circulation as needed and remove any cold, wet clothing (cut clothes off the severely hypothermic patient to avoid excessive movement) to prevent a further drop in core temperature. In addition, nearly all hypothermic patients experience volume depletion. Before administering fluids, warm them to 104°F to 107.6°F (40°C to 42°C). EMS systems that regularly respond to patients with hypothermia should have access to fluid warmers.

Mild Hypothermia Most cases of mild hypothermia (89.6°F to 95°F [32°C to 35°C]) will resolve with passive rewarming techniques (e.g., using blankets to help contain the patient's own body heat). In addition to the aforementioned general management instructions, provide warm oral fluids if there are no airway concerns. Avoid caffeinated beverages, however, because they can encourage diuresis. Alcohol and tobacco should also be avoided. Reassess the patient frequently to evaluate for improvement or decline. Mildly hypothermic patients can quickly deteriorate to become moderately or severely hypothermic.

Moderate Hypothermia Mental status changes become more apparent in patients with moderate hypothermia (82.4°F to 89.6°F [28°C to 32°C]). Management begins with immediate stabilization of airway, breathing, circulation, and core temperature. Start passive rewarming techniques and initiate active rewarming as well, such as forced warm air and administration of warm IV fluids. Do not permit the patient to stand or walk, because movement may precipitate a cardiac arrhythmia. Transport the

Table 9-4 Key Considerations in the Management of Severe Hypothermia
Dependent lividity and fixed, dilated pupils are not dependable criteria for withholding CPR in a hypothermic patient.
Evaluation of vital signs and ECG tracings may be difficult because the patient may have an undetectable pulse. Spend a longer time than usual (up to 60 seconds) to check for signs of circulation. If there is any doubt or you are unable to detect a pulse, start CPR immediately.
Patients with severe hypothermia often have bradycardia. This may be a protective mechanism, because a slow heart rhythm can deliver sufficient oxygen under hypothermic conditions. The use of pacing is rarely indicated.
A patient with severe hypothermia will have a significantly reduced metabolic rate, resulting in a toxic buildup of cardiac resuscitation agents. Consider withholding drugs in a patient with a core temperature < 86°F (< 30°C), because the heart is unlikely to respond to drugs at this temperature.
Consider early endotracheal intubation for ventilation with warm humidified oxygen when available.
Defibrillation may be unlikely to be effective at core temperatures < 86°F (< 30°C). Consider withholding repeated defibrillation attempts until the core temperature can be increased above this point.
Gastric dilation and decreased gastric motility can occur in severe hypothermia. Physical examination of the abdomen is unreliable because of rectus muscle rigidity, so after tracheal intubation, you should place a nasogastric tube in patients with moderate or severe hypothermia.

CPR, Cardiopulmonary resuscitation; *ECG,* electrocardiogram.

patient rapidly and gently to an emergency department for continuous rewarming and observation.

Severe Hypothermia Patients with severe hypothermia (68°F to 84°F [20°C to 28°C]) are usually unconscious. Stabilization of airway, breathing, and circulation is essential to prevent further deterioration. If there is a palpable pulse, handle the patient gently and avoid abrupt movements. If the patient is in cardiac arrest, begin CPR immediately. The priority will be to provide quality compressions during active rewarming. Intravenous medications and defibrillation will have limited benefit at these temperatures. Active rewarming techniques include warming blankets, warm IV fluids, and bladder irrigation. More invasive active rewarming techniques include warm fluid irrigation through tube thoracostomy and extracorporeal membrane oxygenation. In some remote regions, resuscitation efforts for hypothermic patients who are found in cardiac arrest are terminated in the field. However, in most jurisdictions, hypothermia is a contraindication to field termination of resuscitation. Key considerations in treating severe hypothermia are described in Table 9-4.

Heat-Related Illness

Heat-related illness is a unique set of disorders brought on when the body is exposed to heat for extended periods. Heat-related illness may also be triggered by exercising too much and not staying adequately hydrated in hot conditions. An inappropriate amount of exercise for one's age or physical condition is a risk factor for developing a heat-related illness. Certain groups—the very old, the very young, and those with obesity—are at higher risk. Table 9-5 present common heat-related disorders.

Heat Cramps

Heat cramps are a common heat-related emergency among people who work or exercise in hot temperatures. These painful muscle contractions usually occur after physical activity has stopped. The classic history involves a person who has been working in a hot environment who experiences cramps after stopping to rest.

Pathophysiology

Heat cramps cause painful muscular spasms attributable to dehydration and electrolyte imbalances such as hyponatremia and hypokalemia. Such imbalances are characteristic of muscles that are fatigued after engaging in strenuous work. A direct correlation exists between heat cramps and salt depletion. The typical patient is someone who has been working or exercising in a hot, dry environment and losing salt by sweating but drinking hypotonic fluids that replenish fluids but do not replace salt.

Table 9-5 Common Heat-Related Disorders

Disorder	Cause/Problem	Signs/Symptoms	Treatment
Muscle (heat) cramps	Failure to replace sodium chloride (salt, or NaCl) lost through sweating; electrolyte and muscle problems	Painful muscle cramps, usually in legs or abdomen	Move to cool place; massage/stretch muscle; encourage drinking sport drinks with NaCl (e.g., tomato juice). Transport those with signs or symptoms listed below.
Dehydration	Failure to replace lost sweat with fluids	Thirst, nausea, excessive fatigue, headache, hypovolemia, decreased thermoregulation; reduces physical and mental capacity	Replace sweat loss with lightly salted fluids; rest in cool place until body weight and water losses are restored. In some patients, IV rehydration is necessary.
Heat exhaustion	Excessive heat strain with inadequate water intake; cardiovascular problems with venous pooling, decreased cardiac filling time, reduced cardiac output; untreated, may progress to heatstroke	Low urine output, tachycardia, weakness, unstable gait, extreme fatigue, wet clammy skin headache, dizziness, nausea, collapse	Remove from heat source and place in cooler location; cool body with water and fanning; encourage drinking lightly salted fluids (e.g., sports drinks); administer intravenous 0.9% NaCl or lactated Ringer's solution.
Heatstroke	High core temperatures > 105°F (40.6°C); cellular disruption; dysfunction of multiple organ systems common; neurologic disorder with thermoregulatory center failure	Mental status changes; irrational behavior or delirium; possible shivering; tachycardia initially, then bradycardia late; hypotension; rapid and shallow breathing; dry or wet, hot skin; loss of consciousness; seizures and coma	Emergency: Apply rapid, immediate cooling by water immersion, or wet patient or wrap in cool, wet sheets and fan vigorously. Continue until core temperature is < 102°F (38.9°C). Treat for shock if necessary once core temperature is lowered. Immediately transport to emergency department.
Exercise-associated hyponatremia (also referred to as water intoxication)	Low plasma sodium concentration; typically seen in individuals during prolonged activity in hot environments; drinking water (> 4 L/hour) that exceeds sweat rate; failure to replace sodium lost in sweat.	Nausea, vomiting, malaise, dizziness, ataxia, headache, altered mental status, polyuria, pulmonary edema, signs of intracranial pressure, seizures, coma; core temperature < 102°F (39.9°C); mimics signs of heat illness	Restrict water intake; give salty foods/saline. Unresponsive patients receive ABC standard care, 15 L/min of oxygen by nonrebreathing mask. If available, provide hypertonic saline (100-mL bolus of 3% hypertonic saline), which can be repeated twice at 10-minute intervals. Transport immediately with alert patient in sitting position or unresponsive patient in left-lateral position.

Signs and Symptoms

Cramps can occur all over the body, but the legs and abdomen are the most common sites. Patients will be sweaty and sometimes nauseated.

Differential Diagnosis

Heat cramps must not be confused with athletic cramps, which occur during athletic activity and resolve with massage. Heat cramps most often involve several different muscles, whereas athletic cramps typically occur in one muscle due to overexertion or stretching.

Treatment

Heat cramps unaccompanied by associated heat-related illnesses are not a life-threatening emergency. Commercially available oral salt solutions, such as Gatorade or Powerade, are useful in the treatment of mild heat cramps. Oral hydration is best (if the patient is not vomiting). Patients with more severe heat cramps accompanied by vomiting will require IV fluids (0.9% normal saline). Salt tablets are not recommended alone, as they can induce nausea and do not address the issue of volume depletion.

Heat Exhaustion

Heat exhaustion is caused by volume depletion from excessive sweating in hot temperatures. People who work in hot environments, such as laborers, athletes, and military personnel, are at risk if they do not drink enough water. If left untreated, heat exhaustion can progress to heatstroke.

Pathophysiology

Heat exhaustion is characterized by water depletion and salt depletion in the setting of exercise. Core temperature may be normal or elevated up to 104°F (< 40°C). Typically patients who suffer from heat exhaustion are volume depleted and hemoconcentrated.

Signs and Symptoms

The clinical manifestations of heat exhaustion are nonspecific. Central nervous system abnormalities such as seizures, coma, confusion, delirium, or severe **hyperthermia** (> 104.9°F [> 40.5°C]) suggest heatstroke rather than heat exhaustion. Signs and symptoms of heat exhaustion include the following:

- Weakness, malaise, and lethargy
- Headache
- Vertigo
- Nausea and vomiting
- Core temperature often normal or less than 40°C (< 104°F)
- Normal LOC
- Tachycardia, sweating
- Abdominal pain
- Muscle cramps

Treatment

Most patients with heat exhaustion have both water and salt depletion. The principal problem you will encounter is volume deficit. Mild cases can be managed with oral fluid replacement with salt-containing solutions. IV fluid replacement is often necessary, especially if there are any signs of hemodynamic instability. The fluid of choice is 0.9% normal saline, although determination of the patient's electrolyte status should be used to guide treatment if available. In addition, the patient should be moved to a cool, shady, or indoor environment.

Exercise-Associated Hyponatremia

A disorder closely related to sodium-depleted heat exhaustion is **exercise-associated hyponatremia**. This is one of the most common causes of death in young healthy athletes who are involved in endurance sports such as marathon running.

Pathophysiology

The most common cause of exercise-associated hyponatremia is overhydration with hypotonic fluids. Athletes lose both water and sodium through perspiration at a significant rate during exercise. If water is used as a replacement without an adequate sodium ingestion, the patient's serum sodium level is driven down. This can lead to central nervous system edema, neurologic symptoms, and death. Risk factors that have been shown to increase the risk of exercise-associated hyponatremia in the setting of marathons include excessive hydration, nonsteroidal antiinflammatory drug use, female gender, finishing time over 4 hours, and low body mass index.

Signs and Symptoms

Patients should be categorized based on symptoms rather than measured serum sodium concentrations, but relative values are given in parentheses:

- *Mild*: Dizziness, nausea, vomiting, headache (sodium 135–130 mmol/L)
- *Moderate*: Mental status changes (confusion, disorientation) (sodium 130–125 mmol/L)
- *Severe*: Altered consciousness, lethargy, pulmonary edema, seizures, coma (sodium < 125 mmol/L)

Differential Diagnosis

Symptoms of exercise-associated hyponatremia can be nonspecific, as previously discussed. A diagnosis of this type of heat illness can be challenging because there is a great deal of overlap with the signs and symptoms of heatstroke. To help you differentiate between the two conditions, remember that heatstroke always involves an altered mental status with an elevated temperature, whereas exercise–associated hyponatremia may occur without significant hyperthermia.

Treatment

As with most conditions, prevention through education of persons at risk is the best course. Athletes should be instructed to avoid excessive ingestion of hypotonic fluids during exercise. Even commercially available sports drinks do not contain enough sodium to prevent hyponatremia. Salty snacks should be eaten along with fluids.

For patients with mild to moderate symptoms, fluid restriction should be initiated, and salty snacks or broth should be administered while a sodium level is obtained. IV fluids are generally contraindicated. For patients with severe symptoms, prehospital treatment begins as usual with the ABCs. Treatment with hypertonic (3%) saline may be indicated but is extremely dangerous without appropriate expertise and the ability to monitor serum sodium levels. Treatment with hypertonic saline must be done under extremely controlled conditions and only with medical direction, as rapid correction of serum sodium concentration may result in central pontine myelinolysis, an irreversible injury to the central nervous system. Patients with severe symptoms should be transported to a facility with intensive care unit capabilities.

Heatstroke

Heatstroke is a syndrome in which the body loses its ability to regulate temperature, resulting in altered mental status, elevated core body temperature, and multiorgan failure. Core body temperature can climb to 108°F (42°C) or even higher. Consequent damage will depend on how high the body temperature is and how long it stays elevated.

Pathophysiology

An almost universal finding in patients with heatstroke is neurologic dysfunction, including altered mental status, headache, seizures, and cerebral edema. During heatstroke, remarkably increased demands are made on the cardiovascular system, which can be a principal contributor to the ultimate collapse of bodily functions. Continued heat exposure produces peripheral vasodilatation with subsequent splanchnic and renal circulatory vasoconstriction, sometimes accompanied by hepatic dysfunction. Continued heat exposure will cause hemodynamic instability, poor skin perfusion, a further elevation of core temperature, and multiorgan failure.

Heatstroke may be classified as either classic or exertional. Although it is not critical to differentiate these conditions in the field because treatment is similar, they will be discussed separately here.

Classic heatstroke is associated with prolonged exposure to even a moderately high environmental temperature and humidity level. It is classically associated with the chronically ill, bedridden, elderly, or psychiatric patient who lacks air conditioning or is using medications that impair tolerance to heat stress, such as diuretic, anticholinergic, and neuroleptic agents. Anhidrosis (lack of perspiration) is caused by extreme dehydration, skin disorders, or medication side effects.

In contrast, exertional heatstroke is associated with young people, such as athletes who train in conditions of high temperature and humidity, during which the core temperature rises faster than the body can dissipate heat. About 50% of such patients will continue to sweat even as heatstroke becomes imminent.

Signs and Symptoms

The patient with either type of heatstroke will have the following similar signs and symptoms:

- Altered mental status
- Hyperventilation
- Tachycardia
- Hypotension
- High-output cardiac failure (hypotension and tachycardia are warning signs)
- GI bleeding
- Pulmonary edema
- Electrolyte imbalance
- Hepatic dysfunction

Differential Diagnosis

Suspect heatstroke and check the core temperature of any person behaving strangely in a hot environment. The diagnosis of heatstroke is easy to miss. It may develop rapidly in a patient whose heat exhaustion was mistaken for the flu, or it may present as a coma of unknown origin. Unless you keep the possibility of heatstroke in mind during the hot months of the year and assess the patient's temperature as part of the vital signs, you may waste precious time searching for some other cause of the patient's symptoms.

Treatment

The first step in management is to recognize this potentially lethal condition. Maintain airway, ventilation, and circulation, initiate immediate cooling measures, and transport the patient rapidly to the emergency department. Place the patient on a cardiac monitor, establish two peripheral IV lines, and initiate supplemental oxygen therapy.

The patient's clothes must be removed. Check and record core temperature, preferably with a rectal or esophageal probe, every 5 minutes. Once core body temperature drops to 102.2°F (39°C), cooling measures should be stopped to avoid inducing shivering. You can lower temperature by spraying the skin with lukewarm water and fanning. Using cold water is counterproductive because it induces shivering, which elevates core body temperature.

If evidence of hypovolemic shock is present, rehydrate the patient with fluid boluses as needed. Cold IV fluids can be used. Reassess hemodynamic stability and maintain a mean arterial pressure of 60 mm Hg. Avoid fluid overload, because the patient is at risk of developing high-output cardiac failure and pulmonary edema, as described previously. If seizures are present, administer lorazepam or diazepam under medical direction or according to local protocol.

Heat Syncope and Exercise-Associated Syncope

Heat exposure combined with underlying physiologic problems that alter blood return can cause a transient loss of consciousness. This condition is more common among older adults, who are more susceptible to dehydration during heat exposure.

Pathophysiology

When a person is exposed to heat for a significant period, the body responds by dilating cutaneous vessels. Blood tends to pool in peripheral vessels. If a person stands for a prolonged period or suddenly rises from a sitting position in the heat, poor central venous return can cause inadequate cerebral perfusion, manifested as **heat syncope**.

Exercise-associated syncope has a similar pathophysiology but occurs in different circumstances. This condition usually occurs among endurance athletes whose muscles are hyperperfused with blood. The pumping action of the lower extremities facilitates venous return to the central circulation. On cessation of exercise, blood is still disproportionately distributed to skeletal muscle, but its return is no longer aided by the pumping of the legs. Blood quickly pools in the lower extremities, leading to syncope. This mechanism is much different from that of syncope *during* exercise, which suggests a more ominous diagnosis, such as hypertrophic cardiomyopathy, acute coronary syndrome, or arrhythmia.

Signs and Symptoms

Patients with heat syncope have dizziness, light-headedness, and signs of volume depletion. Those with exercise-associated syncope have these signs after cessation of exercise. The patient's body temperature is generally above 104°F (40°C).

Differential Diagnosis

Heat syncope occurs under similar conditions as heatstroke, and therefore it may not be distinguished easily from heatstroke.

Treatment

As with any heat-related illness, the patient should be moved to a cooler environment. Most cases are self-limiting, and lying down offers some relief of symptoms. Monitor the patient for signs of deterioration. People at risk for heat syncope should move frequently. Athletes, for example, should be educated to continue walking after cessation of vigorous activity and to recognize warning symptoms such as light-headedness or weakness so they can move out of the hot environment. This could help avoid potential traumatic injuries or medical sequelae that can occur after syncope.

Other Common Environmental Emergencies

Drowning

Drowning is the process of experiencing respiratory impairment from submersion or immersion in liquid. Drowning outcomes include death, morbidity, and near morbidity. Terminology describing these patients continues to evolve. Terms such as near-drowning, wet, dry, and secondary drowning are confusing and while previously popular appear now to have limited usefulness.

Pathophysiology

The drowning continuum progresses from breath holding, to laryngospasm (severe constriction of the larynx), to the accumulation of carbon dioxide and the inability to oxygenate the lungs, to subsequent respiratory and cardiac arrest from multiple-organ failure due to tissue hypoxia. The patient can be resuscitated at any point along this continuum and, generally, the earlier the resuscitation takes place, the better the success rate.

Signs and Symptoms

Most drownings are not witnessed, and therefore the person's body is found submerged or floating in the water. Toddlers typically drown in bathtubs, school-age children in pools, and teens in lakes or rivers. Comorbidities such as a seizure disorder or medical or physical handicaps may also contribute to drowning in an apparently safe environment such as a bathtub.

Treatment

The resuscitation of a victim of a drowning incident is the same as that for any other patient in respiratory or cardiac arrest, but the victim first must be reached. Providers who have specialized training and experience in water rescue are the best able to accomplish the rescue. The treatment of drowning is given in Table 9-6.

Diving Emergencies

Diving and altitude emergencies can arise from extremes of pressure at altitude or water depth. Divers have long feared the bends, the colloquial name for **decompression sickness**. Decompression sickness, direct barotrauma such as sinus or middle ear injury, and arterial gas emboli are the major illnesses associated with extreme high-pressure environments such as SCUBA diving.

All divers, irrespective of the type of diving they do, are subject to the increased ambient pressures that occur under water. Injury results from the physical effect of these pressures on the body. In order for you to understand these changes, it is important to review how gases act under certain physical conditions.

Table 9-6 **Treatment of Drowning**
Rescuers trained and practiced in performing water rescue should participate in the rescue if appropriate.
Protect the patient's cervical spine in cases of obvious trauma, diving, waterslides, or alcohol intoxication.
Ensure basic life support measures are being carried out with an emphasis on airway and oxygenation.
Anticipate vomiting; have suction immediately available.
Administer supplemental oxygen and intubate if needed.
Establish IV access.
Measure core temperature; prevent or treat hypothermia
Administer a beta-2 adrenergic agent for wheezing.
Monitor ETCO$_2$ and obtain a pulse oximetry reading.
Insert a nasogastric tube in intubated patients.
Transport every drowning patient to the hospital, including patients who seem to recover at the scene.

Pathophysiology

Diving barotrauma is explained by the laws of physics that govern the behavior of gases under pressure. Pressure changes affect the volume in air-filled spaces—in the case of the mostly fluid-filled human body, these spaces are the lungs, bowel, sinuses, and middle ear. According to **Boyle's law**, these spaces compress on descent and expand on ascent because as pressure increases, the gas volume is reduced; conversely, as pressure eases, gas volume increases.

In addition, the solubility of a gas in liquid is governed by the amount of pressure exerted on that gas, so a gas will become decreasingly dissolved in the liquid (i.e., blood) as the body ascends while diving. The body can tolerate this if the amount of gas separating from the blood is small enough to be exhaled. If the ascent is rapid, large amounts of gas are liberated, and life-threatening gas bubbles can block the circulation—the phenomenon known as decompression sickness.

The location and size of the gas bubbles will determine their clinical effects. Bubbles trapped in the muscles or joints cause pain in corresponding areas. In fact, the source of the nickname *the bends* is that this condition leaves the afflicted person doubled over for long periods of time. Gas bubbles in the spinal cord can cause paralysis, paresthesia, and anesthesia. Gas bubbles in the arterial circulation can cause limb ischemia, in the pulmonary arteries can cause pulmonary gas embolism, and in the cerebral arteries can cause stroke.

Nitrogen narcosis, a change in mental status while diving, is a slightly different clinical entity. Its effect is similar to alcohol or benzodiazepine intoxication. The condition may occur at shallow depths, but it typically doesn't set in unless the dive is more than 98 feet (30 meters). The effect is explained by the increased solubility of nitrogen under higher pressure, with consequent impairment of cognition, motor function, and sensory perception. Nitrogen narcosis also impairs judgment and coordination, potentially causing serious errors that can jeopardize underwater safety. The condition, however, is reversible and resolves over several minutes once the diver has ascended.

Signs and Symptoms

The average risk of severe decompression sickness is slightly more than 2 cases per 10,000 dives. Asthma, pulmonary blebs, and patent foramen ovale increase the risk and severity of symptoms. Decompression sickness may begin with sinus and ear pressure, pressure in the back, and joint pain and aches that worsen with motion. More severe decompression sickness may be characterized by dyspnea, chest pain, altered mental status, or shock. The most severe illness is seen with arterial gas embolism. Gas emboli often occur a few minutes after surfacing. Acute-onset dyspnea and severe chest pain are common in people with acute gas emboli, and the condition can be fatal.

Treatment

The physical exam should focus on detecting emergent symptoms, including gas emboli. Pay particular attention to performing a complete cardiovascular exam, looking for decreased breath sounds, muffled heart sounds, and heart murmurs. Jugular venous distention or petechiae on the head or neck can indicate more severe decompression sickness. Palpate the skin to detect crepitus, and palpate all pulses.

Emergency care includes careful attention to maintaining the airway with supplemental oxygen. IV hydration should be given to maintain systolic blood pressure. Placement of a urinary catheter can help in monitoring renal function. Tube thoracostomy is indicated if pneumothorax occurs. Consider hyperbaric therapy in patients having neurologic symptoms, unstable blood pressure, respiratory compromise, or altered mental status. Arrange for transport per protocol to a hyperbaric facility. If you do not know where the facility is, contact the Divers Alert Network for assistance at 919-684-9111.

High-Altitude Illnesses

Pathophysiology

The illnesses associated with ascent to high altitudes are precipitated by a combination of low atmospheric pressure and the resultant low partial pressure of oxygen. That is, although oxygen makes up 21% of atmospheric gas at all altitudes, as you ascend the total pressure of atmospheric gas decreases according to Boyle's Law and the air becomes "thinner," with fewer molecules of oxygen in each liter of air. This condition is sometimes referred to as *hypobaric hypoxia*, which results in hypoxemia. The body attempts to compensate for this decreasing availability of oxygen by increasing respiratory rate, cardiac output, and cerebral vasodilatation. Low atmospheric pressure causes capillary leaking in both the lungs and brain. Hypoxia causes a diffuse pulmonary vasoconstriction (as the body tries to overcome a perceived ventilation/perfusion mismatch), which results in pulmonary hypertension and edema. Together, these adaptive and maladaptive responses may result in the development of acute mountain sickness, high-altitude cerebral edema, and high-altitude pulmonary edema. These illnesses may overlap and coexist.

Rapid rate of ascent, lack of pre-acclimatization, poor physical fitness levels, and many medications and intoxicants may all increase risk for high-altitude emergencies. Surprisingly, people younger than 50 years are at higher risk of experiencing high-altitude illnesses.

Signs and Symptoms

Acute Mountain Sickness Acute mountain sickness (AMS) is nonspecific syndrome that may be confused with general fatigue, dehydration, hangover, or even influenza. The single most common complaint is headache. Symptoms generally begin within 24–48 hours following ascent and resolve in 3–5 days. There are no definitive physical exam findings, making a high index of suspicion critically important.

High-Altitude Cerebral Edema High altitude cerebral edema (HACE) represents a more severe illness that is often preceded by AMS and the symptoms are likewise more severe and include nausea and vomiting, ataxia, altered mental status, seizures, and paralysis. HACE often does not develop until the third day after ascent but may occur much earlier. HACE may be fatal if not appropriately treated.

High-Altitude Pulmonary Edema High-altitude pulmonary edema (HAPE) most commonly occurs on the second night following ascent. In mild cases, a dry cough and decreased tolerance to exercise may be noted. In more severe cases, dyspnea on exertion, hypoxia, and cyanosis may all develop.

Treatment

For all high-altitude illnesses beyond mild AMS, the mainstay of treatment is supplemental oxygen and immediate descent. If descent cannot be accomplished expeditiously, a portable hyperbaric chamber may be employed if available. Other therapies may be employed as follows:

- CPAP, diuretics, and calcium channel blockers may all be used in the treatment of HAPE.
- Dexamethasone and diuretics are used in treating HACE.
- NSAIDs and acetazolamide may be used for symptom control in mild AMS.

Expert consultation should be sought in all cases of high-altitude related illnesses.

Putting It All Together

Assisting patients with environmental emergencies can be among some of the most challenging problems a healthcare provider faces. Similarities and differences in cardinal presentations/chief complaints are sometimes subtle, and the underlying diagnosis can be obscured, delaying appropriate interventions. Utilizing the AMLS assessment pathway will assist in generating an appropriate differential diagnosis, obtaining a comprehensive history and focused physical exam, and refining that differential diagnosis.

SCENARIO SOLUTION

© HunThomas/ShutterStock, Inc.

- Differential diagnoses may include mild, moderate, or severe hypothermia.
- To narrow your differential diagnosis, you'll need to perform a physical examination that includes assessing for trauma injuries. The patient has a weak and rapid radial pulse; therefore, treatment priorities will focus on the treatment of any trauma injuries and passive rewarming.
- The patient has signs that may indicate hypothermia because he is shivering.

Summary

- Body temperature is regulated by neural feedback mechanisms that operate primarily through the hypothalamus; the hypothalamus contains not only the control mechanisms (which maintain a temperature set point) but also the sensory mechanisms necessary to detect and respond to body temperature changes.
- Cold emergencies include frost nip, frostbite, and systemic hypothermia.
- Heat illnesses include heatstroke, heat cramps, heat exhaustion, heat syncope and exercise-associated syncope, and neuroleptic malignant syndrome.
- Drowning is the process of experiencing respiratory impairment from submersion or immersion in liquid. Drowning progresses from breath holding, to laryngospasm, to respiratory and cardiac arrest.
- Barotrauma can result during a dive descent, owing to a pressure imbalance between the inside of the body and the outside atmosphere.
- High-altitude illnesses result from hypobaric hypoxia.

KEY TERMS

© HunThomas/ShutterStock, Inc.

acute mountain sickness Any illness that can effect the body in a high-altitude environment.

barotrauma Injury resulting from pressure disequilibrium across body surfaces.

Boyle's law At a constant temperature, the volume of a gas is inversely proportional to its pressure (if you double the pressure of gas, you halve its volume; written as PV = K, where P = pressure, V = volume, and K = a constant).

decompression sickness A broad range of signs and symptoms caused by nitrogen bubbles in blood and tissues coming out of solution on ascent.

drowning The process of experiencing respiratory impairment from submersion or immersion in liquid.

exercise-associated hyponatremia A condition due to prolonged exertion in a hot environment coupled with excessive hypotonic fluid intake that leads to nausea, vomiting, and, in severe cases, mental status changes and seizures (also known as exertional hyponatremia).

frostbite Localized damage to tissues resulting from prolonged exposure to extreme cold.

frostnip Early frostbite, characterized by numbness and pallor without significant tissue damage.

heat exhaustion A clinical syndrome characterized by volume depletion and heat stress that is thought to be a milder form of heat illness and on a continuum leading to heatstroke.

heat syncope An orthostatic or near-syncopal episode that typically occurs in nonacclimated people who may be under heat stress.

heatstroke The least common and most deadly heat illness, caused by a severe disturbance in thermoregulation, usually characterized by a core temperature of more than 104°F (40°C) and altered mental status.

high-altitude cerebral edema A form of acute mountain sickness where the brain swells and stops functioning normally.

high-altitude pulmonary edema A noncardiogenic form of pulmonary edema (fluid accumulation in the lungs) that occurs in high altitudes.

hyperthermia Unusually elevated body temperature.

hypothermia Core body temperature below 95°F (35°C); at lower temperatures, hypothermia may induce cardiac arrhythmia and precipitate a decline in mental status.

neuroleptic malignant syndrome A condition caused by antipsychotic and even common antiemetic medications that presents with hyperthermia, muscular rigidity, altered mental status, and a hyperdynamic state.

nitrogen narcosis A state resembling alcohol intoxication produced by nitrogen gas dissolved in the blood at high ambient pressure.

thermoregulation The process by which the body compensates for environmental extremes.

BIBLIOGRAPHY

American Academy of Orthopaedic Surgeons: *Nancy Caroline's emergency care in the streets*, ed 7, Burlington, MA, 2013, Jones & Bartlett Learning.

Centers for Disease Control and Prevention: *Trench food or immersion foot*. Disaster recovery fact sheet. Available from http://emergency.cdc.gov/disasters/trenchfoot.asp

Conc D, Brice JH, Delbridge TR, et al: *Emergency medical services: clinical practice and systems oversight*. Hoboken, NJ, 2015, Wiley.

Department of Health and Social Services, Division of Public Health, Section of Community Health and EMS, State of Alaska, 2003, Juneau, AK.

Hamilton GC, Sanders AB, Strange GR: *Emergency medicine*, ed 2, St. Louis, MO, 2003, Saunders.

Kumar G, Sng BL, Kumar S. Correlation of capillary and venous blood glucometry with laboratory determination, *Prehosp Emerg Care*. 8(4):378, 2004.

Mallet ML: Pathophysiology of accidental hypothermia, *QJ Med*. 95:775–785, 2002.

Marx JA, Hockberger RS, Walls RM: *Rosen's emergency medicine*, ed 7, St. Louis, MO, 2009, Mosby.

Mistovich JJ, Krost WS, Limmer DD: Beyond the basics: Endocrine emergencies, Part I, *EMS Mag*. 36(10):123–127, 2007.

Mistovich JJ, Krost WS, Limmer DD: Beyond the basics: Endocrine emergencies, Part II, *EMS Mag*. 36(11):66–69, 2007.

Pagan KD, Pagana TJ: *Mosby's manual of diagnostic and laboratory tests*, ed 4, St. Louis, MO, 2010, Mosby.

Plaisier BR: Thoracic lavage in accidental hypothermia with cardiac arrest—report of a case and review of the literature, *Resuscitation*. 66:95–104, 2005

Sanders MJ: *Mosby's paramedic textbook*, ed 3, St. Louis, MO, 2005, Mosby.

Thomas R, Cahill CJ. Case report: Successful defibrillation in profound hypothermia (core body temperature 25.6°C), *Resuscitation*. 47:317–320, 2000.

U.S. Department of Transportation National Highway Traffic Safety Administration: *EMT-paramedic national standard curriculum*, Washington, DC, 1998, The Department.

U.S. Department of Transportation National Highway Traffic Safety Administration: *National EMS education standards*, Draft 3.0, Washington, DC, 2008, The Department.

Walpoth BH, Walpoth-Aslan BN, Mattle HP, et al.: Outcome of survivors of accidental deep hypothermia and circulatory arrest treated with extracorporeal blood warming, *N Engl J Med*. 337:1500–1505, 1997.

Xu J: Number of hypothermia related deaths—by sex: National Vital Statistics System, United States, 1999–2011, *MMWR*. 61:1050, 2013.

CHAPTER REVIEW QUESTIONS

1. You respond to a call to a local marina for a scuba diver who is complaining of right-sided chest pain. The boat captain tells you the diver made an emergency ascent from a 75-foot dive. On assessment, the patient has a respiratory rate of 36 breaths/min, a pulse rate of 130 beats/min, a blood pressure of 90/50 mm Hg, and an SaO_2 of 82%. Breath sounds are diminished on the right side. The most appropriate immediate treatment is:
   a. Oxygen by nonrebreathing mask
   b. Obtaining an ECG
   c. Needle chest decompression
   d. Transport to a hyperbaric chamber

2. The cardinal feature of heatstroke is:
   a. Tachycardia
   b. Altered mental status
   c. Hypotension
   d. Anhidrosis

3. The most important immediate step in treatment of the hypothermic patient is:
   a. Assess the ECG
   b. Remove from the cold environment
   c. Warm IV fluids
   d. Administer supplemental oxygen

4. Administration of hypertonic saline to the patient with exercise-associated hyponatremia can cause what complication if not done in an extremely controlled manner?
   a. Seizure
   b. Irreversible neurologic injury
   c. Altered mental status
   d. Diuresis

5. Identify a way in which heat cramps are different from athletic cramps.
   a. Heat cramps resolve with massage.
   b. Heat cramps only involve one muscle.
   c. Heat cramps begin during physical activity.
   d. Heat cramps most often involve several different muscles.

6. CNS abnormalities such as seizures, coma, confusion, delirium, or severe hyperthermia (>104.9°F [>40.5°C]) suggest:
   a. Heat exhaustion
   b. Severe salt depletion
   c. Heat stroke
   d. A medication overdose

© HunThomas/ShutterStock, Inc.

7. During mild hypothermia, most people will:
   a. Shiver vigorously
   b. Need CPR
   c. Experience decreased consciousness
   d. Improve with caffeinated beverages

8. An ECG that indicates hypothermia may show which of the following?
   a. Prolonged PR intervals
   b. Bradycardia or Osborne waves and electrolyte abnormalities
   c. Shortened QT intervals
   d. PR segment depression and ST elevation in leads I and II

9. The phenomenon in which life-threatening gas bubbles block a person's circulation is known as:
   a. Nitrogen narcosis
   b. Decompression sickness
   c. Boyle's law
   d. Patent foramen ovale

10. A 62-year-old hunter was lost in a swampy area. When you begin to care for him, he is lethargic, disoriented, and has a body temperature of 87.8°F (31°C). His ECG shows bradycardia. What should be your treatment priority?
    a. Atropine 0.5 mg IV
    b. Epinephrine drip at 2 to 10 mcg/min
    c. Rapid rewarming
    d. Transcutaneous pacing

CHAPTER 10

Toxicology, Hazardous Materials, and Weapons of Mass Destruction

This chapter explores the devastating effects of natural and man-made toxins on the human body. As always, rely on the methodical AMLS assessment pathway approach, at the heart of which is a thorough scene survey, skillful assessment, and rapid stabilization of life threats. Medications as toxins and drugs of abuse will be examined in detail. The chapter covers toxins in the home and workplace and describes how to recognize and respond safely and effectively to hazardous materials exposure. The chapter also discusses land and marine environmental toxicology, which includes arthropod and snake envenomation and plant toxins. Biological, chemical, and radiologic contamination by weapons of terrorism, including incendiary devices and their attendant fire and chemical dangers, are addressed. Essential information is given on regulatory agency notification, setting up staging areas, decontamination, and personal protective equipment.

LEARNING OBJECTIVES

At the conclusion of this chapter, you will be able to:

- Understand the basic approach to a patient who has been poisoned or taken an overdose.

- Identify and describe the most common toxidromes.

- Recognize which patients are at risk of respiratory depression and arrhythmia from poisoning.

- Discuss the chief complaint/cardinal presentation, assessment, and treatment of patients with toxicologic medical emergencies using the AMLS assessment pathway.

- Describe the value of poison control in the treatment of toxicologic emergencies.

- Outline general principles of assessment and management for patients exposed to a variety of hazardous materials and weapons of mass destruction.

- Understand the treatment of toxin-induced arrhythmias.

- Describe the signs and symptoms, assessment, and treatment of patients who encounter chemical, biological, and radiologic agents.

- Specify safety concerns for healthcare providers and patients who are at risk of exposure to hazardous materials or weapons of mass destruction.

- Describe general decontamination procedures for patients and healthcare providers who have been exposed to a toxic agent.

SCENARIO

© HunThomas/ShutterStock, Inc.

A 24-year-old quadriplegic man is anxious and slightly combative. His vital signs include a blood pressure of 188/104 mm Hg; pulse rate, 136 beats/min; and respirations, 28 breaths/min. He was found this way when his roommate returned from work.

- What differential diagnoses are you considering based on the information you have now? (Include any toxidrome or specific drugs you may be considering.)
- What additional information will you need to narrow your differential diagnosis?
- What treatments would you consider for this patient?

Toxicologic emergencies caused by accidental and intentional exposures are a principal cause of morbidity and mortality in the United States. Poisoning has surpassed motor vehicle collisions as the leading cause of unintentional injury death in the United States. In 2013, there were 43,982 drug overdose deaths, more than 80% of which were unintentional. The remaining deaths were the result of suicide attempts or unknown intent. According to the Drug Abuse Warning Network (DAWN), nearly 7,000 patients per day are treated in emergency departments for the misuse or abuse of drugs. The American Association of Poison Control Centers' Annual Report of the National Poison Data System reported a total of 2,188,013 human poison exposures in 2013 as well as a continued increase in cases with serious outcomes.

Toxicologic emergencies are frequently encountered by prehospital professionals and other healthcare providers. These emergencies include intentional overdose, unintentional poisoning, occupational exposure, environmental hazards, envenomation, biological and chemical warfare, and radiation illness. Early recognition of toxicity and identification of the causative agent can help you initiate appropriate management, maintain safe conditions for yourself, the patient, and the public, and provide essential information to your colleagues at all levels.

Such emergencies cause a broad spectrum of illness, yet regardless of the offending agent, early recognition and management of dangerous environments and life-threatening patient presentations necessitates following an orderly, unwavering set of fundamental principles. To diagnose and treat toxicologic disorders efficiently, you must have a solid grasp of nervous system, cardiovascular, and respiratory physiology. This chapter focuses on the body's response to classes of drugs and toxins (toxidromes) and does not analyze numerous particular agents. The following topics are emphasized:

- Obtaining historical information
- Identifying toxins
- Understanding the pathophysiology of toxicity
- Making a preliminary evaluation
- Applying general treatment concepts
- Selecting specific therapy

The AMLS assessment pathway guides you through an efficient but comprehensive assessment of the poisoned patient. In some cases, preventing life-threatening sequelae means immediate initiation of therapy, such as stabilizing the airway or administering cardioactive drugs. After first addressing your patient's critical needs, performing a more detailed history, scene survey, and examination often narrows the diagnosis significantly, allowing you to institute potentially life-saving treatment measures without delay.

AMLS Assessment Pathway

▼ Initial Observations

Once you arrive on scene, you can gather a great deal of useful information at the outset of the encounter. The patient's physical location may lead you to consider toxicity as the primary cause of the illness. For example, finding a patient with altered mental status in a house where heroin abuse has been known to occur can guide appropriate management of that patient. In addition, the position and circumstances in which you find the patient offer clues to the underlying toxicity and prognosis. Finding pill bottles in the room or easily accessible in the house, for example, can give you useful information even before you begin your examination.

Scene Safety Consideration

You must verify that the scene is safe. Patients who have taken an overdose can be extremely dangerous. Do not hesitate to call for law enforcement backup in these situations. A number of gases and toxins can injure or incapacitate medical personnel. The dispatchers should ask thorough questions about scene safety and relay the answers to all responding providers. This information is particularly important when multiple patients are affected. In fact, the involvement of more than one patient suggests that toxicity may be related to a gas, which can rapidly induce symptoms. The causative agent in an exposure is often unknown. When a hazardous material is suspected, consider requesting a hazardous materials (Hazmat) response team. Resources to help you identify toxic materials and handle them safely are given in the *Hazardous Materials* section of this chapter.

Patient Cardinal Presentation/ Chief Complaint

Patients who are experiencing a toxicologic emergency may have an altered mental status. Common signs and symptoms of poisoning are given in Table 10-1.

Primary Survey

As in any emergency situation, evaluation of airway, breathing, circulation, and perfusion forms the backbone of your assessment. The primary survey approach is the same as for all patients. The Rapid Recall box offers a review of the ABCDEE mnemonic.

RAPID RECALL
© HunThomas/ShutterStock, Inc.

ABCDEE Assessment Mnemonic

A Airway
B Breathing
C Circulation
D Disability
E Exposure
E Environment

In addition to checking the ABCs, be sure to check for disability, or D, which refers to perfusion related to altered mental status. Changes in mentation might be caused by a serum glucose derangement, so it is vitally important to take a serum glucose reading in patients who exhibit neurologic symptoms. Also keep in mind E for exposure, which necessitates visualizing your patient for any abnormal skin lesions such as rashes, bumps, or needle marks. In addition, E should prompt you to ensure that the environment is not making your patient too cold (hypothermic) or too hot (hyperthermic).

Table 10-1 Common Signs and Symptoms of Poisoning

Sign or Affected Body Part or System	Type	Possible Causative Agents
Odor	Bitter almonds	Cyanide
	Garlic	Arsenic, organophosphates, phosphorus
	Acetone	Methyl alcohol, isopropyl alcohol, aspirin, acetone, diabetes
	Wintergreen	Methyl salicylate
	Pears	Chloral hydrate
	Violets	Turpentine
	Camphor	Camphor
	Alcohol	Alcohol
Pupils	Constricted	Narcotics, organophosphates, jimsonweed, nutmeg, propoxyphene (Darvon)
	Dilated	Barbiturates, atropine amphetamine, glutethimide (Doriden), lysergic acid diethylamide (LSD), cyanide, carbon monoxide
Mouth	Salivation	Organophosphates, arsenic, strychnine, mercury, salicylates
	Dry mouth	Atropine (belladonna), amphetamines, diphenhydramine (Benadryl), narcotics
	Burns in mouth	Formaldehyde, iodine, lye, toxic plants, phenols, phosphorous, pine oil, silver nitrate, acids
Skin	Pruritus	Jimsonweed, belladonna, boric acid
	Dry, hot skin	Atropine (in belladonna), botulism, nutmeg
	Sweating	Organophosphates, arsenic, aspirin, amphetamines, barbiturates, mushrooms, naphthalene

(continues)

Table 10-1 Common Signs and Symptoms of Poisoning (*continued*)

Sign or Affected Body Part or System	Type	Possible Causative Agents
Respiratory	Depressed respirations	Narcotics, alcohol, propoxyphene, carbon monoxide, barbiturates
	Increased respirations	Aspirin, amphetamines, boric acid, cyanide, kerosene, methyl alcohol, nicotine
	Pulmonary edema	Organophosphates, petroleum products, narcotics, carbon monoxide
Cardiovascular	Tachycardia	Alcohol, amphetamines, arsenic, atropine, aspirin, cocaine, some antiasthma drugs
	Bradycardia	Digitalis, gasoline, nicotine, mushrooms, narcotics, cyanide, mistletoe, rhododendron
	Hypertension	Amphetamines, lead, nicotine, antiasthma drugs
	Hypotension	Barbiturates, narcotics, tranquilizers, house plants, mistletoe, nitroglycerin, antifreeze
Central nervous system	Seizures	Amphetamines, camphor, cocaine, strychnine, arsenic, carbon monoxide, petroleum products, scorpion sting
	Coma	All depressant drugs (such as narcotics, barbiturates, tranquilizers, alcohol), carbon monoxide, cyanide
	Hallucinations	Atropine, LSD, mushrooms, organic solvents, phencyclidine (PCP), nutmeg
	Headache	Carbon monoxide, alcohol, disulfiram (Antabuse)
	Tremors	Organophosphates, carbon monoxide, amphetamine, tranquilizers, poisonous marine animals
	Weakness of paralysis	Organophosphates, botulism, eel, hemlock, puffer fish, pine oil, rhododendron
Gastrointestinal	Cramps, nausea, vomiting, and/or diarrhea	Many, if not most, ingested poisons

▼ First Impression

Determine whether the patient is sick or not sick. In this context, "sick" means that the patient's illness is likely to become life threatening if you do not intervene immediately. Weak or erratic vital signs and a poor mental status evaluation generally contribute to this impression. In patients with toxicologic emergencies, mental status changes can range from agitation and **psychosis** to coma. Either extreme is profoundly dangerous. Coma is associated with respiratory depression and an inability to protect the airway. Agitation and **delirium** may indicate significant metabolic derangements and can provoke violent behavior or trigger acute, severe cardiovascular disorders that may be fatal.

The adage "vital signs are vital" holds true in toxicologic emergencies. Assessing and stabilizing abnormal vital signs is critical in early management. Frequent ongoing evaluation can help you gauge the nature and severity of toxicity in a poisoned patient. Initiate airway support and ACLS protocols in sick patients without delay.

▼ Detailed Assessment

History Taking

Most poisoning and overdose cases involve patients with medical conditions, so you will need to elaborate on their chief complaint using the OPQRST questions and SAMPLER history from the patient or bystanders. Historical information is often critical in the diagnosis and treatment of toxicity. Interviewing family members and witnesses, particularly when treating a child or a patient with altered mental status, can be crucial. When the offending agent has been identified, you must consider and ask about co-ingestions and verify the following:

- Timing of ingestion
- Suspected dose
- Patient's access to the drug or chemical
- Situational information such as the patient's position and location and the presence or absence of nearby drug paraphernalia or other intoxicated patients

As a provider who responds on scene, you are often in a position to gather the most accurate information. Historical information, however, is often untrustworthy. Clues revealed during physical examination may be more reliable.

Secondary Survey

The primary and secondary survey focus on identifying and managing life-threatening emergencies related to the specific toxin exposure. Interventions are aimed at treating the patient's mental status changes and perfusion abnormalities. If there is no trauma as the cause, such as when an overdosed patient falls, evaluate the patient's distal pulse, motor and sensory functions, and range of motion.

Any suspected case of poisoning should be reported to your regional poison control center at 1-(800) 222-1222. Not only will diagnostic and treatment recommendations optimize patient care, notification will allow for near real-time surveillance of poisonings both locally and nationally as well as continued patient follow-up in the emergency department and afterwards when necessary.

▼ Refine the Differential Diagnosis

The range of toxic agents and specific therapies is vast, but the good news is that many drugs, on entering the body, result in similar signs and symptoms. The syndrome-like symptoms of a class or group of similar poisonous agents are termed a toxic syndrome, or toxidrome. Toxidromes are useful for remembering the assessment and management of different substances that fall under the same clinical umbrella. The six major toxidromes are discussed later. The patient's history and physical examination findings in conjunction with the vital signs will help you develop a working diagnosis that will enable you to provide appropriate care.

▼ Ongoing Management

Ongoing management focuses on monitoring the patient's condition and reprioritizing the patient's status if necessary.

After completing your initial evaluation and stabilization of the patient, you must consider treatment strategies to attempt to limit gastrointestinal (GI) absorption of an ingested toxin. **Gastrointestinal decontamination** with syrup of ipecac and activated charcoal has been researched and debated for decades. The current standard of care does not call for administration of ipecac in any patient and rarely indicates administration of activated charcoal. Activated charcoal is recommended only when less than 1 hour has elapsed between the confirmed time of *potentially toxic* exposure and the time of administration. Even then, activated charcoal is contraindicated in patients with any alteration in mental status or with nausea or vomiting, because of the significant documented risk of aspiration.

Body stuffers represent one notable exception to these contraindications to the use of activated charcoal. If good mentation exists after ingestion of a poorly wrapped packet of drugs, administration of single-dose activated charcoal is recommended. Activated charcoal continues to play a role in the treatment of some ingestions (e.g., salicylate), but the risks associated with its use may outweigh the benefits of treatment. Multiple-dose activated charcoal may also be considered in some cases; you should consult with a medical toxicologist or poison control center before initiating such therapy. Whole-bowel irrigation is used in the treatment of body packers, as well as in patients with a proven residual intraluminal toxin (e.g., lithium, lead, or other heavy metals).

En route to the hospital, monitoring the patient's response to therapy is essential, and, as always, early communication with the receiving facility can ensure a fluid continuum of care.

Conditions That Indicate Toxin Exposure

Coma

Coma, a state of unconsciousness or deep sedation from which the patient cannot be aroused by any external stimulus, is a common presentation after intoxication. The term **intoxication** refers to the presence of a poison or toxin in the body, with no specific implication of altered consciousness, but it is often used to describe patients who have an impaired or depressed mental status.

In an unconscious patient, bystanders, family, and a physical examination may provide the only data for arriving at a prehospital diagnosis. Therefore, it is essential that you be proficient in recognizing environmental variables, mechanisms of injury, patient posturing, and odors that may offer insight regarding the cause of the patient's condition.

Treatment of the comatose patient is primarily supportive and may include advanced airway support. Most current recommendations suggest first supporting airway, breathing, and circulation and then considering drug therapy. Therapeutic agents used to reverse coma include thiamine, glucose, naloxone (Narcan), and occasionally flumazenil (Romazicon), a benzodiazepine reversal agent.

Naloxone

Naloxone has a key role in the management of comatose patients. Naloxone is a μ-opioid receptor antagonist that reverses the effects of opioids. The primary indication for its use is respiratory depression as evidenced by a decreased respiratory rate, hypercapnia, or hypoxemia, a late finding. Naloxone therapy restores adequate oxygenation and ventilation. Excessive dosing with naloxone causes acute opioid withdrawal in opioid-dependent patients. Naloxone has also been associated with hypertension and acute lung injury, presumably from catecholamine release associated with abrupt withdrawal. Patients who are known or thought likely to be opioid dependent should be given smaller doses of naloxone to avoid inducing these complications. If the initial dose is ineffective, however, rapid escalation of dosing is recommended. If a patient has already undergone endotracheal intubation, naloxone administration should be withheld because abrupt awakening can place the patient and healthcare provider at risk. Additionally, while naloxone is appropriate treatment for respiratory depression or arrest, cardiac arrest should be managed using ACLS protocols. For patients with known or suspected opioid addiction who are unresponsive with no normal breathing but a pulse, it is appropriate for properly trained lay rescuers and BLS providers to administer IM or intranasal naloxone.

Flumazenil

Flumazenil is a γ-aminobutyric acid (GABA) benzodiazepine receptor antagonist that effectively reverses sedation; however, you should be aware of the danger associated with its use. Many patients being treated for overdose have taken benzodiazepines in combination with other drugs. Benzodiazepines are often protective in this scenario, particularly when the patient has also ingested a tricyclic antidepressant. In such cases, reversal with flumazenil may worsen toxicity and patient outcome. Withdrawal from GABA-agonist medications is associated with severe vital sign abnormalities, seizures, delirium, and death. Many patients who overdose on benzodiazepines are long-term users, and administering flumazenil may precipitate an acute withdrawal syndrome.

Hypoglycemia

Hypoglycemia is a rapidly reversible, life-threatening cause of altered mental status. Availability of bedside glucose testing using rapid reagent strips allows you to test quickly for hypoglycemia before administering glucose. Intravenous (IV) administration of a 50% dextrose in water solution (D_{50}) is safe and advisable.

Thiamine Deficiency

Thiamine deficiency may lead to Wernicke encephalopathy in patients who are chronically malnourished, primarily those who have alcoholism (see Chapter 5 for more information on Wernicke-Korsakoff syndrome). Although this condition is uncommon, a single dose of thiamine may provide some benefit and poses no risk at the standard dose of 100 mg administered intravenously (IV) or intramuscularly (IM). Despite widely propagated concerns, it is not necessary to give thiamine before dextrose. Although encephalopathy due to thiamine deficiency can be exacerbated by chronic hypoglycemia, administration of dextrose in an acute situation has not been shown to induce Wernicke-Korsakoff syndrome in a previously healthy person. You should not delay treatment of hypoglycemia because of concern about thiamine deficiency.

Agitation

Many drugs and toxins can cause central nervous system (CNS) excitation, agitation, or psychosis. Regardless of the cause, however, initial management is the same. The goal of treatment in an agitated patient is to depress the CNS to protect the patient from metabolic derangements associated with agitation, tissue injury from cardiovascular toxicity, and self-injury.

Benzodiazepines

Benzodiazepines are a mainstay of therapy for the agitated patient. Because benzodiazepines have a benign safety profile and a wide therapeutic index, this class of medications is widely used to prevent injury to intoxicated patients and the providers who care for them. Benzodiazepines also have the benefit of preventing seizure activity, attenuating sympathetic hyperactivity, and reducing other causes of morbidity often associated with severe agitation (e.g., rhabdomyolysis).

Benzodiazepines depress the CNS, but physical restraint by law enforcement personnel may be necessary in order to administer them. Take great care to minimize physical restraint in favor of chemical restraint, however, because physical restraint is associated with worsening metabolic acidosis, rhabdomyolysis, and occasionally respiratory compromise.

The benzodiazepines most commonly used for sedation of the acutely agitated patient in the emergency care setting are lorazepam (Ativan) and diazepam (Valium). Midazolam (Versed) is available in IV, IM, and oral forms; diazepam is available in IV, oral, and rectal forms. The amount of the agent required to adequately sedate a patient varies significantly with body size, degree of agitation, history of benzodiazepine tolerance, and amount of stimulant ingested. Although benzodiazepines are associated with sedation and potential loss of airway protective reflexes, they do not, on their own, suppress respiratory drive. When combined with other sedative agents such as opioids, ethanol, and barbiturates, benzodiazepines do synergistically contribute to respiratory depression. Regardless of the situation, any patient receiving sedative therapy requires close cardiorespiratory monitoring.

Antipsychotics

Antipsychotic medications, especially haloperidol (Haldol), ziprasidone (Geodon), and olanzapine (Zyprexa), are also commonly used in emergency care to treat agitated patients. Haloperidol is an antipsychotic agent that potently antagonizes dopamine D_2 receptors. A desired side effect of administration is sedation. Ziprasidone is approved for acute agitation in schizophrenic patients. Its mechanism of action is unknown, but the antipsychotic activity of ziprasidone, like haloperidol, is mediated primarily by antagonism at dopamine D_2 receptors. Olanzapine is also commonly used in the treatment of the acutely agitated patient. The newer atypical antipsychotics, including ziprasidone and olanzapine, have less potent dopamine antagonist effects as well as enhanced effects at alternative receptors such as muscarinic blockade. Haloperidol, however, remains the preferred antipsychotic of choice when use becomes necessary.

If benzodiazepines are not immediately available, use of an antipsychotic agent is preferable to physical restraint. Despite the potential for adverse effects, use of antipsychotics after administration of benzodiazepines has a central role in the treatment of agitated patients. Intoxicated patients with excess dopaminergic stimulation exhibit acute psychosis, often manifested by visual and tactile hallucinations or abnormal repetitive involuntary movements. Once benzodiazepines have been given to improve agitation and cardiovascular instability, haloperidol is effective in treating these specific toxic effects.

Seizures

CNS excitation can also lead to seizures. Most toxin-induced seizures are generalized tonic-clonic seizures that rarely progress to status epilepticus, although exceptions do occur (e.g., isoniazid toxicity). Chapter 5 provides additional information on seizures. Seizure activity should always prompt you to evaluate the patient's blood glucose level or to administer dextrose prophylactically. Otherwise, benzodiazepines are used in both the prevention and treatment of seizures. If a patient shows tremor activity, especially if it is accompanied by tachycardia and anxiety, you should administer benzodiazepines in an effort to prevent seizure activity. Once a seizure has occurred, administration of high-dose benzodiazepines is indicated.

If benzodiazepines are ineffective for seizure activity, you should administer barbiturates, typically phenobarbital (Luminal) 10-20 mg/kg. Be prepared to address airway concerns and correct hypotension in patients who require barbiturate loading doses, although in some extremely agitated patients, intubation may not be necessary. Propofol (Diprivan), a GABA agonist and *N*-methyl-D-aspartate (NMDA) antagonist, is another potent sedative that can be titrated quickly but requires intubation for administration. Phenytoin (Dilantin) and other typical anticonvulsants are ineffective in the treatment of toxin-induced seizures.

Finally, consider pyridoxine (vitamin B_6) in the treatment of refractory seizures. Classically, pyridoxine has been used as an antidote for seizures caused by isoniazid (Nydrazid) toxicity, but it can be used as an adjunct agent in status epilepticus due to any cause. Empirical dosing of 5 g IV is generally recommended, with a maximum dose of 70 mg/kg. Consider continuous electroencephalogram (EEG) monitoring if seizures continue despite an apparent halt in motor activity.

Temperature Alteration

Although often overlooked, particularly in the prehospital setting, obtaining an accurate body temperature is crucial in managing toxicologic emergencies. Stimulant intoxication or poisoning is associated with increased mortality when accompanied by hyperthermia. Temperature alteration is a cardinal feature of some toxicologic diagnoses such as serotonin syndrome, neuroleptic malignant syndrome, and malignant hyperthermia. The therapeutic goal for such patients is rapid normalization of temperature through external cooling techniques and medication administration.

Hypothermia can occur after ingestion of sedative-hypnotic agents or opioids. Whether the patient's temperature has climbed or fallen, you should initiate treatment of any severe temperature alteration as soon as the condition is discovered.

Heart Rate Abnormalities

The pulse irregularities and arrhythmias that often occur during toxicologic emergencies can help you diagnose the patient's condition and select initial therapy. Although the patient's pulse rate may deviate significantly from the norm, you must concentrate on the patient as a whole, rather than focus on treating the number. In many patients, mild tachycardia or bradycardia does not need to be treated aggressively if no evidence suggests end-organ injury as a result of the rhythm disturbance.

Tachycardia

In a toxicologic emergency, tachycardia may be caused directly by the drug effect, rather than by volume depletion. A variety of pharmacologic mechanisms may accelerate the heart rate, including sympathomimetic toxicity, dopamine receptor agonism, and calcium channel blockade, which causes vasodilation and reflex tachycardia (Table 10-2). Many toxins are active at more than one receptor site, which may complicate treatment algorithms. In addition to these pharmacologic effects, toxicity from drugs, plants, or chemicals can cause volume depletion as a result of reduced oral intake, prolonged immobilization, vomiting, diarrhea, or a combination of such factors.

Regardless of the etiology, initial treatment with isotonic IV fluids is indicated and may be all that is required. In many patients, tachycardia is accompanied by agitation and tremulousness. Administration of benzodiazepines in these patients provides sympatholysis, helping to moderate vital signs and quell agitation. Otherwise, treatment depends on assessment of heart rate, blood pressure, and specific drug activity. For example, beta-blockers such as esmolol (Brevibloc) may be used to treat beta-adrenergic toxicity but can worsen hypotension or coronary artery vasospasm in patients with cocaine toxicity.

A degree of tachycardia is acceptable if the patient's blood pressure is controlled and intensive supportive care has been instituted, but give special consideration to patients with underlying coronary artery disease or evidence of myocardial ischemia. More aggressive control of heart rate and blood pressure is required in this patient population.

Bradycardia

A variety of plant and drug toxicities and chemical exposures can cause bradycardia (Table 10-3). Many patients require no treatment. In those who do, the goal is to maintain end-organ perfusion. Patients must be closely monitored, often using invasive techniques such as placement of central venous catheters or pulmonary artery catheters. Urine output, mental status, renal function, and acid–base status serve as markers of perfusion.

Management of toxin-induced bradycardia can be complex. Atropine has little downside but inconsistent success, depending on the toxin, and its effects are often transient. Glucagon is a reasonable option, particularly when treating known beta-blocker toxicity, but its effectiveness is limited. Cardioactive vasopressors such as dopamine and epinephrine are often required. These

Table 10-2 Mechanisms of Toxin-Induced Tachycardia

Mechanism of Toxicity	Examples	Treatment
Sympathomimetic toxicity	Cocaine, amphetamine, ephedrine, phencyclidine	IV fluids, benzodiazepines
Peripheral α-blockade	Antipsychotics, tricyclic antidepressants, doxazosin	IV fluids, phenylephrine
Peripheral calcium channel blockade	Dihydropyridine calcium channel blockers (nifedipine, amlodipine)	IV fluids, phenylephrine
Muscarinic receptor blockade	Tricyclic antidepressants, diphenhydramine, cyclobenzaprine, antipsychotics	IV fluids, benzodiazepines, +/– physostigmine
Nicotinic receptor activation	Tobacco, poison hemlock, betel nut, carbamates, organophosphates	IV fluids, benzodiazepines
Serotonin receptor stimulation	Selective serotonin reuptake inhibitors (SSRIs), tricyclic antidepressants, cocaine, tramadol, meperidine	IV fluids, benzodiazepines, +/– cyproheptadine
Dopamine receptor agonism	Amantadine, bupropion, bromocriptine, amphetamine, cocaine	IV fluids, benzodiazepines, +/– haloperidol
GABA agonist withdrawal/GABA antagonism	Ethyl alcohol or benzodiazepine withdrawal, water hemlock, flumazenil	IV fluids, benzodiazepines, barbiturates
Adenosine receptor antagonism	Methylxanthines (e.g., theophylline, caffeine)	IV fluids, benzodiazepines, esmolol
β-receptor agonism	Albuterol, clenbuterol, terbutaline	IV fluids, esmolol

agents will be discussed in detail later. In patients with bradycardia accompanied by hypertension, boosting the heart rate may precipitate a further spike in blood pressure, causing secondary organ injury by mechanisms such as intracranial hemorrhage.

Heart Rhythm Abnormalities

In addition to monitoring the patient's heart rate, recognizing rhythm and interval changes is also critically important to accurate diagnosis and initial stabilization of an intoxicated patient. Toxin-induced ventricular dysrhythmias can be the result of excess sympathetic activation, increased myocardial sensitivity, or alterations in myocardial action potential and ion channel activity.

Fast-acting sodium channel influx is responsible for rapid depolarization of myocardial cells. This depolarization corresponds to the QRS interval on an electrocardiogram (ECG). The opening of potassium channels allows potassium efflux and repolarization, which is represented on ECG by T waves. Sodium channel blockade results in QRS prolongation, which can eventually devolve into bradycardia, hypotension, ventricular

dysrhythmia, and death. A number of drugs and toxins, including tricyclic antidepressants, induce sodium channel blockade. Some of these agents are listed in Table 10-3.

Indications for treatment include a widened QRS complex (> 120 ms, new right bundle branch block) or evidence of significant cardiovascular toxicity. Treatment consists of serum alkalinization, which is accomplished by administering a bolus of sodium bicarbonate solution (1–2 mEq/kg) over several minutes. Monitoring strips often show a decrease in QRS duration, but repeat boluses may be necessary. Once the necessity of administering sodium bicarbonate has been established, a sodium bicarbonate infusion is generally necessary. Once adequate alkalinization has occurred without desired success in treatment or in the case of ongoing clinical deterioration, hypertonic saline (3%) may be administered, typically 0.5–1 cc/kg/hr.

Potassium chloride may also be given to counter potassium shifts and extracellular hypokalemia caused by alkalinization. Many drugs and toxins have potassium channel–blocking properties. Inhibition of potassium efflux causes prolongation of the QT interval corrected for heart rate (the QTc interval), eventually

Table 10-3 Mechanisms of Toxin-Induced Bradycardia

Mechanism of Toxicity	Examples	Treatment
Cardiac sodium channel opening	Veratrum alkaloids, aconite, grayanotoxin, ciguatera	Atropine, dopamine
Cardiac sodium channel blockade	Tricyclic antidepressants, carbamazepine, yew plant, propranolol	Sodium bicarbonate, hypertonic saline, pressors
β-adrenergic receptor blockade	Atenolol, propranolol, metoprolol	Atropine, glucagon, epinephrine, insulin
Calcium channel antagonism	Verapamil, diltiazem	Atropine, calcium salts, epinephrine, insulin
Na$^+$/K$^+$-ATPase inactivation	Digoxin, foxglove, oleander, lily of the valley	Atropine, digoxin-specific antibody fragments (Fab)
Muscarinic and nicotinic activation	Carbamates, *Clitocybe* mushrooms, organophosphates, nerve agents	Atropine, pressors, +/− pralidoxime
Peripheral α-receptor agonists	Imidazolines (e.g., clonidine initial activity)	Supportive care, +/− phentolamine vs. nitroprusside
Central α-receptor agonists	Imidazolines (e.g., clonidine secondary activity)	Atropine, dopamine when associated with hypotension
Opioids	Oxycodone, heroin, fentanyl	Rarely required; supportive care, +/− pressors

ATPase, Adenosine triphosphatase; *K$^+$,* potassium; *Na$^+$,* sodium.

leading to polymorphic ventricular tachycardia (torsades de pointes). Consider preventive treatment with IV magnesium sulfate when the QTc interval is > 500 ms. If the patient has unstable torsades de pointes, perform defibrillation. The routine use of magnesium sulfate for v-fib or pulseless v-tach is no longer recommended. In patients with recurrent torsades de pointes, overdrive pacing with isoproterenol (Isuprel) or a mechanical pacemaker (transvenous or transcutaneous) is indicated, because the QTc interval shortens as heart rate accelerates.

Evaluation of QRS and QTc intervals in the intoxicated patient, particularly in those with evidence of cardiovascular instability, is critical. If the patient has QTc interval prolongation, administer magnesium sulfate and consider induction of tachycardia. Administer sodium bicarbonate liberally to a patient with any type of toxin-induced ventricular dysrhythmia. Standard therapies alone are unlikely to be effective. Otherwise, follow ACLS protocol.

Notable exceptions to ACLS guidelines within the scope of toxicology are the avoidance of amiodarone (Cordarone) in toxin-induced ventricular dysrhythmia and the avoidance of epinephrine in patients suspected of **huffing**, or abusing, inhalants. Among other mechanisms of action, amiodarone is a potassium channel blocker. As such, it can further prolong the QTc interval thereby exacerbating dysrhythmias in patients with toxic reactions in whom toxins may already be affecting potassium channels. Therefore, lidocaine is recommended as an alternative.

Inhaled halogenated hydrocarbons enhance myocardial sensitivity to catecholamines and can provoke sudden sniffing death syndrome. In this syndrome, the cause of death is ventricular dysrhythmia induced by release of the patient's endogenous catecholamines. Such a dysrhythmia would probably be exacerbated by exogenous administration of epinephrine, and the patient might benefit from administration of a beta-blocker. However, accurate diagnosis of this cause of cardiovascular toxicity is fraught with difficulty. Unless you have overwhelming evidence of inhalant use, you should perform cardiovascular stabilization according to standard ACLS protocols.

Blood Pressure Abnormalities

Because of significant baseline variation in normal blood pressure, as well as the possibility of underlying hypertension, blood pressure variation can be a misleading parameter by which to judge acute toxicity. Nevertheless, blood pressure extremes are of pivotal importance in identifying intoxication and guiding management. Depending on the agent, a toxic exposure may induce extreme hypotension or hypertension. In some cases (e.g., alpha-2 agonists), both hypertension and hypotension may be seen, depending on how long ago the ingestion occurred. The degree of blood pressure derangement dictates care.

Hypertension

Toxin-induced hypertension may be due to a variety of agents. Toxicity of a sympathomimetic agent such as cocaine or amphetamines is most often responsible. These agents induce hypertension by increasing systemic vascular resistance through stimulation of peripheral alpha-adrenergic receptors, both the alpha-1 and alpha-2 subtypes. They also tend to step up cardiac output via beta-adrenergic effects, further elevating blood pressure.

Isolated alpha-receptor stimulation results in hypertension and reflex bradycardia, as seen early in the course of alpha-2 agonist toxicity (e.g., in clonidine [Catapres] and oxymetazoline [Afrin] ingestions). Other agents, such as anticholinergic agents and hallucinogens, can cause mild hypertension but are rarely responsible for severe hypertension.

The treatment of toxin-induced hypertension depends on both the severity and the mechanism of hypertension. Mild hypertension frequently responds to supportive care, including the benzodiazepines that are often administered to agitated patients with sympathomimetic toxicity. However, if the patient has significantly increased blood pressure, further treatment with vasoactive drugs may be necessary.

The precise blood pressure at which treatment is required is unknown and is different for each patient. Many patients can tolerate significant blood pressure elevation without adverse effects, but older patients and patients with underlying hypertension may lack autoregulatory mechanisms when their blood pressure is high. Such patients can have significant adverse sequelae, including intracranial hemorrhage, ischemic stroke, myocardial or intestinal ischemia, and arrhythmia. Evidence of end-organ damage due to hypertension is an indication for rapid initiation of treatment. Arbitrarily, a systolic blood pressure above 180 mm Hg or a diastolic blood pressure above 110 mm Hg is considered a relative indication for treatment and should, at the very least, prompt you to consider taking steps to lower blood pressure.

In general, beta-adrenergic antagonists are a poor choice in the treatment of toxin-induced hypertension, because these medications can generate unopposed alpha-adrenergic stimulation, which can worsen hypertension, result in coronary artery vasospasm, and result in end-organ injury. Short-acting vasodilators with alpha-1 antagonist properties, dihydropyridine calcium channel–blocking activity (e.g., nicardipine [Cardene]), or direct vasodilation properties (e.g., nitroglycerin [Nitro-Dur, Nitrol] or nitroprusside [Nipride]) are typically preferred. Such medications can be titrated as needed to control blood pressure without exacerbating the underlying toxicity. Although toxin-induced hypertension can usually be well controlled with supportive care and adequate sedation, it can cause severe tissue injury and should be addressed with short-acting, titratable vasodilators (Table 10-4).

Hypotension

Treating toxin-induced hypotension is often complicated. The condition can be caused by any of several discrete toxicologic mechanisms or by a combination of several (Table 10-5). Although toxin-directed antidotal therapy is often the preferred approach to treating toxin-induced hypotension, general therapeutic principles are applicable as well.

A common cause of hypotension in the patients with toxic reactions is volume depletion associated with a variety of mechanisms, including decreased oral intake, GI losses from vomiting and diarrhea, excessive insensible losses from diaphoresis, and tachypnea or osmotic diuresis, as is seen in alcohol toxicity. Before you resort to vasopressor administration, aggressive resuscitation with isotonic fluids such as normal saline is an important first step in treating hypotension. Even in patients with toxin-induced heart failure, an initial trial of crystalloid fluids is reasonable. However, you must carefully consider the total volume administered and the risk of exacerbating pulmonary edema, particularly in patients with bradycardia and hypotension. Patients with tachycardia and hypotension can generally tolerate a much larger fluid volume.

Norepinephrine (Levophed) and phenylephrine (Neo-Synephrine) are the agents of choice for the treatment of toxin-induced hypotension. Phenylephrine is preferable in patients with significant tachycardia and hypotension, whereas norepinephrine may be used in patients with low to normal heart rates. Patients with significant bradycardia, depressed ejection fraction, and associated hypotension may be treated with epinephrine (Adrenalin) infusions. A common pitfall with the use of vasopressors is underdosing. In toxin-induced hypotension, high doses of vasopressors are often required to compete with the toxic effects of the drug on which the patient has overdosed. This may entail administering more than the stated maximum dose of these drugs. Do not consider vasopressor treatment to have failed if you administer the so-called maximum dose without achieving the anticipated clinical response. Continue to titrate the original drug rather than switching to an alternative agent.

Another common pitfall is the use of dopamine monotherapy. Dopamine is a mixed-acting sympathomimetic agent whose vasopressor activity depends primarily on presynaptic uptake and subsequent release of endogenous norepinephrine. At low doses, dopamine receptor activation does boost heart rate and contractility but may result in splanchnic vasodilation and worsening hypotension. This is particularly true in the setting of overdose, in which many drugs (e.g., tricyclic antidepressants) block presynaptic uptake channels. Dopamine may be effective in the setting of mild hypotension and bradycardia associated with a sodium channel opener and alpha-2 agonist toxicity or as an adjunctive treatment in combination with a more potent vasopressor after beta-blocker or calcium channel blocker–induced heart failure.

Respiratory Rate Abnormalities

One vital sign that is often overlooked or inaccurately recorded is respiratory rate. This reading can be an important clue in

Table 10-4 Toxin-Induced Hypertension

Drug Class	Examples	Clinical Presentation	Treatment
Sympathomimetics	Cocaine, amphetamines, ephedrine, monoamine oxidase inhibitors, methylphenidate, phentermine	Tachycardia, mydriasis, diaphoresis, hypertension, agitation, tremors, seizure, delirium	Benzodiazepines, barbiturates, phentolamine, nitrates, calcium channel blockers
α_1-agonists	Ergot alkaloids, phenylephrine	Hypertension, reflex tachycardia, limb ischemia	Phentolamine, nitrates, calcium channel blockers
α_2-agonists	Clonidine, oxymetazoline, tetrahydrozoline	Mental status depression, pinpoint pupils, bradycardia with hypertension initially, followed by bradycardia and hypotension	Nitroprusside or nitroglycerin for initial hypertension if needed
α_2-antagonists	Yohimbine	Tachycardia, hypertension, mydriasis, diaphoresis, lacrimation, salivation, nausea, vomiting, and flushing	Benzodiazepines, clonidine, nitrates
Anticholinergic	Diphenhydramine, cyclobenzaprine, benztropine, doxylamine	Tachycardia, flushing, mydriasis, urinary retention, delirium	Supportive care; vasodilators rarely required
Hallucinogens	Dextromethorphan, lysergic acid diethylamide (LSD), mescaline	Mydriasis, tachycardia, mild hypertension, hallucinations	Supportive care; vasodilators rarely required

Table 10-5 Toxin-Induced Hypotension

Drug Class	Examples	Clinical Presentation	Treatment
Sodium channel openers	Veratrum alkaloids, grayanotoxin, aconite	Nausea, vomiting, bradycardia, hypotension, paresthesias, dysesthesias, mental status depression, paralysis, seizures	IV fluids Atropine Dopamine, epinephrine, or norepinephrine
Sodium channel blockers	Tricyclic antidepressants, diphenhydramine, carbamazepine, quinine, taxine	Nausea, vomiting, bradycardia, QRS prolongation, hypotension, coma, seizures (many are also anticholinergic)	IV fluids Sodium bicarbonate Hypertonic saline Epinephrine, norepinephrine, or phenylephrine
α_1-antagonists	Prazosin, doxazosin, tricyclic antidepressants, antipsychotics	Mental status depression, hypotension, reflex tachycardia	IV fluids Norepinephrine or phenylephrine
α_2-agonists	Clonidine, tetrahydrozoline, oxymetazoline	Mental status depression, pinpoint pupils, bradycardia with hypertension initially followed by bradycardia and hypotension	IV fluids, atropine, dopamine, epinephrine, or norepinephrine Case reports of benefit with yohimbine and naloxone

(continues)

Table 10-5 Toxin-Induced Hypotension (*continued*)			
Drug Class	**Examples**	**Clinical Presentation**	**Treatment**
Beta-blockers	Metoprolol, atenolol, sotalol, labetalol, propranolol	Mental status depression, bradycardia, hypotension	Atropine, glucagon, epinephrine, or insulin
Beta-agonists	Albuterol, terbutaline, clenbuterol	Supraventricular tachycardia, hypotension	Esmolol +/– phenylephrine
Adenosine antagonists	Theophylline, caffeine	Supraventricular tachycardia, hypotension, altered mental status, tremor, seizure	Benzodiazepines, esmolol +/– phenylephrine, hemodialysis
Calcium channel blockers	Diltiazem, verapamil, nifedipine, amlodipine, felodipine	Hypotension with bradycardia (diltiazem, verapamil, high-dose-pines) or reflex tachycardia (-pines)	IV fluids Atropine Calcium salts Epinephrine, norepinephrine, or insulin
Sedative hypnotics and opioids	Heroin, morphine, barbiturates	Sedation, pinpoint pupils (with opioids), respiratory depression	IV fluids, supportive care, vasopressors rarely required
Na^+/K^+-ATPase inhibitors	Digoxin, foxglove, oleander, lily of the valley, Bufo toads, Chan su	Nausea, vomiting, atrioventricular node block, premature ventricular contractions, ventricular dysrhythmias	Atropine or digoxin-specific antibody fragments (Fab)
Electron transport chain toxins	Cyanide, cyanogenic glycosides (e.g., amygdalin), carbon monoxide, salicylate	Hypotension, reflex tachycardia, severe metabolic acidosis, hyperthermia (uncouplers), altered mental status, seizures	Dextrose, IV fluids, sodium bicarbonate, amyl nitrite + sodium nitrite + sodium thiosulfate vs. hydroxocobalamin (CN), hyperbaric oxygen (CO), epinephrine vs. norepinephrine vs. phenylephrine
Agents that cause endothelial disruption/ distributive shock	Surfactant-containing herbicides (e.g., glufosinate [Basta]), phenol, caustic agents	Hypotension, tachycardia, pulmonary edema, third spacing of fluid, altered mental status, seizures	IV fluids Benzodiazepines Norepinephrine or phenylephrine

diagnosing intoxicated patients and guiding therapy. Bradypnea (decreased respiratory rate) or hypopnea (decreased tidal volume) can complicate exposure to several different toxins. Opioids, for example, are typically associated with respiratory depression; however, beta-blocker toxicity, severe sedative-hypnotic toxicity, and alpha-2 agonist toxicity have also been associated with respiratory depression. Early recognition of hypoventilation by physical examination, blood gas analysis, or capnography is critical in the appropriate treatment of the intoxicated patient. Reversal of the effects of opioids was discussed earlier in the chapter. In addition, supportive care such as ventilatory assistance or endotracheal intubation may be necessary.

Arterial or venous blood gas measurements can be used to differentiate metabolic acidosis with respiratory compensation from a combined metabolic acidosis and respiratory alkalosis. Toxin-induced metabolic acidosis typically creates an anion gap. Although medications such as carbonic anhydrase inhibitors (e.g., acetazolamide [Diamox] and topiramate [Topamax]) do cause non–anion gap metabolic acidosis, the presence of a high–anion gap metabolic acidosis is more common and carries a broad differential diagnosis that can typically be narrowed rapidly by careful history taking and further laboratory testing. The classic, but perhaps outdated, mnemonic for this differential diagnosis is MUDPILES, which can be expanded to CAT MUDPILES to include a broader range of possible toxicologic causes (see Chapter 7). More recently, updated mnemonics have been proposed including GOLDMARK [glycols (ethylene and propylene), oxoproline (as observed in acetaminophen toxicity), L-lactate, D-lactate, methanol, aspirin, renal failure, and ketoacidosis. CUTE DIMPLES has also been suggested as an expanded toxicologic representation: cyanide, uremia, toluene, ethylene glycol, diabetic ketoacidosis, isoniazid, methanol, propylene glycol, lactic acidosis, ethanol, and salicylates.

Tachypnea

Tachypnea may be an indicator of a significant metabolic acidosis or acute respiratory disease like pneumonia or pneumonitis. In the setting of underlying metabolic acidosis, the exaggerated respiratory rate is a compensatory mechanism that allows the body to decrease the partial pressure of carbon dioxide (Pco_2), thereby raising systemic pH. In some patients, the actual rate of respiration may not accelerate significantly, but an uptick in tidal volume and minute ventilation has the same effect.

Hyperpnea

An increase in the depth of breathing is referred to as *hyperpnea*. Any underlying metabolic acidosis can result in tachypnea, hyperpnea, or both. Patients might or might not be aware of the change in their breathing pattern, depending on the severity of the alteration. Another cause of hyperventilation is direct activation of a patient's respiratory center. Classically, salicylate toxicity may cause tachypnea or hyperpnea in the absence of metabolic acidosis. In fact, early toxicity may be accompanied by an isolated respiratory alkalosis.

Oxygen Saturation Abnormalities

Oxygen saturation should be measured in any acutely ill patient. A normal oxygen saturation is reassuring but does not rule out the possibility of lung disease, hemoglobin dysfunction, or impaired oxygen delivery to body tissues. For example, oxygen saturation measured by noninvasive pulse oximetry may remain normal despite severe carbon monoxide toxicity that prevents delivery of oxygen to tissues. Aspiration often occurs when treating patients with toxicologic emergencies. Toxic emergencies related to ingestion can be accompanied by a high incidence of vomiting, which is a risk factor for aspiration. Noncardiogenic pulmonary edema and pneumonitis can also complicate the course of opioid toxicity and withdrawal, salicylate toxicity, and toxin inhalation, all of which may cause hypoxemia and diffuse alveolar disease. Pneumothorax has also been reported in patients who smoke or inhale toxins. However, oxygen saturation and, more importantly, partial pressure of oxygen (Po_2), can be helpful metrics in sick intoxicated patients.

Abnormal pulse oximetry readings sometimes accompany hemoglobinopathies such as methemoglobinemia and sulfhemoglobinemia. Of these two derangements, the former is the more common. It is generally caused by oxidative stress, which converts the ferrous iron in hemoglobin into the ferric state, allowing more avid binding of oxygen to hemoglobin but resulting in poor oxygen delivery to tissues. Cyanosis, or blue discoloration of the skin, is a common finding. Pulse oximetry typically reveals an oxygen saturation in the high 80s to low 90s regardless of the amount of supplemental oxygen delivered. Treatment with the reducing agent, methylene blue, allows reduction of ferric iron and consequent restoration of tissue-delivery capability. More information on the use of methylene blue in patients with methemoglobinemia is given later in the chapter.

Various toxins may also produce a relative tissue hypoxia without inducing a significant change in hemoglobin binding. Uncouplers and inhibitors of oxidative phosphorylation impede the proper functioning of the electron transport chain, which is responsible for using oxygen during adenosine triphosphate (ATP) synthesis. The result is constrained energy production and cellular injury. Uncouplers such as salicylate invigorate this process with increased oxygen consumption, but they prohibit ATP synthesis. Therefore, the energy created is dissipated as heat. Hyperthermia is a late finding in uncoupler toxicity. Arterial oxygen saturation is generally normal, but venous oxygen content is significantly diminished as a result of the escalating cellular demand for oxygen. Oxidative phosphorylation inhibitors such as cyanide, on the other hand, suppress cellular oxygen demand, raise venous oxygen content, and decrease ATP production. Both classes of toxins cause metabolic acidosis, altered mental status, seizures, and eventual cardiovascular collapse. In either scenario, treating patients with sodium bicarbonate buffers acidosis and, in the case of salicylates, decreases tissue distribution and toxicity.

Cyanide toxicity is treated with a cyanide antidote kit. Historically, the patient is given a series of treatments. Inhaled amyl nitrite and intravenous sodium nitrite induce methemoglobinemia, which draws cyanide out of cells. This treatment is followed by IV sodium thiosulfate, creating thiocyanate, which is renally excreted. More recently, hydroxocobalamin, a vitamin B_{12} precursor, has been approved for the treatment of cyanide toxicity. Cobalt within the hydroxocobalamin moiety binds cyanide to form cyanocobalamin, which is then excreted by the kidneys. Cyanide toxicity is discussed in detail later.

Arterial and venous oxygen content, measured by conventional pulse oximetry and blood gas evaluation, can be altered by various anatomic and physiologic changes in intoxicated patients. Recognizing and identifying the underlying cause and rapidly reversing decreased blood oxygen content and tissue oxygen delivery are critical in the effective treatment of toxicity. Administer high-flow oxygen to any patient with respiratory compromise and abnormal oxygen saturation.

Toxidromes

A **toxidrome** (an abridgement of *toxin* and *syndrome*) is the constellation of symptoms, vital signs, and exam findings typically associated with exposure to a particular toxin. Taken together, a patient's history and toxidrome can often help you identify the class of drug or, in some instances, the specific toxin responsible for the patient's illness. In general, if the class of toxin is known, the specific agent is unimportant, since the treatment will be the same. Descriptions of various toxidromes are given in Table 10-6.

Table 10-6 Major Toxidromes

Toxidrome	Drug Examples	Signs and Symptoms
Stimulant	Amphetamine, methamphetamine, cocaine, diet aids, nasal decongestants, bath salts	Restlessness, agitation, incessant talking; insomnia, anorexia; dilated pupils, tachycardia; tachypnea, hypertension or hypotension; paranoia, seizures, cardiac arrest
Narcotic (opiate and opioid)	Heroin, opium, morphine, hydromorphone (Dilaudid), fentanyl, oxycodone-aspirin combination (Percodan), zolpidem tartrate (Ambien), secobarbital	Constricted (pinpoint) pupils, marked respiratory depression; needle tracks (IV abusers); drowsiness, stupor, coma
Sympathomimetic	Pseudoephedrine, phenylephrine, phenylpropanolamine, amphetamine, and methamphetamine	Hypertension, tachycardia, dilated pupils (mydriasis), agitation and seizures, hyperthermia
Sedative/hypnotics	Phenobarbital, diazepam (Valium), thiopental, midazolam (Versed), lorazepam	Drowsiness, disinhibition, ataxia, slurred speech, mental confusion, respiratory depression, progressive central nervous system depression, hypotension
Cholinergic	Acephate (Orthene), diazinon (Basudin, Knox Out, Spectracide), and malathion (Celthion, Cython), parathion, sarin, tabun, VX	Increased salivation, lacrimation, gastrointestinal distress, diarrhea, respiratory depression, apnea, seizures, coma
Anticholinergic	Atropine, scopolamine, antihistamines, antipsychotics	Dry, flushed skin, hyperthermia, dilated pupils, blurred vision, tachycardia; mild hallucinations, dramatic delirium

Medications as Toxins

A number of prescription medications and over-the-counter (OTC) products can have toxic effects if used improperly, especially by vulnerable individuals such as the very young and those with reduced drug clearance due to renal or liver impairment (Table 10-7).

Acetaminophen

Acetaminophen (*N*-acetyl-*p*-aminophenol [APAP], or Tylenol) is a commonly used OTC antipyretic and analgesic. The benign safety profile of the drug at therapeutic doses has led to its inclusion in a variety of combination medications, including prescription and OTC pain relievers, cough and cold preparations, and allergy medications. The drug is widely available and easy to obtain.

Although acetaminophen is safe at therapeutic levels, overdose ingestions carry significant risk. The primary threat is hepatotoxicity. In fact, acetaminophen-related liver injury is the leading cause of acute liver failure in the United States, making it a far more common cause of liver failure than acute viral hepatitis. Questions about possible acetaminophen toxicity, alone or in combination with other agents, accounted for approximately 130,000 calls to poison control centers in 2013.

Pathophysiology

Acetaminophen is metabolized through several pathways, and most of its metabolites are nontoxic. However, after supratherapeutic dosing, the major metabolic pathways become saturated, resulting in excessive formation of the toxic metabolite *N*-acetyl-*p*-benzoquinone imine (NAPQI). When insufficient glutathione (< 30% of normal stores) is present, NAPQI induces a series of reactions that lead to cell death. Cells with cytochrome P450 enzyme systems (e.g., hepatic and renal cells) are primarily affected, resulting in hepatic centrilobular necrosis and renal proximal tubular necrosis.

Signs and Symptoms

The clinical presentation of APAP toxicity can vary significantly, depending on the dose and timing of ingestion. Single doses of over 150 mg/kg are considered toxic, but dosage history in overdose scenarios is notoriously unreliable, and the dosage threshold fails to account for staggered ingestions or for unintentional repeated supratherapeutic ingestions. Nonetheless, it does give us some idea of what constitutes a worrisome single dose. In a 70-kg person, ingestion of 10.5 g of APAP, or 21 extra-strength tablets, would be enough to confer toxicity. The time of the ingestion is also critical, both for evaluation of symptoms and interpretation of serum levels, which is discussed in the next section. Clinical manifestations can be loosely divided into stages on the basis of the amount of time elapsed from ingestion as follows:

- *Stage I (< 24 hours).* Symptoms are nonspecific and may include nausea, vomiting, and malaise. In severe overdose, patients may have an altered level of consciousness and acidosis. Patients may also have very mild or no symptoms, even after toxic ingestions.

- *Stage II (24 to 36 hours).* This stage is marked by the onset of hepatic injury, characterized by abdominal pain, worsening nausea and vomiting, and elevated liver enzymes and coagulation studies.

- *Stage III (48 to 96 hours).* Peak liver injury, perhaps progressing to fulminant hepatic failure, occurs during this period. Liver enzyme tests typically become significantly elevated, but of greater clinical relevance are the patient's coagulation studies, mental status, acidosis, and renal function. A systemic inflammatory

Table 10-7 Toxic Effects of Drugs

Drug or Toxin	Clinical Presentation of Intoxication	Specific Collaborative Management
Acetaminophen	*Mild/early stage* May be asymptomatic Anorexia, nausea, vomiting Diaphoresis Hypotension Pallor *12 hours to 4 days later* Signs of hepatotoxicity may occur: liver enzymes, bilirubin, prothrombin time increased; right upper quadrant pain Gradual return to normal may occur *Late: indications of hepatic failure* Anorexia, nausea, vomiting Jaundice Hepatosplenomegaly Clinical indications of hepatic encephalopathy: confusion to coma Bleeding Hypoglycemia Acute renal failure may develop Dysrhythmias and shock may occur	Consider activated charcoal if patient arrives within 2 hours after ingestion (although activated charcoal does adsorb *N*-acetylcysteine and reduces its peak serum levels if oral N-acetylcysteine is used, the loading dose of *N*-acetylcysteine does not need to be increased) IV *N*-acetylcysteine (Acetadote) 150 mg/kg loading dose over 1 hour, then 50 mg/kg over 4 hours, then 100 mg/kg over 16 hours (21 hours and 300 mg/kg total). A 16-hour bag should be repeated until end points of therapy met Oral *N*-acetylcysteine (Mucomyst) 140 mg/kg initially, then 70 mg/kg every 4 hours × 17 doses to total of 1330 mg/kg If given PO, dilute in juice or carbonated beverage; if given via nasogastric or duodenal tube, dilute with water May cause anorexia, nausea, vomiting; repeat dose if vomiting occurs within 1 hour Vitamin K may be prescribed, especially if hepatic failure occurs Dextrose (e.g., $D_{50}W$) may be needed Antidysrhythmics may be needed
Amphetamines	Tachycardia Hypertension Tachypnea Dysrhythmias Hyperthermia, diaphoresis Dilated but reactive pupils Dry mouth Urinary retention Headache Paranoid-type psychotic behavior Hallucinations Hyperactivity, anxiety Hyperactive deep tendon reflexes, tremor, seizures Confusion, stupor, coma	Calm, quiet environment Avoid overstimulation of patient Do not speak loudly or move quickly Do not approach from behind Avoid touching the patient unless you speak to the patient first or are sure it is safe Diazepam (Valium) for agitation Phentolamine (Regitine) for hypertension Anticonvulsants (e.g., diazepam, phenytoin, phenobarbital) for seizures Antidysrhythmics (e.g., lidocaine) for ventricular dysrhythmias Haloperidol (Haldol) for acute psychotic reactions Hypothermia blanket, ice packs, ice water sponge baths for hyperthermia

(continues)

Table 10-7 Toxic Effects of Drugs (*continued*)

Drug or Toxin	Clinical Presentation of Intoxication	Specific Collaborative Management
Barbiturates, sedatives, hypnotics, tranquilizers	Bradycardia, cardiac dysrhythmias Hypotension Hypothermia Respiratory depression to respiratory arrest Headache Nystagmus, disconjugate eye movements Dysarthria Ataxia Depressed deep tendon reflexes Confusion, stupor, coma Hemorrhagic blisters Gastric irritation (chloral hydrate) Pulmonary edema (meprobamate)	Phenobarbital: sodium bicarbonate to alkalinize the urine and increase rate of barbiturate excretion; maintain urine pH > 7.50 Monitor potassium, calcium, and magnesium levels. Anticonvulsants (e.g., diazepam, phenobarbital) for withdrawal seizures Hemodialysis or hemoperfusion may be required.
Benzodiazepines	Hypotension Loss of airway protective reflexes Diminished or absent bowel sounds Decreased deep tendon reflexes (DTR) Confusion, drowsiness, stupor, coma	Flumazenil (Romazicon), a benzodiazepine receptor antagonist may be prescribed in rare cases, e.g. pediatric or iatrogenic exposure. Otherwise, its use is contraindicated. Monitor for seizures, agitation, flushing, nausea, and vomiting as side effects of flumazenil. Intubation and mechanical ventilation may be necessary.
Beta-blockers	Sinus bradycardia, arrest, block Junctional escape rhythm, AV nodal block Bundle branch block (usually right) Hypotension Heart failure Cardiogenic shock Cardiac arrest Decreased level of consciousness Seizures Respiratory depression, apnea Bronchospasm Hyperglycemia or hypoglycemia	May consider gastric lavage, activated charcoal within 1 hour of ingestion Glucagon 3–5 mg IV, IM, or SQ, followed by infusion of 1–5 mg/h Epinephrine, dopamine, isoproterenol, or atropine for bradycardia and hypotension; temporary pacing may be required $D_{50}W$ for hypoglycemia Anticonvulsants (e.g., diazepam, phenobarbital) for seizures; phenytoin is contraindicated
Calcium channel blockers	Sinus bradycardia, arrest, block SA blocks (diltiazem) AV blocks (verapamil) Hypotension Heart failure Confusion, agitation, dizziness, lethargy, slurred speech Seizures Nausea, vomiting Paralytic ileus Hyperglycemia	May consider gastric lavage, activated charcoal within 1 hour of ingestion Calcium chloride 5 (500 mg) to 10 (1 g) mL of 10% solution Glucagon 3–5 mg IV, IM, or SQ, followed by infusion of 1–5 mg/h Anticonvulsants (e.g., diazepam, phenytoin, phenobarbital) for seizures Atropine, isoproterenol, temporary pacing for bradycardia Vasopressor therapy with epinephrine, norepinephrine, and/or phenylephrine Hyperinsulinemia euglycemia (HIE) therapy

(continues)

Table 10-7 Toxic Effects of Drugs (*continued*)

Drug or Toxin	Clinical Presentation of Intoxication	Specific Collaborative Management
Carbon monoxide Note: the affinity between carbon monoxide and hemoglobin is approximately 200 times the affinity between oxygen and hemoglobin	Dysrhythmias Impaired hearing or vision Pallor; cherry-red skin coloring may be seen 10%–20%: mild headache, flushing, dyspnea or angina on vigorous exertion, nausea, dizziness 20%–30%: throbbing headache, nausea, vomiting, weakness, dyspnea on moderate exertion, ST-segment depression 30%–40%: severe headache, visual disturbances, syncope, vomiting 40%–50%: tachypnea, tachycardia, chest pain, worsening syncope 50%–60%: chest pain, respiratory failure, shock, seizures, coma 60%–70%: respiratory failure, shock, coma, death	Removal from contaminated area Oxygenation: 100% oxygen via mask initially; CPAP by mask may be utilized Intubation and mechanical ventilation if patient is unresponsive; PEEP may be utilized Fluids, diuretics, urine alkalinization to treat myoglobinuria if present Anticonvulsants (e.g., diazepam, phenytoin, phenobarbital) for seizures Hyperbaric oxygen (at 2–3 atmospheres) as soon as available if: COHb > 25% (relative indication) CO-induced acute ECG changes, or persistent CNS symptoms

Caustic poisoning
Acids (e.g., battery acid, drain cleaners, hydrochloric acid)
Alkalis (e.g., drain cleaners, refrigerants, fertilizers, photographic developers)
	Burning sensation in the oral cavity, pharynx, esophageal area
	Dysphagia
	Respiratory distress: dyspnea, stridor, tachypnea, hoarseness
	Soapy-white mucous membrane
	Acid:
	  Oral ulcerations and/or blisters
	  May have signs of shock
	Alkali:
	  May have signs of esophageal perforation (e.g., chest pain, subcutaneous emphysema)
		Diluent: flush mouth with copious volumes of water; drink water or milk (approximately 250 mL)
		Do not induce vomiting or perform gastric lavage
		Esophagogastroscopy to assess damage

Cocaine, including crack cocaine	Tachycardia, dysrhythmias Hypertension or hypotension Tachypnea or hyperpnea Cocaine-induced MI Pallor or cyanosis Hyperexcitability, anxiety Headache Hyperthermia, diaphoresis Nausea, vomiting, abdominal pain Dilated but reactive pupils Confusion, delirium, hallucinations Seizures Coma Respiratory arrest	Swabbing of inside of nose to remove any residual drug if cocaine was snorted Single dose activated charcoal for body stuffers Bowel irrigation for body packers Anticonvulsants (e.g., diazepam, phenobarbital) for seizures Antidysrhythmics, usually lidocaine; calcium channel blockers may also be used (they may also help with coronary artery spasm) Antihypertensives: alpha-blockers (e.g., phentolamine) or vasodilators (e.g., nitroprusside [Nipride]) Hypothermia blanket, ice packs, ice water sponge baths for hyperthermia Fluids, diuretics, urine alkalinization to treat myoglobinuria if present

(continues)

Table 10-7 Toxic Effects of Drugs (*continued*)

Drug or Toxin	Clinical Presentation of Intoxication	Specific Collaborative Management
Cyanide	Anxiety, restlessness, hyperventilation initially Bradycardia followed by tachycardia Hypertension followed by hypotension Dysrhythmias Bitter almond odor to breath Cherry-red mucous membranes Nausea Dyspnea Headache Dizziness Pupil dilation Confusion Stupor, seizures, coma, death	100% oxygen initially by mask Intubation and mechanical ventilation is frequently necessary Supportive care if only anxiety, restlessness, hyperventilation Discontinuance of causative agent (e.g., nitroprusside) Antidotes for more serious symptoms Hydroxocobalamin may be prescribed Amyl nitrite by inhalation Sodium nitrite IV Sodium thiosulfate IV Consider gastric lavage if cyanide was ingested within the last hour Flushing of eyes and/or skin with water if dermal contamination; removal and isolation of clothing Fluids, vasopressors for blood pressure support Anticonvulsants (e.g., diazepam, phenobarbital) for seizures Antidysrhythmics (e.g., lidocaine) for ventricular dysrhythmia, atropine for bradydysrhythmias
Digitalis preparations	Anorexia Nausea Vomiting Headache Restlessness Visual changes Sinus bradycardia, block, or arrest PAT with AV block Junctional tachycardia AV blocks: 1st, 2nd type I, 3rd PVCs: bigeminy, trigeminy, quadrigeminy Ventricular tachycardia: especially bidirectional Ventricular fibrillation	Activated charcoal if less than 1 hour from ingestion, cholestyramine Correction of hypoxia, electrolyte imbalance (especially potassium) Treatment of dysrhythmias For symptomatic bradydysrhythmias and blocks Atropine External pacemaker For symptomatic tachydysrhythmias Lidocaine Phenytoin Magnesium if hypomagnesemia or hyperkalemia present Cardioversion at lowest effective voltage and only if life-threatening dysrhythmias exist Defibrillation for ventricular fibrillation Digoxin immune Fab (Digibind) if hypoperfusion or life-threatening dysrhythmia Relative indications include: > 10 mg ingested (adult), serum digoxin > 10 mg/mL or serum potassium > 5.0 mEq/L Monitor closely for exacerbation of condition if digitalis was being used for (i.e., increase in heart rate, heart failure)

(*continues*)

Table 10-7 **Toxic Effects of Drugs** (*continued*)		
Drug or Toxin	**Clinical Presentation of Intoxication**	**Specific Collaborative Management**

Ethanol	Ethanol concentration (mg/dL)
	< 25: sense of warmth and well-being, talkativeness, self-confidence, mild incoordination
	25–50: euphoria, decreased judgment and control
	50–100: decreased sensorium, worsened coordination, ataxia, decreased reflexes and reaction time
	100–250: nausea, vomiting, ataxia, diplopia, slurred speech, visual impairment, nystagmus, emotional lability, confusion, stupor
	250–400: stupor or coma, incontinence, respiratory depression
	> 400: respiratory paralysis, loss of protective reflexes, hypothermia, death
	Note: These signs/symptoms and blood ethanol levels vary widely; these signs/symptoms are for a non-alcohol-dependent person
	Also:
	    Alcohol odor to breath
	    Hypoglycemia
	    Seizures
	    Metabolic acidosis
		Fluid and electrolyte replacement (potassium, magnesium, calcium may be needed)
		Glucose for hypoglycemia along with multivitamins including thiamine and folic acid
		Note: Thiamine is necessary for the brain to utilize glucose; thiamine deficiency in patients with alcoholism may cause Wernicke encephalopathy

Ethylene glycol	*First 12 hours after ingestion* Appears drunk without the odor of ethanol on breath Nausea, vomiting, hematemesis Focal seizures, coma Nystagmus, depressed reflexes, tetany Metabolic acidosis with increased anion gap *12–24 hours after ingestion* Tachycardia Mild hypertension Pulmonary edema Heart failure 24–72 hours after ingestion Flank pain, costovertebral tenderness Acute renal failure	10% ethanol in D_5W IV to maintain serum ethanol level at 100–200 mg/dL Fomepizole (Antizol) should be used instead of ethanol where available Fluid and electrolyte replacement (particularly calcium, but potassium and magnesium may also be needed) Sodium bicarbonate for severe metabolic acidosis Glucose for hypoglycemia and multivitamins, including thiamine, folic acid, and pyridoxine Note: Thiamine is necessary for the brain to utilize glucose; thiamine deficiency in patients with alcoholism may cause Wernicke encephalopathy. Anticonvulsants (e.g., diazepam, phenobarbital) for seizures Hemodialysis may be needed.
Hallucinogens (e.g., D-lysergic acid diethylamide [LSD])	Tachycardia, hypertension Hyperthermia Anorexia, nausea Headaches Dizziness Agitation, anxiety Impaired judgment Distortion and intensification of sensory perception Toxic psychosis Dilated pupils Rambling speech Polyuria	Reassurance Quiet environment with soft lighting Benzodiazepines (e.g., diazepam) for anxiety and agitation Anticonvulsants (e.g., diazepam, phenobarbital) for seizures Restraints only if necessary to protect patient

(continues)

Table 10-7 Toxic Effects of Drugs (*continued*)		
Drug or Toxin	**Clinical Presentation of Intoxication**	**Specific Collaborative Management**
Isopropyl alcohol	Gastrointestinal distress (e.g., nausea, vomiting, abdominal pain) Headache CNS depression, areflexia, ataxia Respiratory depression Hypothermia, hypotension	Fluids and vasopressors for hypoperfusion H_2 blockers or proton pump inhibitors for gastritis
Lithium	*Mild* Vomiting, diarrhea Lethargy, weakness Polyuria, polydipsia Nystagmus Fine tremors *Severe* Hypotension Severe thirst Tinnitus Hyperreflexia Coarse tremors Ataxia Seizures Confusion Coma Dilute urine, renal failure Heart failure	Hydration Free water replacement to maintain sodium concentration Anticonvulsants (e.g., diazepam, phenobarbital) for seizures, which are rare Hemodialysis may uncommonly be necessary.
Methanol	Nausea and vomiting Hyperpnea, dyspnea Visual disturbances ranging from blurring to blindness Speech difficulty Headache CNS depression Motor dysfunction with rigidity, spasticity, and hypokinesis Metabolic acidosis with anion gap	Gastric lavage (especially helpful if within 2 hours of ingestion) 10% ethanol in D_5W IV to maintain serum ethanol level at 100–200 mg/dL Fomepizole 15 mg/kg IV loading dose followed by maintenance dosing is preferred to ethanol where available Sodium bicarbonate for severe metabolic acidosis Hemodialysis if visual impairment, metabolic acidosis, renal insufficiency, or blood methanol concentration > 30 mmol/L
Methemoglobin-emia caused by nitrites, nitrate, sulfa drugs, and others	Tachycardia Fatigue Nausea Dizziness Cyanosis in the presence of a normal Pao_2; failure of cyanosis to resolve with oxygen therapy Dark red or brown blood Elevated methemoglobin levels Headache, weakness, dyspnea (30% to 40%) Stupor, respiratory depression (60%)	Oxygen Removal of cause Stop nitroglycerin, nitroprusside, sulfa drugs, anesthetic agents, or other causative agent Methylene blue If stupor, coma, angina, or respiratory depression or if level 30% to 40% or more Administered at 2 mg/kg over 5 min; repeated at 1 mg/kg if patient still symptomatic after 30–60 min Ascorbic acid may be administered in large doses Exchange transfusion if methylene blue is contraindicated

(continues)

Table 10-7 **Toxic Effects of Drugs** (*continued*)		
Drug or Toxin	**Clinical Presentation of Intoxication**	**Specific Collaborative Management**
Opioids and opiates	Bradycardia Hypotension Decreased level of consciousness Respiratory depression to respiratory arrest Hypothermia Miosis Diminished bowel sounds Needle tracks, abscesses Seizures Pulmonary edema (especially with heroin)	Bowel irrigation for body packers Naloxone (Narcan) 0.4–2 mg IV, IM, or transtracheally, or nalmefene (Revex) 0.5 mg IV Duration of action of naloxone is 1–2 hours, whereas nalmefene has a duration of action of 4–8 hours (heroin and morphine 4–6 hours, meperidine 2–4 hours) Anticonvulsants (e.g., diazepam, phenobarbital) for seizures Intubation and mechanical ventilation may be required; PEEP may be needed for pulmonary edema
Organophosphate and carbamate (cholinesterase inhibitors)	Bradycardia Nausea, vomiting, diarrhea Abdominal pain and cramping Increased oral secretions Dyspnea Slurred speech Constricted pupils Visual changes Unsteady gait Urinary incontinence Poor motor control Twitching Change in level of consciousness Seizures	Consider gastric lavage,, cathartic if ingested Removal and isolation of clothing Washing of skin with ethyl alcohol and then soap and water if dermal contamination Atropine 1–5 mg IV or IM; repeated as required Pralidoxime chloride (Protopam) 1–2 grams IV over 15–30 min followed by infusion of 10–20 mg/kg may be used for organophosphates Anticonvulsants (e.g., diazepam, phenobarbital) for seizures
Petroleum distillates	Flushed skin Hyperthermia Vomiting Diarrhea Abdominal pain Tachypnea Dyspnea Cyanosis Coughing Breath sound changes: crackles, rhonchi, diminished breath sounds Staggering gait Confusion CNS depression or excitation	Washing of skin with soap and water if dermal contamination; removal and isolation of clothing Oxygen, bronchodilators, mechanical ventilation may be required Potassium supplementation for toluene-associated hypokalemia Consider beta-blockade for ventricular dysrhythmias presumed to be related to halogenated hydrocarbon toxicity
Phencyclidine (PCP)	Tachycardia Hypertensive crisis Hyperthermia Agitation, hyperactivity Nystagmus Blank stare Hypoglycemia	Quiet environment Benzodiazepines (e.g., diazepam) for anxiety and agitation Beta-blockers for dysrhythmias Antihypertensives: vasodilators (e.g., nitroprusside [Nipride])

(continues)

Table 10-7 Toxic Effects of Drugs (continued)

Drug or Toxin	Clinical Presentation of Intoxication	Specific Collaborative Management
Phencyclidine (PCP) (Continued)	Violent, psychotic behavior Ataxia Seizures Myoglobinuria, renal failure Lethargy, coma Cardiac arrest	Hypothermia blanket, ice packs, ice water sponge baths for hyperthermia Anticonvulsants (e.g., diazepam, phenobarbital) for seizures Haloperidol (Haldol) for acute psychotic reactions Fluids and diuretics for myoglobinuria; urinary alkalinization interferes with urinary elimination of PCP, therefore sodium bicarbonate contraindicated
Salicylates	*Initial:* Hyperthermia Burning sensation in mouth or throat Change in level of consciousness Petechiae, rash, hives *Later:* Hyperventilation (respiratory alkalosis) Nausea, vomiting Thirst Tinnitus Diaphoresis *Late:* Hearing loss Motor weakness Vasodilation and hypotension Respiratory depression to respiratory arrest Metabolic acidosis	May consider gastric lavage if performed within an hour of significant ingestion Activated charcoal early in the treatment or if ongoing gastric absorption Consider bowel irrigation if enteric-coated salicylates ingested and persistent absorption and toxicity Fluids with dextrose (e.g., D_5–½ NS) Hypothermia blanket, ice packs, ice water sponge baths for hyperthermia Sodium bicarbonate to alkalinize the serum to prevent tissue distribution and increase rate of salicylate excretion; maintain serum pH > 7.50 Monitor potassium, calcium, and magnesium levels Vitamin K may be needed Anticonvulsants (e.g., diazepam, phenobarbital) for seizures Hemodialysis may be necessary
Tricyclic antidepressants (TCA)	*Anticholinergic* Tachycardia, palpitations Dysrhythmias Hyperthermia Headache Restlessness Mydriasis Dry mouth Nausea, vomiting Dysphagia Decreased bowel sounds Urinary retention Decreased deep tendon reflexes Restlessness, euphoria Hallucinations Seizures Coma *Anti–alpha adrenergic* Hypotension QT prolongation and quinidine-like dysrhythmias (including torsades de pointes) AV and bundle branch blocks Clinical indications of heart failure	Consider activated charcoal less than 1 hour after ingestion if patient is oriented and willing Sodium bicarbonate to alkalinize serum thereby reducing tissue distribution and toxicity; maintain serum pH > 7.50 Monitor potassium, calcium, magnesium levels Hyperventilation may be used to augment alkalosis Physostigmine (Antilirium) should not be prescribed due to risk of seizure in TCA toxicity Sodium bicarbonate +/– hypertonic saline should be given for QRS prolongation and ventricular dysrhythmias Refractory wide complex ventricular dysrhythmia may be treated with lidocaine Cardioversion, defibrillation, pacemaker as needed for dysrhythmias; avoid quinidine, digitalis Magnesium sulfate and overdrive pacing for torsades de pointes Anticonvulsants (e.g., diazepam, phenobarbital) for seizures Fluids and vasopressors for hypotension

This article was published in Pass CCRN, 3e, Dennison RD, p. 717, Copyright Elsevier 2007.

response syndrome resembling septic shock can occur. Death may occur as a result of multiorgan failure, acute respiratory distress syndrome, sepsis, or cerebral edema.

■ *Stage IV (> 96 hours).* If the patient survives, the liver regenerates quickly and is unlikely to evidence any chronic damage.

Nephrotoxicity (kidney damage) may occur with or without liver injury. Renal failure requiring hemodialysis generally occurs only in patients who have also suffered significant hepatotoxicity, but otherwise, renal injury improves with IV fluids and time. Long-term renal dysfunction is not an expected sequela of acute acetaminophen toxicity.

Another variable that may confound the clinical picture is the presence of a co-ingestion. APAP is often combined with anticholinergic and opioid medications (e.g., hydrocodone [Vicodin]). The toxicity of the other drug may obscure signs of acetaminophen-induced toxicity. Moreover, in an overdose scenario, acetaminophen ingestion must always be considered and specifically queried because of its wide availability and the relative absence of early symptoms. In cases of unintentional overdose, the patient may have taken repeated supratherapeutic doses in an attempt to relieve unremitting pain. Obtaining a thorough, accurate history is vitally important in preventing advanced hepatotoxicity.

Differential Diagnosis

On arrival to the emergency department (ED), diagnostic tests include acetaminophen level, liver function tests, coagulation (PT/INR) studies, and measurement of electrolytes, blood urea nitrogen (BUN), and creatinine. In the setting of severe toxicity, arterial or venous blood gases with lactic acid levels may also be analyzed, since acidemia due to metabolic acidosis is a reliable predictor of morbidity and mortality.

Interpretation of serum acetaminophen level hinges on the time of ingestion. The Rumack-Matthew nomogram can be used to predict which patients will develop serious hepatic injury, defined as an aspartate aminotransferase [AST] level above 1000 IU/L. The nomogram has an established treatment line. On the basis of time since ingestion and serum level, you can plot an individual patient's data on the graph. If the patient's mark is above the line, treatment is required. If it falls below this threshold, no further treatment is required. The gold standard is to initiate treatment at a 4-hour level above 150 µg/mL. Note, however, that this boundary is valid only for assessment of a single, all-at-one-time ingestion. It is not valid for chronic or multiple-dose ingestions.

Treatment

Treatment decisions center primarily on the time of ingestion and obtaining a thorough, accurate history.

Prehospital Setting Offer intensive supportive care, including airway management as needed on the basis of mental status. Provide aggressive IV fluid resuscitation. In rare cases in which your evaluation takes place within 1 hour of ingestion and the patient is awake and oriented without nausea, you may consider using activated charcoal. An IV antiemetic may be administered for symptomatic control.

In-Hospital Setting Treatment of acetaminophen toxicity consists of either IV or oral administration of *N*-acetylcysteine (NAC). NAC acts in a variety of ways to detoxify NAPQI, replenish glutathione stores, decrease inflammatory toxicity, and encourage metabolism of APAP to nontoxic metabolites. If given within 8 hours of ingestion, before glutathione stores have been depleted, severe hepatic injury can be avoided. Once again, this demonstrates the importance of accurately determining the time of ingestion. Regardless of how much time has elapsed, however, NAC does offer benefit compared with placebo. NAC therapy should be continued until one of three end points is reached:

1. Symptomatic and laboratory improvement occurs.
2. A liver transplant is performed.
3. The patient dies.

In patients without progression of toxicity, treatment protocols generally unfold over a minimum of 20 hours. Side effects of NAC therapy are generally minor, uncommon, and easily treated. Oral NAC is associated with a high incidence of nausea and vomiting because it has an odor of rotten eggs. Intravenous NAC has been associated with anaphylactoid reactions, which are not true immunoglobulin E (IgE)-mediated allergic reactions. Symptoms generally include rash, pruritus, and occasionally wheezing and upper airway edema. According to the package insert, the incidence of pruritus is 10%, hypotension 4%, bronchospasm 6%, and angioedema 8%. When these symptoms occur, treatment must be temporarily discontinued while the patient is treated with antihistamines, bronchodilators, and epinephrine if necessary. Infusion may then be continued at a slower rate. If symptoms recur, oral NAC may be used.

Pediatric patients are somewhat protected from acetaminophen toxicity compared with adults because they have an increased capacity for nontoxic metabolism of acetaminophen. Diagnosis and treatment of pregnant women do not differ from standard treatment. Patients with chronic alcohol abuse or malnutrition (who probably have decreased glutathione stores) may be at increased risk of hepatotoxicity. Nevertheless, the Rumack-Matthew nomogram and NAC therapy remain the same in these groups of patients, as no evidence exists to support alteration of treatment.

Salicylates

Salicylates such as aspirin (acetylsalicylic acid) are common OTC analgesics. They are also involved in many toxicologic emergencies. Salicylate overdose is also complicated by the fact that other medications are often co-ingested.

Pathophysiology

Salicylates act therapeutically by inhibiting prostaglandin synthesis by acetylating cyclooxygenases (COX-1 and COX-2). In larger doses, salicylates uncouple oxidative phosphorylation, which leads to decreased ATP production and anion-gap metabolic acidosis. Stimulation of the medullary respiratory center also causes a primary respiratory alkalosis from hyperpnea and/or tachypnea.

Signs and Symptoms

Early symptoms of acute salicylate poisoning include gastric irritation, vomiting, and pain. Symptoms may progress to include tinnitus or diminished hearing, hyperpnea/tachypnea, hyperthermia, altered mental status, and seizures. Chronic poisoning can occur with aspirin, because it is an extremely effective analgesic and is now being prescribed at low doses as a daily preventive agent for cardiac care. Symptoms of chronic poisoning, such as gastric irritation and pain, are similar to the early symptoms of acute poisoning, although alteration in mental status is more commonly present at the time of presentation.

Differential Diagnosis

Laboratory evaluation of salicylate toxicity includes immediate evaluation of salicylate level and blood gas, either arterial or venous. Subsequently, serial levels and blood gases should be checked, initially every 2 hours, in order to adequately monitor the effect of treatment as well as to assess ongoing absorption. In overdose, salicylates exhibit delayed absorption as well as diminished elimination leading to unpredictable pharmacokinetics.

Treatment

Salicylate poisoning has no antidote. The primary treatment is alkalinization through the administration of sodium bicarbonate. Activated charcoal may be considered in select patients in consultation with a poison center or toxicologist given the potential for delayed and prolonged absorption.

Prehospital Setting Administration of IV fluids is essential. If metabolic acidosis develops, aggressively treat the condition with sodium bicarbonate. Supportive care, especially airway management, is of primary importance. Rule out hypoglycemia using a blood glucose test.

In-Hospital Setting Sodium bicarbonate administration alters the distribution of salicylate within the body and limits CNS penetration, which is associated with increasing mortality. A secondary benefit of serum alkalinization is urinary alkalinization and enhanced elimination. Potassium supplementation is critical as bicarbonate-induced hypokalemia allows for enhanced renal reabsorption of hydrogen and worsening acidosis. Hemodialysis is indicated by renal failure, rising serum salicylate assays, severe metabolic acidosis, CNS toxicity, or cardiac dysfunction.

Beta-Blockers

Beta-blockers are frequently prescribed for the treatment of hypertension, coronary artery disease, congestive heart failure, arrhythmias, migraine headache prophylaxis, and anxiety disorders. Commonly prescribed beta-blockers include metoprolol (Lopressor, Toprol), carvedilol (Coreg), propranolol (Inderal), and atenolol (Tenormin). Topical ophthalmic preparations, including timolol (Timoptic), may be prescribed for glaucoma. Systemic toxicity has been reported with ingestion and use of these preparations.

Both intentional and unintentional ingestions leading to beta-blocker toxicity are frequently reported. In 2013, beta-blocker ingestions accounted for more than 24,000 calls to poison control centers, resulting in more than 4000 visits to healthcare facilities. Despite this large number of ingestions, only 11 deaths were attributed to beta-blocker toxicity in 2013. Nevertheless, beta-blocker ingestion is a dangerous condition seen frequently in the prehospital setting.

Pathophysiology

Beta-blockers are often classified as beta 1 specific agents or nonspecific agents on the basis of their respective pharmacologic structures. Examples of beta 1 specific drugs include atenolol (Tenormin) and metoprolol (Lopressor, Toprol). Propranolol (Inderal) is a nonspecific beta-blocker. In general, beta 1 receptor inhibition decreases chronotropy and inotropy by modulating G protein–linked second-messenger systems. These receptors are primarily found in cardiac tissue. Peripheral $beta_2$ receptor agonist action causes vasodilation. Beta blockade may cause respiratory distress in patients with a predisposition to bronchoconstriction, such as those with asthma or COPD.

Signs and Symptoms

In patients with suspected beta-blocker toxicity, as with all ingestions, you must obtain a detailed history of drug exposure, approximate dose, and time of ingestion, as well as possible co-ingestions. In patients who have ingested prescribed beta-blockers, obtaining information about the underlying disorder that required the prescription may aid in determining your treatment. A history of severe coronary artery disease, congestive heart failure, or dysrhythmia, for example, can affect decisions about the patient's long-term management. Remember to ask about previous pulmonary diseases such as asthma and COPD.

Patients typically present with bradycardia and hypotension after ingesting beta-adrenergic antagonists. The bradycardia may be a sinus bradycardia or, uncommonly, it may represent a first-, second-, or third-degree heart block. Mental status depression may or may not be present, depending on the specific drug ingested and its cardiovascular toxicity. If it occurs, the altered mental status may be caused by cerebral hypoperfusion or by the direct CNS depressive effects of the drug, particularly lipophilic drugs such as propranolol. Seizures occur in some patients, particularly in those with propranolol toxicity. Patients with CNS depression may also have respiratory depression.

Differential Diagnosis

In a patient with suspected beta-blocker toxicity, a focused physical examination of the cardiovascular system may reveal a decreased respiratory rate, bilateral crackles secondary to acute pulmonary edema, or wheezing. Evaluation of capillary refill serves as an adjunctive measure to assess tissue perfusion. Beta-blocker toxicity can also cause metabolic derangements like mild hypoglycemia or slightly elevated potassium levels, which may be clinically significant in children. The presence of either mild hypoglycemia or normoglycemia can help you differentiate beta-blocker toxicity from bradycardia and hypotension due to calcium channel blocker toxicity. As discussed in the next section, calcium channel blocker toxicity is usually accompanied by hyperglycemia.

Evaluation of patients with suspected beta-blocker toxicity focuses on identifying end-organ dysfunction and hypoperfusion. Beyond physical examination of mental status, cardiopulmonary function, capillary refill response, and urine output, several ancillary tests are often performed. Arterial or venous blood gases may be obtained as a rapid measure of gas exchange and a possible indicator of metabolic acidosis secondary to tissue hypoperfusion and hypoxia. Electrocardiography is used to evaluate heart rhythm and rule out myocardial ischemia. Elevated cardiac enzymes (troponins) indicate myocardial injury due to hypotension and inadequate myocardial oxygen delivery.

Decreased serum bicarbonate levels and elevated serum urea nitrogen and creatinine are markers of poor tissue perfusion. Catheter insertion and subsequent documentation of urine output often yields the best real-time measurement of perfusion. Invasive hemodynamic monitoring, including placement of an arterial line, central venous pressure monitor, or Swan-Ganz catheter, may be initiated as well, depending on the severity of toxicity.

Treatment

Prehospital Setting After managing the patient's airway and establishing IV access, consider administering activated charcoal if less than 1 hour has elapsed since the ingestion of the beta-blocker and the patient is alert and is not experiencing nausea or vomiting. Inhaled beta-agonists such as albuterol (Proventil, Ventolin) are indicated in patients with wheezing. Use caution when giving normal saline IV boluses in hypotensive patients because of the negative inotropic effects of beta-adrenergic antagonists. Aggressive volume resuscitation can cause pulmonary edema. If the patient remains underperfused, as indicated by altered mental status, decreased capillary refill, or evidence of ischemia, provide pharmacologic support. Atropine is an option for bradycardia associated with hypoperfusion, but its effects may be minimal and transient. Additional therapy is often required.

Glucagon is often referred to as the *antidote* for beta-adrenergic antagonist toxicity. Cardiac glucagon receptors, like beta-adrenergic receptors, are coupled to G proteins, increasing intracellular cyclic adenosine monophosphate (cAMP). At the same time, glucagon inhibits phosphodiesterase. Glucagon is a vasodilator and therefore may not produce a corresponding increase in blood pressure. Human data regarding glucagon efficacy are limited to case reports and a case series. Adverse effects may include vomiting, hyperglycemia, and mild hypoglycemia.

If these therapies fail, progress to administering catecholamine vasopressors and other experimental therapies. Cardiac pacing is rarely effective in patients in whom therapy has failed.

In-Hospital Setting Initial ED treatment of patients with beta-blocker toxicity follows the same algorithm as prehospital management. Failure of first-line treatment strategies necessitates administration of vasoactive medications. Pure beta-adrenergic agonists such as isoproterenol (Isuprel) can be effective, but their beta-agonist action may cause peripheral vasodilation and deteriorating hypotension. Dobutamine (Dobutrex), another beta-agonist, also improves cardiac function and stimulates less peripheral vasodilation than isoproterenol. Epinephrine (Adrenalin) infusions can result in improved cardiac function and peripheral vasopressor effects. Primary vasoconstrictors such as norepinephrine (Levophed) and phenylephrine (Neo-Synephrine) may be less beneficial because they increase afterload but produce relatively little improvement in cardiac function. This intervention poses a risk of worsened heart failure and pulmonary edema. Regardless of the catecholamine used, providers must be aware that very high doses—often higher than the recommended maximum dosage—may be required to have an effect on the ingested drug.

A newer therapy gaining popularity (on the basis of encouraging animal data and limited human data) is high-dose insulin infusion. Insulin infusion at doses of 1–10 unit/kg/hr following a bolus dose of 1–10 units/kg may provide benefit in patients with hypotension as a result of calcium channel blocker or beta-blocker ingestion. Referred to as *hyperinsulinemia-euglycemia (HIE) therapy*, the precise mechanism by which it is theorized to reverse toxicity is unclear. Researchers hypothesize that the therapy may improve glucose utilization and energy production by the poisoned myocardium or have direct vasoconstricting properties, or it may alter fatty acid metabolism or calcium sensitivity. HIE therapy in humans has been studied primarily in the setting of calcium channel blocker toxicity, but animal studies have also demonstrated its benefit in beta-blocker toxicity. As the infusion is administered, blood glucose levels must be checked and corrected every 30 minutes initially, and then at less frequent intervals depending on the patient's response.

Although the basic therapeutic concepts in managing beta-blocker toxicity can be generalized to all beta-blockers, several agents have special properties and thus require customized management strategies. Propranolol (Inderal), for example, possesses the most potent membrane-stabilizing properties among beta blockers. As a result, toxicity may lead to sodium channel blockade, QRS prolongation, and ventricular dysrhythmia.

(Sodium channel blockade is discussed later in more detail in the *Tricyclic Antidepressants* section.) In addition to standard therapy, then, sodium bicarbonate administration may be required in the treatment of propranolol toxicity. Propranolol is the most lipophilic beta-blocker; therefore it causes more significant CNS toxicity than other beta-blockers, including seizures. Benzodiazepines are the first-line treatment for propranolol-induced seizures.

Calcium Channel Blockers

Calcium channel blockers account for about 40% of cardiovascular drug exposures reported to the American Association of Poison Control Centers and more than 65% of deaths from cardiovascular medications. There are three commonly prescribed classes of calcium channel blockers in the United States:

1. Phenylalkylamines (e.g., verapamil [Calan, Isoptin])
2. Benzothiazepines (e.g., diltiazem [Cardizem, Cartia, Dilacor])
3. Dihydropyridines (e.g., amlodipine [Norvasc] and felodipine [Plendil])

Verapamil and diltiazem are often referred to as *nondihydropyridines* because their characteristic cardiovascular activity differs from that of dihydropyridines.

Pathophysiology

Calcium channels are found on cardiac cells, vascular smooth muscle, and pancreatic beta islet cells. Opening of calcium channels contributes to myocardial contractility and vascular smooth muscle constriction. In pancreatic cells, calcium influx triggers insulin release. Reduction of intracellular calcium in cardiac muscle, coronary artery smooth muscle, and peripheral vessels depresses both chronotropy and inotropy and suppresses peripheral vasoconstriction. Because of differences in resting membrane potentials, dihydropyridine calcium channel blockers act preferentially on peripheral vascular calcium channels, decreasing peripheral vascular resistance but having little or no effect on cardiac calcium channels at therapeutic doses. This class of calcium channel blocker typically reduces blood pressure by inducing vasodilation with reflex tachycardia.

Signs and Symptoms

Signs and symptoms of calcium channel blocker–induced toxicity may include chest pain, shortness of breath, light-headedness, syncope, hypotension, and bradycardia or tachycardia, depending on the class of calcium channel blocker ingested. First-, second-, or third-degree heart block may also be present. As discussed in the previous section, hyperglycemia typically accompanies calcium channel blocker toxicity, differentiating it from beta-blocker toxicity.

Differential Diagnosis

The history obtained and physical examination performed after calcium channel blocker ingestion are similar to the history and exam that follow beta-blocker ingestion. It is important to obtain a detailed medical history, particularly regarding cardiovascular disease, and an incident history of dose, time of ingestion, and possible co-ingestions.

After evaluation and stabilization of the patient's airway and breathing, cardiovascular evaluation begins with close, often invasive monitoring of the patient's blood pressure and perfusion status, which may be accomplished with the aid of an arterial line or Swan-Ganz catheter (**Figure 10-1**). In patients with altered mental status or diminished airway reflexes, a chest radiograph is routinely performed to evaluate for pulmonary edema and aspiration pneumonitis. Acute pulmonary edema may cause bilateral crackles on auscultation and a decreased pulse oximetry measurement on room air. Mental status is not usually affected directly by calcium channel blockers, but cerebral hypoperfusion may alter the patient's level of consciousness. Extremity capillary refill examination, as in beta-blocker toxicity, provides a clue to perfusion status. In patients with evidence of toxicity, a catheter is placed and urine output documented as a surrogate marker of renal perfusion. An ECG is obtained to evaluate for rhythm abnormalities and evidence of ischemia. Serial electrolyte, serum urea nitrogen, creatinine, and cardiac enzyme studies

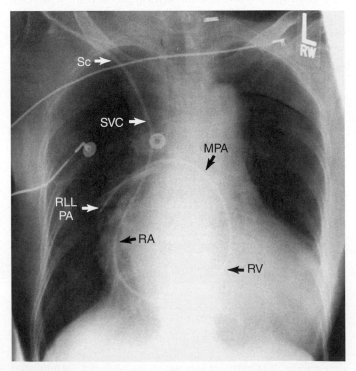

Figure 10-1 Normal course of a Swan-Ganz catheter. A Swan-Ganz catheter inserted on the right goes into the subclavian vein (Sc), into the superior vena cava (SVC), right atrium (RA), right ventricle (RV), main pulmonary artery (MPA), and in this case, the right lower lobe pulmonary artery (RLL PA).

From Mettler F: *Essentials of radiology*, ed 2, Philadelphia, PA, 2005, Saunders.

provide further indicators of possible organ hypoperfusion with resulting kidney injury, metabolic acidosis, and ischemic myocardial injury. Arterial or venous blood gas measurements can also aid in rapid evaluation of acid–base status, but are often not necessary. Patients who are found unresponsive or are known to have been immobile for prolonged periods are evaluated for rhabdomyolysis by serum CPK studies and muscle compartment examination.

Treatment

Prehospital Setting As in beta-blocker poisoning, initial management of calcium channel blocker toxicity centers on controlling the patient's airway and breathing. In appropriate patients, consider using activated charcoal. You may administer IV boluses of normal saline for hypotension, but their effect may be limited by the negative inotropic effects and resultant pulmonary edema associated with calcium channel blockers. You should administer atropine in patients with symptomatic bradycardia, but it is often ineffective or only transiently effective. IV glucagon at doses similar to those studied in beta-blocker toxicity has been used but with less consistent effects. Administration of calcium salts can improve outcomes, but the use of this therapy may be limited by symptomatic hypercalcemia. Administration of IV calcium gluconate poses little risk to the patient and may be beneficial, especially when given in doses of several ampules. Calcium chloride contains more than three times as much elemental calcium as calcium gluconate, but it may provoke more peripheral venous irritation and other adverse effects. For patients taking digoxin, use of calcium salts is contraindicated because of the presumed risk of potentiating digoxin toxicity.

In-Hospital Setting After administration of IV fluid boluses, calcium salts, and atropine or glucagon, patients typically receive IV vasopressors. As in beta-blocker toxicity, the choice of vasopressor has been widely debated, with reports of success and failure of multiple agents. Dopamine remains a poor choice because of its indirect sympathomimetic activity. On the basis of the available data, insulin therapy with maintenance of euglycemia is recommended in patients with severe calcium channel blocker toxicity resistant to vasopressor therapy.

Although severe dihydropyridine calcium channel blocker toxicity can cause bradycardia and hypotension, as with non-dihydropyridine calcium channel blockers, toxic ingestions typically lead to peripheral vasodilation and hypotension with reflex tachycardia. As a result, after administration of IV fluids, the treatment of choice is a peripheral vasoconstrictor such as norepinephrine (Levophed) or phenylephrine (Neo-Synephrine).

When standard therapies fail, an intra-aortic balloon pump, extracorporeal membrane oxygenation, or cardiopulmonary bypass may be considered as temporizing measures. Limited success has been reported.

Tricyclic Antidepressants

Tricyclic antidepressants have historically been a leading cause of toxicologic emergencies, especially intentional overdoses. These medications have a narrow therapeutic index, which means there is a fine line between an ineffectually low dose and an overdose. The use of tricyclic antidepressants has declined recently as newer, safer alternatives have been introduced.

Pathophysiology

Tricyclic antidepressants act therapeutically by increasing the amount of norepinephrine and serotonin available in the CNS. They do so by blocking the reuptake of these neurotransmitters, extending the duration of their action. Additionally, tricyclic antidepressants block cellular ion channels and alpha-adrenergic, muscarinic, GABA-A, and histaminergic receptors. Cardiac toxicity is the hallmark of tricyclic antidepressant poisoning.

Signs and Symptoms

Tricyclic antidepressant toxicity is a result of potassium efflux inhibition and sodium channel inhibition in the myocardium. Early signs and symptoms include classic anticholinergic toxidrome effects like dry mouth, tachycardia, urinary retention, constipation, mydriasis, and blurred vision. Late signs and symptoms include respiratory depression, confusion, hallucinations, hyperthermia, ventricular dysrhythmias (such as torsades de pointes and wide QRS complexes), and seizures.

Differential Diagnosis

Serum levels of tricyclic antidepressants are not well correlated with the severity of intoxication. Evaluation for co-ingestion of additional agents such as acetaminophen and salicylate should be performed. Other lab studies that are indicated include measurement of electrolyte, serum urea nitrogen, and creatinine levels, anion-gap analysis, a complete blood cell count (CBC), and evaluation of arterial blood gases (ABGs). Qualitative urine immunoassays are also available. However, the TCA screen may result in false positive results and should not be relied upon to accurately diagnose toxicity. Clinical and electrocardiographic evaluation of the patient should direct treatment. Chest imaging may be indicated if aspiration has occurred or other respiratory symptoms are noted.

Treatment

Cardiac monitoring is critical in patients with suspected tricyclic antidepressant overdose, because cardiac complications are the primary cause of death. Sudden cardiac arrest may occur days after the overdose. There is no antidote for tricyclic antidepressant poisoning. Activated charcoal, which can be administered in appropriate patients within an hour of ingestion, may have benefit.

Prehospital Setting Provide supportive care, especially cardiac monitoring. Establish IV access, and administer sodium bicarbonate bolus and infusion if there is evidence of QRS prolongation or seizures. Anticipate the potential for administering a large amount of sodium bicarbonate, often more than 4 ampules, to maintain a QRS < 110 ms. Agitation, tremor, and seizures should be treated with escalating doses of benzodiazepines.

In-Hospital Setting Asymptomatic patients should be observed for at least 6 hours to rule out sequelae. Maintaining alkaline serum (pH 7.50 to 7.55) by bicarbonate infusion counteracts cardiac conduction effects. This treatment should be given if QRS widening (> 120 ms) or ventricular ectopy occurs. Tachycardia is anticipated due to anticholinergic effects. Slowing of the rate is indicative of overwhelming sodium channel blockade, worsening cardiotoxicity, and the need for treatment with sodium bicarbonate.

Lithium

Lithium is an agent used to treat bipolar disorder, also known as "manic-depressive illness." Although lithium is an effective treatment, it has a narrow therapeutic index, increasing the likelihood of both accidental and intentional poisonings. To avoid accidental therapeutic poisoning, routine blood tests are necessary to adjust the patient's lithium dosage, as needed.

Several variables affect the drug's toxicity, including acute versus chronic ingestion, dose relative to existing serum levels, and overdose amount. Toxicity is exacerbated by dehydration, diuretic use, and renal dysfunction.

Pathophysiology

Lithium is a small cation (positively charged ion). It is similar to sodium and acts in place of it but has different effects. The precise mechanism by which lithium produces its medicinal benefit is still unknown, although the drug is thought to alter neuronal cell membrane function, cellular sodium and energy balance, and hormonal response. These effects may cause permanent CNS damage. Lithium decreases kidney function and is eliminated almost entirely by the kidneys. This property of the drug sometimes causes inadvertent lithium reabsorption.

Signs and Symptoms

Signs and symptoms of lithium poisoning depend heavily on the dose and whether toxicity is related to an acute, acute on chronic, or chronic ingestion. Serum levels can be misleading in predicting toxicity. Patients who have not previously been exposed to lithium would be expected to have higher serum levels and fewer symptoms because they do not have saturated tissue distribution. However, with chronic ingestion, more significant toxicity can be seen with lower levels. Minor symptoms include nausea, vomiting, excessive thirst, and muscle cramping. Progressive toxicity can result in tremor, myoclonus, diabetes insipidus with resulting hypernatremia, confusion, delirium, coma, and, in rare but serious cases, hypotension, electrocardiographic abnormalities, and dysrhythmias.

Differential Diagnosis

The lab workup of a patient with suspected lithium toxicity should include a urinalysis and periodic monitoring of serum lithium and sodium levels until symptoms resolve. Cardiac monitoring may be indicated. To yield accurate results, the blood sample must be sent in a lithium-free tube. A thyroid function panel, analysis of acetaminophen level, and a lumbar puncture can be useful in eliminating alternative etiologies. Toxic co-ingestion must always be considered as a possibility.

Treatment

Prehospital Setting In the field, treatment is mainly supportive. Maintain airway, breathing, and circulation. Establish IV access. Fluid administration is especially important in patients with lithium poisoning because of the effects of volume depletion on the cardiovascular and renal systems. Some reports indicate that sodium therapy encourages elimination of lithium by the kidneys.

In-Hospital Setting Hospital management of lithium toxicity centers on restoring euvolemia and maintaining a normal sodium level. Chronic lithium toxicity is typically a result of dehydration and associated kidney injury. The majority of patients with lithium toxicity can be treated with volume replacement alone. Acute lithium toxicity is often associated with predominantly GI toxicity and should be treated symptomatically. Hemodialysis is indicated in the rare cases of severe intoxication associated with persistent renal failure, severe cardiovascular effects, or severe neurologic symptoms.

Amphetamines

Amphetamines are a diverse class of commonly abused legal and illicit drugs that can cause significant toxicity. Abuse of these drugs, particularly medications used to treat attention deficit hyperactivity disorder (ADHD), is common, partly because they are being prescribed to an increasing number of adolescents. Since the 1980s, the number of stimulant prescriptions for ADHD has increased fourfold. In one anonymous survey, 15% of 12th-grade students in the United States admitted to having abused prescription amphetamines.

Prescription amphetamines include methylphenidate (Ritalin, Concerta), amphetamine/dextroamphetamine (Adderall), phentermine (Adipex-P), atomoxetine (Strattera), and dexmethylphenidate (Focalin). These medications are generally used to treat ADHD but in some cases are used as diet pills. In addition, selegiline (Eldepryl), an agent used to treat Parkinson's disease, is metabolized to l-methamphetamine.

A wide variety of illicit amphetamines is abused, including amphetamine, methamphetamine, methylenedioxymethamphetamine (MDMA, or "ecstasy"), and methcathinone ("cat" or "Jeff"). Most users are simply trying to get high, but some users take the drugs as physical performance enhancers. Methamphetamine abuse is particularly dangerous because of the drug's astonishing potency. According to the Drug Abuse Warning Network, ED visits related to methamphetamine use rose from 67,954 in 2007 to 102,961 in 2011.

Cathinone is the active compound in khat leaves, which are commonly chewed by people in Eastern Africa for their stimulant effects. The chemical structure of cathinone has been altered to create multiple newer and stronger stimulants such as methyl-methcathinone and methylenedioxypyrovalerone (MDPV), the constituents in the abused stimulants referred to as *bath salts*. Additionally, newer stimulant hallucinogens with amphetamine properties referred to as 2C, 2C-I, 25I and 25C-NBOMe compounds based on their chemical structure are commonly called *acid* or *N-bombs* and are gaining popularity.

Use of a dangerous **synthetic cathinone** drug called alpha-pyrrolidinopentiophenone (alpha-PVP), popularly known as "Flakka," is surging in Florida and is also being reported in other parts of the country.

Alpha-PVP is chemically similar to other synthetic cathinone drugs popularly called "bath salts," and takes the form of a white or pink, foul-smelling crystal that can be eaten, snorted, injected, or vaporized in an e-cigarette or similar device. Vaporizing, which sends the drug very quickly into the bloodstream, may make it particularly easy to overdose.

Like other drugs of this type, alpha-PVP can cause a condition called "excited delirium" that involves hyperstimulation, paranoia, and hallucinations that can lead to violent aggression and self-injury. The drug has been linked to deaths by suicide as well as heart attack. It can also dangerously raise body temperature and lead to kidney damage or kidney failure.

Both prescription and illicit amphetamines are abused in a variety of ways. They can be taken orally or they can be crushed and then snorted, injected, or smoked if sufficiently pure. Street names of some of these drugs are listed in Table 10-8.

Individuals who ingest packets of drugs while evading police, known commonly as **stuffers**, may experience severe toxicity because of the relatively large amount of drug ingested and because its packaging was not designed to traverse the GI tract. They are often identified early by police, who may see them swallow the packets. Administration of activated charcoal is recommended in such patients in order to attenuate potential toxicity. Toxic effects do not always develop, but these patients must undergo extended observation in the ED because of the risk of delayed absorption and toxicity. Otherwise, evaluation and treatment remain the same as for any toxic ingestion.

Packers, people who smuggle large amounts of drugs by ingesting them, require admission to the intensive care unit (ICU) when they are identified. Although the risk of packaging failure is relatively low, such a large amount of drug is present in the GI tract that release of the drug would unleash a torrent of severe toxicity, GI ischemia, and death regardless of treatment. In fact, surgical removal of drug packages is indicated after any sign of toxicity in such patients.

Another concern with illicit amphetamine use and trafficking is the possibility of drug contamination. Many amphetamines are produced by generating chemical reactions that may in themselves cause injury. For example, outbreaks of lead and mercury toxicity have been traced to methamphetamine contamination. Amphetamines are also used in combination with other drugs, such as cocaine, heroin, and marijuana, which may alter their toxicity and clinical presentation.

Pathophysiology

Amphetamines are structurally similar to endogenous catecholamines. They act at presynaptic nerve terminals to prevent reuptake of biogenic amines (norepinephrine, dopamine, and serotonin) from the synaptic cleft and to promote release of these neurotransmitters. The consequent excessive postsynaptic stimulation leads to the clinical manifestations of toxicity as well as to the euphoria associated with use of these drugs. Chemical substitutions alter the potency of amphetamines and confer slight alterations in toxicity. For example, MDMA has predominantly serotonergic properties, which are responsible for the drug's characteristic clinical effects.

Signs and Symptoms

Amphetamine abuse results in sympathomimetic toxicity. Tachycardia, hypertension, agitation, and tremor are typical. Severe toxicity may cause seizures, intracranial hemorrhage, myocardial infarction, ventricular dysrhythmia, or death. Patients may show a marked increase in strength as well as

Table 10-8 **Names of Common Street Drugs**	
Drug	**Street Name**
Methamphetamine	Crank, speed (oral or injected form) Ice, crystal meth (smoked form)
Methylenedioxymethamphetamine (MDMA)	Ecstasy, E, X, XTC, Adam, 007, B-bomb, care bear, Deb, go Jerry Garcia, love pill, playboy, wafer, white diamond
Methcathinone	Cat, khat, Jeff, ephedrine, Flakka

blunted pain perception. Because of excessive dopamine release, amphetamine toxicity may induce psychosis and involuntary movements.

Differential Diagnosis

Although obtaining a history of the dose or time of ingestion may be helpful, this information probably will not significantly affect your management. Identification of the drug is the most important component of the patient's history. Knowing the street names of drugs may help you identify them (see Table 10-8). Gathering additional information about past medical history of cardiovascular disease, seizure disorder, or stroke also aids in management.

Physical examination often reveals mydriasis and diaphoresis, which are a result of sympathetic overstimulation. In patients who have taken MDMA, you may observe bruxism (jaw clenching or chewing). MDMA use, especially in the setting of raves, has also been associated with hyponatremia, which can manifest as altered mental status or seizures. With any amphetamine overdose, hyperreflexia and excessive motor activity can cause muscle breakdown and rhabdomyolysis, raising the specter of possible myoglobinuric renal failure. Hyperthermia is a late and ominous sign. In fact, of all the vital signs, hyperthermia is the most predictive of significant morbidity and mortality in patients with amphetamine overdose.

Treatment

Benzodiazepine administration, IV fluid hydration, and external cooling are the mainstays of treatment in amphetamine toxicity. **Prehospital Setting** Prehospital treatment of patients with sympathomimetic toxicity begins with appropriate airway management and continuous cardiac monitoring. Measurement of blood glucose is critical to rule out hypoglycemia as the cause of altered mental status and tachycardia. Otherwise, initiate IV access and administer fluid boluses. Owing to diaphoresis, increased activity, and insensible fluid losses, patients with amphetamine toxicity are often dehydrated and require volume resuscitation. In addition, administering IV fluids may protect patients from kidney injury as a result of rhabdomyolysis.

In patients who are agitated and combative, administer benzodiazepines. The dose required to achieve sedation varies among individual patients, but the goal of therapy is to achieve sedation and suppress excessive motor activity. Benzodiazepines also act as sympatholytics, thereby treating tachycardia and hypertension. Occasionally, despite adequate sedation, patients may demonstrate rhythmic or involuntary movements as a result of excessive dopaminergic stimulation. Haloperidol (Haldol) may be used to treat this movement disorder, but you should reserve haloperidol treatment until after you administer benzodiazepines whenever possible, because of the risk of seizures.

Perform a 12-lead ECG in patients who complain of chest pain or have evidence of significant toxicity. Consider administering aspirin or nitroglycerin, but in patients with altered mental status, withhold aspirin until a computed tomographic (CT) scan of the brain can be obtained to rule out intracranial hemorrhage. Treating the underlying toxicity with benzodiazepines also treats cardiovascular sequelae. Myocardial ischemia is more commonly related to vasospasm than to vasoocclusive disease. Finally, in patients who are hyperthermic, institute external cooling measures.

In-Hospital Setting After initial stabilization of the patient, evaluation in the ED focuses on identifying end-organ injury from amphetamine toxicity. Most commonly affected are the CNS and cardiovascular system. CT scanning of the brain without IV contrast is often performed to evaluate for hemorrhage, cerebral edema, or early evidence of ischemia. ECG and cardiac enzyme testing may be ordered because of the risk of myocardial ischemia and ventricular dysrhythmia.

Blood tests include a CBC, kidney function tests, and measurement of electrolyte levels and total creatine kinase. An arterial or venous blood gas measurement is obtained in sick patients, because metabolic acidosis is common in severe sympathomimetic toxicity, primarily as a result of increased psychomotor activity. Further testing may be required on the basis of clinical presentation.

Urine drug testing may confirm the presence of amphetamine but should not guide acute management. The patient's clinical presentation/chief complaint, consistent with a sympathomimetic toxidrome, should be a sufficient basis on which to initiate management. Moreover, prescription and OTC medications (e.g., pseudoephedrine [Sudafed]) may cause false-positive results on standard urine drug screens.

ED management is similar to prehospital management. In severe cases, intubation and sedation with propofol (Diprivan) or phenobarbital (Luminal) may be required. In patients with active myocardial ischemia, including ST-segment elevation myocardial infarction (STEMI), cardiology consultation may be obtained, but the decision to perform cardiac catheterization in these patients is not clear. Generally, acute drug toxicity is treated with follow-up cardiac evaluation once the patient is hemodynamically stable. However, focal areas of infarction or myocardial injury on ECG or echocardiogram should raise suspicion for a potential coronary lesion. Because of vascular toxicity, hypertension, and lack of evidence to support thrombosis, thrombolytics are not administered to patients with sympathomimetic toxicity. Patients may require care in an intensive care unit after initial stabilization.

Barbiturates

Barbiturates have been commercially available since 1903. Phenobarbital (Luminal) was used extensively to treat seizure disorders before the advent of newer anticonvulsants, and it is still used to treat refractory, or uncontrolled, seizure disorders. Some patients are treated successfully with phenobarbital for years. Primidone (Mysoline), which is metabolized to phenobarbital, is also used as an anticonvulsant. Butalbital combined with caffeine and either aspirin (Fiorinal) or acetaminophen

(Fioricet) is a barbiturate used as a pain reliever, primarily in the treatment of migraine headaches. Other barbiturates, or "barbs" as they are commonly known, are available but rarely prescribed. Barbiturates have a narrow therapeutic index and are responsible for the highest risk of morbidity and mortality of all sedative-hypnotic agents.

Pathophysiology

Barbiturates act primarily through $GABA_A$ receptor binding. $GABA_A$ receptor agonist action prolongs the duration of chloride influx and hyperpolarizes the cell membrane. Therefore, $GABA_A$ agonists cause neuroinhibition and sedation. This mechanism is primarily responsible for the therapeutic and toxic effects of barbiturates. Sedative activity is further potentiated by inhibition of the excitatory neurotransmitter glutamate at the NMDA receptor.

Signs and Symptoms

Sedation is the primary clinical effect of barbiturate intoxication. Signs of significant barbiturate overdose may include hypothermia, bradycardia, hypotension, and coma. Unlike benzodiazepines, which are discussed later, barbiturates alone do induce hypoventilation, respiratory depression, and sometimes apnea. Co-ingestion of other sedative-hypnotic agents, alcohol, or opioids causes synergistic inhibition of the respiratory drive.

Secondary injury after barbiturate ingestion often occurs as a result of hypoxemia, hypotension, and tissue hypoperfusion. Renal injury and elevated liver enzyme levels are common laboratory findings. Hypoxic brain injury may also occur. Another common effect of barbiturate toxicity is loss of airway reflexes and aspiration pneumonia, which in severe cases can precipitate acute respiratory distress syndrome. In addition, prolonged immobilization while comatose can lead to skin breakdown, rhabdomyolysis, and compartment syndrome, depending on the patient's position. Pressure ulcers found in comatose patients are often still referred to as *barb blisters* because of the historical prevalence of this complication among patients with barbiturate overdose, but the nickname is misleading. These fluid-filled bullae are the indirect effect of protracted pressure on skin during immobilization and can occur in patients immobilized for any reason; they are not a direct result of barbiturate toxicity.

Differential Diagnosis

Associated mental status depression often makes an accurate history difficult to obtain in a patient with barbiturate overdose. In patients who are found unresponsive, the position of the patient on discovery and an estimate of the duration of toxicity may be helpful in guiding treatment and predicting outcome. This information can usually be obtained from friends or family members.

After your initial evaluation of airway, breathing, and vital signs, conduct a thorough neurologic exam, including assessment of cranial nerves and deep tendon reflexes. The absence of these reflexes indicates severe toxicity. The patient may also have decreased bowel sounds and abdominal distention. Pulmonary exam may reveal bradypnea with or without rales, but this exam can be normal in patients with only mild toxicity. Pay special attention to skin bullae during the musculoskeletal exam, and palpate the muscle compartments of the upper and lower extremities. Early identification of compartment syndrome can significantly improve the patient's overall outcome.

Treatment

Prehospital Setting Management of barbiturate toxicity in the prehospital setting consists primarily of supportive care. Ventilatory assistance and airway management are required in patients with significant respiratory depression, refractory hypoxemia despite high-flow oxygen delivery, evidence of hypercapnia on end-tidal carbon dioxide detectors, or inability to protect the airway. If airway patency and ventilatory effort are adequate, give the patient supplemental oxygen, elevate the head to prevent aspiration, and use a nasal trumpet if upper airway soft-tissue obstruction is present and the patient tolerates placement. Establish IV access and give IV fluid boluses with normal saline to treat volume depletion from decreased oral intake, mild hypotension, and possible rhabdomyolysis.

In-Hospital Setting Evaluation of patients with barbiturate intoxication in the ED begins with assessment of airway and breathing, which may include testing of arterial or venous blood gases for hypercapnia and acidosis and a chest radiograph to rule out aspiration pneumonitis. After stabilization of respiratory status, urine drug screening may confirm barbiturate exposure. Quantitative evaluation of serum phenobarbital levels is available in most hospitals, but results won't necessarily correlate with toxicity. Patient tolerance and chronicity of use will indicate the clinical status of the patient, not the drug level. In general, phenobarbital levels above 80 mg/L are considered lethal.

Evaluation of secondary toxicity includes renal and liver function tests, an ECG, analysis of cardiac enzymes, and brain imaging to check for evidence of hypoxic injury. Muscle breakdown and consequent rhabdomyolysis, which often complicates toxicity, is indicated by elevated creatine kinase levels with or without renal injury. Serial creatine kinase measurements and renal function tests are frequently obtained to follow the progression and resolution of the condition. Electroencephalogram tracings may be severely inhibited, resembling findings consistent with the profound sedation of brain death. Evaluation for brain death should not be performed, however, until barbiturate toxicity has resolved.

Airway management, including endotracheal intubation, is often required in significant toxicity, but mild to moderate toxicity may necessitate only supplemental oxygen and continuous pulse oximetry. Hypotension is treated initially with IV boluses of normal saline; refractory hypotension warrants vasopressor administration. The choice of vasopressor generally depends on the physician's preference. Norepinephrine and dopamine are most commonly used, but no randomized controlled study shows benefit of any one pressor compared with others in patients with barbiturate toxicity. Beyond respiratory and circulatory support, general supportive care (hydration, elevation of the head, wound care, prevention of recurrence) is the mainstay of treatment.

Accelerated elimination of barbiturates has been demonstrated with urinary alkalinization, achieved with a sodium bicarbonate infusion. The infusion is prepared by adding 100 to 150 mEq of sodium bicarbonate (2 or 3 ampules) to 1 L of a 5% dextrose-in-water solution (D_5W). The addition of 30 mEq of potassium chloride helps prevent severe hypokalemia associated with bicarbonate administration. The end point of treatment is improvement in mental status rather than a specific serum drug level. In severe cases of toxicity that fail to respond sufficiently to standard therapy, hemodialysis has been effectively employed to hasten recovery.

Healthcare providers must also be cognizant of the effect of barbiturate withdrawal in an agitated patient. As with all GABA-agonist withdrawal syndromes, the patient may have tachycardia, hypertension, tremor, seizure, or delirium. Treatment is the same regardless of the offending agent. Long-acting barbiturates (e.g., phenobarbital [Luminal]) or benzodiazepines (e.g., diazepam [Valium] or lorazepam [Ativan]) are used to prevent and treat withdrawal. Withdrawal from long-acting barbiturates is uncommon because of their long half-life.

Benzodiazepines, Sedative-Hypnotics, and Tranquilizers

Sedative-hypnotic medications include a variety of drug classes in addition to barbiturates. Because of the similarities among these drugs, the term *benzodiazepines* in this text includes all sedative-hypnotics.

Benzodiazepines were introduced in the 1960s, largely replacing barbiturates because of their improved safety profile and lower potential for addiction. As a group, these medications are frequently prescribed and overdose toxicity is common, but significant morbidity or death due to benzodiazepine ingestion alone is rare. The risk of morbidity and mortality is greater when a benzodiazepine is co-ingested with another CNS depressant such as alcohol, an opioid, or a barbiturate. Benzodiazepines do not cause respiratory depression on their own, but they may be responsible for a decreased ability to protect the airway. The other agents just mentioned have similar effects on respiration.

Benzodiazepines are differentiated from one another by half-life of the parent compound, estimated duration of action, and presence of active metabolites. Table 10-9 lists this information for selected common benzodiazepines, as well as for the benzodiazepine-like drug zolpidem (Ambien).

Pathophysiology

Benzodiazepines affect $GABA_A$ receptors, allowing increased frequency of chloride channel opening. This mechanism has CNS depressant effects and produces anxiolysis. More recently, nonbenzodiazepine sleep aids like zolpidem, zaleplon, and eszopiclone (Ambien, Sonata, and Lunesta, respectively) have surpassed benzodiazepines in popularity for treatment of sleep disorders, but they are less potent anxiolytics. The primary activity of all these drugs is $GABA_A$ agonism.

Table 10-9 Duration and Half-Life of Selected Benzodiazepines

Estimated Duration	Benzodiazepine/Benzodiazepine-Like Drug	Half-Life (hours)
Short	zolpidem (Ambien)	1.4–4.5
	triazolam (Halcion)	1.5–5.5
Intermediate	oxazepam (Serax)	3–25
	temazepam (Restoril)	5–20
	alprazolam (Xanax)	6.3–26.9
	lorazepam (Ativan)	10–20
Long	chlordiazepoxide (Librium)	5–48
	clonazepam (Klonopin)	18–50
	diazepam (Valium)	20–80

Signs and Symptoms

Patients with benzodiazepine overdose exhibit a variable clinical picture. Most notable is that depression of the respiratory rate typically does not occur after benzodiazepine ingestion alone, even with massive overdoses. Some patients display mild bradycardia but clinically significant hypotension rarely develops. Hypoxemia may be present, however, in cases of aspiration pneumonitis or concomitant ingestion of another sedative or opioid. Underlying respiratory disease, such as COPD, may also cause respiratory complications. Pressure ulcers may occur after protracted immobilization, but, as with barb blisters, are not specific to benzodiazepines. Firmness of muscle compartments indicates muscle injury and possible compartment syndrome.

Neurologic signs and symptoms vary with the degree of sedation. Mild intoxication with benzodiazepines causes ataxia, slurred speech, somnolence, and nystagmus. Severe toxicity induces deep sedation, but the patient exhibits essentially normal vital signs. Patients may display hyporeflexia and sluggish cranial nerve reflexes. Although patients often respond slightly with noxious stimuli, some have no response.

Benzodiazepine withdrawal is an important syndrome for prehospital providers to recognize. Signs and symptoms are similar to alcohol withdrawal and include tachycardia, hypertension, diaphoresis, tremor, seizure, and delirium. This syndrome is most often seen in patients who are chronically dependent on short- or intermediate-acting benzodiazepines, especially alprazolam (Xanax). Administration of long-acting benzodiazepines followed by tapering doses is the treatment of choice for this disorder.

Toxicity of older nonbenzodiazepine sedative-hypnotics may have unusual features. Carisoprodol (Soma) is prescribed as a centrally acting muscle relaxant. In addition to producing sedation from GABA agonist effects, toxicity may produce sinus tachycardia and myoclonic jerking. The exact mechanism of toxicity is unclear. Chloral hydrate can cause myocardial sensitization to endogenous catecholamines, as can all halogenated hydrocarbons. As a result, patients are at risk for ventricular dysrhythmia that may respond to beta-blocker therapy. Zolpidem, zaleplon, and eszopiclone (Ambien, Sonata, and Lunesta, respectively) are GABA agonists but not benzodiazepines. Nevertheless, their toxic effects are similar, and they are likewise reversible with flumazenil. Overall, these drugs are associated with less severe toxicity and withdrawal.

Differential Diagnosis

As with barbiturate toxicity, history is usually difficult to obtain from a patient suffering from benzodiazepine-induced toxicity. History of medication availability and a scene survey may aid in your diagnosis. A current prescription for a benzodiazepine increases the likelihood of ingestion simply because it confirms that the drug was available.

If the cause of altered mental status is unknown, a broad workup is performed, frequently including a CT scan of the brain, measurement of the ammonia level, liver function tests, CBC, and urine drug screening. Most urine drug screens include benzodiazepine testing, but they may yield false-negative results. For confirmation, the provider must often rely on a history of exposure and a clinical course consistent with benzodiazepine toxicity in the absence of other sedating drugs.

Treatment

Treatment of benzodiazepine toxicity consists primarily of supportive care. Administration of IV fluids, electrolyte repletion, head elevation, supplemental oxygen, and serial evaluation of creatine kinase and kidney function result in favorable outcomes for most patients.

Prehospital Setting The most important prehospital intervention is to protect the patient from aspiration by positioning him or her properly. You should also administer supplemental oxygen. It may be necessary to place an oral airway or nasal trumpet if the patient has evidence of upper airway obstruction such as snoring or an elevated end-tidal carbon dioxide level, but many patients will not tolerate this intervention.

Establishing IV access and infusing normal saline may be helpful, particularly in patients with borderline blood pressure or evidence of prolonged down time. Patients occasionally have mild hypotension, but it is generally responsive to fluid administration. Administration of vasopressors will not likely be required. Activated charcoal is not usually recommended after benzodiazepine ingestion because of progressive mental status deterioration and the accompanying risk of aspiration. If the patient already shows evidence of mental status changes, activated charcoal is contraindicated.

In-Hospital Setting After you have addressed the patient's airway and cardiovascular status, ED evaluation consists of identifying potential co-ingestions, particularly acetaminophen and salicylate, and assessing secondary organ injury due to toxicity. As with all sedatives, kidney injury caused by rhabdomyolysis is a concern. Determination of total creatine kinase, electrolytes, serum urea nitrogen, and creatinine is usually done. Arterial or venous blood gases may be measured if hypoventilation is of concern.

Endotracheal intubation to protect the airway is occasionally required, but patients rarely need prolonged ventilation. The routine use of the GABA antagonist, flumazenil, is not recommended (see earlier discussion of the drug).

Opioids and Opiates

Opiates and opioids (synthetic opiates) are CNS depressants. Fentanyl (Duragesic, Sublimaze), morphine (Duramorph, MS Contin), methadone (Dolophine), oxycodone (Percodan), hydrocodone (Vicodin, Lortab) meperidine (Demerol), propoxyphene (Darvon), heroin, codeine, and opium are included in this drug class. Heroin is a bitter-tasting, white or off-white powder.

It has usually been adulterated, or cut, with various substances such as sugar, baking soda, or starch. The depressant effect of these drugs increases the risk of respiratory failure when an overdose occurs.

Opioids may be administered orally, intranasally (snorting), intradermally (skin popping), intravenously (mainlining), or by inhalation (smoking). A speed ball is a bolus of heroin and cocaine injected IV. Injection track marks can often be seen in abusers who mainline, but the absence of obvious injection sites does not rule out a possible heroin or opioid overdose.

Pathophysiology

Opiates and opioids act on the opiate receptors in the brain and cause CNS depression. Their effects can be agonistic or antagonistic, depending on the opioid in question.

Signs and Symptoms

Signs and symptoms of opioid overdose may include the following:

- Euphoria or irritability
- Diaphoresis
- Miosis (pupil constriction)
- Abdominal cramps
- Nausea and vomiting
- CNS depression
- Respiratory depression
- Hypotension
- Bradycardia or tachycardia
- Pulmonary edema

These signs and symptoms can generally be treated with supportive care. CNS depression, pinpoint pupils, and respiratory depression—the so-called opiate triad—are classic signs. Severe intoxication can cause respiratory arrest, seizures, and coma. Opioid intoxication is distinguished from other causes of toxicity on the basis of euphoria, pinpoint pupils, and hypotension.

Differential Diagnosis

A thorough physical exam and patient history are necessary to narrow down the possible diagnoses. It is especially important to determine the type of opiate, the quantity ingested, the time of ingestion, and whether any other toxins were co-ingested. Lab studies are determined by these findings. Drug screening is not particularly useful in simple intoxications, but it may be helpful in identifying the offending agent in more complicated poisonings. In severe intoxications, a metabolic panel and ABG analysis and determination of the complete blood count and creatine kinase level are indicated. Imaging is useful if you suspect the patient has swallowed drug packages, either for transport or for evasion of law enforcement.

Treatment

Treatment of opiate and opioid overdose consists of supportive care and considering administration of the antidote agent, naloxone (Narcan). Naloxone is structurally similar to opioids but has only antagonistic properties. It displaces the opioid molecules from the opiate receptors, reducing the effective opiate dose. This process reverses miosis, respiratory depression, altered mental status, and even coma. Naloxone is useful in overdose of almost all opioids and opioid-like chemicals. Responsiveness to naloxone is indicative of opioid or other narcotic poisoning. The drug is typically given in small doses. The aim is to relieve respiratory depression, yet leave the patient in a responsive but lethargic state. Users sometimes become agitated or violent when their "high" wears off unexpectedly and they are faced with people in uniform. Seizure activity is a possible side effect, so naloxone should be reserved for patients with respiratory depression.

Prehospital Setting Supportive care, including management of airway, breathing, and circulation, is of primary importance. Airway management is of special concern because of the CNS depressive effects of opiates. Administer naloxone early if significant CNS and respiratory depression is evident, but be cautious when doing so. Increased patient alertness may also lead to escalating combativeness. Consider applying restraints before administration and summoning law enforcement personnel to accompany you during treatment and transport.

In-Hospital Setting In the hospital, supportive care and monitoring are vital to preventing unexpected CNS depression after opiate antagonist treatment wears off. Naloxone acts for 30 to 120 minutes, whereas opioids typically act for 3 to 6 hours. Cardiac monitoring is important, especially for severe intoxication. Patients requiring additional doses of naloxone can be treated with a continuous naloxone infusion while appropriately monitored.

Drugs of Abuse

Although many legally prescribed drugs with legitimate medical uses (e.g., opiates, benzodiazepines) are subject to diversion and intentional misuse or abuse, in the following sections drugs that have few or no legitimate medical uses are discussed. For purposes of classification, they can be considered primarily drugs of abuse; ethanol is included in this section. Of course, alcoholic beverages are enjoyed responsibly by many people, but alcohol is undeniably subject to widespread abuse as well. The toxic alcohols—ethylene glycol, isopropyl alcohol, and methanol—are discussed later in the section on home and workplace toxins.

Methamphetamine

Methamphetamine laboratories pose a particular danger to EMS providers. The chemicals used to manufacture methamphetamine are extremely volatile, and toxic gases such as phosphine can be generated as a by-product of meth production. Exposure to such chemicals can cause mucous membrane irritation, headaches, burns, and death. Of even greater concern is the risk of explosion of improvised explosive devices (IEDs). Meth manufacturers often place IED booby traps in and around their makeshift labs to deter thieves and law enforcement personnel from entering. Never enter such a facility without law enforcement support. If you inadvertently enter a meth lab, exit immediately using the same route by which you entered. If you should come upon a patient while exiting, you should remove him or her as quickly as possible.

Cocaine

Cocaine is derived from the coca plant, which is native to South America. Cocaine is a strong CNS stimulant, causing robust sympathetic discharge that results in increased catecholamine release. The lethal dose in the average adult is estimated to be about 1200 mg. Most fatalities occur from cardiac dysrhythmia, which can occur at a much lower dose in a susceptible person.

The following two forms of cocaine are in common use today:

1. Powdered cocaine, a fine white crystalline substance that is cocaine in its pure form. It is typically inhaled, or snorted, through the nose.
2. Freebase ("crack") cocaine, which takes the form of solid white or off-white lumps, crystals, or rocks. In this form, the drug is much more potent than in its powdered form. The rocks of cocaine are heated in a metal or glass pipe and the fumes are inhaled.

Pathophysiology

Cocaine has a wide variety of effects on the body. It acts as a local anesthetic by reversibly inhibiting sodium channels, blocking nerve conduction. In the myocardium, it decreases the rate of depolarization and the amplitude of the action potential. Cocaine also inhibits the reuptake of norepinephrine and dopamine at the preganglionic sympathetic nerve endings, causing central and peripheral adrenergic stimulation (activation of the brain's pleasure center). It causes catecholamine to accumulate at the postsynaptic membranes by preventing reuptake. This increases intracellular calcium levels and sustains the action potential of neurotransmitters, resulting in vasoconstriction, hypertension, tachycardia, and increased myocardial oxygen consumption. Taken together, these effects stress the heart, sometimes inducing ventricular fibrillation.

Signs and Symptoms

Cocaine produces a high that users say makes them feel euphoric and energetic. Because cocaine is a CNS stimulant, people high on cocaine often appear mentally alert and talkative. Unlike opiates, cocaine stimulates the sympathetic nervous system, causing dilated but sluggish pupils, tachycardia, vasoconstriction, and hypertension. Vasoconstriction and increased motor activity may in turn cause hyperthermia. Because dopamine reuptake is limited, seizures may occur. The risk of stroke is significantly increased. For many reasons, chief among them cardiac stimulation and hypertension, sudden death is not uncommon among people who use cocaine.

Differential Diagnosis

Differential diagnosis of any suspected cocaine overdose should begin with a thorough patient history that includes what substance was used, how it was administered, in what quantity, and how long ago. When a patient has an unremarkable history and mild symptoms, a lab workup is generally not needed. If a history is unavailable or if clinically significant toxicity is noted, however, appropriate lab studies may include a CBC, measurement of glucose, calcium, serum urea nitrogen, creatinine, electrolytes, and troponin (or creatine kinase), a pregnancy test, a urinalysis, and a toxicology screen. The creatine kinase screen may help eliminate rhabdomyolysis as a cause of the patient's signs and symptoms. Serum cocaine levels are unreliable and thus not clinically useful because the drug has a short half-life (30 to 45 minutes). Qualitative urine screens, on the other hand, identify cocaine metabolites and will remain positive with very few false-positive or false-negative test results for an average of 3–4 days after use. Standard cardiac diagnostic protocols should be followed in patients with chest pain.

Imaging studies may be useful to rule out head injuries and respiratory issues, and they may reveal signs of drug abuse (such as granulomatous changes caused by parenteral abuse) or show whether the patient has swallowed packets of drugs.

Treatment

Supportive care, including support of airway, breathing, and circulation, is the primary treatment for cocaine intoxication. Supplemental oxygen, establishing IV access, cardiac monitoring, and pulse oximetry are usually indicated.

Epinephrine should be avoided if possible in patients with cocaine intoxication because its cardiovascular effects are similar to those of cocaine. Vasopressin is often a better alternative. Some evidence also indicates that nonselective beta-blockers should be avoided in these patients.

Prehospital Setting Cocaine users, especially after consuming large doses, can exhibit erratic or violent behavior. Your safety is of paramount importance. Summon help from law enforcement early, and monitor the patient's body language and behavior carefully.

Rule out hypoglycemia by obtaining a serum glucose reading. Patients with dysrhythmias require aggressive cardiac care. Initiate cardiac monitoring with a 12-lead ECG to look for cardiac ischemia due to coronary vasospasm. Use benzodiazepines as necessary to calm the patient, reduce CNS stimulation, and treat seizures.

In-Hospital Setting Hyperpyrexia must be treated aggressively. Hypoglycemia, cardiac symptoms, and trauma should be treated per standard protocols. The effects of cocaine are generally short lived, so the patient can usually be discharged after 2 to 6 hours of uneventful observation.

Ethanol

Ethanol is not a particularly toxic chemical at low doses, as evidenced by its legal use in beer, wine, and distilled spirits, but chronic overuse causes significant morbidity, including cirrhosis and different types of cancer. Because of its wide availability and classification as a food, ethanol causes more toxicologic emergencies than any other kind of alcohol. Most cases are classified as intentional because they involve alcoholic beverages. Ethanol is also used in industrial solvents.

Inhaling powdered ethanol is a dangerous trend. When powdered ethanol is poured over dry ice and the vapors are inhaled, ethanol bypasses the stomach and enters directly into the lungs. Inhaling ethanol is more likely to lead to deadly poisoning than drinking ethanol because when a person drinks ethanol, vomiting usually occurs, which prevents poisoning.

Pathophysiology

Ethanol is readily absorbed into the bloodstream through the GI tract, primarily in the small intestine and stomach. Most of the alcohol consumed is absorbed within an hour. Ethanol passes easily through the blood–brain barrier. This property is responsible for the intoxicating effects of ethanol on the CNS through central $GABA_a$ agonism and NMDA receptor antagonism.

Signs and Symptoms

Signs and symptoms of ethanol intoxication vary by blood alcohol level and may include euphoria, inebriation, confusion, lethargy, CNS depression, ataxia (and associated injuries from falls), stupor, respiratory depression, hypothermia, hypotension, coma, and cardiovascular collapse (Table 10-10).

Extreme intoxication can lead to decreased levels of consciousness, severe respiratory difficulties, or death. Preexisting conditions are often exacerbated by the effects of ethanol. Vasodilation may lead to hypotension and hypothermia. The latter may be severe, depending on the patient and the ambient conditions. Vasodilation may also dangerously reduce cardiac output in predisposed individuals.

Differential Diagnosis

The laboratory workup of a patient with suspected ethanol intoxication should include the following:

- Serum glucose level to rule out hypoglycemia
- Serum ethanol level
- Serum electrolytes (e.g., calcium, magnesium)
- Serum osmolality to calculate the osmolar gap
- Electrolyte levels to determine the size of the anion gap
- Pregnancy testing
- Testing for toxic levels of drugs that may have been co-ingested, such as acetaminophen, salicylates, and methanol
- Imaging studies in patients with severely altered mental status or possible trauma suggested by history or physical exam

Table 10-10 **Effects of Ethanol Related to Blood Alcohol Concentration**	
Concentration (%)	**Effects**
0.02	Few obvious effects, slight intensification of mood
0.05	Loss of emotional restraint, feeling of warmth, flushing of skin, mild impairment of judgment
0.10	Slight slurring of speech, loss of fine motor control, unstable emotions, inappropriate laughter
0.12	Coordination and balance difficult, distinct impairment of mentation and judgment
0.20	Responsive to verbal stimuli, very slurred speech, staggering gait, diplopia (double vision), difficulty standing upright, memory loss
0.30	Briefly aroused by painful stimuli; deep, snoring respirations
0.40	Unresponsiveness, incontinence, hypotension, irregular respirations
0.50	Death possible from apnea, hypotension, or aspiration of vomitus

From Aehlert B: *Paramedic practice today: above and beyond*, St. Louis, MO, 2009, Mosby.

Treatment

A thorough patient history must be obtained to determine the type and amount of alcohol consumed and the time of consumption. Treatment is mainly supportive: maintaining airway, breathing, and circulation and establishing IV access. Cardiac monitoring is especially indicated if the patient has a preexisting heart condition. Hypoglycemia should be ruled out by performing a serum glucose test. If the patient is unresponsive or demonstrates respiratory depression, a trial dose of naloxone should be considered to evaluate for potential opioid toxicity. Thiamine, a cofactor needed to process ethanol, may be indicated after heavy alcohol use, and hemodialysis may be considered in significant ethanol toxicity.

Prehospital Setting The airway is vulnerable because of the CNS depressive effects of ethanol. As a result, airway management may be necessary if the patient is severely intoxicated.

In-Hospital Setting In the ED, the patient's body temperature should be monitored. Endotracheal intubation is rare, but may be necessary in severely intoxicated patients. Activated charcoal is not effective for ethanol and is contraindicated due to alteration in mental status and risk of aspiration.

Hallucinogens

Hallucinogens cause visual disturbances (hallucinations) and alter the user's perception of reality. They include substances such as L-lysergic acid diethylamide (LSD), peyote, mescaline, and psychedelic mushrooms. Hallucinogens can be grouped into the following four major classes:

1. Indole alkaloids (e.g., LSD, lysergic acid amide [LSA], psilocin, and psilocybin)
2. Piperidines (e.g., PCP and ketamine)
3. Phenylethylamines (e.g., mescaline, MDMA, methylenedioxyamphetamine [MDA], and methoxymethylenedioxyamphetamine [MMDA])
4. Cannabinoids (e.g., marijuana or tetrahydrocannabinol [THC])

Synthetic marijuana, or "Spice," refers to a wide variety of herbal mixtures that produce experiences similar to marijuana (cannabis) and that are marketed as "safe," legal alternatives to that drug. Sold under many names, including K2, fake weed, Yucatan Fire, Skunk, Moon Rocks, and others—and labeled "not for human consumption"—these products contain dried, shredded plant material and chemical additives that are responsible for their psychoactive (mind-altering) effects.

Spice users report experiences similar to those produced by marijuana—elevated mood, relaxation, and altered perception—and in some cases the effects are even stronger than those of marijuana. Some users report psychotic effects like extreme anxiety, paranoia, and hallucinations.

So far, there have been no scientific studies of Spice's effects on the human brain, but it is known that the cannabinoid compounds found in Spice products act on the same cell receptors as THC, the primary psychoactive component of marijuana. Some of the compounds found in Spice, however, bind more strongly to those receptors, which could lead to a much more powerful and unpredictable effect. Because the chemical composition of many products sold as Spice is unknown, it is likely that some varieties also contain substances that could cause dramatically different effects than the user might expect.

Spice abusers who have been taken to poison control centers report symptoms that include rapid heart rate, vomiting, agitation, confusion, and hallucinations. Spice can also raise blood pressure and cause reduced blood supply to the heart (myocardial ischemia), and in a few cases it has been associated with heart attacks. Regular users may experience withdrawal and addiction symptoms.

Pathophysiology

The pathophysiology of hallucinogenic drugs is only imperfectly understood, but the principal effects of the drugs are concentrated in the CNS. It is generally believed that hallucinogens alter both serotonin and norepinephrine concentrations in the brain. Indole amine derivatives are thought to act on serotonin receptors. Piperidine derivatives are thought to block serotonin, dopamine, and norepinephrine reuptake. Phenylethylamine derivatives block serotonin and norepinephrine reuptake and even increase their presynaptic release.

In the case of cannabinoids, the component delta (9)-tetrahydrocannabinol (THC) is the source of pharmacologic effects at cannabinoid receptors. The chemical causes maximum plasma concentration within minutes and psychotropic effects in 2 to 3 hours.

Signs and Symptoms

Patients who have ingested hallucinogens can exhibit dangerous and sometimes bizarre behavior. They have altered mental status, which may include behavioral disturbances such as aggressiveness, delusional or paranoid thinking, and visual illusions (hallucinations). CNS effects of the drug can include stimulation or depression, depending on the causative agent, the dose, and the time elapsed since poisoning. Other possible effects include hypertension and tachycardia. Hallucinogen toxicity is distinguished from other possible causes on the basis of behavioral abnormalities and hallucinations.

Differential Diagnosis

A lab workup is not particularly helpful for hallucinogen intoxication. Selected studies may be needed to differentiate it from other etiologies. A comprehensive drug screen may be indicated to rule out co-ingestion or to confirm a questionable diagnosis. Imaging studies are useful only to assess other possible causes of the patient's symptoms.

Treatment

Persons who use hallucinogens may seek medical attention to treat traumatic injuries associated with hallucinogen use or to alleviate unpleasant or distressing psychotropic effects of the drug—a so-called bad trip. Hallucinogens typically have minimal acute side effects. Some patients become violent, and physical or chemical restraints and law enforcement assistance may be needed. LSD is skin absorptive, and every effort should be made to avoid cross-contamination. Primary treatment consists of calming the patient and providing reassurance that the drug's effects are temporary.

Prehospital Setting Manage traumatic injuries per protocol. Acquire a thorough patient history to help determine the correct etiology and ultimately to identify the hallucinogen.

In-Hospital Setting After thorough patient evaluation is done, patients intoxicated with LSD should be isolated to help them remain calm. They may require sedation with benzodiazepines. In severe psychotic episodes, haloperidol may be indicated. LSD intoxication lasts about 8 to 12 hours, but the psychotic effects of the drug may persist for days.

Phencyclidine

The most common hallucinogen is phencyclidine (PCP), which was originally developed as a general anesthetic and later used as a veterinary tranquilizer. When its potential for abuse was discovered, it was replaced with safer alternatives. PCP has CNS stimulatory and depressant properties. It is available as a white crystalline powder, a liquid, or a tablet.

Pathophysiology

PCP is a dissociative anesthetic with hallucinogenic properties. It has both stimulant and depressant effects on the CNS. Its sympathomimetic effects are probably due to dopamine and norepinephrine reuptake inhibition. The drug also acts at nicotinic and opioid receptors, has cholinergic and anticholinergic effects, is a glutamate antagonist at NDMA receptors, and affects the dopamine pathway. Clearly, PCP produces some very complicated interactions that researchers are still attempting to understand. PCP is metabolized in the liver and has a half-life of about 15 to 20 hours.

Signs and Symptoms

At low doses (10 mg or less), PCP produces a combination of psychoactive effects, including euphoria, disorientation and confusion, and sudden mood swings (such as rage). Signs of PCP use may include flushing, diaphoresis, hypersalivation, and vomiting. The pupils generally remain reactive. Facial grimacing and nystagmus, or involuntary eye movement, are identifiable effects of low-dose PCP use.

Persons who use PCP are much less sensitive to pain, which may give them the appearance of having superhuman strength as they overexert themselves. In fact, at low doses, mortality is associated with self-destructive behavior related to the analgesic and CNS depressant effects of PCP. Remember, patients under the influence of hallucinogens pose a threat to themselves and others, including the providers on scene.

High doses of PCP (> 10 mg) may produce extreme CNS depression, including coma. Respiratory depression, hypertension, and tachycardia are common. The hypertension may cause cardiac difficulties, encephalopathy, intracerebral hemorrhage, and seizure. High-dose overdoses may require management of respiratory arrest, cardiac arrest, and status epilepticus. Such patients must be rapidly transported to the hospital.

Acute onset of PCP psychosis may occur even at low doses. This condition is a true psychiatric emergency that may persist for days or weeks after the exposure. Behavior can range from unresponsiveness (a catatonic state) to violent and enraged. Such patients can be extremely dangerous, and law enforcement should accompany you as you transport the patient to an appropriate medical facility.

Differential Diagnosis

Patient history is critical to making a diagnosis of PCP intoxication. The lab workup should include urine toxicology screening, a metabolic panel, measurement of serum glucose level, a CBC, and analysis of arterial blood gases. An elevated WBC count and increased serum urea nitrogen and creatinine levels are often seen in patients with PCP intoxication. Rhabdomyolysis can be assessed by monitoring serum creatine kinase and urine myoglobin levels. Providers should be aware that dextromethorphan is a common cause of positive results on qualitative urine drug screening for PCP.

Treatment

Primary treatment consists of calming the patient and providing reassurance that the drug's effects are temporary. You must obtain a thorough patient history to determine the etiology of the patient's signs and symptoms and to identify the hallucinogen ingested. The history should include the type and amount of drug ingested and the time at which the ingestion occurred. Endotracheal intubation will probably be necessary in severely intoxicated patients.

Prehospital Setting Treatment is mainly supportive, including maintaining airway, breathing, and circulation and establishing IV access. Manage traumatic injuries per protocol. Agitation should be treated with escalating doses of benzodiazepines.

In-Hospital Setting Cardiac monitoring is indicated in any patient with a suspected PCP overdose who has a preexisting heart condition. The patient should be kept calm, and abrupt movements, bright lights, and noise should be avoided. Physical or chemical restraints may be necessary if the patient becomes erratic or violent. Benzodiazepines work well for this purpose. Antipsychotic agents such as haloperidol should not be given to patients with PCP intoxication because they may increase the risk of cardiac dysrhythmia or seizure. Opiate use and hypoglycemia should be ruled out.

Toxins in the Home and Workplace

In the following sections, common causes of toxic exposure in the home and workplace are discussed. Some poisons, such as carbon monoxide, are inhaled. Others, such as antifreeze, are swallowed. Toxins such as pesticides and corrosives are absorbed through the skin or cause dermal irritation and burns. Many of the poisons discussed have important industrial uses and may even be capable of causing mass-casualty disasters (e.g., during a train derailment). But on a day-to-day basis, as a prehospital provider you're most likely to encounter these toxins in a patient's home or workplace.

Ethylene Glycol

Ethylene glycol, one of the toxic alcohols, is found in automotive antifreeze, windshield-washer fluid, and deicers. It is used to prevent overheating and freezing of elements found in these substances. Because it tastes sweet, it is more likely to be ingested accidentally and in larger quantities by children and pets. However, 70% of cases of ethylene glycol poisoning occur in adults, and most such exposures are accidental. The toxicity results from conversion of the alcohol to metabolites. According to the annual 2013 report of the American Association of Poison Control Centers' National Poison Data System, there were 5,419 human exposures to ethylene glycol with nearly 2,000 requiring treatment at a healthcare facility.

Ingestion is the primary route of exposure, since ethylene glycol is not readily absorbed through the skin and has a low vapor pressure that prevents its aerosolization during inhalation.

Pathophysiology

Ethylene glycol is metabolized into glycolic acid and oxalic acid by the enzyme, alcohol dehydrogenase, in the liver. These two metabolites cause most of the significant toxicity, acidosis, and kidney damage associated with ethylene glycol ingestion. The oxalic acid sequesters and binds calcium in the body to form calcium oxalate, which precipitates out and forms crystals. This process has two detrimental effects. First, it causes hypocalcemia, which increases the risk of cardiac dysrhythmia. Second, it can cause severe joint pain, peripheral nerve dysfunction, and cardiomyopathy at the sites of crystal deposition. These oxalic acid crystals can have a detrimental effect on the liver and kidneys, but the destruction usually does not become evident until a sufficient amount of the toxic metabolite has accumulated to cause damage. Glycolic acid also contributes to nephrotoxicity though the mechanism has yet to be elucidated. The threshold for ethylene glycol toxicity has been reported to be 1 to 2 mL/kg.

Signs and Symptoms

Ethylene glycol toxicity typically occurs in the following three stages:

- *Stage 1 (1 to 12 hours after ingestion).* Characterized by CNS effects, including signs of intoxication such as slurred speech, ataxia, sleepiness, nausea and vomiting, convulsions, hallucinations, stupor, and coma.
- *Stage 2 (12 to 36 hours after ingestion).* Characterized by cardiopulmonary effects, which may include tachypnea secondary to metabolic acidosis, cyanosis, pulmonary edema, or cardiac arrest.
- *Stage 3 (24 to 72 hours after ingestion).* Affects the renal system and may include flank pain, oliguria, crystalluria, proteinuria, anuria, hematuria, or uremia.

Not all patients go through all stages. Depending on the patient's physiology, any preexisting conditions, and the quantity ingested, some patients experience life-threatening symptoms early. Life-threatening signs and symptoms include intoxication, headache, CNS depression, respiratory difficulty, metabolic acidosis, hypocalcemia, cardiovascular collapse, renal failure with or without hyperkalemia, seizures, and coma.

Differential Diagnosis

Patients with ethylene glycol ingestion may initially have an unremarkable physical examination until enough toxic metabolites build up to cause signs and symptoms. Serum osmolality may be used to calculate the osmolar gap. Alternatively, a qualitative colorimetric test may be used to detect the presence of ethylene glycol in serum. Ideally, a quantitative level will be obtained, but the equipment required to perform the test is unavailable at most nonacademic hospitals. In addition, a urinalysis and measurement of serum calcium levels and arterial blood gases are indicated. Urinalysis may reveal the presence of calcium oxalate crystals, a late-stage sign.

Treatment

Supportive care, antidote administration, and hemodialysis are the core treatments for ethylene glycol poisoning. Supportive care should focus on airway management. Either ethanol or fomepizole (Antizol) can be administered as an antidote. Both are competitive inhibitors of alcohol dehydrogenase. Cofactor therapy consisting of pyridoxine (vitamin B_6) and thiamine (vitamin B_1) administration may be given to boost the metabolism of ethylene glycol. However, hemodialysis is the definitive treatment for ethylene glycol poisoning.

Prehospital Setting In addition to basic treatment, obtain a detailed patient history, especially regarding the time of ingestion. Establish IV access for rehydration and for antidote therapy in extreme cases. Administer sodium bicarbonate for metabolic acidosis and diazepam (Valium) for seizures as necessary. Transport the patient rapidly to a hospital for hemodialysis.

In-Hospital Setting The antidote for ethylene glycol poisoning has traditionally been ethanol, which is usually administered intravenously but can also be delivered orally. The antidote fomepizole (Antizol) is more effective, easier to dose, and safer than ethanol and should be the preferred treatment where available. Ethanol and fomepizole are competitive inhibitors of alcohol dehydrogenase and prevent the formation of toxic metabolites. Ethylene glycol itself is harmlessly excreted by the kidneys. In the body, the half-life of ethylene glycol is normally 5 hours, but with fomepizole or ethanol treatment it is 17 hours. This allows prolonged excretion time.

Magnesium and pyridoxine are cofactors in the detoxification of ethylene glycol poisoning. Cofactor therapy has been reported to reduce morbidity associated with ethylene glycol toxicity by converting glyoxylic acid to the nontoxic amino acid, glycine.

Hypocalcemia may be present in severe poisoning and requires treatment because insoluble calcium oxalate forms when the toxic metabolite oxalic acid binds with free calcium in the body. Sodium bicarbonate administration is indicated for metabolic acidosis.

Hemodialysis, which offers definitive treatment by removing toxic metabolites from the blood, is indicated by renal failure, serum assays, and severe acidosis.

Isopropyl Alcohol

Isopropyl alcohol is one of the toxic alcohols, but it is significantly less toxic than either methanol or ethylene glycol. Isopropyl alcohol (isopropanol or rubbing alcohol) is a common household and industrial solvent and is involved in many toxic exposures. It is also a common household item, found in items such as mouthwash, skin lotion, and hand disinfectant. Annually, thousands of isopropyl alcohol exposures are reported, although few result in fatalities. Isopropyl alcohol is often abused as an alternative to ethanol. In high doses, it can cause gastritis, vomiting, and hypotension.

Pathophysiology

Isopropanol is quickly absorbed in the stomach and metabolized into acetone, which is not particularly toxic. Isopropyl alcohol toxicity is similar to that of ethanol toxicity. As such, it's twice as strong a CNS depressant as ethyl alcohol and is also a vasodilator. The hypotension caused by vasodilation is typically responsive to fluid and vasopressor administration.

Signs and Symptoms

The typical route of entry is oral. Isopropyl alcohol is metabolized to acetone, a ketone that can be measured in blood and urine. Signs and symptoms include confusion, lethargy, CNS depression, respiratory depression, ketonemia, mild hypothermia,

hypotension, and coma. As a result of acetone production, you may notice a fruity breath odor similar to that of a person with diabetes.

Differential Diagnosis

A thorough physical exam and patient history are necessary to determine the etiology of the toxicity. Lab studies are dictated by the findings, but in severe intoxication, the workup may include measurement of arterial blood gases and analysis of electrolytes and serum alcohol and bicarbonate levels primarily to rule out ingestion of other toxic alcohols such as ethylene glycol and methanol because isopropanol ingestion would not be expected to cause an acidosis. However, acetone may interfere with serum creatinine testing, resulting in an inaccurate elevation that resolves when acetone is cleared.

Treatment

As with other drug intoxications, a serum glucose test should be performed to rule out alternative etiologies. Consider administration of naloxone if the patient exhibits respiratory depression, which may be due to concurrent opiate ingestion. Because of the low toxicity of the metabolites of isopropyl alcohol, fomepizole therapy is not indicated. In fact, such therapy may actually exacerbate CNS depression and hypotension, the primary life-threatening complications associated with isopropyl alcohol toxicity.

Prehospital Setting In the field, treatment is mainly supportive. Maintain airway, breathing, and circulation, and establish IV access.

In-Hospital Setting Hospital treatment is similar to prehospital treatment. Supportive care is of primary importance. Volume resuscitation and aspiration prevention are the mainstays of treatment. Proton pump inhibitors or H_2 blockers may be given in the case of hemorrhagic gastritis.

Methanol

Methanol (methyl alcohol or wood alcohol), a common household solvent, is a component of windshield-washer fluid, paint, gasoline treatments, and canned tabletop fuels such as Sterno. Methanol is used extensively in industry as a solvent and reagent. Intoxication usually follows oral ingestion; just a mouthful can be highly toxic. Methanol has been intentionally ingested as an ethanol substitute, although most poisonings appear to be accidental or suicidal. Methanol is also absorbed through the skin but not particularly well. In addition, because of its high volatility, it is readily inhaled.

Pathophysiology

Methanol is a protoxin that is readily excreted by the kidneys if it escapes liver conversion. In the liver, it is converted by the enzyme, alcohol dehydrogenase, into formaldehyde, a short-lived intermediate metabolite. Formaldehyde is then converted by the enzyme, aldehyde dehydrogenase, into formic acid, which causes most of the significant toxicity, including metabolic acidosis and blindness. Formic acid inhibits the electron transport chain thereby inhibiting adenosine triphosphate synthesis, causing lactate-associated metabolic acidosis, as well as neurologic and cardiovascular toxicity. Methanol is metabolized to formic acid by enzymes within the eye to cause retinal injury. Onset of symptoms of toxicity is usually delayed 12 to 24 hours until the toxic metabolites have accumulated.

Signs and Symptoms

Methanol initially causes inebriation but to a lesser degree than the other alcohols. Early signs and symptoms mimic ethanol intoxication, including slurred speech, ataxia, drowsiness, and nausea and vomiting. Signs and symptoms of more severe toxicity include sedation, ataxia, headache, vertigo, nausea and vomiting, abdominal pain, respiratory difficulty, seizures, and coma. Vision complaints such as blurred vision and visual haziness are an initial hallmark of methanol poisoning. The initial onset of symptoms can be rapid, occurring in as little as 30 minutes, or delayed up to 30 hours, depending on the dose and route of entry. After the initial symptoms have passed, a second set of symptoms can occur 10 to 30 hours after exposure. Complete loss of vision and snow blindness–like symptoms, acidosis, and respiratory failure can occur, especially when ethanol is co-ingested. A long asymptomatic phase does not necessarily preclude later toxicity. Mortality is associated with severe acidosis and cerebral edema.

Visual impairment indicates the need for an eye exam. The pupils may be dilated, with little response. The optic disc may be inflamed, and blindness can ensue over several days as the optic disc bleaches.

Differential Diagnosis

A thorough physical exam and patient history are necessary to determine the etiology of the toxicity. Lab studies are indicated by the findings. In severe methanol intoxication, analysis of the serum alcohol level, electrolytes, arterial blood gases, lactic acid, and serum bicarbonate level is indicated. The serum methanol level can be measured directly in some labs, or it can be estimated by calculating the osmolar gap and the anion gap.

Treatment

As with other drug intoxications, a serum glucose test should be performed to rule out alternative causes. Consider administration of naloxone if the patient exhibits respiratory depression, which may be due to concurrent opiate ingestion.
Prehospital Setting Treatment consists of maintaining the patient's airway, breathing, and circulation. Airway management is particularly important. Activated charcoal does not adsorb methanol significantly and should not be used.
In-Hospital Setting Hospital treatment consists of supportive care, antidote administration, and hemodialysis as indicated. Supportive care should focus on maintaining an airway. IV ethanol or fomepizole (Antizol) are given to minimize further production of toxic metabolites. Ethanol and fomepizole are both competitive inhibitors of alcohol dehydrogenase. Cofactor therapy consisting of tetrahydrofolate should be given to encourage the elimination of formic acid. If the ingestion occurred within the last hour, gastric lavage may be helpful but is associated with significant risk. Hemodialysis is indicated in severe exposures in which the patient complains of visual symptoms, severe acidosis is present, or serum methanol levels are found to be high. Folate is a cofactor in the enzymatic detoxification of toxic methanol metabolites, and folate therapy has been reported to reduce morbidity.

Carbon Monoxide

In the United States, carbon monoxide is a leading cause of morbidity and mortality from poisoning. In 2013, approximately 14,000 people reported carbon monoxide exposure to U.S. poison centers. Carbon monoxide is a colorless, odorless gas produced by incomplete combustion of organic fuels. Sources include household furnaces, space heaters, generators, gas stoves, motor vehicles, and smoke from house fires. Any gasoline- or propane-powered engine, not only vehicle engines, can produce carbon monoxide.

In addition, methylene chloride, a chemical used as a paint stripper, degreaser, and industrial solvent, is metabolized to carbon monoxide in the liver. Ingestion or significant inhalation exposure to methylene chloride can therefore cause delayed carbon monoxide toxicity.

Pathophysiology

Carbon monoxide induces toxicity in a variety of ways. The most obvious is its effect on the function of hemoglobin. Carbon monoxide has greater affinity than oxygen for the oxygen-binding sites of heme. It also inhibits the release of oxygen from hemoglobin. This combination results in decreased oxygen delivery to tissues despite a normal partial pressure of dissolved oxygen in the blood. Mitochondrial cytochrome oxidase is also bound by carbon monoxide, decreasing cellular activity and thus impairing energy production by oxidative phosphorylation. The effects of carbon monoxide toxicity are similar to those of cyanide. Myocardial myoglobin binding by carbon monoxide decreases oxygen extraction by cardiac myocytes, contributing to cardiac toxicity. Finally, carbon monoxide toxicity unleashes a volley of tissue injury by free-radical formation, inflammatory mediators, delayed lipid peroxidation, and cellular apoptosis (programmed cell death).

Signs and Symptoms

Symptoms of carbon monoxide toxicity range from mild to fatal, depending on the concentration of the gas and the duration of exposure. Patients often have fatigue, headache, myalgia, nausea, and vomiting. Severe toxicity can cause chest pain, shortness of breath, syncope, ataxia, seizure, and coma. In high concentrations, carbon monoxide is considered a knockdown agent, meaning that it causes rapid toxicity and loss of consciousness. In addition to primary cellular toxicity, the combined toxic effects of carbon monoxide can induce myocardial ischemia, decreased contractility, vasodilation, and hypotension. It's important to obtain a detailed past medical history because patients with underlying cardiovascular disease are at increased risk of these adverse effects.

The vital signs of a patient with carbon monoxide toxicity may be normal. However, the patient may have tachycardia, tachypnea, or hypotension. Oxygen saturation is usually normal, because pulse oximetry cannot differentiate between carboxyhemoglobin and oxyhemoglobin (see Chapter 2). Blood pressure and peripheral perfusion can be gauged by capillary refill evaluation. Cherry-red skin, a classically described examination finding, is explained by the presence of oxygenated venous blood as a result of the combined inability of hemoglobin to unload oxygen and of tissue to extract it. This finding is rare, though, and is typically a late sign. Pallor is more common. Pulmonary exam may reveal pulmonary edema caused by either cardiogenic failure or primary pulmonary toxicity. The abdominal exam is generally unremarkable except for nausea and vomiting.

On neurologic examination, mild abnormalities in gait and balance indicate significant exposure, whereas altered mental status and seizure coincide with severe toxicity. The patient may have focal neurologic deficits attributable to carbon monoxide–induced stroke. In some patients with carbon monoxide poisoning, the cascade of cytotoxicity and delayed injury leads to delayed neurologic sequelae. In contrast to focal deficits caused by localized tissue hypoxia, these sequelae often involve memory, personality, and behavior. Symptoms may not develop for several weeks after recovery from the acute event. Patients who have lost consciousness or had periods of hypotension are at risk for such delayed adverse effects, but it is not possible to predict their occurrence or severity.

Differential Diagnosis

Mild carbon monoxide toxicity is probably underrecognized because its symptoms are either nonspecific or resemble those of a flulike illness. The diagnosis may be further complicated by the fact that unintentional carbon monoxide exposures tend to occur in cold-weather months, when furnaces are in use and the incidence of viral illness increases. Because carbon monoxide has no color or odor, its presence often goes undetected.

Diagnosis of carbon monoxide toxicity, then, depends heavily on gathering accurate information from the scene. Obviously, a history of running a motor vehicle or other engine is telling. The patient may have been in an enclosed space such as a garage, with a motor running from a space heater, power generator, or other appliance. Household poisoning from a faulty furnace can provoke symptoms in several family members at once. Another historical clue might be the resolution of symptoms when the patient leaves the exposure source and the return of symptoms on reentering. Animals are often affected by carbon monoxide poisoning earlier and more severely than humans who are exposed to the same source. The patient may report that a pet has been acting strangely. Most fire departments are now equipped with carbon monoxide meters, which can be used to detect elevated levels of the dangerous gas at the scene, thereby accelerating diagnosis and treatment. Newer technology is now available for EMS providers that allows field measurement of a patient's carbon monoxide levels using a noninvasive oximetry device.

In addition to the physical examination, supplemental laboratory and radiographic data are used to evaluate patients with carbon monoxide toxicity. The patient's carboxyhemoglobin level can be measured with the oximetry device and confirmed with a venous or arterial blood sample. The documentation of an elevated carboxyhemoglobin level aids in diagnosis, but for a variety of reasons, the specific level does not necessarily predict toxicity or outcome. A patient with severe carbon monoxide toxicity who has been managed with high-flow oxygen for a prolonged period before evaluation could have a normal carboxyhemoglobin level, whereas a patient with only mild symptoms may have a significantly elevated level. In fact, patients who are habitual tobacco smokers can have levels as high as 10%. Normal carboxyhemoglobin levels in nonsmokers range from 0% to 5%.

In patients with direct carbon monoxide exposure, carboxyhemoglobin is measured only once, because the level cannot increase after the patient is removed from the source of carbon monoxide. Patients with suspected exposure to methylene chloride, however, require prolonged observation and repeated testing to ensure that toxicity has peaked, because the carboxyhemoglobin level rises as the body metabolizes methylene chloride.

Supplemental evaluation of the patient with suspected carbon monoxide exposure includes assessment of acid–base status. Metabolic acidosis may be accompanied by elevated serum lactate as a result of impaired oxygen delivery and anaerobic respiration. An ECG is performed to assess myocardial ischemia. Cardiac enzyme studies are performed and followed serially in patients with demonstrated toxicity. Brain imaging with unenhanced CT or magnetic resonance imaging (MRI) may be obtained. Early changes, particularly on CT, portend a poor neurologic outcome. MRI is more sensitive than CT to cerebral changes after carbon monoxide toxicity and is useful in identifying areas of ischemia and infarct.

Treatment

Prehospital Setting The most important treatment for the patient, as well as for the provider, is immediate removal from the source of carbon monoxide. Even a brief exposure can be toxic if the gas is sufficiently concentrated. After moving the patient to a safe location, place the patient on high-flow oxygen delivered through a nonrebreathing mask. Increasing the fractional concentration of oxygen in inspired gas (FIO_2) decreases the half-life of carbon monoxide binding, allowing it to be exhaled. In room air, the average half-life of carbon monoxide on hemoglobin is roughly 5 hours, but at 100% FIO_2, the half-life drops to 1 to 2 hours.

Employ standard airway management. If endotracheal intubation is required, maintain the patient on 100% FIO_2. Use of CPAP may also be beneficial. Treat cardiac arrhythmias as you normally would after administration of oxygen. Hypotension often responds to IV boluses of normal saline; however, you may need to administer vasopressors. Otherwise, provide supportive care and symptomatic treatment. Whenever practical, a patient who shows evidence of significant carbon monoxide toxicity (loss of consciousness, neurologic deficits, myocardial ischemia) should be transported to a medical center that can deliver hyperbaric oxygen.

In-Hospital Setting In the ED, the administration of high-flow oxygen is continued to hasten the dissociation of carbon monoxide from hemoglobin. Support of airway, breathing, and circulation is continued.

After hemodynamic stabilization, hyperbaric oxygen therapy may be indicated. Hyperbaric oxygen chambers are called either *monoplace* or *multiplace*, in reference to the number of patients each can accommodate. A monoplace chamber is roughly the size of a casket and can accommodate only one person at a time. A multiplace chamber is a small room in which several patients or providers can be treated at once. Oxygen is pumped into the room at increasing pressure. Because pressurized oxygen is used, patients are screened carefully to remove any flammable objects. Hyperbaric oxygen further decreases the half-life of carbon monoxide to roughly 20 minutes. On the basis of data that exist, hyperbaric oxygen therapy for severe carbon monoxide toxicity is recommended, but its benefit in less severely poisoned patients is unclear.

Specific criteria for determining the need for hyperbaric oxygen have been poorly defined. Recommendations vary, depending on the source. Severe, persistent symptoms, including altered mental status, coma, seizure, focal neurologic deficits, and hypotension, are widely accepted indications for hyperbaric oxygen therapy; symptoms such as syncope are less obvious indications. In patients with milder toxicity, high-flow oxygen should be administered until symptoms resolve.

The most common complications of barotrauma are sinus pain and tympanic membrane irritation or rupture. Patients undergoing hyperbaric oxygen therapy who are unable to decompress their own tympanic membranes receive temporary bilateral myringotomy incisions.

In treating carbon monoxide exposure, pregnant women represent a special patient population. Fetal hemoglobin may bind carbon monoxide with more affinity than maternal hemoglobin, leading to a high concentration of carboxyhemoglobin in the fetus, which is compounded by decreased oxygen delivery from the pregnant woman. Maternal carboxyhemoglobin levels do not necessarily reflect fetal levels. Severe fetal toxicity, long-term neurologic deficits, and fetal demise have been reported with maternal exposure. These adverse outcomes seem to occur most frequently when the woman exhibits significant symptoms. Children born to women with mild carbon monoxide toxicity have done well.

Hyperbaric oxygen therapy presents a theoretical threat to the fetus, but the risk has not been substantiated. Pregnant women with carbon monoxide toxicity should undergo hyperbaric oxygen therapy if significant symptoms develop. As with nonpregnant patients, the specific carboxyhemoglobin level at which therapy should be initiated is not known, but 20% has been suggested.

Corrosives

Corrosives are a broad category of chemicals that corrode metal and destroy tissue on contact. Several U.S. agencies, such as the Department of Transportation (DOT) and the Environmental Protection Agency (EPA), define precise parameters for corrosive solutions. The corrosivity of a solution—that is, its ability to oxidize and chemically disintegrate materials it comes into contact with—is determined by, at least in part, its pH. The standard pH scale runs from an acidic low of 0 to an alkaline high of 14. A neutral or normal pH is 7.0. Both acids and alkalis are corrosives. Acids have low pH: the DOT defines a strong acid as a solution with a pH below 2. Bases have high pH: the DOT defines a strong base as a solution with a pH above 12.5. These pH thresholds are, of course, approximate. A solution with a pH of 4 does not meet the strict definition of a strong acid but is nevertheless extremely destructive if it enters the eye and isn't flushed out immediately.

Acids and bases are incompatible. This means they react violently when concentrated acid and base solutions come into contact with each other. Usually heat is generated, but the reaction may also give rise to toxic gases. For example, mixing household bleach (hypochlorite) with an ammonia-based cleaner generates chloramine gas. Examples of acids and bases are given in Table 10-11.

Acids are a ubiquitous presence in our lives. At home, we use them to open clogged drains, treat swimming pools, polish metal, and clean everything from toilet bowls to wheel rims. Acids are also found in the foods we eat. Vinegar, for instance, is composed of about 5% to 10% acetic acid, and many soft drinks contain phosphoric acid.

In industry, acids are used as chemical reagents, catalysts, industrial cleaning agents, and neutralizing agents. Sulfuric acid is used in such great quantities that some countries set their

Table 10-11 Selected Acids and Bases	
Acids	**Alkalis (Bases)**
Battery acid	Drain cleaners
Drain cleaners	Refrigerants
Hydrochloric acid	Fertilizers
Hydrofluoric acid	Anhydrous ammonia
Sulfuric acid	Lye
Nitric acid	Sodium hydroxide
Phosphoric acid	Bleach
Acetic acid	Sodium hypochlorite
Citric acid	Lime
Formic acid	Calcium oxide
Trichloroacetic acid	Sodium carbonate
Phenol	Lithium hydride

gross domestic product (GDP) by the quantity of sulfuric acid produced and used each year.

Alkaline solutions, also called *caustics* and *bases*, are as ubiquitous as acids. At home and in industrial processes, they serve many of the same functions as acid solutions. They are used in toilet bowl cleaners, drain openers, household bleach, and ammonia-based cleaning solutions. In industry, they are used as reagents, neutralizing agents, and cleaning solutions.

Ammonia is a widely used and available corrosive and flammable chemical. It is used in agriculture as a fertilizer and in industry as a refrigerant (in the form of a liquefied gas) and chemical reagent. In addition to these legitimate uses, ammonia is a primary ingredient in methamphetamine production. An increasing number of injuries occur each year from the illicit possession and use of ammonia. Several people have died of chemical burns sustained when this flammable gas ignited while they were manufacturing ("cooking") meth. Utmost caution is required if you respond to an ammonia injury under suspicious circumstances. Examples of such calls may include a chemical-related injury in the middle of the night in a rural area, or a chemical-related injury in a primarily residential area. Allow law enforcement to secure the scene and rule out the presence of other chemical hazards before you proceed.

Pathophysiology

The pathophysiology of various acid and base exposures varies widely. First, acid burns and alkali burns are distinctly different. Acids tend to produce necrosis by denaturing proteins, forming an eschar that limits the penetration of the acid, a process called *coagulation necrosis*. Bases, on the other hand, tend to produce *liquefaction necrosis*. (Hydrofluoric acid, which tends to produce liquefaction necrosis like an alkali, is an exception to this rule.) Liquefaction necrosis is a more penetrating injury in which cell membranes break down and dissolve, essentially forming soap. Consequently, a hallmark of caustic exposure is that the skin feels slick or slimy. This process, called *saponification*, results in a deeper burn that is more difficult to decontaminate. Pain is often delayed in these types of exposures.

Second, the severity of the burn depends on a number of variables such as pH, surface area, contact time, concentration, and physical form (solid, liquid, or gas) of the corrosive. Ingestion of solid pellets of alkalis such as lye causes severe burns because the pellets remain in prolonged contact with the esophagus and stomach. Full-thickness or circumferential esophageal burns can be complicated by strictures that form as the burns heal.

Signs and Symptoms

Hydrofluoric acid, or hydrogen fluoride, is dangerous because it is a strong acid that not only has corrosive properties but also induces acute systemic toxicity. Burns caused by hydrofluoric acid penetrate much deeper than those of most acids. The fluoride ion (F^-) contributes to binding and sequestering calcium and magnesium in the body. A white or yellowish-white precipitate of calcium fluoride salt may form beneath the skin in patients with hydrofluoric acid burns. Severe exposures can cause systemic hypocalcemia and hypomagnesemia. Disruption of cellular membranes induced by hydrofluoric acid also causes hyperkalemia as intracellular potassium is released. Cardiac dysrhythmias attributed to either hyperkalemia and/or hypocalcemia are the likely causes of most deaths not directly attributable to caustic injury.

Diagnosis

Lab workups may be necessary following corrosive exposures. The extent of the workup depends on the type of corrosive, the surface area of the burn, and the route of exposure. Localized burns don't typically require lab workups because of the circumscribed effects of the exposure. Severe burns, however, warrant a CBC including hemoglobin/hematocrit, blood glucose level, electrolyte studies, creatinine, serum urea nitrogen and creatine kinase, a coagulation profile, and a urinalysis. Hydrofluoric acid burns require calcium, magnesium, and potassium levels to ascertain the extent of toxicity and identify any systemic effects, in addition to broader lab workups that may be indicated by the severity of the exposure. Phenol exposure requires a CBC, electrolyte studies, creatinine, liver function tests, and a urinalysis.

In addition, pulse oximetry and an arterial blood gas analysis should be performed if the patient has respiratory symptoms. Endoscopy (specifically, esophagoscopy and gastroscopy) should be performed for corrosive ingestions within the first 24 hours and preferably as soon as possible, because significant esophageal injury can occur even in the absence of visible oral burns. Finally, chest radiography is indicated in patients with respiratory symptoms, and abdominal radiography is indicated in patients with signs of peritonitis.

Treatment

Prehospital Setting An acid creates a chemical burn at the site of contact. The longer the acid remains in contact with the skin, eyes, or GI tract, the more severe the burn will be. External decontamination is effective in removing acids. Although acids are considered water reactive, the most effective decontaminating agents are large volumes of plain soap and water or just water alone. This method of decontamination is safe because a relatively small quantity of acid is being washed away by a large quantity of water. The heat generated by the chemical reaction is absorbed by the cool water; take care to not induce hypothermia when decontaminating patients for more than a few minutes.

Carry out decontamination procedures in an area with good ventilation and adequate space. The amount of time to irrigate depends on the corrosive, its concentration, and the size of the body surface area affected. For ocular decontamination, there are two typical approaches that should be guided by the potential damage of the chemical agent: (1) irrigate the eyes for 15 minutes with water or normal saline, or (2) extend irrigation time to 30 to 60 minutes with a Morgan irrigation lens or IV tubing and topical anesthetic. Initial pH of the cornea should be obtained using litmus paper. Irrigation should continue until pH is neutral. Assess eye acuity after decontamination.

Flush the skin with water for at least 5 minutes. Flushing can continue during transport, so long as contaminated water is isolated in a reservoir such as an emesis basin. Testing the area with litmus paper (pH paper) is the best way to determine whether decontamination is complete.

Gastrointestinal decontamination should not be attempted following presumed caustic ingestion given the risk of further GI injury or aspiration. The poison center or medical control may advise you to dilute the acid by giving the patient milk or water to drink following a minor ingestion.

If decontamination is not rapidly completed, the acid produces intense pain at the site of contact. This site becomes a necrotic sore, and eschar may or may not form, depending on the nature of the exposure. Eye exposures produce immediate and severe pain. The thin layer of cells of the corneal epithelium is rapidly destroyed, and the acid begins denaturing the proteins in the cornea, which may lead to permanent visual impairment. GI damage from ingestion of an acid may include burns of the mouth, esophagus, and stomach. Since their severity depends largely on contact time, the stomach is usually the most severely affected part of the GI tract. Injury ranges from local burns to ulceration or perforation of the stomach or esophagus, causing severe abdominal pain. The acid may be absorbed into the vasculature, inducing acidosis.

Hydrofluoric acid burns require special consideration. Fluoride ions can be bound by either calcium or magnesium, so for any hydrofluoric acid burns, administer calcium gluconate or calcium chloride and magnesium to forestall cardiac effects. The antidote for hydrofluoric acid skin burns is thorough decontamination with water, followed by application of topical calcium gluconate gel. Because of the penetrating nature of fluoride burns, you must apply calcium gluconate to the burn site repeatedly and continuously even after initial decontamination and treatment has been completed. Deeper burns may require subcutaneous injections of calcium gluconate. Cover burns and wounds with dry, sterile dressings.

For eye exposures involving hydrofluoric acid, irrigate the eyes with normal saline. Even patients with minor hydrofluoric acid burns or suspected burns should be transported to an appropriate medical facility for evaluation. The primary goal of local burn therapy is pain control. Evaluation of systemic illness will be determined by surface area of the burn, concentration of the acid, and laboratory studies. Analgesics may be provided.

In the case of alkali (base) burns, copious and continuous flushing en route to the emergency room is needed. Alkali exposures burn longer and deeper, causing greater tissue damage. Typical alkali substances, such as drain cleaners, lye ammonia, and household bleaches, are caustic.

In-Hospital Setting Thorough patient decontamination needs to be done first in any corrosive exposure (details in the *Hazardous Materials* section). In addition, because many corrosives are volatile, the airway may need to be secured. Endotracheal intubation may be indicated for ingestion or facial burns. Corrosive burns affecting a large body surface area require fluid therapy analogous to fluid resuscitation given after thermal burns. As with most skin injuries, infection can complicate long-term recovery.

Elemental forms of lithium, potassium, sodium, and magnesium react with water to form alkalis. Therefore, *do not irrigate with water*. Instead, coat the area with mineral oil and remove the caustic material manually with forceps.

Nitrites and Sulfa Drugs That Cause Methemoglobinemia

Compounds such as nitrites and nitrates, which can oxidize the iron in hemoglobin, cause the condition known as **methemoglobinemia**. These types of poisonings can be attributed to a number of different chemicals, some of which are listed in Table 10-12.

Overuse of certain medications such as nitroprussides and benzocaine sprays can cause methemoglobinemia. In rural areas,

Table 10-12 Selected Chemicals That Cause Methemoglobinemia	
Aniline Dyes	**Nitrites (Such as Butyl Nitrite and Isobutyl Nitrite)**
Aromatic amines	Nitroaniline
Arsine	Nitrobenzene
Chlorates	Nitrofurans
Chlorobenzene	Nitrophenol
Chromates	Nitrosobenzene
Combustion products	Nitrous oxides
Dimethyl toluidine	Resorcinol
Naphthalene	Silver nitrate
Nitric acid	Trinitrotoluene
Nitric oxides	

biological processes such as fermentation can create nitrites after silos are filled with grain. Peak toxicity occurs about a week after filling. Agricultural groundwater contamination with fertilizers such as ammonium nitrate can cause methemoglobinemia cyanosis in infants, known as "blue baby syndrome" in some Midwestern states.

Pathophysiology

The pathophysiology of methemoglobinemia can be inferred from its antidote, methylene blue, which was first used by Dr. Madison Cawein in the Appalachian mountains of Kentucky in the early 1960s. Oxygen and other oxidizers naturally convert a small percentage of hemoglobin to methemoglobin on a continuous basis. NADH methemoglobin reductase dispatches this constant threat, and people with active enzymes do not suffer from even mild methemoglobinemia. The "Kentucky blue" people, as they are known, have a mutation in the enzyme NADH methemoglobin reductase, which converts ferric methemoglobin back to ferrous hemoglobin. Affected individuals have a blue skin tone that makes them appear cyanotic; this coloring is not caused by oxygen-deprivation cyanosis but by methemoglobin, which is a dark bluish-brown color. Cawein empirically administered methylene blue to these patients, correctly surmising that it would eliminate their blue pallor by acting as an electron donor (reducing agent) to convert methemoglobin to hemoglobin.

Signs and Symptoms

Patients with methemoglobinemia due to nitrate and nitrite poisoning have altered levels of consciousness, including anxiety, confusion, and stupor. They have a slate-gray cyanosis caused by methemoglobin production. Nausea and vomiting, dizziness, and headache are common. Severe signs and symptoms may include cerebral ischemia, hypotension, and respiratory distress, which can lead to cardiovascular collapse and asphyxiation.

Differential Diagnosis

Recognition of methemoglobinemia can be challenging because the patient may have only mild complaints. Pulse oximetry is inaccurate with methemoglobinemia because the methemoglobin interferes with measurement of oxyhemoglobin (the wavelengths are too close together). Typically, pulse oximetry will give a reading in the high 80s that is unresponsive to additional oxygen supplementation. As noted in the earlier discussion of carbon monoxide poisoning, pulse oximeters sensitive to methemoglobin are available. A thorough history and physical assessment are crucial to discovering the correct etiology. Serum methemoglobinemia and arterial blood gas levels should be analyzed in serious exposures.

Methemoglobinemia can be diagnosed quickly in the field with a blood-drop test. Place a drop of blood on a 4×4-inch gauze pad. If it is chocolate brown and does not turn red in a few minutes with exposure to atmospheric oxygen, you can make a diagnosis of methemoglobinemia with confidence because carboxyhemoglobin turns red when it oxidizes, whereas methemoglobin does not.

Treatment

As previously mentioned, the antidote to nitrate and nitrite poisoning is methylene blue, a thiazine dye that reduces methemoglobin to hemoglobin by boosting the action of a second enzyme, NADPH methemoglobin reductase. Paradoxically, at high concentrations, methylene blue acts as an oxidizing agent. In the body, methylene blue must first be converted to its bioactive form, leukomethylene blue. At higher dosages, the body cannot keep up with this conversion process.

Prehospital Setting Provide supportive care, including maintenance of airway, breathing, and circulation. Administer supplemental oxygen. Ensure that the patient has been removed from the offending environment and thoroughly decontaminated. Decontamination is also important to prevent cross-contamination.

In-Hospital Setting Treatment is selected on the basis of the severity of symptoms. External decontamination is extremely important to prevent continued intoxication and avoid cross-contamination of healthcare personnel and of the ED environment.

Mild exposures resolve on their own, whereas more severe exposures require intervention with supportive care and antidote therapy. Supplemental oxygen is crucial to ensure that the remaining hemoglobin becomes fully saturated with oxygen. Patients in whom methylene blue is contraindicated may benefit from hyperbaric oxygen therapy or exchange transfusion.

Cholinesterase Inhibitors

Cholinesterase inhibitors (organophosphates and carbamates), examples of which are given in Table 10-13, are classes of widely used pesticides. They are found in insect sprays as a liquid, in rose-dusting formulations as a solid, and in mist preparations for application over larger areas. The dangers these agents pose vary widely, depending on the chemical structure of the pesticide and the carrier in which the pesticide is dissolved. Most of these pesticides are not water soluble and are enveloped in a hydrocarbon solvent that acts as a carrier. These two characteristics make most of them highly skin absorbent. However, most organophosphate pesticides are designed to be toxic by ingestion or on contact, rather than poisonous by inhalation, to reduce the risk to the applicator. In addition, household formulations are typically more dilute, and the chemical agents they contain are often less potent. Pesticides intended for commercial use can be highly concentrated and deadly.

Table 10-13 Selected Organophosphates and Carbamates	
Organophosphates	**Carbamates**
Acephate	Sevin
Azinphos-methyl	Aldicarb
Chlorpyrifos	Carbaryl
Demeton	Carbofuran
Diazinon	Methomyl
Dichlorvos	Propoxur
Ethyl 4-nitrophenyl phenylphosphonothioate (EPN)	
Ethion	
Malathion	
Parathion	
Ronnel	
Tetraethyl pyrophosphate	

Organophosphates were first developed as nerve agents in Germany prior World War II, so they were designed as agents of chemical warfare first and adapted for agricultural use as pesticides only later. Nerve agents have been optimized for human toxicity, whereas pesticides have been optimized for toxicity to targeted pests such as wasps or aphids. Some mushrooms also have similar effects through direct receptor stimulation rather than enzyme inhibition.

Pathophysiology

Organophosphates and carbamates overstimulate the parasympathetic and sympathetic nervous systems by interfering with degradation of the neurotransmitter, acetylcholine. The nerve signal travels along the neuron through an electrochemical channel and stops at synapses, the junctions between neurons, where a chemical neurotransmitter—in this case acetylcholine—must be released from the neuron for the signal to travel across the junction. At the target, acetylcholine binds to the cholinergic receptor. Acetylcholine binds to nicotinic receptors on muscles and in both the sympathetic and parasympathetic nervous systems as well as muscarinic receptors found primarily in the parasympathetic system. The electrochemical impulse continues in the next neuron, or contraction begins in the muscle.

Once the signal has been conducted, the neurotransmitter must be removed. Enzymes, proteins that carry out vital metabolic processes, are the workhorses of the cell. Acetylcholinesterase is the enzyme that breaks down acetylcholine into acetate and choline after impulse conduction. Organophosphates inhibit carboxyl ester hydrolases in general and the enzyme acetylcholinesterase specifically.

However, organophosphates and carbamates inhibit acetylcholinesterase in slightly different ways. Organophosphates and nerve agents contain an organic phosphate group, whereas carbamates do not. The phosphate portion of the pesticide binds to the acetylcholinesterase. Over a variable period of time, these two molecules form a permanent bond, a process referred to as aging, which permanently inactivates the enzyme. The shorter the aging time, the faster the antidote, particularly pralidoxime, must be administered.

Signs and Symptoms

The signs and symptoms of organophosphate and carbamate poisoning are the same. The "wet" patient has symptoms that can be summarized using the mnemonic SLUDGE BBM, expanded in the Rapid Recall box. The *M* in this mnemonic stands for *miosis*, which is the most commonly identified physical finding seen in toxicity from these pesticides and nerve agents, making it one of the stronger clues in narrowing the differential diagnosis. Other symptoms include early, nonspecific flulike symptoms, sweating, and muscle fasciculations (twitching). Severe poisoning can lead to severe pulmonary edema, seizures, coma, paralysis, and respiratory failure. The DUMBBELS mnemonic is used to describe muscarinic signs and symptoms brought on by these agents, and their nicotinic effects can be recalled by the mnemonic MTWtHF. Details of these two mnemonics also appear in the Rapid Recall box.

Differential Diagnosis

Organophosphate and carbamate intoxication are recognizable primarily by signs and symptoms. Cholinesterase assays can aid diagnosis, but they are not always reflective of the severity of intoxication if preexisting conditions such as pernicious anemia and use of antimalarial drugs skew results. There are two types of cholinesterase assays: RBC and plasma. The RBC cholinesterase assay is a more accurate reflection of CNS enzyme inactivation, but results take longer to obtain than plasma cholinesterase activity. Because of delays in results as well as limitations in interpretation, therapy should be initiated prior to laboratory confirmation of toxicity.

Treatment

When treating a patient with organophosphate poisoning, you must take great care to avoid cross-contamination from the victim (Table 10-14). The patient's clothing must be removed and isolated (bagged or removed from the immediate area). You must wear personal protective clothing, including gloves, a gown, and eye protection, while treating the patient. In addition, some organophosphates and carbamates are volatile, and respiratory protection may be required. Emesis may also contain significant amounts of poison and must be isolated and handled carefully.

Supportive care, including management of airway, breathing, and circulation, is of paramount importance. Airway management must be a priority because of the increased bronchial secretions and muscle paralysis associated with the cholinergic effects of these agents. Cardiac monitoring is also necessary. Gastric lavage and activated charcoal may be indicated if less than 1 hour has elapsed since the exposure, though commonly the patient will be already vomiting.

Prehospital Setting Prehospital treatment consists of supportive care and antidote administration. The antidotes for organophosphate poisoning are atropine and pralidoxime (2-PAM). Atropine treats the wet symptoms, while 2-PAM reactivates acetylcholinesterase. Atropine can be given in 1- to 5-mg doses every 5 minutes, depending on symptoms. Note that these doses are significantly higher than those used for cardiac conditions. As a cholinesterase antidote, the atropine binds to the muscarinic acetylcholine receptor, inhibiting the parasympathetic stimulation caused by the organophosphate or carbamate. The end point of atropine administration is drying of the secretions and improved respiratory function. There is no maximum dose.

To be most effective, 2-PAM should be administered before the aging process occurs. In contrast, carbamates (such as the pesticide Sevin) do not contain an organophosphate group but can still bind to the acetylcholinesterase enzyme. Because

RAPID RECALL
© HunThomas/ShutterStock, Inc.

Mnemonics for Signs and Symptoms of Organophosphate and Carbamate Poisoning

SLUDGE BBM:

S Salivation
L Lacrimation
U Urination
D Defecation
G Gastrointestinal distress
E Emesis
B Bradycardia
B Bronchoconstriction/bronchorrhea
M Miosis

DUMBBELS:

D Diarrhea
U Urination
M Miosis
B Bradycardia
B Bronchorrhea/bronchoconstriction
E Emesis
L Lacrimation
S Salivation

MTWtHF:

M Muscle weakness and paralysis
T Tachycardia
W Weakness
tH Hypertension
F Fasciculations

carbamates do not have an organophosphate group, they do not require 2-PAM as an antidote. Only atropine is given to dry out the patient's SLUDGE symptoms (see the Rapid Recall box). However, if the substance responsible for exposure is not known and the symptoms are consistent with cholinesterase inhibition, it is appropriate to administer pralidoxime given the potential danger of delay in treatment of an organophosphate agent. Routine medical care includes high-flow oxygen and IV therapy.

In-Hospital Setting If seizures occur, benzodiazepine therapy of 0.1 to 0.2 mg/kg IV is appropriate. A continuous infusion of 2-PAM at 8 mg/kg/h for adults is administered. If the patient

Table 10-14 **Treatment of Pesticide (Organophosphate/Carbamate) Exposure**
■ Adequate decontamination is essential to limit the patient's exposure and the chance of secondary exposure to the caregiver.
■ Establish an open airway. Consider orotracheal or nasotracheal intubation for airway control in the patient who is unconscious, has severe pulmonary edema, or is in severe respiratory distress.
■ Ventilate as necessary. Positive-pressure ventilation with a bag-mask device may be beneficial.
■ Monitor for pulmonary edema and treat as necessary.
■ Monitor cardiac rhythm and treat dysrhythmias as necessary.
■ Start an IV line and infuse at 30 mL/h. For hypotension with signs of hypovolemia, administer fluid cautiously. Consider vasopressors if the patient is hypotensive with a normal fluid volume, per local protocol. Watch for signs of fluid overload.
■ Administer atropine per local protocol. Correct hypoxia before giving atropine.
■ Mydriasis should not be used to determine the end point of atropine administration; the end point for atropine administration is the drying of pulmonary secretions.
■ Administer pralidoxime chloride per local protocol.
■ Treat seizures with adequate atropinization and correction of hypoxia. In rare cases, diazepam (Valium) or lorazepam (Ativan) may be necessary per local protocol.
■ Succinylcholine, other cholinergic agents, and aminophylline are contraindicated.
■ For eye contamination, immediately flush eyes with water. Continuously irrigate each eye with normal saline during transport.

From Currance PL, Clements B, Bronstein AC: *Emergency care for hazardous materials exposure*, ed 3, St. Louis, MO, 2005, Mosby.

arrives within one hour of ingestion, gastric lavage with careful disposition of stomach contents may be considered due to the potential severity of ongoing absorption and toxicity. However, activated charcoal has no role in the treatment of organophosphate toxicity owing to the likelihood of aspiration.

Petroleum Distillates

Hydrocarbons are a broad class of combustible or flammable liquids derived from oil. These liquids are not water soluble and generally float on water. Hydrocarbons are found in small quantities around the home and in large quantities in industry. At home, most of us have small quantities of gasoline, mineral spirits, paint thinner, and other solvents in the garage or shed. In industry, large quantities of hydrocarbons are used as fuels (including diesel fuel), solvents, and reagents for chemical processes (especially in the plastics industry). Examples of other petroleum distillates are toluene, xylene, benzene, and hexane.

Huffing is a form of chemical abuse in which abusers intentionally inhale various halogenated or aromatic hydrocarbons to produce a euphoric high. These effects, which can include severe CNS depression and respiratory depression, can have a rapid onset.

Pathophysiology

Hydrocarbons generally affect the CNS. They are readily absorbed through the skin and are thought to change the properties (such as fluidity) of cell membranes in CNS neurons as they dissolve. Some hydrocarbons cause cancer, whereas others are protoxins, and their metabolites are harmful. The volatility of a substance, which is a measure of vapor pressure, indicates the degree of threat it poses to the respiratory system. The higher the vapor pressure, the greater the concentration of the chemical in the air and the more volatile it is said to be. Higher volatility also equates with greater flammability.

The viscosity of a hydrocarbon affects the likelihood of aspiration during an ingestion. Thinner, less viscous hydrocarbons are more likely to be aspirated than thicker ones. For example, gasoline is more likely than motor oil to cause pulmonary damage. Some hydrocarbon derivatives such as phenol possess anesthetic properties. Phenol burns may therefore go unnoticed for longer periods, which will result in more severe burns with possible systemic effects.

A good scene size-up is critical in determining the level of risk associated with a particular exposure. Many hydrocarbons require specialized personal protective equipment (PPE) to approach the victim. The National Institute of Occupational Safety and Health (NIOSH) guide can be used to determine the degree of danger a particular hydrocarbon poses to both prehospital provider and victim.

Signs and Symptoms

Signs and symptoms of petroleum distillate toxicity vary greatly depending on the specific properties of the hydrocarbon, the route of entry, and the quantity of the chemical ingested. Inhalation typically results in temporary euphoric effects. Dermal exposure can cause skin irritation and a defatting dermatitis. The most common toxicity associated with hydrocarbon ingestion or inhalation is acute lung injury ranging from mild symptoms, such as cough and wheezing, to acute respiratory distress syndrome. Some hydrocarbons have resulted in significant mucosal caustic injuries when ingested. Chronic inhalation abuse of hydrocarbons that contain toluene found in many spray paints, particularly metallic colors, is associated with acidosis and severe hypokalemia that can cause symptomatic muscular weakness. Finally, halogenated hydrocarbons such as 1,1 difluoroethane (DFE) found in air dusters have been associated with myocardial sensitization to catecholamines, cardiac dysrhythmias, and death referred to as *sudden sniffing death syndrome.*

Differential Diagnosis

A lab workup is indicated in petroleum distillate intoxication. A CBC should be performed, because chronic benzene exposure leads to leukemia or aplastic anemia. A basic metabolic panel, including glucose level, serum urea nitrogen, creatinine, and electrolyte studies, is indicated. Hepatic transaminase studies and serum creatine kinase levels (to identify rhabdomyolysis) are also indicated. Chest imaging may be necessary when aspiration of petroleum distillates results in persistent symptoms.

Treatment

Prehospital Setting A thorough patient history and complete external decontamination are crucial. It is important to observe the patient to pinpoint which specific hydrocarbon has been ingested and the quantity. Generally, the most pronounced effects of toxicity are on the CNS. In rare cases of ventricular dysrhythmia known to be the result of inhaled halogenated hydrocarbons, initial treatment would be with an IV beta-blocker rather than standard ACLS. Because of myocardial sensitization to catecholamines, administration of additional epinephrine may exacerbate the underlying cause. However, when the cause of dysrhythmia is not certain, standard ACLS protocols apply. Activated charcoal does adsorb some hydrocarbons but is not indicated in the treatment of hydrocarbon ingestion given the inherently high risk of vomiting and aspiration.

In-Hospital Setting A good patient history should be obtained to determine the type of hydrocarbon, the amount, and time of consumption. In addition, questions should focus on co-ingestants and the possibility of aspiration. Treatment is mainly supportive, including maintaining airway, breathing, and circulation, providing supplemental oxygen, and establishing IV access. The airway is vulnerable to aspiration. Gastric lavage may be indicated in patients who have ingested camphor, halogenated hydrocarbons, aromatic hydrocarbons, heavy metal–containing hydrocarbons, or pesticide-containing hydrocarbons (CHAMP). The physical exam should include a thorough neurologic exam, including cranial nerves, to rule out any traumatic injury.

Environmental Toxins: Poisoning by Envenomation

Environmental toxicology studies the effects of chemicals in the environment. A wide variety of environmental toxins, such as animal venom and microbial and plant toxins, can have adverse effects on humans. Many of the cardiovascular and neurologic effects of natural toxins are treated in ways similar to those used to treat other toxic exposures, as outlined in the preceding sections. However, several specific toxic mechanisms and clinical manifestations require directed therapy.

In the United States, you may treat patients for envenomation by *Latrodectus* (black widow spider), *Loxosceles* (brown recluse spider), or *Buthidae* (scorpion). Although envenomation by any of these arthropods can be painful, death is rare. The linchpins of treatment are supportive care and symptomatic management with opioids and anxiolytics. Table 10-15 summarizes toxicity, mechanism of action, and recommended treatment for each type of arthropod envenomation.

There are thousands of exposures to venom by snakebite in the United States annually, very few of which are fatal. Poisonous snakes can be found throughout the continental United States and Alaska (**Figure 10-2**). There two families of poisonous snakes are as follows:

1. The *Crotalidae* (pit vipers), a family that comprises rattlesnakes (including the eastern and western diamondback, pygmy and massasauga varieties), cottonmouths (water moccasins), and copperheads
2. The Elapidae (coral snakes)

Snake venom toxicity and mode of action vary between the families.

Many marine creatures deliver venom via bites or stings, producing intense pain at the site of envenomation (**Figure 10-3**). Some of these organisms—jellyfish, fire coral, and sea anemones—inject toxin with stinging cells called *nematocysts*. Other organisms such as sea urchins and stingrays have spines that inject venom deeper into the tissue, causing trauma as well as envenomation.

Black Widow Spider

The black widow spider lives in all parts of the continental United States. It is usually found outdoors in woodpiles, brush, sheds, or garages, and it may hitchhike into the home on outdoor-stored items such as firewood or Christmas trees.

Identification

The female black widow is recognizable by its bulbous, shiny black abdomen and red hourglass marking on the ventral side (**Figure 10-4**). The spider is usually an inch or

Table 10-15 Arthropod Toxicity

Arthropod	Toxin	Toxic Mechanism	Clinical Manifestations	Treatment
Latrodectus mactans (black widow)	Alpha-latrotoxin	Presynaptic calcium channel opening with release of multiple vasoactive and myoactive neurotransmitters	Nausea, vomiting, sweating, tachycardia, hypertension, muscle cramping	Diazepam, fentanyl Consider antivenin for severe toxicity
Loxosceles recluse (brown recluse)	Sphingo-myelinase-Dhyaluronidase	Sphingomyelinase-D: Local tissue destruction, intravascular clotting Hyaluronidase: promotes tissue penetration	Local: tissue necrosis and ulcer formation Systemic: loxoscelism, including fever, vomiting, rhabdomyolysis, disseminated intravascular coagulation, hemolysis	Local wound care, tetanus prophylaxis, and analgesia Supportive care for systemic toxicity
Centruroides exilicauda (bark scorpion)	Neurotoxin I-IV	Sodium channel opening with repeated depolarization and neurotransmitter release	Local paresthesias, tachycardia, hypertension, salivation, diaphoresis, muscle fasciculations, opsoclonus, roving eye movements	Tetanus prophylaxis, wound care, anxiolysis, analgesia Severe toxicity may be treated with antivenin where available

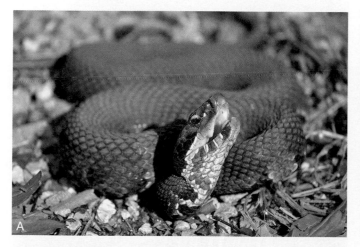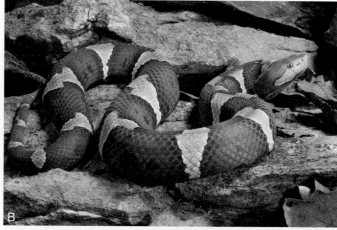

Figure 10-2 A. Water moccasin (cottonmouth) snake. **B.** Southern copperhead (*Agkistrodon contortrix contortrix*) has markings that make it almost invisible when lying in leaf litter. (A., courtesy Michael Cardwell and Carl Barden, Venom Laboratory. B., courtesy Sherman Minton, MD.)
A © James DeBoer/Shutterstock, Inc.; B © Dennis W. Donohue/Shutterstock, Inc.

less in length. Its venom is a potent neurotoxin. The male black widow is brown, about half the size of the female, and nonvenomous.

Signs and Symptoms

Signs and symptoms of black widow envenomation include muscle spasms, nontender abdominal rigidity, and immediate severe, localized pain, redness, and swelling with papule formation at the site. The patient may describe the bite as a bee sting–like

sensation. You might observe two small fang marks spaced 1 mm apart. Systemic effects of envenomation may include nausea and vomiting, diaphoresis (sweating), a decreased level of consciousness, seizures, and paralysis.

Treatment

Prehospital treatment is mainly supportive. Treat muscle spasms with muscle relaxants such as diazepam (Valium) or calcium gluconate. Monitor and treat hypertension aggressively to prevent

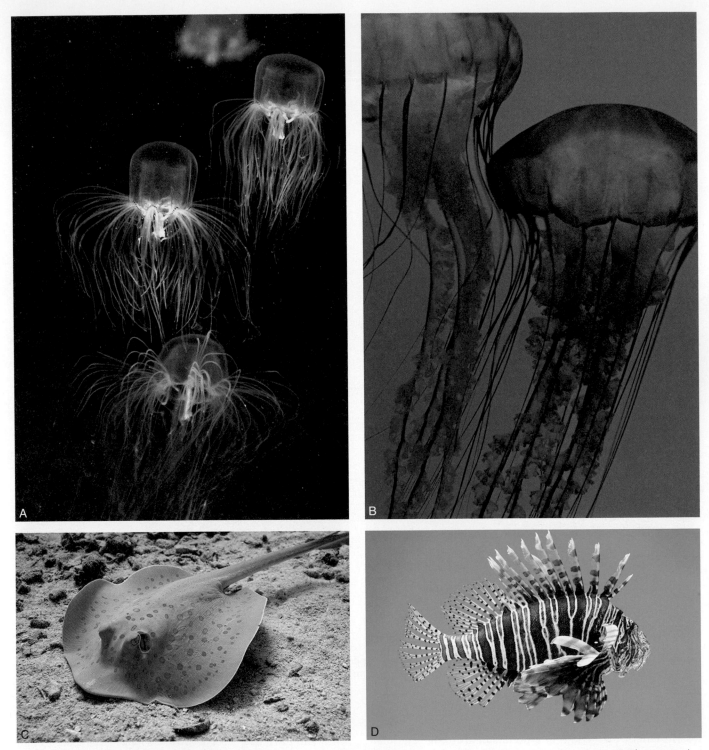

Figure 10-3 A. Box jellyfish (*Chironex fleckeri*) swimming just beneath surface of water. **B.** Atlantic Portuguese man-of-war. **C.** Blue-spotted stingray. **D.** Adult lionfish. (A., courtesy John Williamson, MD. B., courtesy Larry Madin, Woods Hole Oceanographic Institution. C., and D., photos by Paul Auerbach, MD.)

hypertensive crisis. Antivenin is available for black widow envenomation, making identification of the spider and rapid transport to the facility important. Antivenin may be administered in the emergency department.

Brown Recluse Spider

The brown recluse spider lives in dark, dry locations, including inside houses, in relatively warm climates. In the United States,

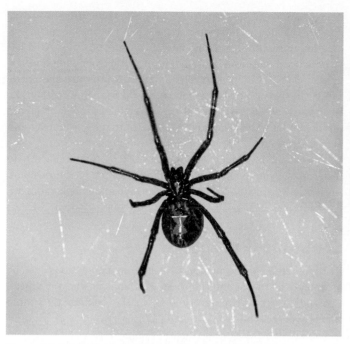

Figure 10-4 Female black widow spider with red hourglass marking on underside of abdomen.
© Brian Chase/Shutterstock

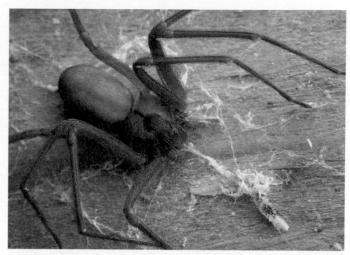

Figure 10-5 Brown recluse spider. Note the dark, violin-shaped marking on spider's back.
© Miles Boyer/Shutterstock

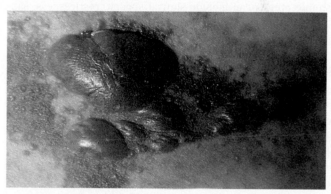

Figure 10-6 Brown recluse spider bite. A severe reaction in which infarction, bleeding, and blistering have occurred.
From Habif TP: *Clinical dermatology: a color guide to diagnosis and therapy*, ed 5, St Louis, 2009, Mosby.

the recluse is found in Hawaii and in the South, the Midwest, and the Southwest. Most envenomations occur in states in the south-central part of the country.

Identification

The recluse is tan to brown, with a distinctive violin-shaped marking on its back (it is also known as the "violin spider" or the "fiddle-back spider"; **Figure 10-5**). Its body can be up to three fourths of an inch long. Another identifying feature is that it has six eyes, rather than the usual eight. The eyes are arranged in a semicircle in pairs of three.

Signs and Symptoms

Systemic symptoms of brown recluse envenomation include malaise, chills, fever, nausea and vomiting, and joint pain. Life-threatening symptoms may include bleeding disorders such as disseminated intravascular coagulation and hemolytic anemia.

The venom of the brown recluse is a pernicious cocktail of at least 11 peptides that possess a variety of cytotoxic properties. The necrotic venom produces a classic bull's-eye lesion at the injection site. Many envenomations occur at night while the patient is asleep. The bite is painless and initially begins as a small blister (papule), sometimes surrounded by a white halo. Over the next 24 hours, localized pain, redness, and swelling develop (**Figure 10-6**). During the next few days or weeks, tissue necrosis develops at the site,

and the redness and swelling begin to spread. The necrosis makes the wound slow to heal, and it may be visible months after the bite.

Treatment

Prehospital care should focus on airway management and pain control. Treatment is supportive because no approved antivenin is available. Clean and dress the wound, apply a cold compress to the envenomation site, and transport the patient for medical evaluation.

Fentanyl is the opioid of choice in the treatment of envenomation because it does not produce the histamine release associated with other opioids. Specific antidotes to brown recluse envenomation have been investigated, but because of serious potential adverse effects and lack of effectiveness, their use is not recommended.

Scorpions

More than 14,000 scorpion stings were reported in 2003, with no fatalities. More than 600 scorpion species are found in the United States, but only the bark or sculptured scorpion of the desert Southwest is dangerous to humans. Scorpions are nocturnal and hide under objects and buildings during the day. They may enter buildings, especially at night.

Identification

Scorpions are yellowish-brown, may be striped, and are about 1 to 3 inches long (**Figure 10-7**). The scorpion injects venom stored in a bulb at the base of a stinger on the end of its tail. It usually injects only a small amount of poison. The sculptured scorpion is active from April to August and hibernates during the winter.

Signs and Symptoms

Systemic effects can include slurred speech, restlessness, salivation, abdominal cramping, nausea and vomiting, muscle fasciculations (twitching), and seizures. Symptoms typically peak within 5 hours of injection. If redness and swelling are present at the injection site, a bark scorpion is probably not responsible for the sting, because its venom does not induce localized inflammation. The venom of the bark scorpion is a neurotoxin that initially produces a burning or tingling sensation followed by numbness. The toxin is a mixture of proteins and polypeptides that affect voltage-dependent ion channels, especially the sodium channels involved in nerve signaling. A secondary effect of envenomation is CNS stimulation through sympathetic neurons.

Treatment

Begin treatment by managing airway, breathing, and circulation and by calming the patient. Offer supportive care for respiratory

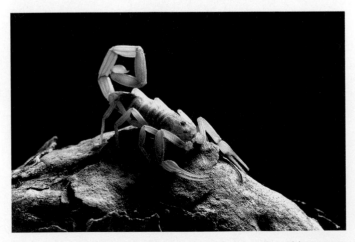

Figure 10-7 Arizona bark scorpion (*Centruroides exilicauda*).
© K Lorenz Craig/Photo Researchers RM/Getty Images

depression. Clean the wound and apply a cold compress. You may consider placement of a constricting band over the site of envenomation to restrict lymphatic flow if transport time is expected to be long. The band should be at least 2 inches wide and not tighter than a watch band. The amount of pressure should be similar to that of an elastic bandage used for a sprained ankle. Be aware that this technique is controversial, however. It should *not* be confused with application of a tourniquet, which should never be placed.

Avoid giving analgesics because they may exacerbate respiratory symptoms. Provide rapid transport to the hospital. Antivenin is available for scorpion stings in endemic locations.

Crotalids (Pit Vipers)

In the United States, nearly all snake envenomations can be attributed to the *Crotalidae* family of snakes, the pit vipers. Crotalids are native to every state in the continental United States except Maine.

Identification

Pit vipers are named for the distinctive pits that form grooves in the maxillary bone on each side of their triangular heads. They have vertical elliptical pupils and long, hinged fangs.

Signs and Symptoms

Signs and symptoms of crotalid envenomation include distinctive fang marks at the injection site, accompanied by redness, pain, and swelling that may precede compartment syndrome. Systemic effects can include the following:

- Thirst
- Sweating
- Chills
- Weakness
- Dizziness
- Tachycardia
- Nausea and vomiting
- Diarrhea
- Hypotension
- Clotting defects
- Respiratory distress
- Numbness and tingling around the head (with some species)

Despite coagulation abnormalities, significant bleeding complications of envenomation are rarely reported though certainly possible. The primary morbidity is associated with local tissue injury. Neurotoxicity such as paresthesias and weakness are associated with only select species of crotalids, primarily the Mojave rattlesnake (*Crotalus scutulatus*) in the United

States. Crotalid envenomation is associated with injury and significant morbidity, but fatalities related to crotalid envenomations are rarely reported. Pit viper venom consists of multiple peptides and enzymes, the aggregate effect of which primarily leads to tissue and muscle injury as well as consumption and depletion of clotting factors including platelets and fibrinogen. While disseminated intravascular coagulopathy has been reported with severe envenomation, coagulopathy, thrombocytopenia, and hypofibrinogenemia develop in most patients without the microangiopathic clotting and associated tissue injury seen in disseminated intravascular coagulopathy. Intravascular envenomation can lead to disseminated intravascular coagulopathy, hypotension, and death. Allergic reactions to crotalid venom have also been reported. Approximately 25% of bites are considered dry, meaning that little or no venom is delivered with the bite.

Treatment

Treatment consists of supporting airway, breathing, and circulation; and elevating the affected limb to ameliorate the degree of local tissue injury.

Immobilize the limb by elevation with a splint, but do *not* suction, incise, or apply cold packs to the wound. No attempt should be made to constrict the affected area. The primary morbidity associated with crotalid envenomation is local tissue injury and the potential for compartment syndrome, whereas systemic toxicity is relatively minor by comparison. Therefore, the goal of prehospital care should be to extend and elevate the affected extremity to prevent further tissue injury associated with sequestration of venom in smaller distal extremities.

Antivenin is available for crotalid envenomation, so rapid transport to an appropriate medical facility is critical.

Using snakebite kits or attempting to suck out the venom has never been proved beneficial and should be avoided due to potential for causing further local tissue injury. Give fentanyl as needed for analgesia.

Once the patient is at a healthcare facility, antivenin may be administered in consultation with a medical toxicologist if evidence of local or systemic toxicity is apparent. The patient must be closely observed for a possible allergic reaction to the antivenin.

Tissue injury and limb dysfunction may take weeks or months to resolve, and physical therapy may be necessary. In rare cases, surgical intervention and fasciotomy may also be necessary to treat compartment syndrome or other complications.

Elapids

In the United States, snakes of the elapid genus *Micrurus*, the coral snakes, are found in the Southeast (Eastern variety) and Southwest (Arizona variety).

Identification

Coral snakes are smaller than pit vipers, have round pupils, a narrow head, small fixed fangs, and no pits on the head (**Figure 10-8**). They can be identified by their distinctive alternating horizontal bands of black, pale yellow or white, and deep orange or red. Some nonpoisonous snakes (such as the king snake) mimic this color pattern, but imperfectly. The old saying "Red on yellow, kill a fellow; red on black, venom lacks" can be helpful in distinguishing between the coral snake and its imposters. However, the rhyme applies only to coral snakes native to the United States.

Signs and Symptoms

Coral snake envenomation is uncommon because of the snake's docile nature, its short fixed teeth, and its small size, but severe envenomations can cause respiratory and skeletal muscle paralysis. Signs and symptoms include fang marks and swelling, redness, and localized numbness at the injection site. Systemic effects, some of which may be delayed for 12 to 24 hours, include the following:

- Weakness
- Drowsiness
- Slurred speech or salivation
- Ataxia
- Paralysis of the tongue and larynx
- Drooping eyelids
- Dilated pupils
- Abdominal pain
- Nausea and vomiting
- Seizures
- Respiratory distress
- Hypotension

The venom of a coral snake contains a mixture of hydrolytic toxins and a neurotoxin that blocks acetylcholine receptor sites. It has more significant neurologic effects than pit viper venom and may induce paralysis and respiratory failure, but only 40% of bites cause envenomation.

Treatment

Prehospital Setting Initial management of elapid envenomation differs from that of crotalid envenomation. The primary concern after elapid envenomation is systemic neurotoxicity rather than local limb injury, so pressure immobilization to prevent lymphatic drainage is recommended. Do *not* apply a tourniquet, however, because of the risk of limb ischemia. Decontaminate the wound with water or normal saline, keep the affected extremity below the heart, and encourage the patient to remain quiet and still. Immobilize the limb with a splint, apply a loose-fitting constricting band (see earlier description), and start an IV line with a volume expanding crystalloid fluid.

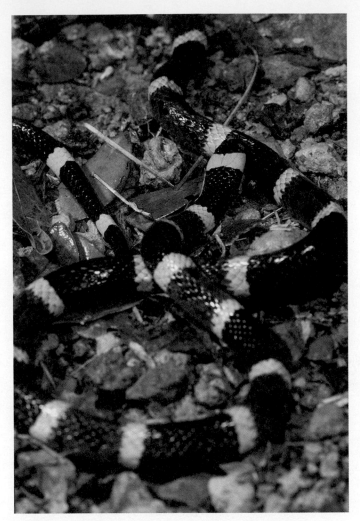

Figure 10-8 Texas coral snake (*Micrurus tener,* formerly *M. fulvius tenere*) has a highly potent venom but is secretive, and bites are uncommon.
© Joe McDonald/Visuals Unlimited, Inc.

Do not incise or apply cold packs to the wound. Antivenin is available, so rapid transport to an appropriate medical facility is critical.

In-Hospital Setting Because of the severity of toxicity and the lack of distinctive symptoms associated with early coral snake envenomation, treatment consists of specific antivenin therapy, where available, if there is any evidence of skin penetration. Alternatively, the patient may be admitted to the hospital and observed for 24 hours for any sign of delayed neurologic toxicity, which may last days or weeks if it develops.

Jellyfish

Many jellyfish stings cause only minor local dermal irritation and pain, but some species, such as *Chironex fleckeri* (the "box jellyfish"), produce more severe symptoms and systemic toxicity. Jellyfish have long tentacles equipped with nematocysts that discharge and deposit venom on contact with skin. Drowning deaths have been reported when victims incapacitated by severe pain have been unable to swim to shore.

Signs and Symptoms

Jellyfish envenomation can cause the following signs and symptoms:

- Intense localized pain
- Swelling and skin discoloration along the line of tentacle contact
- Nausea and vomiting
- Respiratory difficulty
- Cardiovascular toxicity that infrequently results in cardiac dysrhythmia and death

Treatment

The primary recommendations for treating jellyfish stings are to administer opioids and antihistamines, apply salt water, and place the affected area in warm (110°F to 113°F [43°C to 45°C]) water.

Researchers have studied various methods of removing nematocysts, including flushing the area with water, vinegar, urine, or ethanol and applying commercially available products such as StingEze. Do not use fresh water, because the difference in osmolarity (compared with salt water) causes embedded nematocysts to fire. Vinegar is beneficial in some species but intensifies symptoms in others. Antivenin is of uncertain benefit and, in any case, is available only for box jellyfish stings and only in Australia.

Spinous Sea Creatures

Many species of fish and echinoderms have venomous spines. Venom from such spinous sea animals produces similar symptoms of varying severity, but the treatment of envenomation is standard.

A stingray tail is armed with a serrated spine within an integumentary sheath that not only delivers venom but can also deliver significant traumatic injuries. The tail reflexively whips dorsally and may penetrate deeply into tissue, causing intrathoracic and intra-abdominal injuries that have sometimes been fatal to divers.

Sea urchins and other echinoderms have spines of varying lengths that typically envenomate humans when stepped on. Fish of the Scorpionida family have venomous spines as well. This family includes the scorpion fish, the lionfish, and the stonefish, which is responsible for the most severe toxicity.

Signs and Symptoms

Toxicity from spinous marine animals causes severe local irritation and pain that may radiate proximally. Systemic symptoms can include nausea, vomiting, and cardiovascular instability. Envenomations are occasionally fatal.

Treatment

All venom from spinous creatures is heat labile, which means that it is neutralized by heat. Prolonged immersion in hot water is associated with improvement in toxicity. The water temperature and the duration of immersion should be limited only by the patient's tolerance. Surgical intervention may be required to repair traumatic damage after stingray impalement.

The spines and stingers of all these fish and rays are brittle, often breaking off during exposure and attempted removal. Plain radiography is generally suggested to ensure that all fragments have been completely removed. Treat lacerations from spines. Update tetanus prophylaxis, and consider giving antibiotic therapy covering normal skin flora and selected marine bacteria (e.g., *Vibrio parahaemolyticus*). Antivenin therapy is available and recommended for only a few species, including the stonefish, because of the potency of its venom.

Biting Sea Creatures

Sea snakes, cone snails, and the blue-ring octopus are all capable of delivering venom through bites. Sea snake venom contains several toxins that primarily produce myotoxicity and neurotoxicity. Severe rhabdomyolysis and paralysis may occur.

Treatment

Supportive care and antivenin administration are the primary therapies recommended for marine envenomation. Because the venom is chiefly neurotoxic, pressure immobilization may be advisable, as with elapids. The following are specific recommendations:

- Blue-ring octopus venom consists of tetrodotoxin, a peripheral nervous system sodium channel blocker that causes paresthesia, paralysis, and respiratory depression in severe toxicity. Treatment is supportive.
- Cone snail bites may cause severe local pain and systemic sequelae of muscle weakness, coma, and cardiovascular collapse. Again, supportive therapy is indicated.
- Ingestion of certain fish may cause systemic toxicity. **Table 10-16** summarizes marine food-borne toxicity

Plant Toxicity

Most plants and mushrooms are nontoxic or only slightly toxic, but plant ingestion can cause GI, cardiovascular, and neurologic toxicity through various mechanisms. Of the thousands of exposures annually, fatalities blamed on plants or mushrooms are rare.

Most plant poisonings are accidental and involve household plants or ornamentals ingested by children. The categories of plant poisonings are GI irritants, dermatitis inducers, and oxalate-containing plant ingestions. The specific toxins involved include cyanogenic glycosides, cardiac glycosides, and solanine.

It is not possible to become familiar with all the different poisonous plants and mushrooms in North America or with the mosaic of signs and symptoms they cause, but it is helpful to know how to approach a patient suspected of having ingested a toxic plant or mushroom. Irritating chemicals in the plant may produce redness or irritation at the site of contact, so begin by examining the patient's oropharynx for redness, irritation, swelling, or blistering. Excessive salivation, lacrimation, and diaphoresis may also be present. Abdominal effects of toxicity may include nausea and vomiting, cramps, and diarrhea. Severe exposures may diminish the patient's level of consciousness or induce a coma.

In any toxic plant or mushroom ingestion, it is critical to gather a good patient history and collect a sample of the ingested material for later identification or laboratory analysis. Poison control centers and wilderness medicine resources can help you identify specific species and gauge their level of toxicity.

Treatment of plant ingestions is mainly supportive. GI toxicity is managed with fluid resuscitation, antiemetics, and electrolyte repletion as needed. Cardiovascular and neurologic toxicity is mediated by altering the activity of neurotransmitters, receptors, and ion channels. Clinical presentation and management will depend on the toxin's specific activity and are summarized in detail in the following pages.

Cardiac Glycoside Plants

Cardiac glycoside plants contain naturally occurring toxins similar to digoxin (also known as "digitoxin" or "digitalis" and sold under the proprietary names Digitek and Lanoxin). Digitalis is a cardiac glycoside heart medication derived from the foxglove plant. Plants containing cardiac glycosides, such as the lily of the valley, are popular as ornamental flowers and sometimes accidentally ingested, especially by children. The digoxin-like property of these plants increases the force of myocardial contraction and decreases the conduction rate of the atrioventricular (AV) node. Toxicity after ingestion of these plants is similar to toxicity after acute digoxin ingestion.

The incidence of plant-induced cardiac glycoside toxicity is low, with only 1% of plant exposures attributable to cardiac

Table 10-16 Mechanisms of Marine Food-Borne Intoxication

Toxin	Source	Mechanism	Description	Clinical Manifestations	Treatment
Brevetoxin	Shellfish	Neuromuscular sodium channel opening	Neurotoxic shellfish poisoning	GI upset, paresthesias, hot/cold reversal	Supportive
Ciguatoxin	Reef fish (e.g., amberjack, barracuda, grouper, snapper)	Neuromuscular sodium channel opening	Seafood poisoning from ingestion of fish that ingested other fish that were toxic (dinoflagellates)	Paresthesias, GI upset, hot/cold reversal, bradycardia, hypotension	Supportive Tricyclic antidepressants for prolonged neuropathy
Saxitoxin	Shellfish	Neuromuscular sodium channel blockade	Paralytic shellfish poisoning	Numbness, paresthesia, muscle weakness, paralysis, respiratory failure	Supportive
Tetrodotoxin	Puffer fish (fugu), blowfish	Neuromuscular sodium channel blockade	Neurotoxin that blocks nerve cell action potential	GI upset, paresthesia, numbness, ascending paralysis, respiratory failure	Supportive
Domoic acid	Mussels	Glutamate and kainic acid analogues	Amnestic shellfish poisoning	GI upset, memory loss, coma, seizures	Supportive
Histidine	Tuna, mackerel, skipjack	Histamine production due to improper cooling	Scombroid fish poisoning	Upper body erythema, pruritus, bronchospasm, angioedema	Antihistamines

glycoside plants. Mortality from plant cardiac glycoside toxicity is rare, and the rate is much lower than that associated with pharmaceutical digitalis toxicity.

Identification

Following are examples of common plants that contain digoxin-like glycoside toxins (**Figure 10-9**):

- Foxglove (*Digitalis purpurea*)
- Lily of the valley (*Convallaria majalis*)
- Oleander (*Nerium oleander*)
- Red squill (*Urginea maritima*)
- Yellow oleander (*Thevetia peruviana*)

Signs and Symptoms

Acute toxicity from plants containing cardiac glycosides often causes nonspecific GI symptoms like abdominal pain, nausea, and vomiting within a few hours. It may also induce hyperkalemia and neurologic symptoms such as altered mental status and weakness. Chronic toxicity likewise manifests with GI symptoms but can also cause weight loss, diarrhea, anorexia, hypokalemia, and hypomagnesemia.

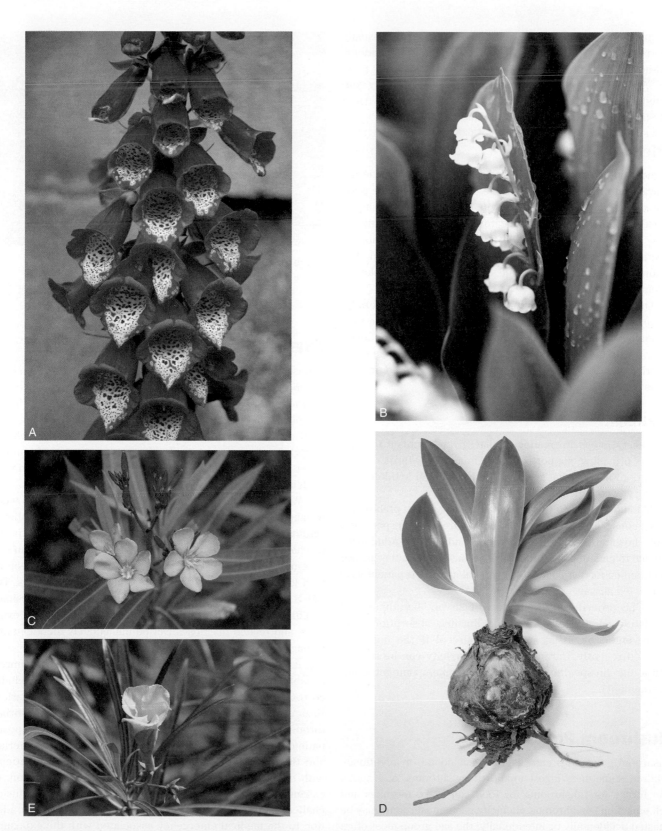

Figure 10-9 A. *Digitalis purpurea* (foxglove). **B.** Lilly of the valley (*Convallaria majalis*). **C.** *Nerium oleander* (common oleander) plants have white or pink flowers and long, narrow seedpods. **D.** *Urginea* species (squill or sea onion) have broad leaves and a red underground bulb (some varieties have a white bulb). **E.** *Thevetia peruviana* (yellow oleander) has yellow flowers with smooth seedpods known as "lucky nuts," which are composed of green flesh surrounding a hard brown seed.

In both acute and chronic exposures, the patient usually reports a variety of cardiac symptoms, including palpitations, light-headedness, dizziness, shortness of breath, and chest pressure. Almost any type of dysrhythmia other than a rapidly conducted atrial dysrhythmia may occur and can rapidly evolve into a life-threatening ventricular tachycardia.

Differential Diagnosis

Diagnosis of cardiac glycoside toxicity depends on gathering accurate information from the scene and the patient. The presence of cardiac glycoside plants in the environment should arouse suspicion if you detect a cardiac dysrhythmia during the physical exam. Ask whether the exposure was accidental or intentional and whether other people were also exposed. The poisoning may represent a suicide attempt, which may make the patient history unreliable.

On physical exam, you may find the patient to be bradycardic or tachycardic, with a weak, irregular pulse. The skin is usually pale, cold, and clammy (diaphoretic). Lung sounds are typically normal. Examination of emesis may reveal plant material. The neurologic exam may reveal altered mental status.

Treatment

The general steps in treating cardiac glycoside plant toxicity include providing supportive care, minimizing further toxin absorption, neutralizing absorbed toxin using an antidote, and treating any complications.

Management of cardiac glycoside toxicity in the prehospital setting consists primarily of supportive care and transportation to the hospital for further evaluation and testing. Administer atropine to patients with bradycardia. Consider initiating gastric decontamination with activated charcoal in an alert patient with a protected airway.

ACLS procedures for support of airway, breathing, and circulation should be followed. Further absorption may be prevented by using activated charcoal if the ingestion occurred recently. Cardiac glycoside toxicity can be treated with a digoxin-specific antibody Fab fragment (antigen binding fragment).

Mushroom Poisoning

Mushroom poisonings can be either accidental or intentional. Children sometimes ingest unknown mushrooms, and adults who forage for mushrooms for food can make mistakes and pick poisonous mushrooms. Hallucinogenic mushrooms may be ingested accidentally or intentionally; the age group most often affected seems to be children and young adults between the ages of 6 and 19. The cyclopeptide group of mushrooms, which includes the *Amanita* and *Galerina* genera, contains potent hepatotoxins (liver toxins) and accounts for most lethal exposures (**Figure 10-10**).

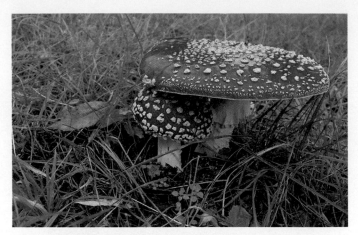

Figure 10-10 *Amanita muscaria* mushroom.
© Chris Hellyar/Shutterstock

Hazardous Materials

Exposure to hazardous materials poses a threat to all the communities we serve as healthcare providers. Hazardous materials are found, for example, in local refineries, factories, and industrial plants that produce a variety of chemicals. These dangerous goods pass along our highways and railways and through our airports as they are transported across the country. Hazardous materials are also manufactured in illicit neighborhood and rural meth labs.

We must maintain a keen awareness of these threats when we approach a perilous scene or situation or when a patient's cardinal presentation indicates he or she may have been exposed to a hazardous material. Continuing education will help you stay informed about the risks in your geographic area and keep up with local protocols and national management guidelines. The AMLS assessment provides a systematic approach to obtaining an efficient and thorough history so that life-threatening exposures and related diagnoses can be immediately identified and managed.

A hazardous material is any substance that poses an unreasonable threat to health, safety, or the environment. It includes corrosives, **radioactive** matter, and flammable materials. Hazardous substances can be inhaled, ingested, or absorbed through the skin. The cardinal presentation of an exposed patient is as varied as the myriad types of hazardous materials and their routes of exposure and levels of toxicity. Patients with underlying medical conditions, immunosuppression, or extremes of age are all at higher risk because of their perfusion challenges. Many patients sustain traumatic injuries in addition to the medical emergency associated with the exposure, providing daunting assessment and treatment challenges for us in the field.

An efficient primary survey that allows immediate identification and management of life threats is essential, not only to ensuring your safety but to reducing the likelihood of morbidity and mortality for the patient. Through the AMLS assessment process, emergent/critical and non–life-threatening diagnoses are quickly revealed and decisively treated.

Regulatory Agency Notification

It is important to ensure that you notify receiving facilities and local, state, and national agencies of hazardous materials and possible weapons of mass destruction as soon as you recognize them. Chief among these agencies are the **Occupational Safety and Health Administration (OSHA)** and the Environmental Protection Agency (EPA). These agencies develop and mandate personnel training and local, state, and federal emergency plans. An OSHA regulation known as the **Standard on Hazardous Waste Operations and Emergency Response (HAZWOPER)** provides guidelines for the development of and compliance with safety protocols and procedures for governmental and nongovernmental personnel who make, store, or dispose of, or are first responders to cleanup of hazardous materials. For first-response personnel such as firefighters, EMTs, and paramedics, the **National Fire Protection Association (NFPA)** identifies standards for safety competency related to scene management.

Incident Recognition

In general, patients with medical emergencies often have subtle or nondescript clinical presentations for a variety of conditions. The occurrence of a hazardous materials incident can be equally difficult to identify. For prehospital providers, dispatch information regarding the number of patients and any similarities in the signs and symptoms they exhibit can indicate the need for immediate identification of appropriate safety precautions and additional resources.

At the scene, low-lying clouds, smoke, or unusual fog patterns or air density should heighten your awareness that a hazardous materials incident may have occurred. Significant skin or eye irritation, respiratory difficulties, and unfamiliar odors are all descriptors that warrant taking special precautions. If you recognize an unsafe scene before making patient contact, view the area with binoculars to look for evidence of hazards. This practice allows you to avoid contamination and deploy resources efficiently.

Once you recognize that an area or patient may have been subject to a hazardous materials exposure, you must immediately don personal protection devices and notify the appropriate agencies. Transportation destinations may be altered, depending on the number of patients and available resources.

Identification and Labeling

The presence of a hazardous material is identified by the use of placards, shipping papers, labels, or pictographs that specify the type of hazardous agent present, the nature and degree of the

medical compromise expected if an exposure were to occur, and the signs and symptoms of exposure. All healthcare providers must be able to interpret hazardous materials labeling or have immediate access to guides or agencies that can assist in identification. Providers who cannot recognize the labeling on hazardous products risk unintentionally entering a contaminated area or beginning treatment of an exposed patient without first completing proper decontamination procedures.

In the United States, the DOT regulates the transportation of hazardous materials, including the labeling of such materials during transport. The agency sets the following standards specifying:

- Which types of containers must be used to transport various kinds of hazardous materials
- How the containers must be labeled
- By which modes of transportation they may be moved
- What kind of documentation must accompany the transport container

First-response personnel must be available at the delivery destination, such as a laboratory, refinery, or factory, to take safety precautions before the shipment arrives. Appropriate PPE must be used by all personnel if the threat of a hazardous materials exposure incident exists.

A **placard** is a diamond-shaped sign affixed to a transport vehicle (**Figure 10-11**). The placard is color coded to identify the hazardous agent as being flammable, combustible, poisonous,

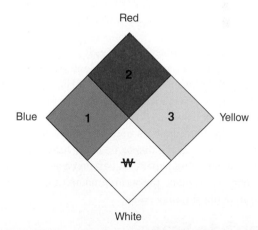

Figure 10-11 National Fire Protection Association placard consists of four diamonds within a larger diamond. Red (flammability) diamond is at the 12 o'clock position; yellow (instability) diamond is at 3 o'clock; white (special hazards) diamond is at 6 o'clock; and blue (health) hazard diamond is at 9 o'clock. Degree of hazard severity is indicated by a numerical rating that ranges from 4, indicating the most severe hazard, to 0, indicating no hazard. Special hazards are indicated in the white section and refer to chemicals that react with water (W), and those that are oxidizers (OX).

radioactive, gaseous, explosive, oxidizing, infectious, or corrosive. Each placard carries a four-digit identification number that allows the agent to be looked up quickly in print and online reference sources.

OSHA requires chemical manufacturers to create material safety data sheets (MSDS) for every chemical developed, stored, and used in the United States. These sheets provide instructions for safe handling and storage of the chemical and outline emergency actions to take if an exposure occurs. These sheets must remain with the chemical at all times.

A number of published guides and books offer detailed instructions regarding the safe handling and transport of various types of hazardous materials. They include the following:

- The DOT publishes the **North American Emergency Response Guidebook**.
- A poison control center can be accessed by calling 1-800-222-1222. The center can provide a list of toxic substances and appropriate medical interventions.
- The Chemical Manufacturers Association offers a public service known as the *CHEMical TRansportation Emergency Center (CHEMTREC)*, which provides scene advice on hazardous materials identification. CHEMTREC can be accessed by dialing 800-424-9300.
- Transport Canada's CANUTEC (1-613-996-6666) is a good resource.
- Web-based services include the National Library of Medicine's Wireless Information System for Emergency Responders (WISER). WISER is available free of charge on the web, and the information can be downloaded to a computer or PDA (www.webwiser. nlm.nih.gov).

Take advantage of these resources if you anticipate or have identified a hazardous materials incident. Tables 10-17 and 10-18 present the Classification System for Hazardous Materials. Table 10-19 lists selected agencies that assist in hazardous material incidents.

Class or division numbers may be displayed in the bottom of placards, or they may be displayed in the hazardous materials description on shipping papers. In certain cases, a class or division number may replace the written name of the hazard class description on the shipping paper.

Dispatch to Scene

At the time of dispatch and while en route to the scene of a hazardous materials incident, begin assessing information and taking stock of your resources as follows:

- Note weather conditions and wind direction.
- Gauge the proximity of highly populated areas relative to the exposure area.
- Determine the number and location of receiving facilities.

- Review the type of hazardous material and the amount to which victims are thought to have been exposed.
- Estimate the number of people who have been exposed or are at risk of exposure.

Approach all external scenes uphill and upwind. Be sure the scene has been secured. Deploy the appropriate mutual aid agencies before accessing the scene.

Staging Areas

The incident command system will assume control of the incident and direct responders to the appropriate safe staging zones for decontamination and patient triage and care. These zones must be clearly marked and well circumscribed to prevent further contamination and maintain an organized approach to patient access. Safety zones are identified as follows:

- **Hot (red) zone.** This is where the hazardous material is located and contamination has occurred. Access to this zone is limited to protect rescuers and patients from further exposure. Specific protective gear worn by trained personnel is required for access.
- **Warm (yellow) zone.** This is usually the area surrounding the contaminated hot zone. Properly protected healthcare providers are allowed to access this zone for rapid assessment and management of emergent or life-threatening conditions. Decontamination occurs in this zone.
- **Cold (green) zone.** This is a support zone for general triage, stabilization, and management of illness or injuries. Patients and uncontaminated personnel are given access to this zone. However, healthcare personnel must wear protective clothing while in the green zone and properly discard it in predetermined areas on exiting.

Hazardous materials incidents can be emotionally and physically challenging for rescue personnel and healthcare providers. Your health history should be evaluated and your vital signs assessed before you're allowed to enter staging areas. In events that involve many patients and resources, rescuers often remain at the scene or in transport vehicles for long hours while wearing heavy and constricting protective clothing. Rescuers can become drained by dehydration, heat or cold exposure, and exhaustion. All healthcare personnel should receive a medical evaluation and rehydration after the incident or after each shift.

Decontamination

A final safety component in management of hazardous materials incidents is the decontamination process. Staged decontamination areas should be clearly identified by incident

Table 10-17 International Classification System for Hazardous Materials

Class 1	Explosives
Division 1.1	Explosives with a mass explosion hazard
Division 1.2	Explosives with a projection hazard
Division 1.3	Explosives with predominantly a fire hazard
Division 1.4	Explosives with no significant blast hazard
Division 1.5	Very insensitive explosives
Division 1.6	Extremely insensitive explosive articles
Class 2	Gases
Division 2.1	Flammable gases
Division 2.2	Nonflammable gases
Division 2.3	Poison gases
Division 2.4	Corrosive gases (Canadian)
Class 3	Flammable Liquids
Division 3.1	Flashpoint below 0°F (−18°C)
Division 3.2	Flashpoint 0°F (−18°C) and above but less than 73.4°F (23°C)
Division 3.3	Flashpoint of 73°F (23°C) and up to 141°F (61°C)
Class 4	Flammable Solids, Spontaneously Combustible Materials, Materials That Are Dangerous When Wet
Division 4.1	Flammable solids
Division 4.2	Spontaneously combustible materials
Division 4.3	Materials that are dangerous when wet
Class 5	Oxidizers and Organic Peroxides
Division 5.1	Oxidizers
Division 5.2	Organic peroxides
Class 6	Poisonous and Etiological (Infectious) Materials
Division 6.1	Poisonous materials
Division 6.2	Etiological (infectious) materials
Class 7	Radioactive Materials
Class 8	Corrosives
Class 9	Miscellaneous Hazardous Materials

Data from U.S. Department of Transportation, National Highway Traffic Safety Administration: EMT-Paramedic national standard curriculum, Washington DC, 1997, The Department.

Table 10-18 **Classes of Hazardous Materials**

Class/Division	Notes
Class 1: Explosives	Explosive placards and labels are orange and have a symbol showing an exploding ball with fragments on the top and a division number (1.1 to 1.6) on the bottom. The word *explosive* or a four-digit ID number appears in the center of the symbol.
Division 1.1: Mass detonation hazard	
Division 1.2: Mass detonation hazard with fragments	
Division 1.3: Fire hazard with minor blast or projectile hazard	
Division 1.4: Explosive substances that present no significant hazard	
Division 1.5: Very insensitive explosives	
Division 1.6: Extremely insensitive explosives	
Class 2: Gases	Compressed or liquefied gas placards and labels are red (flammable), green (nonflammable), or white (poison); have a fire symbol, gas cylinder symbol, or a skull and crossbones on the top; and have a division number (2.1 to 2.3) on the bottom. These symbols have *flammable gas*, *nonflammable gas*, or *poison gas* labeling or a four-digit ID number in the center.
Division 2.1: Flammable gases	
Division 2.2: Nonflammable gases	
Division 2.3: Poisonous gases	
Class 3: Flammable or Combustible Liquids	Flammable or combustible liquids placards and labels are red, have a flame symbol on the top, and a division number (3.1 to 3.3) on the bottom. They have the wording *flammable liquid* or *combustible liquid* or a four-digit ID number in the center.
Division 3.1: Liquids with flash points <0°F	
Division 3.2: Liquids with flash points from 0°F to 73°F	
Division 3.3: Liquids with flash points from 73°F to 141°F	
Combustible liquids	
Class 4: Flammable Solids	Flammable solid placards and labels are red-and-white striped (flammable solids), red over white (spontaneously combustible solids and liquids), or blue (dangerous when wet); have a flame symbol on the top; and have a division number (4.1 to 4.3) on the bottom. They have the wording *flammable solid*, *spontaneously combustible*, or *dangerous when wet* or a four-digit ID number in the center.
Division 4.1: Flammable solids	
Division 4.2: Spontaneously combustible or pyrophoric solids and liquids	
Division 4.3: Dangerous when wet	
Class 5: Oxidizing Substances	Oxidizing substances placards and labels are yellow, have a symbol showing an *O* with flames on the top, and a division number (5.1 to 5.2) on the bottom. They have the wording *oxidizer* or *organic peroxide* or a four-digit ID number in the center.
Division 5.1: Oxidizing substances	
Division 5.2: Organic peroxides	

(continues)

Table 10-18 Classes of Hazardous Materials (*Continued*)

Class/Division	Notes
Class 6: Poisonous and Infectious Substances Division 6.1: Poisons Division 6.2: Infectious substances	Poison liquid and solid material and infectious material placards and labels are white; have either a skull and crossbones, biomedical symbol, or grain stock with an *X* through it (depending on material) on the top; and a division number (6.1 to 6.2) on the bottom. These symbols have the wording *poison*, *infectious material*, *keep away from foodstuffs"* or a four-digit ID number in the center.
Class 7: Radioactive Substances	Radioactive materials placards and labels are yellow over white, have the radioactive propeller symbol on the top, and the number 7 on the bottom. Labels must identify the radionuclide and the amount of activity in the package. They will have the Roman numerals I, II, or III in the center to identify the level of hazard and type of container and space to write in specific information. The I, II, or III numbering designates the amount of radiation detectable from outside the package. Labels have the wording *radioactive material* or a four-digit ID number in the center.
Class 8: Corrosive Materials	Corrosive materials placards and labels are white over black, have a symbol showing a test tube spilling liquid onto a human thumb, and a piece of steel on the top and have the number 8 on the bottom. The word *corrosive* or a four-digit ID number appears in the center.
Class 9: Miscellaneous Hazardous Materials	Miscellaneous hazardous materials placards and labels are black and white striped over white and have the number 9 on the bottom. They have a four-digit ID number in the center.

Table 10-19 Agencies That Assist in Hazardous Materials Incidents

Federal Agencies
Centers for Disease Control and Prevention
Department of Transportation
Environmental Protection Agency
Federal Aviation Administration
National Response Center
U.S. Armed Forces (Army, Navy, Air Force, Marines)
U.S. Coast Guard
U.S. Department of Energy
Regional and State Agencies
National Guard
State emergency management agencies
State Environmental Protection Agency
State health departments
State police

Local Agencies
Emergency management
Fire service (hazardous materials units)
Law enforcement agencies
Poison control centerv
Public utilities
Sewage and treatment facilities
Commercial Agencies
American Petroleum Institute
Association of American Railroads and Hazardous Materials Systems
Chemical Manufacturers Association
Chevron (provides assistance with Chevron products)
HELP (the Union Carbide Emergency Response System for company shipments)
Local industry
Local contractors
Local carriers and transporters
Railway industry

Note: This list is a sample and does not include all agencies.

From Sanders MJ: *Mosby's paramedic textbook*, ed 3, St. Louis, MO, 2005, Mosby.

command personnel at the scene and at all receiving facilities. Decontamination procedures should be implemented for patients, rescuers, and equipment.

Decontamination may be dry or wet. Dry decontamination procedures are appropriate for minimal exposures. These procedures call for careful and systematic removal and disposal of all clothing. For wet decontamination procedures, use copious amounts of warm (90°F to 95°F [32°C to 35°C]) water and mild soap to cleanse exposed equipment and clothing. Remove clothing and personal items, and place them in designated labeled bags. Contain runoff water to keep it from entering irrigation or sewer systems. Use small wading pools or commercially purchased containers to house runoff particles and water.

Take care during the primary decontamination process to ensure that the hazardous material has been completely removed. Secondary decontamination should be performed at the receiving facility if remnants of the contaminant remain in transport vehicles or on your clothing. After the incident, dispose properly of contaminated clothing. Thoroughly decontaminate rescue and transport vehicles. The measures of toxicity and levels that identify potentially dangerous exposure are explained as follows:

- *Lethal dose 50% (LD$_{50}$):* The oral or dermal exposure dose that kills 50% of the exposed animal population in 2 weeks' time.
- *Lethal concentration 50% (LC$_{50}$):* The air concentration of a substance that kills 50% of the exposed animal population. This also is commonly noted as LCt50. This denotes the concentration and the length of exposure time that results in 50% fatality in the exposed animal population.
- *Threshold limit value:* The airborne concentrations of a substance; represents conditions under which nearly all workers are believed to be repeatedly exposed day after day without adverse effects.
- *Permissible exposure limit:* Allowable air concentration of a substance in the workplace as established by OSHA. These values are legally enforceable.
- *Immediately dangerous to life or health concentrations (IDHLs):* Maximal environmental air concentration of a substance from which a person could escape within 30 minutes without symptoms of impairment or irreversible health effects.

Personal Protective Equipment

OSHA and the EPA classify protective clothing on the basis of its ability to seal exposed skin. These agencies identify protection by levels:

- Level A is the highest level of skin and respiratory protection. It necessitates a fully encapsulating, airtight outer garment and self-contained breathing apparatus (SCBA), completely sealing off the wearer from the environment. A NIOSH-certified positive-pressure respirator must be worn. This level of protection is worn by first responders who enter the contaminated site.
- Level B provides the highest level of respiratory/breathing protection. It consists of an SCBA plus protective clothing. This level is typically worn by decontamination crews.
- Level C protection consists of an air-purifying respirator plus protective clothing.
- Level D is for less worrisome exposures. This level requires standard work gear, gloves, and goggles or a facemask, as appropriate.

The proper sequence for donning PPE is outlined in Table 10-20, and the order in which you should remove PPE is summarized in Table 10-21.

Severity and Symptoms of Exposure

Several factors determine the severity of a hazardous materials exposure. The type of hazardous material, its chemical components, the route of entry, and the individual's general health all affect the severity of the signs and symptoms exhibited. Some symptoms appear immediately, whereas others may be delayed, making it difficult to obtain an accurate patient history. General symptoms of exposure to a hazardous material include the following:

- Dyspnea and chest tightness
- Nausea and vomiting
- Diarrhea
- Excessive salivation and drooling
- Tingling and numbness of the extremities
- Altered mentation
- Skin discoloration

Types of Hazardous Materials Exposure
Oral and Inhalation

OSHA, along with the EPA and NIOSH, has used animal studies to ascertain the levels of exposure considered to be dangerous for each type of hazardous material. This level is expressed using metrics known as the **lethal dose, 50% (LD$_{50}$)** and the **lethal concentration, 50% (LC$_{50}$)**. The LD$_{50}$ is the level of oral or dermal exposure dose that kills 50% of an exposed animal population in 2 weeks. The LC$_{50}$ is the air concentration of an agent that kills 50% of the exposed animal population. LD$_{50}$ applies to hazardous materials that are dangerous when swallowed or

Table 10-20 Sequence for Donning Personal Protective Equipment

Gown

Fully cover torso from neck to knees, arms to end of wrists, and wrap around the back.

Fasten in back of neck and waist.

Mask or Respirator

Secure ties or elastic bands at middle of head and neck.

Fit flexible band to nose bridge.

Fit snug to face and below chin

Fit-check respirator.

Goggles or Face Shield

Place over face and eyes and adjust to fit.

Gloves

Extend to cover wrist of isolation gown.

Safe Work Practices

Use safe work practices to protect yourself and limit the spread of contamination

Keep hands away from face.

Limit surfaces touched.

Change gloves when torn or heavily contaminated.

Perform hand hygiene.

Note: The type of PPE used will vary based on the level of precautions required (e.g., standard precautions and contact, droplet, or airborne infection isolation).

Data from Centers for Disease Control and Prevention.

Table 10-21 Sequence for Removing Personal Protective Equipment

Gloves

Outside of glove is contaminated!

Grasp outside of glove with opposite gloved hand; peel off.

Hold removed glove in gloved hand.

Slide fingers of ungloved hand under remaining glove at wrist.

Peel glove off over first glove.

Discard gloves in waste container.

Goggles

Outside of goggles or face shield is contaminated!

To remove, handle by head band or ear pieces.

Place in designated receptacle for reprocessing or in waste container.

Gown

Gown front and sleeves are contaminated!

Unfasten gown ties.

Pull away from neck and shoulders, touching inside of gown only.

Turn gown inside out.

Fold or roll into a bundle and discard.

Mask or Respirator

Front of mask/respirator is contaminated—do not touch!

Grasp bottom, then top ties or elastics, and remove.

Discard in waste container.

Wash hands or use an alcohol-based hand sanitizer immediately after removing PPE

Note: Except for the respirator, remove PPE at the doorway or in an anteroom. Remove respirator after leaving the patient's room and closing the door.

Data from Centers for Disease Control and Prevention.

absorbed through the skin, whereas LC_{50} applies to agents that are toxic when inhaled.

Exposure to agents with low water solubility can seriously damage lung tissue, resulting in irreversible pulmonary edema and long-term chronic lung disease. Exposure to agents with high water solubility, such as ammonia, causes only benign symptoms in the upper airway, because such agents are absorbed in the mucous membranes before reaching the lungs. The patient will complain of eye irritation, skin burns, respiratory tract irritation, and a nonproductive cough.

On your initial physical assessment, identify and manage any increased work of breathing. If the patient is wheezing, administer bronchodilators such as albuterol (Proventil). Give fluids and vasopressors for hypotension. Because of the potential for pulmonary edema, monitor IV fluids closely to avert fluid overload. Once you have completed decontamination protocols, initiate routine supportive care.

Ingestion

Ingestion of hazardous materials is not common, but it can occur if decontamination is not thorough. If a hazardous material is still present and you or the patient places the hands near the mouth, as when drinking a cup of coffee, contamination can occur.

Injection

For medication administration, the IV route offers the fastest rate of absorption compared with intramuscular and subcutaneous routes. However, penetrating contaminated skin tissue can allow the toxic substance to be absorbed by the body where it may damage organs. Many injected substances are metabolized by the liver and are capable of causing debilitating damage. Identifying a patient's or provider's risk for this route of exposure is essential in preventing contamination.

Weapons of Mass Destruction

Acts of terrorism involving biological, chemical, or radiologic agents threaten military personnel and civilians alike. Response to these types of disasters poses a significant safety risk to healthcare providers and rescue personnel. Although providers often respond to natural disasters such as earthquakes, avalanches, and floods and to mass-casualty accidents such as building collapses and crashes involving mass-transportation vehicles, the focus of the following section is to increase your awareness of common Category A weapons of terrorism and the implications of such incidents for patients and healthcare providers.

Biological, chemical, or radiologic **contamination** by a terrorist attack results in a crime scene designation for the affected area. In addition, the Department of Homeland Security must be notified of all suspected terrorist attacks. As is the case with hazardous materials, weapons of mass destruction can be biological, chemical, incendiary, or explosive agents or devices. The difference is that when used by terrorists, these agents are released with the intent to destroy or to cause injury and death when inhaled, ingested, or absorbed. In 2000, the CDC established categories of bioterrorism agents to assist in identifying those that are lethal (Table 10-22).

Biological Agents

Agents of bioterrorism do not call attention to themselves. There is no dramatic implosion, no blazing cone of fire, no hail of shrapnel to announce their presence. That insidious quality makes **biological agents** all the more threatening, because it gives them time to infect many people in a wide geographic area before health officials recognize a pattern of illness. Public health authorities eventually begin to notice a high incidence of certain signs and symptoms or similar chief complaints within a given geographic area. Perhaps they're tipped off by an unorthodox disease presentation, a heavy load of cases within a circumscribed area, or reports of unusual routes of exposure.

Regardless of how the incident finally comes to light, the recognition that a biological exposure has occurred is almost invariably delayed. Healthcare providers can help compress the time from exposure to awareness by promptly reporting any unexpected influx of patients or other atypical patient trend. The biological agents of greatest concern follow.

Anthrax

Anthrax is an acute infectious disease caused by the gram-positive, spore-forming bacterium *Bacillus anthracis*. The most common route of entry is by direct skin contact and absorption of spores, which causes a localized red, itchy ulcer (cutaneous anthrax).

Signs and Symptoms

Workers and farmers who are in frequent direct contact with animals are highly susceptible to this route of exposure. Within 2 weeks, skin begins to necrose, and a black eschar forms. Anthrax spores can also be inhaled, which may initially cause apparently benign symptoms similar to those of the common cold. In the early **prodromal** stage, the patient complains of a nonproductive cough, fever, and nausea. The disease then progresses to the **fulminant** stage, which is characterized by high fever, cyanosis, shock, diaphoresis, and severe respiratory distress.

Treatment

Prehospital Setting Supportive care with supplemental oxygen, IV therapy for fluid replacement, and application of dry, sterile dressing to wounds is appropriate. You must notify

Table 10-22 **Critical Biological Agents for Public Health Preparedness**	
Biological Agent	**Disease**
Category A	
Variola major	Smallpox
Bacillus anthracis	Anthrax
Yersinia pestis	Plague
Clostridium botulinum (botulinum toxins)	Botulism
Francisella tularensis	Tularemia
Filoviruses and arenaviruses (e.g., Ebola, Lassa fever)	Viral hemorrhagic fevers
	(continues)

Table 10-22 Critical Biological Agents for Public Health Preparedness (*continued*)

Biological Agent	Disease
Category B	
Coxiella burnetii	Q fever
Brucella spp.	Brucellosis
Burkholderia mallei	Glanders
Burkholderia pseudomallei	Melioidosis
Alphaviruses (VEE, EEE, WEE)	Encephalitis
Rickettsia prowazekii	Typhus fever
Toxins (e.g., ricin, staphylococcal enterotoxin B)	Toxic syndromes
Chlamydia psittaci	Psittacosis
Food safety threats (e.g., *Salmonella* spp., *Escherichia coli* O157:H7)	
Water safety threats (e.g., *Vibrio cholerae, Cryptosporidium parvum*)	
Category C	
Emerging threat agents (e.g., Nipah virus, hantavirus)	

EEE, Eastern equine encephalomyelitis; *VEE,* Venezuelan equine encephalomyelitis; *WEE,* western equine encephalomyelitis.

Reprinted from Rotz L, Khan A, Lillibridge SR, et al.: *Public health assessment of potential biological terrorism agents.* 2000. http://www.cdc.gov.

the receiving facility of the exposure. **Emergency decontamination** is not necessary unless the exposure has just occurred. You are at risk only if you have direct contact with lesions.

In-Hospital Setting Care in the hospital includes blood cultures to identify the toxin and determine appropriate antibiotics. Scientists doing anthrax research and military personnel can receive vaccinations to prevent anthrax.

Botulism

Clostridium botulinum, the bacterial agent that causes botulism, produces a nerve toxin that causes paralysis. Types of exposure include ingestion of contaminated food and contamination of wounds with the bacterium (**Figure 10-12**). All forms are considered medical emergencies and can be lethal. In the case of

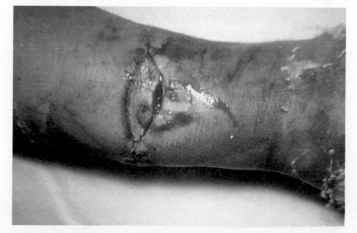

Figure 10-12 Wound botulism.
Courtesy of CDC.

bioterrorism, infiltration of food sources or the water supply can cause many people to become sick. Even small amounts of the bacteria can devastate large populated areas.

Signs and Symptoms

The patient with botulism usually has nausea, blurred vision, fatigue, slurred speech, muscle weakness, and paralysis. Symptoms can occur within hours or several days after exposure. Report any increase in patients with similar complaints to the appropriate receiving facilities and agencies.

Treatment

Prehospital Setting Provide routine medical care, with continuous monitoring for signs of respiratory distress due to respiratory muscle paralysis. Cover wounds to prevent further infection.

In-Hospital Setting Blood cultures to determine the type of toxin will allow the most effective antitoxin to be identified. Hospitals may not have antitoxin immediately available, so local protocols must include a process for obtaining the appropriate therapies. Mechanical ventilation may become necessary in patients with respiratory failure.

Plague

Yersinia pestis is the bacterium that causes plague. Transmission occurs through the bites of fleas from rodents such as mice, groundhogs, squirrels, and chipmunks. In terrorist attacks, the bacteria can be aerosolized, which is considered a pulmonic category of exposure (pneumonic plague). Assessment reveals difficulty breathing, productive cough, bloody sputum, and an associated complaint of chest pain. If not treated, these symptoms are followed by respiratory and cardiovascular collapse.

Signs and Symptoms

Bubonic plague occurs when a person is bitten by a flea infected by a rodent. Patients with this form of plague have enlarged lymph nodes, altered mentation, agitation, anuria, tachycardia, and hypotension. Untreated bubonic plague can progress to a third type of plague known as *septicemic plague*. Patients with this form of the illness have nausea and vomiting, diarrhea, necrotic skin lesions, and gangrene.

Treatment

Everyone who has come into contact with the patient should also be evaluated for symptoms. Initiate routine supportive medical care. Use PPE to avoid contact with airborne droplets. Early intervention with antibiotics and antimicrobial agents is appropriate. Providers must take respiratory precautions, using N-95 respirators.

Ricin

Ricin is a cytotoxic protein derived from the bean of the castor plant (*Ricinus communis*). Terrorist applications include extracting this toxin into an aerosol, powder, or pellet form.

Signs and Symptoms

Within 8 hours of inhalation, severe respiratory compromise will develop. Hypoxia will become evident within 36 to 72 hours of exposure. Symptoms are flulike and vague but typically include nausea, vomiting, cough, weakness, fever, and hypotension. Fortunately, it is difficult to aerosolize and typically requires subcutaneous injection to cause severe toxicity. Ingestion typically results in GI complaints, but a large amount needs to be ingested to cause systemic life-threatening toxicity. Trends in symptoms within a population can be easily overlooked because of the vagueness of their presentation, until high numbers of patients with similar symptoms indicate reason for concern and evaluation.

Treatment

Remove contaminated clothing and secure it in a bag. Decontaminate the patient, your equipment, and yourself if necessary. If exposure occurred by inhalation, the vehicle should remain well ventilated during transport. Continuous assessment and management of airway, breathing, and circulation are the initial interventions. Monitor the patient for respiratory and cardiovascular abnormalities. Because there is no antidote for ricin exposure, hospital interventions are aimed at elimination of the toxin and avoidance of secondary contamination.

Viral Hemorrhagic Fevers

Filoviruses, flaviviruses, and arenaviruses can all be categorized as viral hemorrhagic fevers. Arthropods and other animals are common hosts for these highly infectious viruses. Contact with the urine, feces, or saliva of an infected rodent and bites from infected arthropods such as fleas or ticks are typical routes of transmission.

Signs and Symptoms

The infected person will have fever, fatigue, and muscle aches. If exposure is undetected, severe symptoms such as bleeding from the ears, nose, and mouth and bleeding of internal organs develop. Altered mentation and collapse of the cardiovascular and renal systems may result.

Treatment

Provide routine supportive medical care and continuous monitoring of airway, breathing, circulation, and perfusion status. Don appropriate PPE for infection control.

No vaccine or antidote is currently available unless there is a diagnosis of yellow fever. Initial and continuing interventions focus on support of vital organ function. Isolation rooms should be used for contaminated patients. Air-purifying respirators should be worn by all immediate caregivers.

Radiologic Weapons

Nuclear radiation comprises particles and energy released when atoms break up (fission) or combine (fusion). *Ionizing radiation* refers to radiation (alpha, beta, gamma, and neutrons) whose energy is sufficient to strip electrons from atoms or molecules. Essentially all types of radiation from the atomic nucleus are ionizing.

Absorbed ionizing radiation is expressed in units called *rads*. One rad is equal to an absorbed dose of 0.01 gray (Gy). Assessment of a patient exposed to ionizing radiation requires determining the dose of rad he or she has absorbed. The greater the dose of rad absorbed, the greater the potential for serious illness and injury, as shown here:

- *100 rad*: Nausea, vomiting, and abdominal cramping within hours of exposure
- *600 rad*: Dehydration and gastroenteritis; death within a few days
- *1000+ rad*: Cardiovascular and neurologic complications, altered mentation, ataxia, arrhythmia, cardiovascular collapse, and shock

Management principles that can be implemented during a radiologic attack are given in Table 10-23.

Types of Ionizing Radiation

Nonionizing radiation includes visible light, microwaves, radio waves, ultrasound, and other types. Ionizing radiation can be classified as alpha, beta, gamma, or neutron particles.

Alpha Radiation

Alpha particles (protons and neutrons) generally do not pass through the skin. In fact, they travel only a few feet and can be blocked by a simple barrier such as a piece of paper. They present a significant biohazard, then, only when radioactive material is inhaled or ingested.

Beta Radiation

Beta particles (electrons) are smaller and faster than alpha particles and thus can travel farther, penetrating tissue to a depth of about 8 mm. They can cause significant burns to the skin's surface, although these burns are not usually visible immediately after the exposure. Since clothing effectively shields covered areas, the primary danger is to exposed skin. Standard skin-cleansing procedures remove most of contamination from beta particles. The only means of detection is a radiation-sensing instrument called a *Geiger-Mueller counter*, which all hospitals should have. If exposure continues, significant exposure to gamma radiation can occur, because most radioisotopes decay by emitting beta radiation followed by gamma emission.

Gamma Rays

Gamma rays are photons emitted from the nucleus of the atom. They are electromagnetic waves that travel quickly and penetrate deeply through skin, soft tissue, and bone. Gamma rays are involved in nearly all accidents involving external irradiation. X-rays are relatively lower-energy photons that are occasionally involved in radiation accidents arising from improper use of industrial or medical equipment. Gamma rays are emitted

---

Table 10-23 Principles of Management During a Radiologic Disaster

1. Assess the scene for safety.
2. All patients should be medically stabilized from their traumatic injuries before radiation injuries are considered. Patients are then evaluated for their external radiation exposure and contamination.
3. An external source of radiation, if great enough, can cause tissue injury, but it does not make the patient radioactive. Patients with even lethal exposures to external radiation are not a threat to medical staff.
4. Patients can become contaminated with radioactive material deposited on their skin or clothing. More than 90% of surface contamination can be removed by removal of clothing. The remainder can be washed off with soap and water.
5. Protect yourself from radioactive contamination by observing, at a minimum, standard precautions, including protective clothing, gloves, and a mask.
6. Patients who develop nausea, vomiting, or skin erythema within 4 hours of exposure have probably received a high dose of external radiation.
7. Radioactive contamination in wounds should be treated as dirt and irrigated as soon as possible. Avoid handling any metallic foreign body.
8. Potassium iodide (KI) is of value only if there has been a release of radioactive iodine. KI is not a general radiation antidote.
9. The concept of time/distance/shielding is key in the prevention of untoward effects from radiation exposure. Radiation exposure is minimized by decreasing time in the affected area, increasing distance from a radiation source, and using metal or concrete shielding.

Modified from Department of Homeland Security Working Group on Radiological Dispersion Device Preparedness/Medical Preparedness and Response Subgroup. 2004. www1.va.gov/emshg/docs/Radiologic_Medical_Countermeasures_051403.pdf.

from radioisotopes after beta decay and are the primary cause of acute radiation syndrome. Phases of this syndrome are outlined in Table 10-24. Delayed effects occur in symptom clusters (Table 10-25).

Neutrons

The fourth classification, neutron, easily penetrates surfaces and can cause significant damage to body systems. Neutrons are unique. When they are stopped, or "captured," after emission, they cause previously stable atoms to become radioactive. This is the source of radioactive fallout. The surface burst of a thermonuclear weapon instantly vaporizes tons of soil, transforming it by intense neutron bombardment into highly radioactive material. This cloud—the so-called mushroom cloud we associate with the nuclear bomb—rises with the fireball and is carried away by the prevailing winds at high altitudes. Its radioactive particles ultimately descend as fallout. A nuclear reactor harnesses this same powerful form of radiation by creating a controlled, sustained neutron chain reaction in order to generate energy.

Some gamma exposure also occurs with neutron exposure. Quantification of the radioactive material generated by neutron irradiation is helpful in estimating neutron exposure

Table 10-24 Phases of Acute Radiation Syndrome

Feature	Effects of Whole-Body Irradiation From External Radiation or Internal Absorption by Dose Range in Rad (1 Rad = 1 cGy; 100 Rad = 1 Gy)					
	0–100	100–200	200–600	600–800	800–3000	> 3000
Prodromal Phase						
Nausea, vomiting	None	5%–50%	50%–100%	75%–100%	90%–100%	100%
Time of onset		3–6 h	2–4 h	1–2 h	<1 h	Minutes
Duration		< 24 h	< 24 h	< 48 h	48 h	N/A
Lymphocyte count	Unaffected	Minimally decreased	< 1000 at 24 h	< 500 at 24 h	Decreases within hours	Decreases within hours
Central nervous system (CNS) function	No impairment	No impairment	Routine task performance Cognitive impairment for 6–20 h	Simple, routine task performance Cognitive impairment for > 24 h	Rapid incapacitation May have a lucid interval of several hours	
Latent Phase						
No symptoms	> 2 wk	7–15 days	0–7 days	0–2 days	None	None
Manifest Illness						
Signs/symptoms	None	Moderate leukopenia	Severe leukopenia, purpura, hemorrhage, pneumonia Hair loss after 300 rad	Diarrhea, fever, electrolyte disturbance	Convulsions, ataxia, tremor, lethargy	
Time of onset		> 2 wk	2 days–4 wk		1–3 days	
Critical period		None	4–6 wk; greatest potential for effective medical intervention	2–14 days	1–46 hr	

(continues)

Table 10-24 Phases of Acute Radiation Syndrome (*continued*)

Feature	Effects of Whole-Body Irradiation From External Radiation or Internal Absorption by Dose Range in Rad (1 Rad = 1 cGy; 100 Rad = 1 Gy)					
	0–100	100–200	200–600	600–800	800–3000	> 3000
Organ system	None		Hematopoietic; respiratory (mucosal) systems		GI tract Mucosal systems	CNS
Hospitalization duration	0%	< 5% 45–60 days	90% 60–90 days	100% 100+ days	100% Weeks to months	100% Days to weeks
Mortality	None	Minimal	Low with aggressive therapy	High	Very high; significant neurologic symptoms indicate lethal dose	

Modified from Armed Forces Radiobiology Institute: *Medical management of radiological casualties*, 2003, Bethesda, MD.

Table 10-25 Symptom Clusters as Delayed Effects* of Radiation Exposure

1	2	3	4
Headache Fatigue Weakness	Anorexia Nausea Vomiting Diarrhea	Partial-thickness and full-thickness skin damage Depilation (hair loss) Ulceration	Lymphopenia Neutropenia Thrombocytopenia Purpura Opportunistic infections

*The effects may appear from days to weeks after exposure.

and, sometimes indirectly, the dose of gamma radiation. The radioactivity generated is primarily sodium-24, which can be detected by a Geiger-Mueller counter or in a blood sample. If neutron exposure is suspected, save and refrigerate all feces and urine. In addition, save all clothing, especially items containing metal parts such as belt buckles for analysis of neutron-induced radioisotopes.

Radiologic Exposure

Radioactive materials used by terrorists are easily accessible and can be found in research laboratories, hospitals, facilities with radiograph capabilities, and industrial complexes. Radioactive devices that are combined with explosives can be employed as terrorist weapons.

A terrorist can intentionally detonate an explosive device such as a so-called **dirty bomb** in a highly populated area. Contamination of humans, animals, buildings, and the environment occurs when radioactive materials such as cobalt-60 and radium-226 are released. The initial blast will cause traumatic injury. If early recognition of the radiologic exposure does not occur, prolonged exposure can cause emergent medical problems. Inhalation of radioactive particles can provoke respiratory distress, and ingestion can induce GI discomfort.

The components necessary to construct an actual nuclear weapon of mass destruction—namely, plutonium and uranium—are much more difficult to obtain than the readily available components of a dirty bomb.

The extent of injury and illness from the initial blast of a radioactive device is related to the duration (time) of exposure, distance from the explosion or blast, and the amount of the person's protection. Exposed persons may contaminate others if gas, liquid, or dust particles on their bodies or clothing are transferred to others. It is essential for first-response providers to ascertain accurate information regarding time, distance, and shielding. Table 10-26 offers additional important information for dealing with a terrorist attack involving ionizing radiation.

Table 10-26 Terrorism With Ionizing Radiation: General Guide

Diagnosis
Be alert to the following:
1. The acute radiation syndrome follows a predictable pattern after substantial exposure or catastrophic events (see Table 10-24).
2. Individuals may become ill from contaminated sources in the community and may be identified over much longer periods based on specific syndromes (see Table 10-25).
3. Specific syndromes of concern, especially with a 2- to 3-week prior history of nausea and vomiting, are the following:
  ❑ Thermal burn–like skin effects without documented thermal exposure
  ❑ Immunologic dysfunction with secondary infections
  ❑ Tendency to bleed (epistaxis, gingival bleeding, petechiae)
  ❑ Marrow suppression (neutropenia, lymphopenia, and thrombocytopenia)
  ❑ Depilation (hair loss)
Understanding Exposure
Exposure may be known and recognized or clandestine through the following mechanisms:
1. Large recognized exposures, such as a nuclear bomb or damage to a nuclear power station.
2. Small radiation source emitting continuous gamma radiation, producing group or individual chronic intermittent exposures (e.g., radiologic sources from medical treatment devices or environmental, water, or food contamination).
3. Internal radiation from absorbed, inhaled, or ingested radioactive material (internal contamination).

Modified from Department of Veterans Affairs pocket guide produced by Employee Education System for Office of Public Health and Environmental Hazards. This information is not meant to be complete but to be a quick guide; please consult other references and expert opinion.

Treatment

Prehospital Setting Initial interventions center on ensuring scene safety and donning appropriate PPE (see Table 10-23). Avoid direct contact with radioactive materials. Decontaminate only patients who were exposed to liquids or gases that were combined with the explosive materials. If contamination is questionable or undetermined, wrap the patient in a blanket or sheet to minimize possible contamination of others. Notify the receiving facility of the contamination from the scene to allow for appropriate precautions on your arrival. Keep in mind the psychological effects of sustaining a sudden, violent injury and illness from the blast.

In mass-casualty situations, local medical and response-team resources can easily become overwhelmed. Verbal communication is an important part of the team effort to minimize contamination efficiently and to assess and manage multiple patients effectively.

In-Hospital Setting Once decontamination and appropriate mass-casualty protocols have been implemented, initial patient interventions can proceed. Consider administration of sodium bicarbonate, calcium gluconate, or ammonium chloride. Administer the chelating agents and potassium iodide.

Incendiary Weapons

Terrorists use incendiary threats such as firebombs to create panic in heavily populated areas. These types of devices produce large conflagrations.

Incendiary Devices

A typical example of an incendiary device is the Molotov cocktail, which consists of a fuel-soaked rag placed in a bottle or other container. The rag is ignited and the container thrown into a populated area or building. The explosion causes a fire, creating panic and injuries. As with any fire, cyanide poisoning is a medical emergency of concern.

Treatment

Attention to scene safety, including use of the appropriate PPE, is essential in treating victims of incendiary devices. When safe to do so, notify receiving facilities from the scene that multiple patients will be arriving. Initial care consists of stabilizing airway, breathing, and circulation and treating related injuries. Consider instituting internal protocols to prepare for a mass casualty.

Chemical Agents
Chemical Asphyxiants

Exposure to chemical asphyxiants can occur through inhalation, absorption, or ingestion. One of the most common asphyxiants is hydrogen cyanide, which carries the military designation *AC*. Notable for its bitter almond-like odor when found in a solid form, cyanide can also take the form of a liquid or a colorless gas. It's often used to treat metals and is a byproduct of gas combustion. Another chemical asphyxiant used as an agent of warfare is cyanogen chloride, which carries the military designation CK. Once these chemicals enter the bloodstream, they decrease the ability of cells to absorb oxygen and manufacture adenosine triphosphate. Initial exposure causes respiratory distress, headaches, and tachycardia. If exposure is undetected or prolonged, seizures and respiratory failure result.

Carbon monoxide is an inhaled chemical asphyxiant that binds with hemoglobin, reducing the oxygen-carrying capacity of the red blood cells and inducing hypoxia.

Treatment

Assessment of respiratory and cardiovascular status is the key to determining treatment interventions. Routine medical care includes providing supplemental oxygen, administering IV therapy, and monitoring for cardiac dysrhythmias. Cyanide toxicity requires administration of a cyanide antidote kit or hydroxocobalamin. If seizure activity occurs, benzodiazepines are administered (Table 10-27). Remember that pulse oximetry readings will not reflect delivery of oxygen to cells with chemical asphyxiant exposure.

If the contaminant is a known liquid, initiate the decontamination processes immediately. Stabilizing airway, breathing, and circulation and treating presenting signs and symptoms are the initial medical interventions. Use a cyanide antidote kit on each patient exposed to that chemical. These kits include amyl nitrite, sodium nitrite, and sodium thiosulfate. The first two medications combine with hemoglobin to form methemoglobin. Methemoglobin binds cyanide ions more avidly than cytochrome oxidase within the electron transport chain to create cyanomethemoglobin. The third medication, sodium thiosulfate,

binds cyanide from cyanomethemoglobin to create thiocyanate, which is easily excreted by the kidneys. A recently approved and simpler therapeutic agent is hydroxocobalamin. Cobalt moieties within hydroxocobalamin bind cyanide to form cyanocobalamin, or vitamin B_{12} structurally. Cyanocobalamin is the excreted by the kidneys. Administration of hydroxocobalamin is associated with deep red to purple staining of body excretions and secretions. Hydroxocobalamin also interferes with determination of some colorimetric laboratory studies including chemistries for several days.

In the ED, the patient is observed and given continued supportive care.

Nerve Agents

The most toxic agents in chemical warfare are nerve agents. These agents disrupt nerve transmission in the central and peripheral nervous systems by inhibiting acetylcholinesterase release, exciting the cholinergic response and overstimulating the parasympathetic nervous system. Although minimal exposure has no long-term devastating results, high amounts and long duration of exposure are associated with high rates of mortality and morbidity. Nerve agents are similar to organophosphates (discussed earlier) but much more potent and destructive. Nerve agents can also be classified as G and V agents.

The G agents include tabun (GA), sarin (GB), soman (GD), and cyclohexyl methylphosphonofluoridate (GF). Developed in the United Kingdom, VX is the most common V agent. G agents are very volatile, limited-action, colorless liquids. When aerosolized or released into warm environments or closed buildings, they become more volatile. V liquids are usually not volatile and are longer acting.

Table 10-27 Treatment of Chemical Asphyxiant Exposure

- Patients exposed to carbon monoxide usually do not require decontamination. Because of cyanide's toxicity, patients should undergo decontamination. With liquid or solid cyanide exposure, adequate decontamination is essential.
- Establish an open airway. Consider orotracheal or nasotracheal intubation for airway control in the patient who is unconscious, has severe pulmonary edema, or is in severe respiratory distress.
- Ventilate as necessary. Positive-pressure ventilation with a bag-mask device may be beneficial.
- Do not induce vomiting or use emetics.
- Monitor for pulmonary edema, and treat as necessary.
- Monitor cardiac rhythm, and treat dysrhythmias as necessary.
- Start an IV line, and infuse at 30 mL/h. For hypotension with signs of hypovolemia, give fluid cautiously. Consider vasopressors if the patient is hypotensive with a normal fluid volume, per local protocol. Watch for signs of fluid overload.
- Administer cyanide antidote kit per local protocol for symptomatic patients with cyanide exposure.
- Treat seizures with diazepam (Valium) or lorazepam (Ativan) per local protocol.
- For eye contamination, immediately flush the eyes with water. Continuously irrigate each eye with normal saline during transport.
- Pulse oximetry readings may not be accurate in these exposures.
- Hyperbaric oxygen may be required for optimal treatment.

From Currance PL, Clements B, Bronstein AC: *Emergency care for hazardous materials exposure*, ed 3, St. Louis, MO, 2005, Mosby.

- *Sarin (GB)*. In its liquid state, sarin is colorless, odorless, and tasteless. It can infiltrate into waterways and reach toxic levels in drinking water or water used for bathing. Sarin can also be converted to a gas and released as a vapor into the air, contaminating large geographic areas. People exposed to sarin complain of headache, increased salivation, abdominal cramping, and respiratory distress with wheezing. Symptoms begin minutes to hours after exposure.

- *Soman (GD)*. Soman is also a clear, colorless, tasteless liquid, but it can have a camphor odor similar to mentholated rubs and cough drops. More volatile than sarin, this liquid provokes symptoms within seconds or minutes, rather than hours after exposure. Signs and symptoms are similar to those associated with sarin exposure.

- *Tabun (GA)*. Tabun, also a clear, colorless, and tasteless liquid, has a minimal fruity odor. It can vaporize and thus be inhaled. Exposure can also occur through ingestion or absorption. Since the liquid mixes easily with water, it can be ingested, causing GI discomfort. Absorption can cause skin and eye irritation. If the liquid remains on clothing, it can cause secondary contamination of those who touch it. Symptoms begin within seconds when a person is exposed to the vapor and within several hours when a person is exposed to tabun in liquid form. Patients exhibit altered mentation, seizures, watery eyes, cough, and excessive sweating. Cardiac arrhythmia sometimes occurs.

- *VX*. VX, a V agent, is an odorless, slightly amber liquid. This liquid is more toxic when inhaled or absorbed through the skin than when ingested. It mixes easily with water, causing abdominal discomfort when ingested. Signs and symptoms begin to appear within seconds or hours of exposure and are similar to those provoked by other nerve agents. Victims may have muscle twitching and miosis. Unrecognized and untreated, the twitching can progress to status epilepticus and can be difficult to stop.

Treatment

Your initial response must be to secure scene safety. Because nerve agent vapors are heavier than air, park vehicles uphill and upwind. Prevention of secondary contamination is essential; appropriate PPE is required. Removal of contaminants by decontamination procedures may be necessary, since chemicals can stay on clothing 30 to 40 minutes after exposure. It is essential that you move patients to a well-ventilated area. Use the SLUDGE BBM mnemonic in the Rapid Recall box to identify presenting symptoms. Supportive care for airway, breathing, and circulation are the initial medical interventions. Provide continual monitoring of blood pressure alterations. Manage cardiac arrhythmias per American Heart Association (AHA) ACLS protocols.

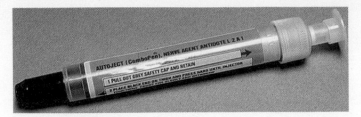

Figure 10-13 Mark I antidote kit.
From Miller R, Eriksson L, Fleisher L, et al: *Miller's anesthesia*, ed 7, New York, 2009, Churchill Livingstone.

Use nerve agent autoinjector antidote kits, known as *Mark 1 antidote kits*, containing atropine and pralidoxime (**Figure 10-13**). Newer kits, known as *DuoDote kits*, combine the two medications in one autoinjector. A detailed explanation of how these agents work to reverse toxicity was given earlier. If seizures develop, administer diazepam (Valium) or lorazepam (Ativan).

Pulmonary Agents

Poisonous gases, known as **pulmonary agents**, pose a grave threat to the safety of first responders and prehospital personnel. These gases, which include chlorine, phosgene, and anhydrous ammonia, are easily obtained, and victims can be quickly contaminated by inhaling them.

- *Chlorine*. Chlorine is a yellow-green gas that has a slight odor some describe as smelling like a combination of pepper and pineapple. It's commonly found in plastics and solvent manufacturing plants. When pressurized, chlorine easily vaporizes into a gas. Chlorine can be inhaled, absorbed through the skin, or ingested if water is contaminated. Signs and symptoms include eye and throat irritation, burns from skin exposure, and respiratory distress caused by inhalation. Severe respiratory complications such as pulmonary edema can become evident within 20 to 24 hours of exposure.

- *Phosgene (CG)*. Phosgene appears in gaseous form as a gray-white cloud with the vague odor of freshly baled hay. This agent is commonly found in pesticides, pharmaceuticals, and dyes. Another potential source of phosgene gas is the heating of Freon as is seen with soldering refrigeration pipes. When cooled, it converts to a liquid. When released into the air, it vaporizes quickly. Early symptoms of exposure may be minimal as phosgene is far less irritating to mucosal membranes than chlorine, for instance. However, delayed pulmonary injury and edema may develop 24 or more hours later and can be fatal. The agent can cause significant cardiovascular compromise and hypotension. If the exposure is not identified and managed, death can occur within a few days.

■ *Anhydrous ammonia.* Anhydrous ammonia is a colorless gas commonly found in agricultural settings, where it's used as fertilizer. Industrial factories use this gas for cooling and freezing foods like meat and poultry. Anhydrous ammonia is considered volatile and, when present in high concentrations, forms a white cloud. Symptoms occur within several hours of exposure.

Treatment

Unfortunately, no antidote exists. Contaminated clothing must be removed and properly packaged per local protocol. Decontamination must be performed promptly by trained personnel.

Putting It All Together

When you are a first responder to a patient with a toxicologic exposure or a situation involving hazardous materials or possible weapons of mass destruction, the initial scene and patient assessment challenges can be daunting. If you can maintain a heightened level of awareness for situations and patients that may present safety issues, your AMLS training and skills can then help you organize a methodical healthcare plan. First you have to know the extent of the threat of the toxic exposure to yourself and your patient, and then you have to be able to implement appropriate safety precautions in addition to treating your patient's medical emergency.

Become familiar with local, regional, state, and federal agencies that can offer support in these situations. If mutual aid is required, those agencies should be contacted immediately for activation. As always, the AMLS assessment pathway provides the appropriate approach to evaluating the patient's presenting signs and symptoms, determining a working diagnosis, and arriving at an effective treatment plan. In toxicologic emergencies in particular, the patient's historical information can provide key clues to medical management that will stabilize the patient and improve outcomes.

SCENARIO SOLUTION

© HunThomas/ShutterStock, Inc.

■ Differential diagnoses may include sympathomimetic intoxication (cocaine, amphetamine, ephedrine, phencyclidine), stroke, autonomic hyperreflexia, or alcohol withdrawal.

■ To narrow your differential diagnosis, you need to complete a more thorough history of past and present illness. Question his roommate about the use of alcohol or other drugs. Perform a physical examination that includes vital sign assessment, stroke scale, pupil assessment, evaluation of heart and breath sounds, ECG monitoring and a 12-lead ECG, Sao$_2$, capnography, and blood glucose analysis. If you suspect autonomic hyperreflexia, look for a trigger such as a full bladder that could be the source of the problem.

■ The patient has signs that indicate an exaggerated sympathetic response. Administer oxygen if indicated. Establish vascular access. Continue to monitor the ECG. Further treatment will depend on the rest of your assessment findings. If you suspect sympathomimetic overdose or alcohol withdrawal, treat with a benzodiazepine and IV fluid administration. If the patient has signs of stroke, transport him to the closest appropriate center. If the patient's exam points to autonomic hyperreflexia, transport if the source of the problem is not immediately resolved.

Summary

■ Ensure safety before entering any scene that may be contaminated, and consider airborne toxins that could be dangerous.

■ Obtain a thorough history, including available drugs/toxins, time of ingestion, and dose. Ask bystanders and witnesses for additional information.

■ Maintain supportive care for comatose patients, including airway management and administration of glucose, thiamine, and small doses of naloxone if necessary.

■ Obtain an accurate core temperature, and institute temperature normalization strategies if necessary.

■ Gauge perfusion status by monitoring mental status, urine output, blood pressure, capillary refill time, and acid–base status. Initiate invasive monitoring as time allows.

Summary (CONTINUED)

- Contact a poison control center early in the encounter to aid appropriate diagnosis and treatment of any toxicologic disorder.
- Scene assessment of an environment compromised by a hazardous material or a biological, chemical, or radiologic agent is a key component in preserving the safety of healthcare personnel and patients.
- Incident command should establish hot, warm, and cold zones to maintain scene control and safety.
- Identification of the proper personal protective devices needed for unstable scenes and patient exposures is critical to ensuring the safety of personnel and patients and containing the spread of a toxin or hazardous material.
- Decontamination must occur before entering a hot zone, and it must be performed again before and after transport to the receiving facility.
- Understanding various procedures for responder, patient, and equipment decontamination is essential to maintaining the safety of all healthcare providers and patients and to preventing secondary contamination.
- The potential for exposure is reduced when providers make use of references for the identification of possible hazardous materials. These references also specify associated signs and symptoms and outline appropriate treatment modalities, should an exposure occur.
- Disaster response preparedness is essential in the emergent assessment and management of patients and scenes with possible exposure to toxic agents, hazardous materials, or chemical, biological, or radiologic weapons.
- Weapons of mass destruction include biological, nuclear, incendiary, chemical, and radiologic agents.
- Identifying chemical, biological, and radiologic agent cardinal presentations/chief complaints and safety and management strategies reduces morbidity and mortality in individuals and reduces the potential for exposure.
- Performing a thorough assessment and obtaining a complete history can help eliminate secondary exposure by identifying contamination early.
- Presentation of signs and symptoms of exposure varies with different contaminants, on the basis of volatility, duration, and route of exposure.
- Early recognition of hazardous materials and bioterrorist incidents can reduce exposure and promote timely implementation of treatment strategies for all involved agencies.
- Report all suspected hazardous materials and bioterrorist incidents to the appropriate local, state, and federal authorities so that disaster response protocols can be implemented.

KEY TERMS

© HunThomas/ShutterStock, Inc.

biological agent   Disease-causing pathogen or toxin that may be used as a weapon to cause disease or injury to humans.

cold (green) zone   A support zone for general triage, stabilization, and management of illness or injuries. Patients and uncontaminated personnel are given access to this zone, but healthcare personnel must wear protective clothing while in the green zone and properly discard it in predetermined areas on exiting.

contamination   Condition of being soiled, stained, touched, or otherwise exposed to harmful agents, making an object potentially unsafe for use as intended or without barrier techniques. An example is entry of infectious or toxic materials into a previously clean or sterile environment.

delirium   An acute mental disorder characterized by confusion, disorientation, restlessness, clouding of consciousness, incoherence, fear, anxiety, excitement, and often illusions.

dirty bomb   A conventional explosive device used to disperse radiologic agents.

emergency decontamination   Process of decontaminating people exposed to and potentially contaminated with hazardous materials; focuses on rapidly removing the contamination to reduce their exposure and save lives, with secondary regard for completeness of decontamination.

fulminant   Describes a sudden intense occurrence that creates a hazardous environment

KEY TERMS (CONTINUED)

© HunThomas/ShutterStock, Inc.

gastrointestinal decontamination Any attempt to limit absorption or hasten elimination of a toxin from a patient's gastrointestinal tract. Examples include activated charcoal, gastric lavage, and whole-bowel irrigation. While these methods do have a small role in toxicology, their use is not routinely recommended and should be discussed with a poison control center or medical toxicologist.

hot (red) zone An area where the hazardous material is located and contamination has occurred. Access to this zone is limited so as to protect rescuers and patients from further exposure. Specific protective gear worn by trained personnel is required for access.

huffing The act of pouring an inhalant onto a cloth or into a bag and inhaling the substance, usually in an attempt to alter one's mental status.

intoxication The state of being poisoned by a drug or other toxic substance; the state of being inebriated as a result of excessive alcohol consumption.

lethal concentration 50% (LC$_{50}$) The air concentration of an agent that kills 50% of the exposed animal population. This denotes the concentration and the length of exposure time of that population.

lethal dose 50% (LD$_{50}$) The oral or dermal exposure dose that kills 50% of an exposed animal population in 2 weeks.

methemoglobinemia The presence of methemoglobin in the blood, which prevents the ability of hemoglobin to carry and transport oxygen to the tissues. Hemoglobin is converted to methemoglobin by nitrogen oxides and sulfa drugs.

National Fire Protection Association (NFPA) A national and international voluntary membership organization that promotes improved fire protection and prevention and establishes safeguards against loss of life and property by fire. The NFPA writes and publishes national voluntary consensus standards.

North American Emergency Response Guidebook A book published by the U.S. Government Printing Office that provides a quick reference to hazardous materials emergencies for first responders.

Occupational Safety and Health Administration (OSHA) The U.S. federal agency that regulates worker safety.

packer A person who ingests a large quantity of well-packed drugs for the purpose of smuggling. These carefully prepared packages are less likely to rupture than those ingested by stuffers, but toxicity can be severe if they do because of the large amount of drug present.

placards Diamond-shaped signs placed on containers that identify hazardous materials.

prodromal Early symptoms that mark the onset of a disease.

psychosis Any major mental disorder characterized by a gross impairment in reality testing, in which the individual incorrectly evaluates the accuracy of perceptions and thoughts and makes incorrect references about external reality. It is often characterized by regressive behavior, inappropriate mood and affect, and diminished impulse control. Symptoms include hallucinations and delusions.

pulmonary agent An industrial chemical used as a weapon to kill those who inhale the vapor or gas; lung damage causes asphyxiation. Also known as a "choking agent."

radioactive Giving off radiation as the result of the disintegration of atomic nuclei.

Standard on Hazardous Waste Operations and Emergency Response (HAZWOPER) (CFR 1910.120) Occupational Safety and Health Administration (OSHA) and Environmental Protection Agency (EPA) regulation intended to protect the safety of employees who respond to emergency incidents related to storage and disposal of hazardous materials.

stuffer A person who hastily ingests small packets of poorly packaged drugs to avoid apprehension and drug confiscation. The dose is much lower than that seen with packers, but the likelihood of toxicity is much greater because the packages, meant for distribution, are likely to open in the patient's stomach or bowel.

toxidrome A specific syndrome-like group of symptoms associated with exposure to a given poison.

warm (yellow) zone The area surrounding a contaminated hot zone. Properly protected healthcare providers are allowed to access this zone for rapid assessment and management of emergent or life-threatening conditions. Decontamination occurs in this zone.

BIBLIOGRAPHY
© HunThomas/ShutterStock, Inc.

Acetadote [package insert]. Nashville, TN: Cumberland Pharmaceuticals, Inc., March 2004.

Auerbach P: *Wilderness medicine*, ed 5, St. Louis, MO, 2007, Mosby.

Bailey B: Glucagon in beta-blocker and calcium channel blocker overdoses: A systematic review, *J Toxicol Clin Toxicol.* 41:595–602, 2003.

Baltarowich L: Barbiturates, *Top Emerg Med.* 7:46–53, 1985.

Brent J, Wallace K, Bukhart K: *Critical care toxicology*, St. Louis, MO, 2004, Mosby.

Bronstein AC, Spyker DA, Cantilena LR, et al.: 2006 annual report of the American Association of Poison Control Centers National Poison Data System, *Clin Toxicol.* 45:815–917, 2007.

Bronstein AC, Spyker DA, Cantilena LR, et al.: 2007 annual report of the American Association of Poison Control Centers National Poison Data System: 25th annual report. American Association of Poison Control Centers, *Clin Toxicol.* 46:927–1057, 2008.

Buchanan JF, Brown CR: "Designer drugs": A problem in clinical toxicology, *Med Toxicol.* 3:1–17, 1988.

Budisavljevic MN, Stewart L, Sahn SA, et al.: Hyponatremia associated with 3,4-methylenedioxy-methylamphetamine ("ecstasy") abuse, *Am J Med Sci.* 326:89–93, 2003.

Cai Z, McCaslin PP: Acute, chronic, and differential effects of several anesthetic barbiturates on glutamate receptor activation in neuronal culture, *Brain Res.* 611:181–186, 1993.

Campbell NR, Baylis B: Renal impairment associated with an acute paracetamol overdose in the absence of hepatotoxicity, *Postgrad Med J.* 68:116–118, 1992.

Caravati EM: Hallucinogenic drugs. In *Medical toxicology*, ed 3, Philadelphia, PA, 2004, Lippincott, pp. 1103–1111.

Cater RE: The use of sodium and potassium to reduce toxicity and toxic side effects from lithium, *Med Hypotheses.* 20:359–383, 1986.

Centers for Disease Control and Prevention. *Web-based Injury Statistics Query and Reporting System (WISQARS).* 2014. http://www.cdc.gov/injury/wisqars/fatal.html

Chan P, Chen JH, Lee MH, et al.: Fatal and nonfatal methamphetamine intoxication in the intensive care unit, *J Toxicol Clin Toxicol.* 32:147–155, 1994.

Chance BC, Erecinska M, Wagner M: Mitochondrial responses to carbon monoxide, *Ann NY Acad Sci.* 174:193–203, 1970.

Chandler DB, Norton RL, Kauffman J: Lead poisoning associated with intravenous methamphetamine use—Oregon, 1988, *MMWR Morb Mortal Wkly Rep.* 38:830–831, 1989.

Chyka PA, Seger D: Position statement: Single-dose activated charcoal, *J Toxicol Clin Toxicol.* 35:721–741, 1997.

Coburn RF, Mayers LB: Myoglobin oxygen tension determines from measurements of carboxyhemoglobin in skeletal muscle, *Am J Physiol.* 220:66–74, 1971.

Coupey SM: Barbiturates, *Pediatr Rev.* 18:260–264, 1997.

DeWitt CR, Waksman JC: Pharmacology, pathophysiology, and management of calcium channel blocker and beta blocker toxicity, *Toxicol Rev.* 23:223–238, 2004.

Doyon S, Roberts JR: The use of glucagon in a case of calcium channel blocker overdose, *Ann Emerg Med.* 22:1229–1233, 1993.

Eddleston M, Ariaratnam CA, Meyer WP, et al.: Multiple-dose activated charcoal in acute self-poisoning: A randomised controlled trial, *Lancet.* 371:579–587, 2008.

Emerson TS, Cisek JE: Methcathinone ("cat"): A Russian designer amphetamine infiltrates the rural Midwest, *Ann Emerg Med.* 22:1897–1903, 1993.

Fingerhut LA, Cox CS: Poisoning mortality, 1985–1995, *Public Health Rep.* 113:218–233, 1998.

Finkle BS, McCloskey KL, Goodman LS: Diazepam and drug-associated deaths. A survey in the United States and Canada, *J Am Med Assoc.* 242:429–434, 1979.

Flomenbaum NE, Goldfrank LR, Hoffman RS, et al.: *Goldfrank's toxicologic emergencies*, ed 8, New York, NY, 2006, McGraw-Hill.

Frierson J, Bailly D, Shultz T, et al.: Refractory cardiogenic shock and complete heart block after unsuspected verapamil—SR and atenolol overdose, *Clin Cardiol.* 14:933–935, 1991.

Garnier R, Guerault E, Muzard D, et al.: Acute zolpidem poisoning—analysis of 344 cases, *J Toxicol Clin Toxicol.* 32:391–404, 1994.

Graham SR, Day RO, Lee R, et al.: Overdose with chloral hydrate: A pharmacological and therapeutic review, *Med J Aust.* 149:686–688, 1988.

Greenblatt DJ, von Moltke LL, Harmatz JS, et al.: Acute overdosage with benzodiazepine derivatives, *Clin Pharmacol Ther.* 21:497–514, 1977.

Hariman RJ, Mangiardi LM, McAllister RG, et al.: Reversal of the cardiovascular effects of verapamil by calcium and sodium: Differences between electrophysiologic and hemodynamic responses, *Circulation.* 59:797–804, 1979.

Hendren WC, Schreiber RS, Garretson LK: Extracorporeal bypass for the treatment of verapamil poisoning, *Ann Emerg Med.* 18:984–987, 1989.

Hesse B, Pedersen JT: Hypoglycaemia after propranolol in children, *Acta Med Scand.* 193:551–552, 1973.

Hoegholm A, Clementson P: Hypertonic sodium chloride in severe antidepressant overdosage, *J Toxicol Clin Toxicol.* 29:297–298, 1991.

Horowitz AL, Kaplan R, Sarpel G: Carbon monoxide toxicity: MR imaging in the brain, *Radiology.* 162:787–788, 1987.

Kaim SC, Klett CJ, Rothfeld B: Treatment of the acute alcohol withdrawal state: A comparison of four drugs, *Am J Psychiatry.* 125:1640–1646, 1969.

Kerns W II, Schroeder D, Williams C, et al.: Insulin improves survival in a canine model of acute beta-blocker toxicity, *Ann Emerg Med.* 29:748–757, 1997.

Kitchens CS, Van Mierop LHS: Envenomation by the eastern coral snake *(Micrurus fulvius fulvius)*, *J Am Med Assoc.* 258:1615–1618, 1987.

Kleinman ME, Brennan EE, Zachary D, et al. Part 5. Adult BLS and CPR Quality. 2015 American Heart Association Guidelines for Cardiopulmonary Resuscitation and Emergency Cardiovascular Care. *Circulation.* 132 (18 Suppl 2): S414–S436, 2015.

Kline JA, Tomaszewski CA, Schroeder JD, et al.: Insulin is a superior antidote for cardiovascular toxicity induced by verapamil in the anesthetized canine, *J Pharm Exp Ther.* 267:744–750, 1993.

Kunkel DB, Curry SC, Vance MV, et al.: Reptile envenomations, *J Toxicol Clin Toxicol.* 21:503–526, 1983–1984.

Lange RA, Cigarroa RG, Yancy CW, et al.: Potentiation of cocaine-induced coronary vasoconstriction by beta-adrenergic blockade, *Ann Intern Med.* 112:897–903, 1990.

Leonard LG, Scheulen JJ, Munster AM: Chemical burns: Effect of prompt first aid, *J Trauma.* 22:420–423, 1982.

BIBLIOGRAPHY (CONTINUED)

© HunThomas/ShutterStock, Inc.

Lindberg MC, Cunningham A, Lindberg NH: Acute phenobarbital intoxication, *South Med J.* 85:803–806, 1992.

Long H, Nelson LS, Hoffman RS: A rapid qualitative test for suspected ethylene glycol poisoning, *Acad Emerg Med.* 15:688–690, 2008.

Love JN, Sachdeva DK, Curtis LA, et al.: A potential role for glucagon in the treatment of drug-induced symptomatic bradycardia, *Chest.* 114:323–326, 1998.

Lundborg P: The effect of adrenergic blockade on potassium concentrations in different conditions, *Acta Med Scand Suppl.* 672:121–126, 1983.

Makin AJ, Williams R: The current management of paracetamol overdosage, *Br J Clin Pract.* 48:144–148, 1994.

Marques I, Gomes E, de Oliveira J: Treatment of calcium channel blocker intoxication with insulin infusion: Case report and literature review, *Resuscitation.* 57:211–213, 2003.

McCarron MM, Schulze BW, Thompson GA, et al.: Acute phencyclidine intoxication: Clinical patterns, complications, and treatment, *Ann Emerg Med.* 10:290–297, 1981.

Mehta AN, Emmett JB, Emmett M: GOLD MARK: An anion gap mnemonic for the 21st century. *Lancet,* 2008;372(9642):892.

Mitchell JR, Jollow DJ, Potter WZ, et al.: Acetaminophen-induced hepatic necrosis. I. Role of drug metabolism, *J Pharmacol Exp Ther.* 187:185–194, 1973.

Miura T, Mitomo M, Kawai R, et al.: CT of the brain in acute carbon monoxide intoxication: Characteristic features and prognosis, *AJNR Am J Neuroradiol.* 6:739–742, 1985.

Monitoring the Future: 2003 Data from in-school surveys of eighth, tenth, and twelfth grade students. Drug and alcohol press release: Trends in use of various drugs. Available from www.monitoringthefuture.org/data/03data/pr03t1.pdf.

Moon RE, DeLong E: Hyperbaric oxygen for carbon monoxide poisoning, *Med J Aust.* 170:197–199, 1999.

Mowry JB, Spyker DA, Cantilena LR, et al.: 2013 Annual report of the American Association of Poison Control Centers' National Poison Data System (NPDS): 31st annual report, *Clin Toxicol.* 52:1032–1283, 2013.

NAEMT: *PHTLS prehospital trauma life support,* ed 7, St. Louis, MO, 2010, Mosby.

National Institute on Drug Abuse. "Flakka" (alpha PVP). 2015. http://www.drugabuse.gov/emerging-trends/flakka-alpha-pvp

National Institute on Drug Abuse. K2/Spice ("Synthetic Marijuana"). 2015. http://www.drugabuse.gov/publications/drugfacts/k2spice-synthetic-marijuana

Ostapowicz G, Fontana RJ, Schiodt FV, et al.: Results of a prospective study of acute liver failure at 17 tertiary care centers in the United States, *Ann Intern Med.* 137:947–954, 2002.

Palmer BF: Effectiveness of hemodialysis in the extracorporeal therapy of phenobarbital overdose, *Am J Kidney Dis.* 36: 640–643, 2000.

Pena BM, Krauss B: Adverse events of procedural sedation and analgesia in a pediatric emergency department, *Ann Emerg Med.* 34:483–491, 1999.

Pentel PR, Benowitz NL: Tricyclic antidepressant poisoning—management of arrhythmias, *Med Toxicol.* 1:101–121, 1986.

Peterson JE, Stewart RD: Absorption and elimination of carbon monoxide by inactive young men, *Arch Environ Health.* 21:165–171, 1970.

Prescott LF: Paracetamol overdosage: Pharmacological considerations and clinical management, *Drugs.* 25:290–314, 1983.

Raphael JC, Elkharrat D, Jars-Guincestre MC, et al.: Trial of normobaric and hyperbaric oxygen for acute carbon monoxide intoxication, *Lancet.* 1989:414–419, 1989.

Reith DM, Dawson AH, Epid D, et al.: Relative toxicity of beta blockers in overdose, *J Toxicol Clin Toxicol.* 34:273–278, 1996.

Roth BA, Vinson DR, Kim S: Carisoprodol-induced myoclonic encephalopathy, *J Toxicol Clin Toxicol.* 36:609–612, 1998.

Seger DL: Flumazenil—treatment or toxin? *J Toxicol Clin Toxicol.* 42:209–216, 2004.

Sieghart W: Structure and pharmacology of gamma-aminobutyric acid$_A$ receptor subtypes, *Pharmacol Rev.* 47:181–234, 1995.

St. Onge M, Dubé PA, Gosselin S, et al. Treatment for calcium channel blocker poisoning: A systematic review. *Clin Toxicol.* 52(9):926–944, 2014.

Stewart R, Baretta ED, Platte LR, et al.: Carboxyhemoglobin levels in American blood donors, *J Am Med Assoc.* 229:1187–1195, 1974.

Substance Abuse and Mental Health Services Administration. Highlights of the 2011 Drug Abuse Warning Network (DAWN) findings on drug-related emergency department visits. The DAWN report. Rockville, MD: US Department of Health and Human Services, Substance Abuse and Mental Health Services Administration; 2013. Available from http://www.samhsa.gov/data/2k13/DAWN127/sr127-DAWN-highlights.htm

Substance Abuse and Mental Health Services Administration, Center for Behavioral Health Statistics and Quality. *The DAWN report: Emergency department visits involving methamphetamine: 2007 to 2011.* 2014. http://www.samhsa.gov/data/sites/default/files/DAWN_SR167_EDVisitsMeth_06-12-14/DAWN-SR167-EDVisitsMeth-2014.pdf

Vale JA: Position statement: Gastric lavage, *J Toxicol Clin Toxicol.* 35:711, 1997.

Van Hoesen KB, Camporesi EM, Moon RE, et al.: Should hyperbaric oxygen be used to treat the pregnant patient for acute carbon monoxide poisoning? A case report and literature review, *J Am Med Assoc.* 261:1039–1043, 1989.

Vollenweider FX, Gamma A, Liechti M, et al.: Psychological and cardiovascular effects and short-term sequelae of MDMA ("ecstasy") in MDMA-naive healthy volunteers, *Neuropsychopharmacology.* 19:241–251, 1998.

Wason S, Lacouture PG, Lovejoy FH: Single high-dose pyridoxine treatment for isoniazid overdose, *J Am Med Assoc.* 246: 1102–1104, 1981.

Weaver LK, Hopkins RO, Chan KJ, et al.: Hyperbaric oxygen for acute carbon monoxide poisoning, *N Engl J Med.* 347: 1057–1067, 2002.

Wiley CC, Wiley JF II: Pediatric benzodiazepine ingestion resulting in hospitalization, *J Toxicol Clin Toxicol.* 36:227–231, 1998.

Yildiz S, Aktas S, Cimsit M, et al.: Seizure incidence in 80,000 patient treatments with hyperbaric oxygen, *Aviat Space Environ Med.* 75:992–994, 2004.

Zuvekas S, Vitiello B: Recent trends in stimulant medication use among U.S. children, *Am J Psych.* 163:579–585, 2006.

CHAPTER REVIEW QUESTIONS

1. Your patient is agitated and sweaty. Her vital signs include a blood pressure of 170/108 mm Hg; pulse rate, 132 beats/min; and respirations, 20 breaths/min. Her pupils are dilated, and her hands are trembling. These signs and symptoms may be associated with:
   a. Alcohol withdrawal
   b. Carbamates
   c. Diazepam
   d. Tramadol

2. Which source provides the most detailed information related to hazardous materials?
   a. Location of the emergency
   b. Material safety data sheets
   c. Pictographs
   d. Placards

3. A 2-year-old male is found chewing on berries from a lily of the valley plant. Predict his vital signs.
   a. BP 130/72, P 128 bpm
   b. BP 100/60, P 100 bpm
   c. BP 70/50, P 128 bpm
   d. BP 70/50 P 70 bpm

4. A 24-year-old woman took 24 diphenhydramine tablets. Her vital signs include a blood pressure of 86/54 mm Hg; pulse rate, 110 beats/min; respirations, 20 breaths/min. What other sign or symptom should you anticipate?
   a. Drooling
   b. Pale skin
   c. Pinpoint pupils
   d. Seizures

5. The family of a 72-year-old man is worried about their father. His blood glucose level is 80 mg/dL (4.4 mmol/L). His rate and depth of breathing are increased, and he is sleepy and weak. He takes metformin (Glucophage). You suspect his signs and symptoms may be related to:
   a. Diabetic ketoacidosis
   b. Hyperosmolar hyperglycemic nonketotic coma
   c. Lactic acidosis
   d. Pulmonary embolus

6. A farmer was spraying his barn when he became ill. His heart rate is 60 beats/min, and his blood pressure is 88/50 mm Hg. Tears are streaming down his cheeks, and he is vomiting. What toxidrome does this clinical picture fit?
   a. Anticholinergic
   b. Cholinergic
   c. Opioid
   d. Sympathomimetic

7. Which of the following biological warfare agents causes serious neurologic symptoms that may include paralysis?
   a. Botulism
   b. Plague
   c. Ricin
   d. Viral hemorrhagic fever

8. A 22-year-old woman is found at a party unresponsive and breathing approximately 8 breaths/min. Her skin is gray. Which of the following signs or symptoms will confirm your suspicion that the opioid toxidrome is causing her emergency?
   a. Blood pressure, 170/110 mm Hg
   b. Pupils, 2 mm and equal
   c. QRS duration, 0.24 sec.
   d. Tremors

9. Your patient is reported to have taken an overdose. She has a history of anxiety disorder and depression. She is unresponsive, and her vital signs include a blood pressure of 100/70 mm Hg; pulse rate, 128 beats/min; respirations, 20 breaths/min. Her ECG shows right bundle branch block. You expect she has taken:
   a. Amitriptyline
   b. Lorazepam
   c. Paroxetine
   d. Quetiapine

10. You respond to a warehouse for multiple patients with difficulty breathing. From a hallway, you see a patient lying in a room with two other people who don't seem to be breathing. He calls out to you, saying he can't breathe. You should first:
    a. Administer oxygen by nonrebreathing mask.
    b. Drag him out of the room.
    c. Examine the shipping papers.
    d. Stage at a safe distance.

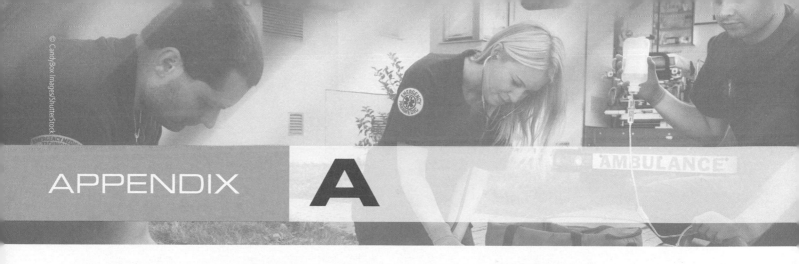

AMLS Patient Assessment Pathway

INITIAL OBSERVATIONS

Scene/Situation
Safety threats
Situational clues

Patient
Cardinal presentation/Chief complaint
Primary survey

FIRST IMPRESSION

Identify and treat life threats immediately
Sick/Not sick?
Generate initial differential diagnosis

DETAILED ASSESSMENT

History
OPQRST, SAMPLER

Secondary survey
Vital signs, full-body or focused physical exam

Diagnostics
Glucose, ECG, O$_2$ saturation, ETCO$_2$

Continually reassess.

REFINE THE DIFFERENTIAL DIAGNOSIS
(BASED ON ASSESSMENT AND CLINICAL REASONING)

Life threatening

Critical

Nonemergent

ONGOING MANAGEMENT

Reassess, further refine the diagnosis, modify treatment

Patient disposition

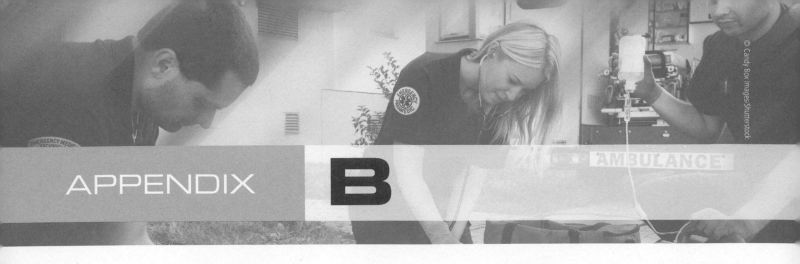

Chapter Review Answers

Chapter 1

1. b. Clinical reasoning

Rationale: Healthcare providers must integrate good judgment based on strong knowledge and clinical experience to perform a comprehensive assessment and determine working diagnoses and treatment modalities. Clinical reasoning filters out nonessential historical information to efficiently assess and treat the patient.

2. d. A life threat

Rationale: The AMLS assessment pathway begins with the initial observation. This observation entails identifying scene or situation safety concerns, using all the senses (vision, auditory, olfactory) to understand the patient's chief complaint/cardinal presentation and begin the primary survey. All of these tasks occur rapidly to immediately recognize and manage life threats.

3. c. Blood glucose analysis

Rationale: The detailed assessment includes the history, vital signs, focused physical exam, and obtaining and interpreting relevant diagnostic information. Obtaining blood glucose levels will assist the provider in ruling in or ruling out endocrine and neurologic diagnoses.

4. b. Increase in systolic blood pressure

Rationale: The aging process results in changes in the cardiovascular system. Large arteries become less elastic, creating more pressure in the arteriole system during systole, raising the systolic blood pressure.

5. c. Identify and manage life threats

Rationale: Identifying and managing life threats are essential in improving the outcome of the patient. Early, appropriate interventions, contacting the appropriate receiving facility, and transport decisions are determined in the initial observation component of the AMLS assessment pathway. Throughout the patient encounter it is essential to continue to assess for life threats and manage them as they are identified.

6. a. Is this patient likely to die now?

Rationale: Using the primary survey to identify life threats is the key to establishing immediate management strategies. Anticipating the worst underlying medical problem by asking what may cause a poor outcome in the patient will improve awareness of the patient's presentation and identify life threats in the initial observation of the AMLS assessment pathway.

7. a. Cardinal presentation/chief complaint

Rationale: The patient's cardinal presentation/chief complaint is the reason the patient called for medical assistance. The presentation includes areas of pain, discomfort, and onset. This information assists the provider in prioritizing obtaining the history, focused physical exam, and other secondary survey components. The cardinal presentation may be symptoms, such as chest discomfort or a sign, such as observed syncopal event. Observation and active listening skills allow efficiency in determining the underlying condition and formulating an initial impression.

8. c. Oropharyngeal airway

Rationale: While unconsciousness demonstrates urgency in maintaining the patient's airway, the provider's assessment determines the most appropriate airway adjunct. Always beginning with BLS adjuncts and progressing to ALS adjuncts allows efficient patient stabilization. Unconscious patients with a gag reflex would not tolerate an oropharyngeal BLS airway. The lack of a gag reflex identifies a life threat.

9. b. Chemotherapy regimens

Rationale: The importance of the focused physical exam in patients with medical complaints cannot be overemphasized. Identification of implanted devices, such as a pacemaker, defibrillator, or vascular access device identifies the acuity of the patient's disposition and determines the most immediate diagnostic information to obtain. The physical exam augments the historical and vital sign information to continue to rule in and rule out working diagnoses to determine a differential diagnosis.

10. b. Chronic obstructive pulmonary disease

Rationale: Using all the components of the detailed assessment in the AMLS pathway assists the provider in obtaining a comprehensive assessment. The detailed assessment includes the history, focused physical exam, vital signs, and obtaining and interpreting diagnostic information. All of these components provide the information needed to accurately determine the working diagnosis and begin appropriate treatment and transport decisions. Understanding the difference between a life threat and emergent and nonemergent cardinal presentations/chief complaints assists in determination of management strategies.

Chapter 2

1. a. Anaphylaxis

Rationale: *Ventilation* is movement of air into and out of the lungs. Airway swelling and bronchoconstriction related to anaphylaxis can obstruct airflow and impair ventilation.

2. d. Sleepiness

Rationale: Fatigue is an indication of respiratory failure. All other signs may be present during an asthma attack without respiratory failure.

3. a. Pulmonary edema

Rationale: Pulmonary edema is more likely to present with a sudden onset, no fever, and bilateral lung findings. Status asthmaticus is more likely to include generalized wheezes and no fever. Pneumothorax is characterized by sudden onset and absent breath sounds; fever is unlikely.

4. a. Capnography

Rationale: Capnography assesses carbon dioxide levels, which measure ventilation. Carbon monoxide detectors measure carboxyhemoglobin levels in the blood. A chest radiograph assesses structural changes in the lung. Oxygen saturation measures oxygen levels in the blood, which may decline with a severe decline in ventilation, but this occurs slowly.

5. c. Ludwig's angina

Rationale: Fever and swelling do not accompany FBAO. The jaw is not swollen in tonsillitis, and laryngotracheobronchitis (croup) is found in children.

6. c. Tobacco smoker

Rationale: Tobacco use is strongly associated with spontaneous pneumothorax.

7. b. Jugular venous distention

Rationale: Right-sided heart failure can develop as a consequence of each of these disease processes, which may result in jugular venous distention.

8. a. Apply oxygen

Rationale: The patient's condition indicates respiratory failure that requires oxygen administration.

9. c. Pneumonia

Rationale: Guillain-Barré syndrome is a respiratory disease caused by a dysfunction of the nervous system. The loss of nerve impulses to the muscles that control respiration diminish the tidal volume. Many patients have compromised immune systems, which result in an opportune condition for bacteria to grow and respiratory infections to develop.

10. a. Expiratory time

Rationale: The risk of barotrauma increases as PEEP and tidal volume increase.

Chapter 3

1. c. Increased respiratory rate

Rationale: Clot formation in the vessels causes diminished blood flow through the pulmonary circulation. Blood flow is also redirected, which has an impact on the lungs and causes dyspnea, hypoxia, and an increase in respiratory rate.

2. a. Boerhavve's syndrome

Rationale: A person with chronic alcoholism is at risk for forceful vomiting, which places the patient at risk for acute rupture of the esophagus, known as "Boerhaave's syndrome." Mediastinitis, sepsis, and shock are frequent signs of this syndrome. Swallowing often aggravates the pain. *Cholecystitis* refers to inflammation of the gallbladder and presents with right shoulder pain. Esophageal varices typically present with dull pain and are related to portal hypertension, often associated with cirrhosis. *Pleurisy* is inflammation of the lining of the lungs and/or chest wall. Typical presentations have sharp pain on inhalation.

3. c. Left-sided heart failure

Rationale: Left ventricular failure leads to congestion in the pulmonary vessels, causing crackles. Hypertension is often an underlying etiology. Orthopnea occurs during rest or sleep and results in greater tidal volume and air exchange in a tripod or upright position. Reactive airway disease results from inflammation and constriction of the airways, such as in asthma. This presents with wheezing rather than crackles.

4. d. The renal arteries are involved

Rationale: The renal arteries are off to the side of the abdominal aorta. If these arteries are blocked, this can lead to hypertension. Hypertension causes renin to be released and an increase in blood pressure to continue to perfuse the kidneys.

5. **a.** A 55-year-old with end-stage lung cancer
Rationale: Fluid accumulation caused by cancerous lesions and tissue destruction and fluid leakage due to chest radiation therapy place the 55-year-old patient at the highest risk for pericardial tamponade.

6. **a.** Administer a bolus of normal saline if the blood pressure drops
Rationale: Nitroglycerin will dilate the coronary arteries, thus decreasing preload. It may be necessary to increase the fluid volume to increase the right ventricular filling pressures.

7. **a.** Administer nitroglycerin, 0.4 mg sublingually
Rationale: Nitroglycerin decreases the pain of ischemia and can be administered if the patient's systolic blood pressure is 90 mm Hg or above.

8. **d.** Pulmonary embolism
Rationale: Chest discomfort, hypotension, and clear lung fields are typical presentations of pulmonary embolism.

9. **b.** Lorazepam, 2 mg IV
Rationale: Benzodiazepines such as lorazepam will reduce the anxiety caused by the pain and cocaine.

10. **d.** ST-segment elevation is apparent in every lead
Rationale: Involvement of more than one coronary vascular area is typical of pericarditis and rarely happens in a myocardial infarction.

Chapter 4

1. **d.** Pulse pressure, 32 mm Hg
Rationale: The original pulse pressure is 40 mm Hg and has now narrowed to 32 mm Hg. The $ETCO_2$ is normal, the heart rate has decreased and should be expected to increase if the patient's shock was getting more severe. The MAP is within normal limits.

2. **c.** Angiotensin II
Rationale: Angiotensin II is a potent vasoconstrictor. Beta 1 stimulates the heart and increases cardiac rate and contractility. Beta 2 causes bronchial dilation and vasodilation. Renin is released by the kidneys and causes the release of angiotensin 1, which is converted to angiotensin 2.

3. **c.** $PaCO_2$ less than 32 mm Hg
Rationale: A $PaCO_2$ of less than 32 mm Hg suggests a compensation for a metabolic acidosis. In sepsis, the pulse rate is usually elevated, and the levels of lactate and glucose are elevated.

4. **d.** Neurogenic
Rationale: Warm, dry skin indicates a vasodilation, and a slow heart rate is indicative of a neurologic disruption of the messages through the spinal cord. Hypovolemic and obstructive shock present with cool, moist skin and an increase in heart rate. Cardiogenic shock

may present with a slow heart rate, but the skin is cool and diaphoretic.

5. **c.** Class III, decompensated shock
Rationale: Because the blood pressure is low, the heart rate is elevated and the capillary refill is >3 seconds. To have class I or II, the blood pressure would still be within normal ranges. For Class IV, the capillary refill would be >5 seconds.

6. **a.** Capnography and lactic acid
Rationale: Capnography and lactic acid provide an insight into the acidotic status of the patient and the presence of anaerobic metabolism.

7. **a.** A 26-year-old man
Rationale: This patient is showing signs of a tension pneumothorax, which is a condition that results in obstructive shock. Vomiting and diarrhea are associated with hypovolemic shock. Chest pain and crackles suggest cardiogenic shock. Tarry stools suggest hemorrhagic shock, which is a type of hypovolemic shock.

8. **c.** Intramuscular epinephrine
Rationale: Epinephrine should be administered due to the respiratory component. The other drugs are treatments for anaphylaxis and allergic reactions, but should only be considered after the epinephrine has been administered.

9. **b.** A 250- to 500-mL isotonic fluid bolus
Rationale: Fluids should be considered. Because the patient's skin is warm, her heart rate is elevated, and her blood pressure is low, sepsis should be considered. She is at risk because she is elderly and in a long-term care facility. Acetaminophen is not indicated until a temperature has been taken, and then treatment would be dependent on local protocol. A pressor or volume expander may be indicated later, but not at this time. An isotonic crystalloid is indicated until more history and assessment and lab results are obtained.

10. **d.** Pressure on the heart
Rationale: Pressure on the heart from the fluid in the pericardial sac is not allowing the heart to fill and empty adequately. Pericardial tamponade is not a volume problem. The tissues may become hypoxic, but that is not the primary problem. Afterload is not affected; the heart can pump blood out, but there is inadequate filling due to the pressure surrounding the heart.

Chapter 5

1. **c.** Is drowsy and slow to respond after awakening from a nap
Rationale: The patient responds after a normal event with appropriate answers; this patient would need to

be evaluated for continued drowsiness. Repetitive questions suggest altered mental status and a disruption of short-term memory. Deep pain is required to elicit a response of localizing pain; this is indicative of altered mental status. A patient who is experiencing auditory hallucinations has a disturbance of perception. Care should be taken with this person, as the behavior may be unpredictable and unsafe.

2. b. Cincinnati Prehospital Stroke Scale

Rationale: Only the Cincinnati Prehospital Stroke Scale assesses cranial nerves. Cranial nerve VII (facial nerve) is evaluated when the patient is asked to smile or show his or her teeth.

3. a. Did he fall or hit his head recently?

Rationale: The question rules trauma in or out as a possible cause. Confirming the presence of allergies is important but not likely a factor that assists with the differential diagnosis in this setting. Although it's important to confirm the patient is compliant with his medications, missing one dose of either of these medications is unlikely to cause a syncopal incident. The onset of Alzheimer's is useful information, but it's not vital in generating an initial differential diagnosis.

4. d. Specialized neurologic and vascular capability

Rationale: This patient is showing signs and symptoms of a possible stroke. It would be best to transfer the patient to a stroke center or a facility with specialized neurologic and vascular capabilities.

5. a. Abnormal gaze

Rationale: The abnormal gaze and pupil size are strong indicators of an intracerebral hemorrhage. Migraines tend to cause disturbances in vision but not changes in gaze or pupil size. The key findings for intracerebral bleeds or hemorrhage are alteration in vital signs (hypertension, pulse and respiration changes), altered LOC, stiff neck or headache, focal neurologic deficits (weakness, gaze preference/deviation of the eyes), difficulty with gait and fine motor control, nausea, vomiting, dizziness or vertigo, or abnormal eye movements. Migraine headaches are severe, recurrent headaches accompanied by incapacitating neurologic symptoms such as cognitive or visual disturbances, dizziness, nausea, and vomiting. The headache may be either unilateral or bilateral. The eyes usually do not deviate, but the patient may complain of photophobia, flashing lights, phonophobia, or zigzagging lines in the visual field. Migraines tend to occur in younger people, but intracerebral bleeds can occur in any age group.

6. b. End-tidal CO_2 of 60 mm Hg

Rationale: A patient with an end-tidal CO_2 should have ventilations assisted to bring $ETCO_2$ readings down to 40 mm Hg. Supplemental oxygen should be applied to return the oxygen saturations to at least 95%. Simply adding oxygen may increase the O_2 sats, but if this doesn't improve them, ventilatory assistance may be necessary. If a patient with a Glasgow Coma Scale score of 10 is ventilating and oxygenating adequately, assisting ventilations is not required. A patient with an elevated blood glucose level may be acidotic due to diabetic ketoacidosis, and ventilation may be used, but an elevated blood glucose level in itself is not a reason for ventilation.

7. d. Stiff neck

Rationale: A stiff neck in the presence of sudden onset of an explosive headache is consistent with a subarachnoid bleed. The stiff neck is associated with irritation of the meninges from the bleeding.

8. d. Unilateral blown pupil

Rationale: A pupil that is dilated, fixed, or slow to respond on the same side of the injury may indicate herniation due to increased intracranial pressure. The classic symptoms of an increasing herniation are coma, fixed and dilated pupil, and decerebrate posturing.

9. b. Proprioception

Rationale: Proprioception is information that comes to the brain from the body to help determine where the body is in space. She may still be able to feel but cannot identify the position of her thumb.

10. b. Insert a nasopharyngeal airway

Rationale: This patient is likely to recover his level of consciousness. The nasal airway will help maintain his airway, but more invasive techniques are not indicated at this time. He does not need intubation at present. Placing him in a supine position puts him at risk for aspiration and potentially increases the difficulty of managing his airway. He is breathing and has adequate oxygen saturation, so ventilation is unnecessary at this time.

Chapter 6

1. d. Vagal stimulation

Rationale: The vagus nerve plays a role in GI stimulation. It also exerts parasympathetic stimulation on the SA node and AV node in the heart.

2. a. Appendix

Rationale: Visceral pain in the periumbilical area often relates to the appendix, small bowel, or cecum.

3. b. Bilirubin

Rationale: Jaundice occurs in patients who have excessive bilirubin. This is often seen in advanced hepatitis.

4. c. Normal saline, 250 mL bolus

Rationale: The patient has signs of impending shock. Fluid resuscitation has the highest priority.

5. c. Illness began about 10 minutes after eating

Rationale: The sudden onset of illness may indicate an allergic reaction. The patient should be carefully questioned about allergies and the foods she ate.

6. a. Ask her to take a deep breath as you press upward into her right upper quadrant

Rationale: Severe right upper quadrant pain that increases with a deep breath suggests gallbladder or liver disease.

7. c. Mallory-Weiss syndrome

Rationale: Esophageal varices are more common in chronic alcoholism. Eating disorders can cause severe vomiting that may precipitate a Mallory-Weiss tear.

8. c. Infuse normal saline at 250 mL/h

Rationale: Visual observation and physical exam indicate fluid loss. Immediate treatment would be IV therapy with normal saline.

9. c. Grey Turner sign

Rationale: Grey Turner and Cullen's signs are indicators of hemorrhagic pancreatitis.

10. c. Famotidine

Rationale: Famotidine (Pepcid) is prescribed for stomach and duodenal ulcers to decrease pain and heal inflammation.

Chapter 7

1. c. Hypoparathyroidism

Rationale: Trousseau's sign, a carpal pedal spasm in response to the inflation of a blood pressure cuff, along with hypocalcemia, bradycardia, and malnutrition are seen in hypoparathyroidism. Congestive heart failure, myxedema, hyponatremia, and hypoglycemia are seen in hypothyroidism. Addison's disease, as seen in adrenal insufficiency and lack of cortisol production, presents with hypoglycemia, hypotension, hyperkalemia, hyponatremia, and emaciation. Cushing's disease, which results in an excess of the production of cortisol, results in hyperglycemia, obesity, hypertension, and electrolyte imbalances.

2. c. Intravenous fluids

Rationale: Exophthalmos (protrusion of the eyeball) is a common presentation in hyperthyroidism. In this patient, resultant dehydration from excessive sweat and diarrhea requires aggressive IV therapy. Amiodarone can cause autoimmune destruction of the thyroid gland. Aspirin is associated with decreased protein binding of thyroid hormones and increased unbinding of T_3 and T_4.

3. b. Dry, yellow skin

Rationale: Dry, yellow skin, hypotension, bradycardia, and low blood glucose levels are typical presentations of myxedema related to hypothyroidism. Chvostek's sign, hyperactive reflexes, and exophthalmos are symptoms of hyperthyroidism.

4. d. Hydrocortisone

Rationale: Typical clinical findings of Addison's disease are hyponatremia, hypoglycemia, and hyperkalemia. The adrenal glands are unable to produce sufficient amounts of corticosteroids to meet the body's demand, so administration of corticosteroids is necessary. If blood glucose levels are low, it may be appropriate to administer glucose.

5. a. Blood glucose, 180 mg/dL (10 mmol/L)

Rationale: The metabolic alkalosis associated with Cushing's syndrome causes hypernatremia, hypocalcemia, hypertension, and hyperglycemia. Typical presentations are obesity and facial puffiness, often referred to as a *moon face*. A high blood glucose reading is common.

6. a. Epinephrine secretion increases

Rationale: Central nervous system dysfunction, tachycardia, confusion, and secretion of epinephrine are typical presentations in hypoglycemia. Patients experiencing hypoglycemia may have a medical history of hypopituitarism and diminished growth hormone secretion. Insulin production decreases.

7. c. Infuse normal saline rapid IV

Rationale: Hyperglycemia, which results in fluid shifts that cause dehydration, abdominal pain, and metabolic acidosis, requires fluid replacement with IV therapy. Performing a 12-lead ECG provides important diagnostic information, as cardiac dysrhythmias may occur.

8. d. A 45-year-old

Rationale: Acute metabolic acidosis, as seen in prolonged cardiac-arrest resuscitation, may require the administration of sodium bicarbonate.

9. a. Hypocalcemia

Rationale: The patient's cardinal presentation of facial twitching (as seen in Chvostek's sign), general weakness, and seizures can signify hypocalcemia. Hypercalcemia can result from thiazide diuretics, hyperthyroidism, adrenal insufficiency, and hyperparathyroidism. Hyperkalemia is often seen in Addison's disease, renal failure, rhabdomyolysis, and digitalis toxicities. Hyponatremia results from hyperglycemia, CHF, excessive sweating, and Addison's disease.

10. d. Glucose, 406 mg/dL; $ETCO_2$, 25 mm Hg

Rationale: DKA is characterized by an elevated glucose level and a decreased $ETCO_2$ level, reflecting metabolic acidosis.

Chapter 8

1. **b.** Thousand die or become ill from an influenza outbreak on all 7 continents

   Rationale: Diseases that are considered pandemic sweep the globe as opposed to an isolated area. Pandemics will usually have a high death toll and are often associated with a virulent new pathogen or a new form of a pernicious old pathogen.

2. **c.** Communicability period

   Rationale: This patient is showing signs and symptoms of having active tuberculosis and is infectious at this time and would be able to infect another individual.

3. **a.** Participate in vaccination/immunization programs

   Rationale: Keeping immunizations up to date will decrease the chance of becoming infected. You should report an exposure as soon as possible. Wearing gloves is the minimum standard for all patient care if there is any possibility for exposure to blood or body fluids. It is important to wash hands prior to caring for a patient so as not to spread an infection to the patient. To prevent spread to yourself, wash your hands after caring for patients.

4. **a.** Antigens

   Rationale: The body's immune system makes antibodies in response to being exposed to an antigen. An antigen is a substance the body recognizes as foreign, causing the body to react with an immune response.

5. **d.** Blood-borne

   Rationale: Hepatitis C is transmitted via the blood-borne route.

6. **d.** Use standard precautions

   Rationale: Meningococcal meningitis occurs by direct contact with droplets from the nose or mouth of an infected person. Standard precautions are encouraged.

7. **a.** Wash your hands with soap and water and vigorous scrubbing

   Rationale: Hand washing should include vigorous scrubbing to increase effectiveness. There is no need to expose to air or light. A chlorine bleach solution is recommended to kill the spores. Alcohol-based gels do not eradicate the spores.

8. **b.** Pertussis

   Rationale: Pertussis is the only disease listed with a vaccine available at this time.

9. **c.** A 14-year-old with lesions that are all crusted and dry

   Rationale: A patient is contagious until all lesions have crusted over and are dry.

10. **c.** Chikungunya

   Rationale: Chikungunya is a disease transmitted by mosquitoes and causes the victim to be bent over. The patient presents with a sudden onset of fever and joint pain. The patient can have long-term joint pain.

Chapter 9

1. **c.** Needle chest decompression

   Rationale: Although the patient would benefit from high-flow oxygen and hyperbaric therapy, this patient is presenting with a tension pneumothorax that requires immediate intervention to decompress the chest and prevent further cardiovascular collapse.

2. **b.** Altered mental status

   Rationale: While heat-related illnesses represent a continuum of disease, progression to altered mental status is the hallmark feature of heatstroke.

3. **b.** Remove from the cold environment

   Rationale: A core tenet of prehospital care and rescue operations in general is to remove the patient from the hazardous situation. In this case, rewarming efforts and other treatments will likely be ineffective until the patient is removed from the cold environment.

4. **b.** Irreversible neurologic injury

   Rationale: Overly rapid shifts in osmotic pressure from hypertonic saline administration can cause physical injury to neurons from excessive fluid shifts.

5. **d.** Heat cramps most often involve several muscles

   Rationale: Athletic cramps involve only one muscle.

6. **c.** Heat stroke

   Rationale: Heat stroke occurs when the body temperature rises above 104°F (>40.5°C)

7. **a.** Shiver vigorously

   Rationale: Shivering mechanisms are still intact during mild hypothermia. Mild hypothermia does not usually cause cardiac arrest or altered mental status. Caffeine, alcohol, and tobacco should all be avoided in the hypothermic patient.

8. **b.** Bradycardia or Osborne waves and electrolyte abnormalities

   Rationale: Although hypothermic patients may show a range of ECG changes, bradycardia and Osborne waves are most characteristic.

9. **b.** Decompression sickness

   Rationale: As the pressure a person is exposed to changes, gases may come out of solution as bubbles in the blood according to Boyle's law. These bubbles cause a variety of symptoms together referred to as decompresssion sickness. Patients with a PFO (patent foremen ovale) are at risk of stroke if the bubbles cross from the right to the left side of circulation and lodge in the cerebral arteries instead of the pulmonary circulation. Nitrogen narcosis refers to the mental status effects from excess nitrogen that can accumulate in the blood under pressure.

10. c. Rapid rewarming

Rationale: The first step is rewarming as the other therapies would be ineffective and possibly harmful with ongoing hypothermia.

Chapter 10

1. a. Alcohol withdrawal

Rationale: These signs and symptoms are consistent with the sympathomimetic toxidrome.

2. b. Material safety data sheets

Rationale: The material safety data sheet (MSDS) is a comprehensive reference for hazardous materials. It includes information on routes of entry, health effects, first aid, firefighter measures, handling, storage, exposures, and the chemical and physical properties of hazardous substances.

3. d. BP 70/50 P 70 bpm

Rationale: The digitalis-like properties of this plant cause bradycardia.

4. d. Seizures

Rationale: Benadryl overdose signs and symptoms include dry mouth, fever, ringing in the ears, sleepiness, blurred vision, large pupils, and the potential for seizures.

5. c. Lactic acidosis

Rationale: Metabolic acidosis related to metformin is associated with high mortality.

6. b. Cholinergic

Rationale: Anticholinergic drugs cause ataxia, decreased production of mucus, dry mouth, and perspiration. Cholinergic medications cause an increase of secretions in the saliva, tears, and digestive acids. Sympathomimetics are used in decongestants to decrease histamine responses.

7. a. Botulism

Rationale: *Clostridium botulinum* is a nerve toxin.

8. b. Pupils, 2 mm and equal

Rationale: Pinpoint pupils are consistent with opiate toxidrome. Establishing adequate ventilation is the first priority.

9. a. Amitriptyline

Rationale: Tricyclic antidepressant overdose causes the characteristic ECG change with tachycardia.

10. d. Stage at a safe distance

Rationale: Do not enter until appropriate authorities deem it is safe.

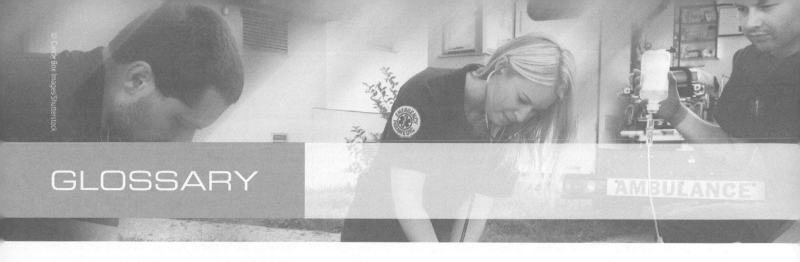

abscess (peritonsillar) An abscess in which a superficial soft-tissue infection progresses to create pockets of purulence in the submucosal space adjacent to the tonsils. This abscess and its accompanying inflammation cause the uvula to deviate to the opposing side.

acidosis An abnormal increase in the hydrogen ion concentration in the blood, resulting from an accumulation of an acid or the loss of a base, indicated by a blood pH below the normal range.

acute coronary syndrome (ACS) An umbrella term that covers any group of clinical symptoms consistent with acute myocardial ischemia (chest pain due to insufficient blood supply to the heart muscle that results from coronary artery disease). ACS covers clinical conditions including angina, unstable angina, ST-segment elevation myocardial infarction (STEMI), and non–ST-segment elevation myocardial infarction (NSTEMI).

acute lung injury/acute respiratory distress syndrome (ALI/ARDS) A systemic disease that causes lung failure.

acute mountain sickness Any illness that can effect the body in a high-altitude environment.

acute myocardial infarction (AMI) Commonly known as a "heart attack," AMI occurs when the blood supply to part of the heart is interrupted, causing heart cells to die. This is most commonly due to blockage of a coronary artery following the rupture of plaque within the wall of an artery. The resulting ischemia and decreased supply of oxygen, if left untreated, can cause damage and/or death of heart muscle tissue.

Addison's disease An endocrine disease caused by a deficiency of corticosteroid hormones produced by the adrenal cortex. The disease is characterized by nausea, vomiting, abdominal pain, and tanning of the skin.

adrenal crisis An endocrine emergency caused by a deficiency of corticosteroid hormones produced by the adrenal cortex. The disease is characterized by nausea, vomiting, abdominal pain, hypotension, hyperkalemia, and hyponatremia.

Advanced Medical Life Support (AMLS) assessment pathway A dependable framework to support the reduction of morbidity and mortality by using an assessment-based approach to determine a differential diagnosis and effectively manage a broad range of medical emergencies.

aerobic metabolism Metabolism that can proceed only in the presence of oxygen.

afterload In the intact heart, the pressure against which the ventricle ejects blood. It is impacted by peripheral vascular resistance and the physical characteristics and volume of blood in the arterial system.

altered mental status Any decrease in normal level of wakefulness, change in mentation or behavior that is not normal for a particular patient.

amyotrophic lateral sclerosis (ALS) The disease characterized by degeneration of the upper and lower motor neurons, which causes voluntary muscles to weaken or atrophy. Also known as Lou Gehrig disease.

anaerobic metabolism The metabolism that takes place in the absence of oxygen; the principal byproduct is lactic acid.

angioedema A vascular reaction that may have an allergic cause and may result in profound swelling of the tongue and lips.

antibodies Immunoglobulins produced by lymphocytes in response to bacteria, viruses, or other antigenic substances.

antiemetic A substance that prevents or alleviates nausea and vomiting.

antigens Substances, usually proteins, that the body recognizes as foreign and that can evoke an immune response.

apneustic center A portion of the pons that assists in creating longer, slower respirations.

assessment-based patient management Utilizing the patient's cardinal presentation; historical, diagnostic, and physical exam findings; and one's own critical thinking skills as a healthcare professional to diagnose and treat a patient.

ataxia Loss of coordination of muscle control, which can lead to gait disturbance or extremity clumsiness. May be due to many causes, including peripheral nerve, spinal cord, or brain dysfunction, often of the cerebellum, which controls coordination.

atelectasis The collapse of the alveolar air spaces of the lungs.

barotrauma Injury resulting from pressure disequilibrium across body surfaces.

biological agent Disease-causing pathogen or toxin that may be used as a weapon to cause disease or injury to humans.

blood-borne pathogens Pathogenic microorganisms that are transmitted via human blood and cause disease in humans; examples include hepatitis B virus (HBV) and human immunodeficiency virus (HIV).

blood brain barrier (BBB) A filtering mechanism of the capillaries that carry blood to the brain and spinal cord tissue, blocking the passage of certain substances.

blood pressure The tension exerted by blood on the arterial walls. Blood pressure is calculated using the following equation: Blood pressure = Flow × Resistance.

Boyle's law At a constant temperature, the volume of a gas is inversely proportional to its pressure (if you double the pressure of gas, you halve its volume; written as PV = K, where P = pressure, V = volume, and K = a constant).

carboxyhemoglobin Hemoglobin loaded with carbon monoxide.

cardiac cycle A complete cardiac movement or heartbeat. The period from the beginning of one heartbeat to the beginning of the next; from diastole through systole.

cardiac output The effective volume of blood expelled by either ventricle of the heart per unit of time (usually volume per minute); it is equal to the stroke volume multiplied by the heart rate.

cardiac tamponade Also known as "pericardial tamponade," this is an emergency condition in which fluid accumulates in the pericardium (the sac that surrounds the heart). If the amount of fluid increases slowly (such as in hypothyroidism), the pericardial sac can expand to contain a liter or more of fluid prior to tamponade occurring. If the fluid increases rapidly (as may occur after trauma or myocardial rupture), as little as 100 mL can cause tamponade.

cerebral perfusion pressure (CPP) Represents the pressure gradient driving cerebral blood flow (CBF) and therefore oxygen and metabolite delivery; it is the difference between the mean arterial pressure (MAP) and the intracranial pressure (ICP). CPP=MAP-ICP.

cerebrospinal fluid (CSF) A transparent, slightly yellowish fluid in the subarachnoid space around the brain and spinal cord.

cerebrovascular accident (CVA) Another term for *stroke*.

chemoreceptors Chemical receptors that sense changes in the composition of blood and body fluids. The primary chemical changes registered by chemoreceptors are those involving levels of hydrogen (H^+), carbon dioxide (CO_2), and oxygen (O_2).

clinical decision making The ability to integrate assessment findings and test data with experience and evidence-based recommendations to make decisions regarding the most appropriate treatment.

clinical reasoning The second conceptual component underpinning the AMLS assessment pathway, which combines good judgment with clinical experience to make accurate diagnoses and initiate proper treatment. This process assumes the provider has a strong foundation of clinical knowledge.

cold (green) zone A support zone for general triage, stabilization, and management of illness or injuries. Patients and uncontaminated personnel are given access to this zone, but healthcare personnel must wear protective clothing while in the green zone and properly discard it in predetermined areas on exiting.

communicable diseases Any disease transmitted from one person or animal to another either directly, by contact with excreta or other discharges from the body; or indirectly, by means of substances or inanimate objects such as contaminated drinking glasses, toys, water, or by vectors such as flies, mosquitoes, ticks, or other insects.

contaminated A condition of being soiled, stained, touched, or otherwise exposed to harmful agents, making an object potentially unsafe for use as intended or without barrier techniques; for example, entry of infectious or toxic materials into a previously clean or sterile environment.

contamination Condition of being soiled, stained, touched, or otherwise exposed to harmful agents, making an object potentially unsafe for use as intended or without barrier techniques. An example is entry of infectious or toxic materials into a previously clean or sterile environment.

convulsion The visual clinical manifestation of a seizure.

Cushing's triad Hypertension, bradycardia, and rapid, deep, or irregular respirations.

decompression sickness A broad range of signs and symptoms caused by nitrogen bubbles in blood and tissues coming out of solution on ascent.

decontamination The process of removing foreign material such as blood, body fluids, or radioactivity; it does not eliminate microorganisms but is a necessary step preceding disinfection or sterilization.

delirium An acute mental disorder characterized by confusion, disorientation, restlessness, clouding of consciousness, incoherence, fear, anxiety, excitement, and often illusions.

diabetic ketoacidosis (DKA) An acute endocrine emergency caused by a lack of insulin. The condition is characterized by an elevated blood glucose level, ketone production, metabolic acidosis, dehydration, nausea, vomiting, abdominal pain, and tachypnea.

differential diagnosis The possible causes of the patient's cardinal presentation.

dirty bomb A conventional explosive device used to disperse radiologic agents.

disseminated intravascular coagulation (DIC) A disturbance of blood coagulation as a result of activation of the coagulation mechanism and simultaneous clot lysis.

drowning The process of experiencing respiratory impairment from submersion or immersion in liquid.

dysarthria Garbled speech (but of one's intended words) due to cranial nerve dysfunction (distinguish from expressive and receptive aphasia).

embolus A particle that travels in the circulatory system and obstructs blood flow when it becomes lodged in a smaller artery. A blood clot is the most common type of embolus, but fat (after long bone fracture), atherosclerotic, and air (diving) emboli can also occur.

emergency decontamination Process of decontaminating people exposed to and potentially contaminated with hazardous materials; focuses on rapidly removing the contamination to reduce their exposure and save lives, with secondary regard for completeness of decontamination.

end-tidal carbon dioxide ($ETCO_2$) monitoring Analysis of exhaled gases for CO_2; a useful method of assessing a patient's ventilatory status or lung perfusion. In cardiac arrest it may indicate the effectiveness of chest compressions or return of spontaneous circulation.

epidemic A disease that affects a significantly large number of people at the same time and spreads rapidly through a demographic segment of the human population.

epidemiology The study of the determinants of disease events in populations.

exercise-associated hyponatremia A condition due to prolonged exertion in a hot environment coupled with excessive hypotonic fluid intake that leads to nausea, vomiting, and, in severe cases, mental status changes and seizures (also known as exertional hyponatremia).

exposure incident A state of being in the presence of or subjected to a force or influence (e.g., viral exposure, heat exposure).

expressive aphasia Inability to speak intended words due to dysfunction of the cerebral speech center (Broca's area) in the left frontal lobe (distinguish from dysarthria).

frostbite Localized damage to tissues resulting from prolonged exposure to extreme cold.

frostnip Early frostbite, characterized by numbness and pallor without significant tissue damage.

fulminant Describes a sudden intense occurrence that creates a hazardous environment

fulminant hepatic failure A rare condition that occurs when hepatitis progresses to hepatic necrosis (death of the liver cells); classic symptoms include anorexia, vomiting, jaundice, abdominal pain, and asterixis (flapping tremor).

gas exchange The process in which oxygen from the atmosphere is taken up by circulating blood cells and carbon dioxide from the bloodstream is released to the atmosphere.

gastrointestinal (GI) Pertaining to the organs of the GI tract. The GI tract links the organs involved in consumption, processing, and elimination of nutrients. It begins at the mouth, moves to the esophagus, travels through the chest cavity into the abdomen, and terminates in the pelvic girdle at the rectum.

gastrointestinal decontamination Any attempt to limit absorption or hasten elimination of a toxin from a patient's gastrointestinal tract. Examples include activated charcoal, gastric lavage, and whole-bowel irrigation. While these methods do have a small role in toxicology, their use is not routinely recommended and should be discussed with a poison control center or medical toxicologist.

gastroparesis A medical condition consisting of a paresis (partial paralysis) of the stomach, resulting in food remaining in the stomach for an abnormally long time.

heat exhaustion A clinical syndrome characterized by volume depletion and heat stress that is thought to be a milder form of heat illness and on a continuum leading to heatstroke.

heatstroke The least common and most deadly heat illness, caused by a severe disturbance in thermoregulation, usually characterized by a core temperature of more than 104°F (40°C) and altered mental status.

heat syncope An orthostatic or near-syncopal episode that typically occurs in nonacclimated people who may be under heat stress.

hematemesis Vomiting of bright red blood, indicating upper GI bleeding.

hematochezia Passage of red blood through the rectum.

hemiparesis Unilateral weakness, usually occurring on the opposite side of the body from the stroke.

hemiplegia Paralysis or severe weakness on one side of the body.

hemorrhagic stroke Damage to the brain from bleeding in the brain tissue (intracerebral) or into the subarachnoid space, usually due to rupture of an aneurysm or arteriovenous malformation.

high-altitude cerebral edema A form of acute mountain sickness where the brain swells and stops functioning normally.

high-altitude pulmonary edema A noncardiogenic form of pulmonary edema (fluid accumulation in the lungs) that occurs in high altitudes.

history of the present illness (HPI) The most important element of patient assessment. The primary elements of the HPI can be obtained by using the OPQRST and SAMPLER mnemonics.

hospital-acquired infection (HAI)/healthcare-associated infections An infection acquired from exposure to an infectious agent at a healthcare facility, defined as at least 72 hours after hospitalization.

hot (red) zone An area where the hazardous material is located and contamination has occurred. Access to this zone is limited so as to protect rescuers and patients from further exposure. Specific protective gear worn by trained personnel is required for access.

huffing The act of pouring an inhalant onto a cloth or into a bag and inhaling the substance, usually in an attempt to alter one's mental status.

hypercapnia A condition of abnormally elevated carbon dioxide (CO_2) levels in the blood, caused by hypoventilation, lung disease, or diminished consciousness. It may also be caused by exposure to environments containing abnormally high concentrations of carbon dioxide, or by rebreathing exhaled carbon dioxide. Usually defined as a carbon dioxide level over 45 mm Hg.

hyperosmolar hyperglycemic nonketotic coma (HHNC) An endocrine emergency characterized by a high plasma glucose concentration, absent ketone production, and increased serum osmolality (> 315 mOsm/kg). The syndrome causes severe dehydration, nausea, vomiting, abdominal pain, and tachypnea.

hyperthermia Unusually elevated body temperature.

hypoglycemia A plasma glucose concentration of less than 70 mg/dL. This condition is often associated with signs and symptoms such as sweating, cold skin, tachycardia, and altered mental status.

hypothermia Core body temperature below 95°F (35°C); at lower temperatures, hypothermia may induce cardiac arrhythmia and precipitate a decline in mental status.

hypovolemia Abnormally decreased volume of circulating blood in the body; the most common cause is hemorrhage.

infectious diseases Diseases caused by another living organism or virus, which may or may not be transmissible to another person.

initial patient presentation The patient's primary presenting sign or symptom; often this is the accompanied by the patient's chief complaint, but it may be an objective finding such as unconsciousness or choking.

intoxication The state of being poisoned by a drug or other toxic substance; the state of being inebriated as a result of excessive alcohol consumption.

intussusception Prolapse of one segment of the bowel into the lumen of another segment. This kind of intestinal obstruction may involve segments of the small intestine, colon, or terminal ileum and cecum.

ischemia A restriction in oxygen and nutrient delivery to muscle caused by physical obstruction to blood flow, increased demand by the tissues, or hypoxia, which leads to damage or dysfunction of tissue.

ischemic stroke A stroke that occurs when a thrombus or embolus obstructs a vessel, diminishing blood flow to part of the brain.

Korsakoff's syndrome Chronic and irreversible condition involving cognitive dysfunction, especially memory loss, due to prolonged thiamine deficiency.

lethal concentration 50% (LC$_{50}$) The air concentration of an agent that kills 50% of the exposed animal population. This denotes the concentration and the length of exposure time of that population.

lethal dose 50% (LD$_{50}$) The oral or dermal exposure dose that kills 50% of an exposed animal population in 2 weeks.

Lou Gehrig disease *See* amyotrophic lateral sclerosis (ALS).

Ludwig's angina A deep-space infection of the anterior neck just below the mandible. The name derives from the sensation of choking and suffocation reported by most patients with this condition.

mean arterial pressure (MAP) The average pressure in a patient's arteries during one cardiac cycle, an indicator of perfusion to vital organs; to calculate MAP, double the diastolic blood pressure and add the sum to the systolic blood pressure, then divide by 3.

melena Abnormal black, tarry stool that has a distinctive odor and contains digested blood.

methemoglobinemia The presence of methemoglobin in the blood, which prevents the ability of hemoglobin to carry and transport oxygen to the tissues. Hemoglobin is converted to methemoglobin by nitrogen oxides and sulfa drugs.

myxedema Severe hypothyroidism associated with cold intolerance, weight gain, weakness, and declining mental status.

National Fire Protection Association (NFPA) A national and international voluntary membership organization that promotes improved fire protection and prevention and establishes safeguards against loss of life and property by fire. The NFPA writes and publishes national voluntary consensus standards.

neuroleptic malignant syndrome A condition caused by antipsychotic and even common antiemetic medications that presents with hyperthermia, muscular rigidity, altered mental status, and a hyperdynamic state.

neurotransmitter A chemical substance that is released at the end of a nerve fiber by the arrival of a nerve impulse (action potential) and, by diffusing across the synapse or junction, causes the transfer of the impulse to another nerve fiber, a muscle fiber, or some other structure.

nitrogen narcosis A state resembling alcohol intoxication produced by nitrogen gas dissolved in the blood at high ambient pressure.

noninvasive positive-pressure ventilation (NPPV) A procedure in which positive pressure is provided through the upper airway by some type of mask or other noninvasive device.

non–ST-segment elevation myocardial infarction (NSTEMI) A type of MI caused by a blocked blood supply that causes nontransmural infarction in an area of the heart. There is no ST-segment elevation on electrocardiogram (ECG) recordings, but other clinical signs of MI are present. NSTEMI is diagnosed on the basis of positive laboratory tests for cardiac enzymes and other products of myocardium damage and death.

North American Emergency Response Guidebook A book published by the U.S. Government Printing Office that provides a quick reference to hazardous materials emergencies for first responders.

nosocomial infection *See* hospital-acquired infection (HAI).

Occupational Safety and Health Administration (OSHA) The U.S. federal agency that regulates worker safety.

ophthalmoplegia Abnormal function of the eye muscles.

packer A person who ingests a large quantity of well-packed drugs for the purpose of smuggling. These carefully prepared packages are less likely to rupture than those ingested by stuffers, but toxicity can be severe if they do because of the large amount of drug present.

pandemic A disease occurring throughout the population of a large part of the world.

parenteral Pertaining to treatment other than through the digestive system.

pattern recognition A process of recognizing and classifying data based on past knowledge and experience.

perfusion The act of pouring over or through, especially the passage of a fluid through the vessels of a specific organ.

pericarditis A condition in which the tissue surrounding the heart (pericardium) becomes inflamed. This can be caused by several factors but is often related to a viral infection. Accompaniment by cardiac dysfunction or signs of congestive heart failure (CHF) suggests a more serious myocarditis or involvement of the heart muscle.

peritonsillar abscess *See* abscess (peritonsillar).

pharmacokinetics The absorption, distribution, metabolism, and excretion of medications.

placards Diamond-shaped signs placed on containers that identify hazardous materials.

pleura A thin membrane that surrounds and protects the lungs (visceral pleura) and lines the chest cavity (parietal pleura)

pneumotaxic center Located in the pons, this center generally controls the rate and pattern of respiration.

preload The mechanical state of the heart at the end of diastole, it reflects venous return and the stress or stretch on the ventricular wall.

primary survey The process of initially assessing the airway, breathing, circulation, and perfusion status to identify and manage life-threatening conditions and establish priorities for further assessment, treatment, and transport.

prodromal Early symptoms that mark the onset of a disease.

proprioception Sensory function that provides the awareness of the location of body parts relative to the rest of the body.

psychosis Any major mental disorder characterized by a gross impairment in reality testing, in which the individual incorrectly evaluates the accuracy of perceptions and thoughts and makes incorrect references about external reality. It is often characterized by regressive behavior, inappropriate mood and affect, and diminished impulse control. Symptoms include hallucinations and delusions.

pulmonary agent An industrial chemical used as a weapon to kill those who inhale the vapor or gas; lung damage causes asphyxiation. Also known as a "choking agent."

pulmonary embolism (PE) The sudden blockage of a pulmonary artery by a blood clot, often originating from a deep vein in the legs or pelvis, that embolizes and travels to the lung artery, where it becomes lodged. Symptoms include tachycardia, hypoxia, and hypotension.

pulse pressure The difference between the systolic and diastolic blood pressures; normal pulse pressure is 30 to 40 mm Hg.

pulsus paradoxus An exaggeration of the normal inspiratory decrease in systolic blood pressure, defined by an inspiratory fall of systolic blood pressure of greater than 10 mm Hg.

radioactive Giving off radiation as the result of the disintegration of atomic nuclei.

referred pain Pain felt at a site different from that of an injured or diseased organ or body part.

respiration The reciprocal passage of oxygen into the blood and carbon dioxide into the alveoli.

respiratory failure A disorder in which the lungs become unable to perform their basic task of gas exchange, the transfer of oxygen from inhaled air into the blood and the transfer of carbon dioxide from the blood into exhaled air.

retrovirus Any of a family of ribonucleic acid (RNA) viruses containing the enzyme, reverse transcriptase, in the virion; examples include human immunodeficiency virus (HIV1, HIV2) and human T-cell lymphotropic virus.

secondary survey An in-depth systematic evaluation of the patient's history, physical exam, vital signs, and diagnostic information used to identify additional emergent and nonemergent conditions and modify differential diagnoses and management strategies.

seizure A transient occurrence of abnormal excessive or synchronous neuronal activity in the cerebral cortex of the brain that can cause loss of or alteration in consciousness, convulsions or tremors, incontinence, behavior changes, subjective changes in perception (taste, smell, fears), and other symptoms.

shock A condition of profound hemodynamic and metabolic disturbance characterized by failure of the circulatory system to maintain adequate perfusion of oxygen and nutrients to vital organs. It may result from inadequate blood volume, cardiac function, or vasomotor tone.

signs Objective evidence that a healthcare professional observes, feels, sees, hears, touches, or smells.

somatic (parietal) pain Generally well-localized pain caused by an irritation of the nerve fibers in the parietal peritoneum or other deep tissues (e.g., musculoskeletal system). Physical findings include sharp, discrete, localized pain accompanied by tenderness to palpation, guarding of the affected area, and rebound tenderness.

ST-segment elevation myocardial infarction (STEMI) Anginal symptoms at rest that result in myocardial necrosis as identified by elevated cardiac biomarkers with ST-segment elevation on the 12-lead electrocardiogram. These attacks carry a substantial risk of death and disability and call for a quick response by a STEMI system geared for reperfusion therapy.

stable angina Symptoms of chest pain, shortness of breath, or other equivalent symptoms that occur predictably with exertion, then resolve with rest, suggesting the presence of a fixed coronary lesion that prevents adequate perfusion with increased demand.

Standard on Hazardous Waste Operations and Emergency Response (HAZWOPER) (CFR 1910.120) Occupational Safety and Health Administration (OSHA) and Environmental Protection Agency (EPA) regulation intended to protect the safety of employees who respond to emergency incidents related to storage and disposal of hazardous materials.

standard precautions Guidelines recommended by the Centers for Disease Control and Prevention for reducing the risk of transmission of blood-borne and other pathogens in hospitals. Standard precautions apply to (1) blood; (2) all body fluids, secretions, and excretions except sweat, regardless of whether or not they contain blood; (3) nonintact skin; and (4) mucous membranes.

stroke center designation There are currently 4 levels of stroke center designation: Basic Stroke Capable Hospital, Advanced Stroke Capable Hospital, Primary Stroke Center, and Comprehensive Stroke Center. Both Primary and Comprehensive stroke centers are certified by The Joint Commission to be fully capable of delivering acute stroke treatment and rehabilitation services, and are held to higher standards of care and reporting. A Comprehensive Stroke Center is the highest level of stroke center designation and provides, including those services of a Primary Stroke Center, the following: (1) availability of advanced imaging techniques, including MRI/MRA, CTA, DSA, and TCD, (2) availability of personnel trained in vascular neurology, neurosurgery, and endovascular procedures, (3) 24/7 availability of personnel, imaging, operating room, and endovascular facilities, (4) ICU/neuroscience ICU facilities and capabilities, (5) experience and expertise treating patients with large ischemic strokes, intracerebral hemorrhage, and subarachnoid hemorrhage.

stroke Sometimes called a *brain attack* or *cerebrovascular accident* (CVA), a stroke is a brain injury that occurs when blood flow to a part of the brain is obstructed or interrupted, or when bleeding in the brain damages brain cells from increased pressure.

stroke volume The amount of blood ejected by the ventricle at each heartbeat. It varies with age, sex, and exercise.

stuffer A person who hastily ingests small packets of poorly packaged drugs to avoid apprehension and drug confiscation.

The dose is much lower than that seen with packers, but the likelihood of toxicity is much greater because the packages, meant for distribution, are likely to open in the patient's stomach or bowel.

symptoms The S in SAMPLER; subjective perceptions by patients indicating what they feel, such as nausea, or have experienced, such as a sensation of seeing flashing lights.

tension pneumothorax A life-threatening condition that results from progressive worsening of a simple pneumothorax, the accumulation of air under pressure in the pleural space. This can lead to progressive restriction of venous return, which leads to decreased preload, then systemic hypotension.

therapeutic communication A communication process in which the healthcare provider uses effective communication skills to obtain information about the patient and his or her condition, including the use of the four *E*s: engagement, empathy, education, and enlistment.

thermoregulation The process by which the body compensates for environmental extremes.

thoracentesis A procedure to remove fluid or air from the pleural space.

thoracic duct Located in the left upper thorax; the thoracic duct is the largest lymph vessel in the body. It returns the excess fluid that is not collected by the veins from the lower extremities and abdomen to the venae cavae.

thoracostomy A procedure in which a tube may be connected to a Heimlich valve, a one-way valve that lets air escape but not enter the pleural space.

thrombus A blood clot that forms in a blood vessel.

thyroid storm An endocrine emergency characterized by hyperfunction of the thyroid gland. This disorder is associated with fever, tachycardia, nervousness, altered mental status, and hemodynamic instability.

thyrotoxicosis A condition of elevated thyroid hormone levels, which often leads to signs and symptoms of tachycardia, tremor, weight loss, and high-output heart failure.

toxidrome A specific syndrome-like group of symptoms associated with exposure to a given poison.

ultrasound Also called *sonography* or *diagnostic medical sonography*, this imaging method uses high-frequency sound waves to produce precise images of structures within the body.

unstable angina (UA) Angina of increased frequency, severity, or occurring with less intensive exertion than the baseline. This suggests the narrowing of a static lesion, causing further limitation of coronary blood flow with increased demand.

virulence The power of a microorganism to produce disease.

visceral pain Poorly localized pain that occurs when the walls of the hollow organs are stretched, thereby activating the stretch receptors. This kind of pain is characterized by a deep, persistent ache ranging from mild to intolerable and commonly described as cramping, burning, and gnawing.

viscus (*pl.* viscera) The internal organs enclosed within a body cavity, including the abdominal, thoracic, pelvic, and endocrine organs.

volvulus A condition in which the stomach rotates more than 180 degrees; this twisting seals the stomach on both ends, blocking the flow of blood and the passage of fluid and food. The condition is characterized by an acute onset of abdominal pain, severe vomiting, and shock.

warm (yellow) zone The area surrounding a contaminated hot zone. Properly protected healthcare providers are allowed to access this zone for rapid assessment and management of emergent or life-threatening conditions. Decontamination occurs in this gone.

Wernicke's encephalopathy A disorder often caused by deficiency of thiamine, or vitamin B_1, and characterized by a triad of symptoms: acute confusion, ataxia, and ophthalmoplegia.

working diagnosis The presumed cause of the patient's condition, arrived at by evaluating all assessment information thus far obtained while conducting further diagnostic testing to definitively diagnose the illness.

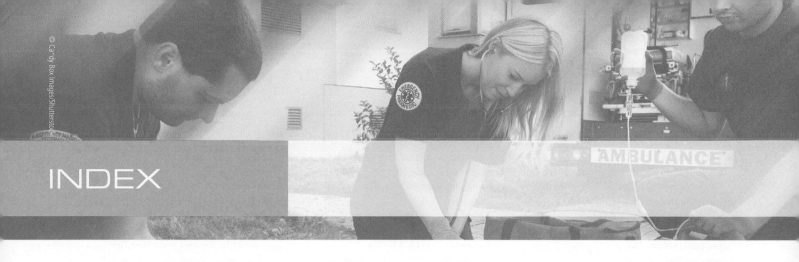

INDEX

Note: Page numbers followed by *f* or *t* indicate material in figures or tables, respectively.